Current Therapies and Treatments of Non-small Cell Lung Cancer

Current Therapies and Treatments of Non-small Cell Lung Cancer

Editor: Rex White

AMERICAN
MEDICAL PUBLISHERS
www.americanmedicalpublishers.com

AMERICAN
MEDICAL PUBLISHERS
www.americanmedicalpublishers.com

Cataloging-in-Publication Data

Current therapies and treatments of non-small cell lung cancer / edited by Rex White.
p. cm.
Includes bibliographical references and index.
ISBN 979-8-88740-570-4
1. Lungs--Cancer. 2. Small cell lung cancer. 3. Lungs--Cancer--Diagnosis. 4. Lungs--Cancer--Treatment,
5. Lungs—Diseases. I. White, Rex.
RC280.L8 N66 2023
616.994 24--dc23

American Medical Publishers,
41 Flatbush Avenue,
1st Floor, New York,
NY 11217, USA

ISBN 979-8-88740-570-4 (Hardback)

Contents

Preface

Non-small cell lung cancer (NSCLC) is a type of cancer characterized by the development of malignant cells in the tissues of the lung. The major signs and symptoms of NSCLC are shortness of breath, cough, chest discomfort, hoarseness, problem in swallowing, tiredness, etc. Some risks factors of this type of cancer include chronic obstructive pulmonary disease, asbestos exposure, pulmonary exposure, HIV or AIDS, and air pollution. There are five main ways of treating NSCLC, namely, surgery, radiation therapy, chemotherapy, targeted therapy and immunotherapy. Surgical procedures including lobectomy, segmentectomy, a wedge resection and pneumonectomy are used for treating this cancer. Chemotherapy utilizes drugs for destroying cancer cells by preventing the cancer cells from proliferating, dividing and replicating. This book is a compilation of chapters that discuss the current therapies and treatments of non-small cell lung cancer. It will also provide interesting topics for research which interested readers can take up. With state-of-the-art inputs by acclaimed experts, this book targets students and professionals.

Various studies have approached the subject by analyzing it with a single perspective, but the present book provides diverse methodologies and techniques to address this field. This book contains theories and applications needed for understanding the subject from different perspectives. The aim is to keep the readers informed about the progresses in the field; therefore, the contributions were carefully examined to compile novel researches by specialists from across the globe.

Indeed, the job of the editor is the most crucial and challenging in compiling all chapters into a single book. In the end, I would extend my sincere thanks to the chapter authors for their profound work. I am also thankful for the support provided by my family and colleagues during the compilation of this book.

Editor

1

Immune-Stromal Score Signature: Novel Prognostic Tool of the Tumor Microenvironment in Lung Adenocarcinoma

Xiaoguang Qi[1†], Chunyan Qi[2†], Boyu Qin[1], Xindan Kang[1], Yi Hu[1] and Weidong Han[3*]*

[1] Department of Oncology, Chinese PLA General Hospital, Beijing, China, [2] Department of Health Management, Chinese PLA General Hospital, Beijing, China, [3] Department of Bio-therapeutic, Chinese PLA General Hospital, Beijing, China

***Correspondence:**
Yi Hu
huyi0401@aliyun.com
Weidong Han
hanwdrsw69@yahoo.com

† These authors have contributed equally to this work

Background: Immune and stromal cells in the tumor microenvironment (TME) significantly contribute to the prognosis of lung adenocarcinoma; however, the TME-related immune prognostic signature is unknown. The aim of this study was to develop a novel immune prognostic model of the TME in lung adenocarcinoma.

Methods: First, the immune and stromal scores among lung adenocarcinoma patients were determined using the ESTIMATE algorithm in accordance with The Cancer Genome Atlas (TCGA) database. Differentially expressed immune-related genes (IRGs) between high and low immune/stromal score groups were analyzed, and a univariate Cox regression analysis was performed to identify IRGs significantly correlated with overall survival (OS) among patients with lung adenocarcinoma. Furthermore, a least absolute shrinkage and selection operator (LASSO) regression analysis was performed to generate TME-related immune prognostic signatures. Gene set enrichment analysis was performed to analyze the mechanisms underlying these immune prognostic signatures. Finally, the functions of hub IRGs were further analyzed to delineate the potential prognostic mechanisms in comprehensive TCGA datasets.

Results: In total, 702 intersecting differentially expressed IRGs (589 upregulated and 113 downregulated) were screened. Univariate Cox regression analysis revealed that 58 significant differentially expressed IRGs were correlated with patient prognosis in the training cohort, of which three IRGs (*CLEC17A*, *INHA*, and *XIRP1*) were identified through LASSO regression analysis. A robust prognostic model was generated on the basis of this three-IRG signature. Furthermore, functional enrichment analysis of the high-risk-score group was performed primarily on the basis of metabolic pathways, whereas analysis of the low-risk-score group was performed primarily on the basis of immunoregulation and immune cell activation. Finally, hub IRGs *CLEC17A*, *INHA*, and *XIRP1* were considered novel prognostic biomarkers for lung adenocarcinoma. These hub genes had different mutation frequencies and forms in lung adenocarcinoma and participated in different signaling pathways. More importantly, these hub genes were significantly correlated with the infiltration of CD4+ T cells, CD8+ T cells, macrophages, B cells, and neutrophils.

Conclusions: The robust novel TME-related immune prognostic signature effectively predicted the prognosis of patients with lung adenocarcinoma. Further studies are required to further elucidate the regulatory mechanisms of these hub IRGs in the TME and to develop new treatment strategies.

Keywords: tumor microenvironment, lung adenocarcinoma, prognostic model, TCGA database, ESTIMATE algorithm

INTRODUCTION

Lung cancer is still the leading disease worldwide in terms of the threat to human life and health (1, 2), and lung adenocarcinoma is the most common pathological subtype. Studies in the past decade have reported that tyrosine kinase inhibitors (TKIs) targeting epidermal growth factor receptor (EGFR), anaplastic lymphoma kinase (ALK), and ROS proto-oncogene 1 (ROS1) are potential therapeutic targets for lung adenocarcinoma, upon genotyping (3–5). Molecular-targeted therapy based on these sensitive targets has considerably enhanced overall survival (OS) among patients with lung adenocarcinoma; however, this therapy is not suitable for all patients with lung adenocarcinoma. Furthermore, drug resistance is common among patients receiving molecular-targeted therapy, and their prognosis is poor (6, 7). Nonetheless, numerous studies have led to the advancement of immunotherapy for several cancers, including lung adenocarcinoma. Immunotherapy is different from targeted therapy; it has more durable clinical benefits. Furthermore, some antibodies used for immunotherapy have been successfully approved as first- and second-line treatments for advanced lung adenocarcinoma (8). In particular, the immune system reportedly plays an important role in the pathogenesis and prognosis of lung adenocarcinoma (9). Therefore, it is essential to understand the immune prognostic signature of lung adenocarcinoma.

Previous studies have investigated the prognostic role of immune-related genes (IRGs) in lung adenocarcinoma from the ImmPort database (10, 11); however, this database contains published data on IRGs, thus potentially not accounting for all IRGs. Moreover, these studies have reported no correlation between prognostic factors and OS among certain subgroups of patients with lung adenocarcinoma, indicating that this association is largely unknown. One of the important reasons may be the complex prognostic behavior of tumors; furthermore, when considering the characteristics of IRGs directly associated with tumors, it is also important to focus on the tumor microenvironment (TME) (12). The TME is closely associated with tumorigenesis and patient prognosis (13, 14). Moreover, accumulating evidence indicates that tumor-infiltrating immune cells and stromal cells (15, 16), as the primary nontumor components of the TME, play a significant role in lung cancer prognosis. These findings highlight the importance of understanding the association between the TME and lung adenocarcinoma prognosis. The development of a prognostic model of IRGs based on the TME might provide novel insights into the generation of a more accurate prognostic system.

Accurate management and appropriate personalized therapies for lung adenocarcinoma are required in accordance with prognostic stratification. Moreover, an enhanced understanding of IRGs involved in the TME would help elucidate their regulatory mechanisms in the TME and develop new treatment strategies. With advancements in machine learning, the ESTIMATE algorithm has been used to investigate IRGs in the TME, based on the immune and stromal scores of the TME, and to generate a TME-related immune prognostic model (17). Moreover, this algorithm can effectively predict the prognosis of patients with various cancers. Accordingly, in this study, we determined the immune and stromal scores of tumors using the ESTIMATE algorithm and developed a novel TME-related immune prognostic model of lung adenocarcinoma.

Abbreviations: IRGs, immune-related genes; TME, tumor microenvironment; TCGA, The Cancer Genome Atlas data; DAVID, Database for Annotation, Visualization and Integrated Discovery.

MATERIALS AND METHODS

Acquisition of TCGA Data

Normalization of RNA sequence data, in terms of level 3 fragments per kilobase of exon per million fragments mapped (FPKM) reads, was performed for 594 samples obtained from The Cancer Genome Atlas (TCGA) database, including 535 adenocarcinoma and 59 normal lung samples, before December 15, 2019. Thereafter, the Ensemble IDs were converted to gene symbols in accordance with human gene annotations. Furthermore, clinical data of lung adenocarcinoma patients were obtained and merged into a single matrix for subsequent analysis. Patients with an incomplete follow-up duration or recorded date of death of any cause were excluded. Finally, 494 lung adenocarcinoma patients with expression profiles and clinical data were included.

Immune Score and Stromal Score in the TME

Estimation of STromal and Immune cells in MAlignant Tumor tissues using Expression data (ESTIMATE) is a tool for predicting and estimating infiltrating immune and stromal cells in tumor tissues based on gene expression profiles. Herein, the ESTIMATE algorithm was used to analyze the characteristics of specific gene expression in immune and stromal cells for each tumor sample to predict their immune and stromal scores. Thereafter, the immune and stromal scores were analyzed using the estimate package in R software.

Screening of Differentially Expressed IRGs

Based on the median immune and stromal scores, patients with lung adenocarcinoma were divided into two groups: high and low immune/stromal score groups. Significant differences in OS between the high and low immune/stromal score groups were analyzed. On the basis of the significant differences in patient prognosis, differentially expressed IRGs between the two groups were assessed using the Limma package in R software. Finally, intersecting differentially expressed IRGs in both groups were considered for further analysis. A log(fold change) of >2 and an adjusted p-value of <0.05 were considered cutoffs. Heat maps and Venn diagrams were generated using R.

GO and KEGG Pathway Enrichment Analyses of Differentially Expressed IRGs

Gene Ontology (GO) and Kyoto Encyclopedia of Genes and Genomes (KEGG) pathway enrichment analyses were performed to understand gene functional annotation and functional enrichment, respectively. Common differentially expressed IRGs of GO and KEGG annotation were performed using Database for Annotation, Visualization, and Integrated Discovery (DAVID), an online database (https://david.ncifcrf.gov/), to predict functional domains and their biological implications. Fisher's exact test was performed to analyze pathways, diseases, and functions. A p-value of <0.05 indicated the significance of GO terms and KEGG pathway enrichment in genes herein. Furthermore, the top 10 GO terms and KEGG pathway enrichment results were mapped using Hmisc and ggplot2 in R software.

Construction of Prognostic Model for Lung Adenocarcinoma in the Training Set

A total of 494 patients with lung adenocarcinoma in the TCGA dataset were randomly divided into a training set and testing set at a ratio of 7:3 (training cohort, 346 patients; testing cohort, 148 patients).

First, univariate Cox proportional hazard regression analysis was performed to screen out prognostic IRGs in the training cohort (iteration = 1,000), with $p < 0.05$ indicating statistical significance. Second, the key IRGs were further selected from among significant prognostic IRGs on univariate analysis, through least absolute shrinkage and selection operator (LASSO) regression, a powerful tool for developing refined prognostic models, fitting generalized linear models, selecting variables, and regularizing complexity, using R software. Key IRGs were subjected to multivariate Cox regression analysis. Finally, the risk score formula was developed in accordance with the key IRGs identified through LASSO analysis.

Evaluation of the Prognostic Model in the Training Set

After the expression value of each specific gene was included, the risk score formula for each patient was weighted by its estimated regression coefficient on LASSO regression analysis. On the basis of the best separation of risk score, patients were divided into high-risk-score and low-risk-score groups. Survival differences between the two groups were assessed by Kaplan–Meier survival curves using log-rank tests. ROC curves were used to assess the accuracy of model prediction. Furthermore, LASSO regression analysis was performed to examine the role of the risk score in predicting clinical outcomes. Furthermore, the association between risk score and clinical stage was analyzed.

To further determine whether the independent prognostic model could be used as an independent prognostic factor, univariate and multivariate Cox regression analyses were performed to analyze the predictive value of age, sex, stage, TNM stage, and predictive model. In the univariate analysis, the correlation between some independent variables and dependent variables was considered, and some correlations might be masked by the influence of confounding factors. To avoid omitting important predictors of prognosis, the threshold in univariate analysis was relaxed to $p < 0.1$, while the p-value in multivariate analysis was still 0.05.

GSEA Analysis of Differences in Pathway Enrichment in the Training Set

To investigate the differences in the putative mechanism between the high-risk-score and low-risk-score groups, gene set enrichment analysis (GSEA) was performed to comprehensively analyze the differences in function enrichment. GSEA is a computational method of determining whether an a priori defined set of genes is significantly different between two biological states. The number of permutations was set to 1,000, and the permutation type was set to phenotype. In this study, all genes in the training set were sequenced according to the degree of differential expression in the high-risk-score group and the low-risk-score group. GSEA was used to comprehensively analyze differences in gene pathway enrichment between the two groups.

Validation of the Prognostic Model in the Testing Cohort

The prognostic model was further validated for the testing cohort ($n = 148$).

Similarly, the risk score of each patient was weighted on the basis of the risk score. Thereafter, based on the best separation of the risk score, patients in the testing cohort were divided into high-risk-score and low-risk-score groups. A Kaplan–Meier survival curve and ROC curve analysis were performed in the testing however.

Functional Analysis of IRG Signatures in the Model

To further analyze the mutation characteristics and the putative functional mechanisms of these hub IRGs in lung adenocarcinoma, gene expression profiles of patients with lung adenocarcinoma were imported from the following datasets: TCGA database (Broad, Cell 2012), Lung Adenocarcinoma (MSKCC, Science 2015), Lung Adenocarcinoma (TCGA, Firehose Legacy), Lung Adenocarcinoma (TSP, Nature 2008), and Non-Small-Cell Cancer (MSKCC, Cancer Discov 2017). A

TABLE 1 | Baseline characteristics of patients with lung adenocarcinoma.

	Training set		Testing set		*p*-value
	High score (*N* = 194)	**Low score (*N* = 152)**	**High score (*N* = 91)**	**Low score (*N* = 57)**	
Age (years)					
≥60	132	116	68	42	0.131
<60	62	36	23	15	0.767
Gender					
Male	92	67	55	14	0.002
Female	102	85	36	42	0.213
AJCC stage					
Stage I	95	99	35	34	0.802
Stage II	47	29	28	13	0.488
Stage III	41	17	18	4	0.312
Stage IV	9	4	9	4	1.000
NA	2	3	1	2	0.850
T stage					
T1	53	70	22	22	0.429
T2	108	68	52	28	0.577
T3	22	9	11	3	0.593
T4	9	5	5	0	0.257
TX	2	0	1	0	NA
N stage					
N0	114	115	50	39	0.305
N1–3	74	34	40	16	0.701
NX	6	3	1	2	0.523
M stage					
M0	133	92	60	40	0.880
M1	8	4	9	4	1.000
MX	51	54	23	13	0.112
NA	2	2	0	0	NA
Survival Time (days)	653.45 ± 36.96	840.44 ± 82.79	714.41 ± 95.64	953.81 ± 118.03	NA
Survival status					
Alive	113	124	51	44	0.323
Dead	81	28	40	13	0.873

combined study of five datasets including 1,825 patients were included in this study.

GSCALite is an online cancer genomic analysis tool that integrates cancer genomics data for 33 cancer types from the TCGA and normal tissue data from GTEx (http://bioinfo.life.hust.edu.cn/web/GSCALite/), enabling gene set pathway analysis in data analysis. In this study, GSCALite was used to analyze the pathway of hub genes.

The TIMER database is a comprehensive tool for analyzing the immune cell infiltrates in tumors. The abundances of six immune infiltrates (B cells, CD4+ T cells, CD8+ T cells, neutrophils, macrophages, and dendritic cells) were estimated using the TIMER algorithm. In this study, the TIMER database was further applied to analyze the correlation between hub genes and immune cells. The correlation of hub gene expression with immune infiltration level was visualized in lung adenocarcinoma using the Gene module. The scatterplots were generated and displayed after hub genes and cancer type were submitted successfully, showing the purity-corrected partial Spearman's correlation and statistical significance.

Statistical Analysis

All statistical analyses were conducted with the R language (version 3.6.1). All statistical tests were bilateral, and $p < 0.05$ was statistically significant.

RESULTS

Study Design and Workflow Overview

A total of 594 samples were obtained, including 535 adenocarcinoma and 59 normal lung samples. Data for a total of 494 lung adenocarcinoma patients with clinical information were retrieved (**Table 1**). The workflow for constructing and

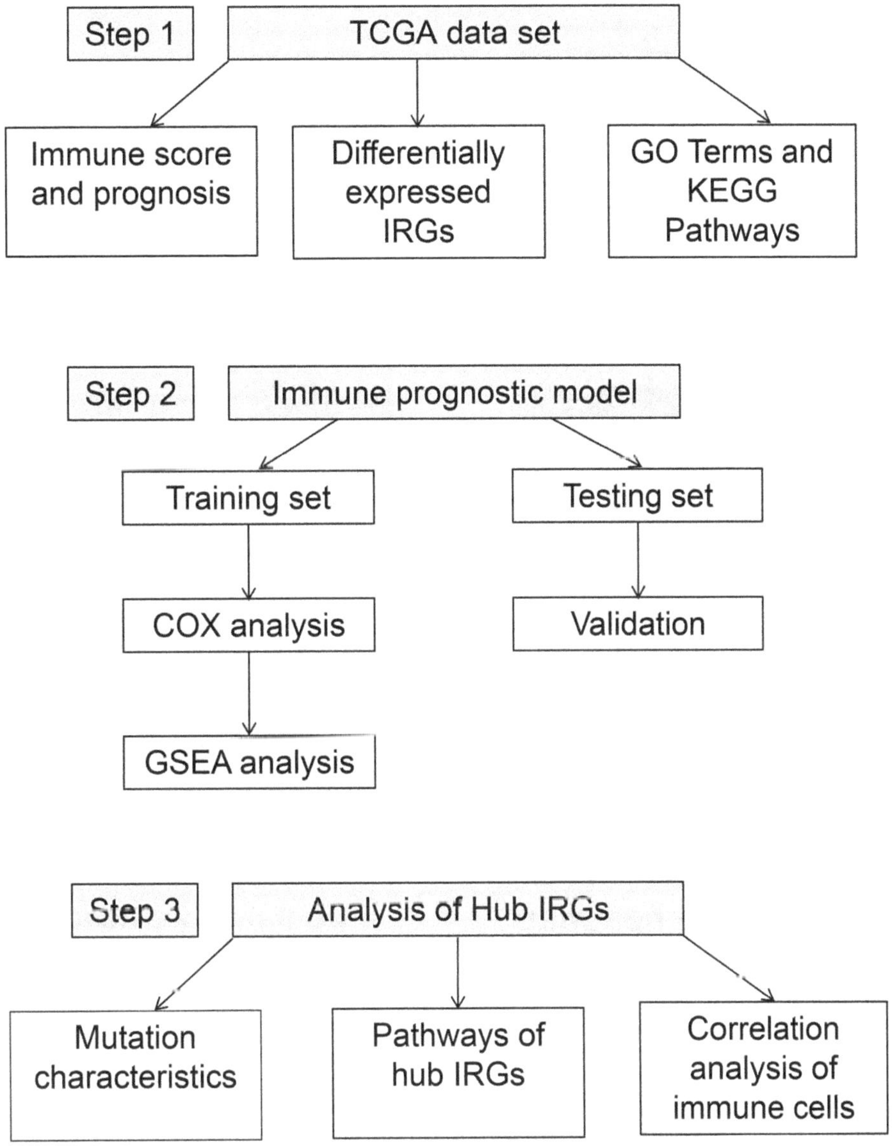

FIGURE 1 | Workflow of the construction and verification of the immune-stromal score prognostic signature.

verifying the immune-related prognostic model is shown in **Figure 1**.

Immune Score and Stromal Score in the TME

The immune and stromal scores were analyzed using the ESTIMATE algorithm. The immune and stromal scores of lung adenocarcinoma are shown in **Supplementary Table 1**. On the basis of the median value of immune and stromal scores, patients with lung adenocarcinoma were divided into two groups: the high immune/stromal score group and the low score group. These results show that the high immune score group had better OS than the low immune score group for lung adenocarcinoma. In terms of stromal score, although patients with high stromal score had better prognosis than those with low stromal score, the difference was not statistically significant (**Figures 2A–C**).

Screening of Differentially Expressed IRGs

According to the criteria of a log(fold change) of >2 and an adjusted p-value of <0.05, our results showed that a total of 3,034 genes with significant differentially expressed IRGs were screened, including 2,521 upregulated IRGs and 513 downregulated IRGs. Among them, 1,394 differentially expressed IRGs (1,092 upregulated IRGs and 302 downregulated IRGs) were included in the immune score group (**Supplementary Table 2**), and 1,640 differentially expressed IRGs (1,429 upregulated IRGs and 211 downregulated IRGs) were included in the stromal score group (**Supplementary Table 3**). Heat maps and

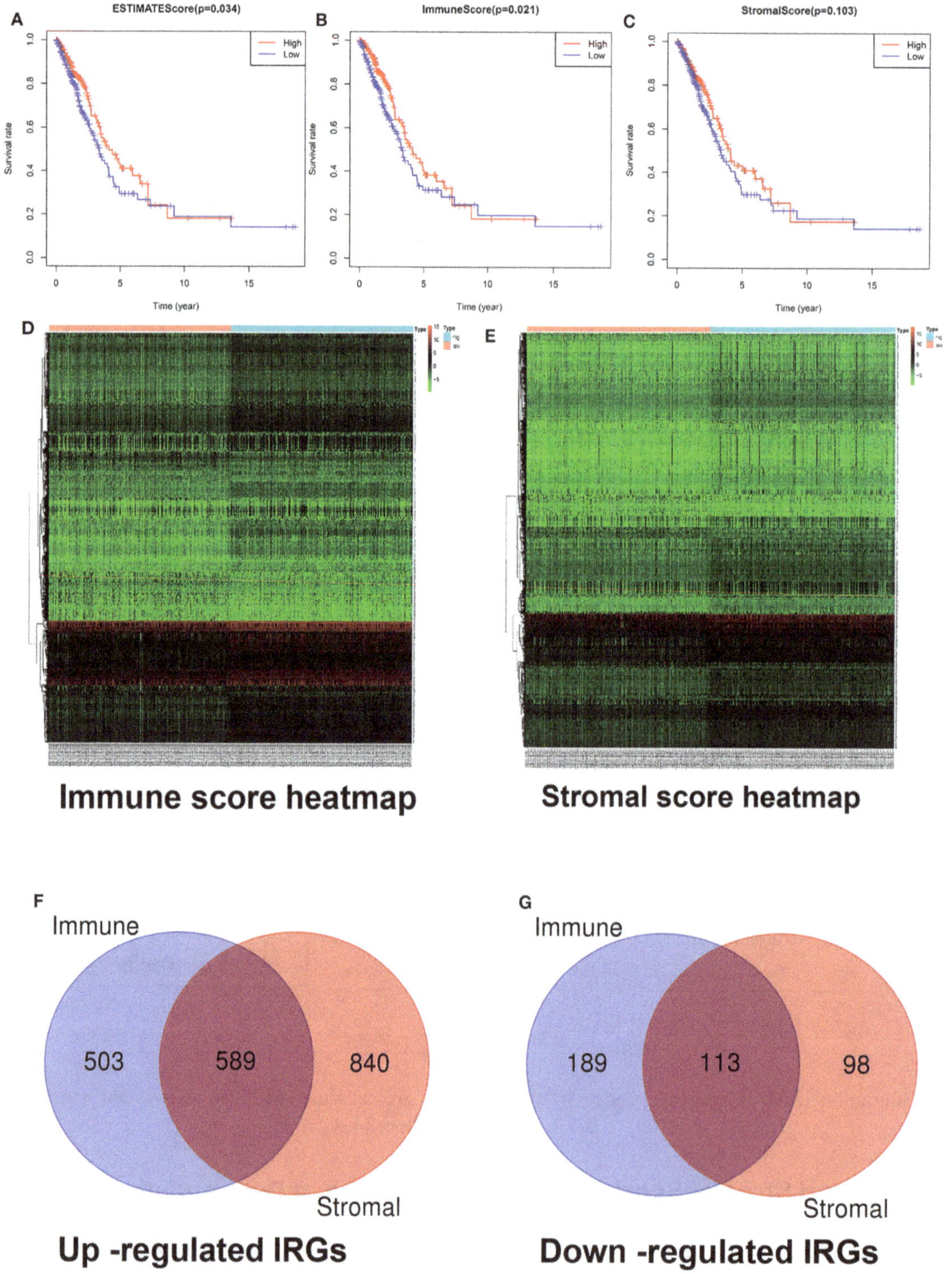

FIGURE 2 | Screening and identification of differentially expressed IRGs. **(A)** Relationship between comprehensive immune score and OS. **(B)** Relationship between immune score and OS. **(C)** Relationship between stromal score and OS. **(D)** Heatmap of immune score groups. **(E)** Heatmap of stromal score groups. **(F)** The Venn diagram of the intersection of up-regulated IRGs between the immune and stromal score groups. **(G)** The Venn diagram of the intersection of down-regulated IRGs between the immune and stromal score groups. OS, overall survival; IRGs, immune-related genes.

Venn diagrams are displayed in **Figures 2D–G**. In total, 702 intersecting differentially expressed IRGs (589 upregulated and 113 downregulated) in both groups are indicated in **Figures 2F,G** (**Supplementary Table 4**).

GO Terms and KEGG Pathway Enrichment Analysis of Differentially Expressed IRGs

GO terms are divided into three parts: biological processes, cellular components, and molecular functions. GO analysis

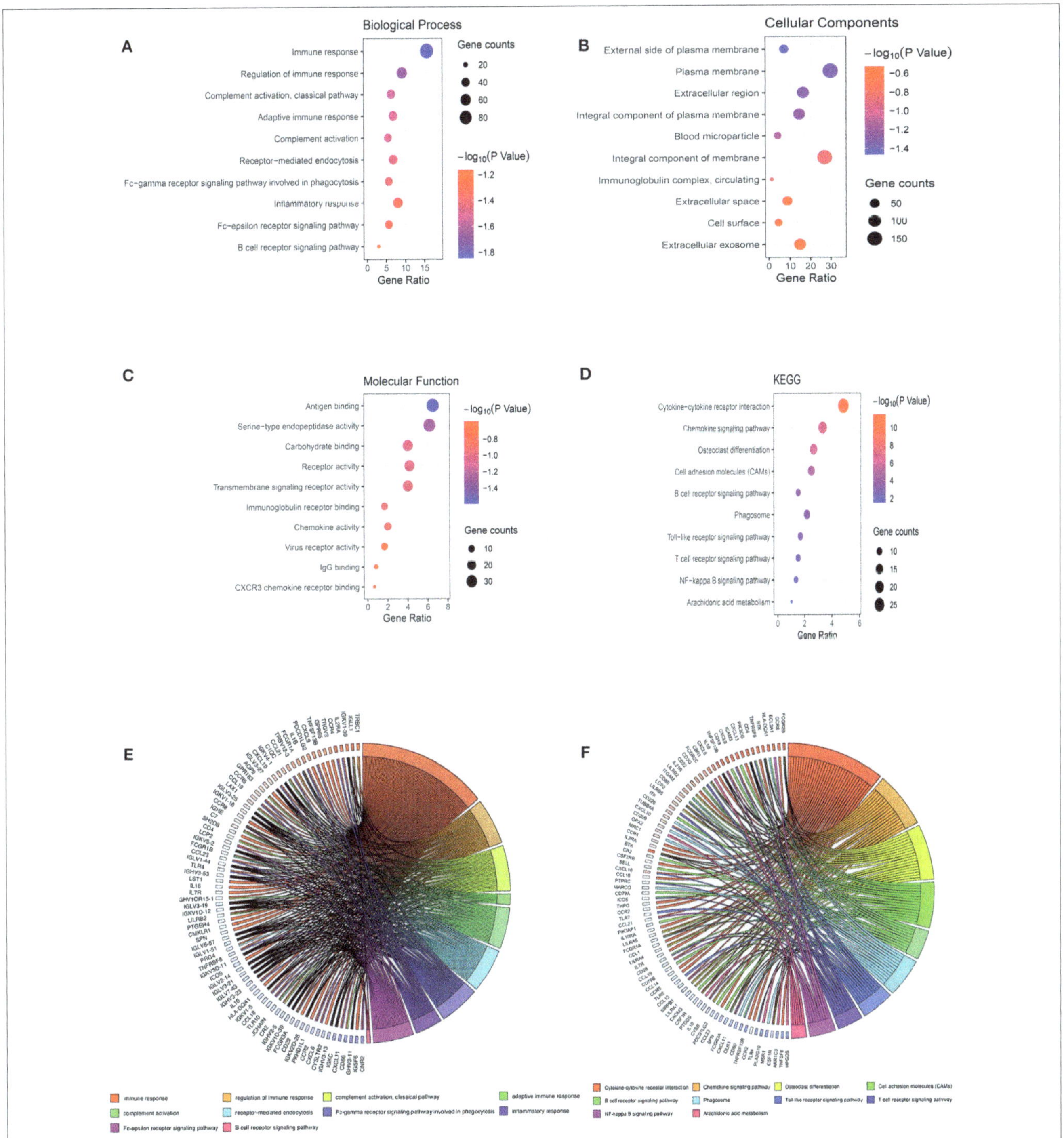

FIGURE 3 | Bubble map of the top 10 GO terms and KEGG pathway enrichment analysis data of differentially expressed IRGs. **(A)** GO analysis of differentially expressed IRGs in biological processes. **(B)** GO analysis of differentially expressed IRGs in cellular components. **(C)** GO analysis of differentially expressed IRGs in terms of molecular function. **(D)** KEGG enrichment analysis of differentially expressed IRGs. A high gene ratio represents a high level of enrichment. The size of the dot indicates the number of target genes in the pathway, and the color of the dot reflects the *p*-value range. **(E)** GO chord plot of differentially expressed IRGs. **(F)** KEGG chord plot of differentially expressed IRGs.

TABLE 2 | Top five GO terms.

Category	ID	Term	Count	%	*p* value	FDR
Upregulated IRGs						
GOTERM_BP_DIRECT	GO:0006955	Immune response	93	17.95366795	4.59E−75	7.47E−72
GOTERM_BP_DIRECT	GO:0050776	Regulation of immune response	55	10.61776062	1.14E−51	1.86E−48
GOTERM_BP_DIRECT	GO:0002250	Adaptive immune response	41	7.915057915	4.73E−36	7.69E−33
GOTERM_BP_DIRECT	GO:0006956	Complement activation	33	6.370656371	6.95E−34	1.13E−30
GOTERM_BP_DIRECT	GO:0006898	Receptor-mediated endocytosis	40	7.722007722	1.48E−30	2.40E−27
GOTERM_CC_DIRECT	GO:0009897	External side of plasma membrane	43	8.301158301	1.52E−31	1.86E−28
GOTERM_CC_DIRECT	GO:0005886	Plasma membrane	167	32.23938224	5.95E−29	7.29E−26
GOTERM_CC_DIRECT	GO:0005887	Integral component of plasma membrane	85	16.40926641	2.95E−23	3.61E−20
GOTERM_CC_DIRECT	GO:0005576	Extracellular region	86	16.6023166	3.11E−20	3.81E−17
GOTERM_CC_DIRECT	GO:0072562	Blood microparticle	24	4.633204633	4.61E−15	5.71E−12
GOTERM_MF_DIRECT	GO:0003823	Antigen binding	39	7.528957529	6.92E−41	9.44E−38
GOTERM_MF_DIRECT	GO:0004252	Serine-type endopeptidase activity	36	6.94980695	1.11E−21	1.52E−18
GOTERM_MF_DIRECT	GO:0004872	Receptor activity	25	4.826254826	4.79E−13	6.53E−10
GOTERM_MF_DIRECT	GO:0004888	Transmembrane signaling receptor activity	24	4.633204633	2.73E−12	3.72E−09
GOTERM_MF_DIRECT	GO:0030246	Carbohydrate binding	23	4.44015444	3.43E−12	4.68E−09
Downregulated IRGs						
GOTERM_BP_DIRECT	GO:0071395	Cellular response to jasmonic acid stimulus	3	3.75	7.50E−05	0.106090023
GOTERM_BP_DIRECT	GO:0044598	Doxorubicin metabolic process	3	3.75	3.47E−04	0.489670004
GOTERM_BP_DIRECT	GO:0044597	Daunorubicin metabolic process	3	3.75	3.47E−04	0.489670004
GOTERM_BP_DIRECT	GO:0030855	Epithelial cell differentiation	4	5	0.002002754	2.797891239
GOTERM_BP_DIRECT	GO:0055114	Oxidation–reduction process	8	10	0.004999641	6.849000785
GOTERM_CC_DIRECT	GO:0043025	Neuronal cell body	6	7.5	0.00495641	5.157580931
GOTERM_CC_DIRECT	GO:0008076	Voltage-gated potassium channel complex	3	3.75	0.038309612	34.05203615
GOTERM_CC_DIRECT	GO:0005576	Extracellular region	11	13.75	0.053136406	44.11602637
GOTERM_CC_DIRECT	GO:0005892	Acetylcholine-gated channel complex	2	2.5	0.081015685	59.35918267
GOTERM_MF_DIRECT	GO:0016655	Oxidoreductase activity, acting on NAD(P)H, quinone or similar compound as acceptor	4	5	2.36E−06	0.002915475
GOTERM_MF_DIRECT	GO:0047086	Ketosteroid monooxygenase activity	3	3.75	3.72E−05	0.045918231
GOTERM_MF_DIRECT	GO:0047115	trans-1,2-dihydrobenzene-1,2-diol dehydrogenase activity	3	3.75	7.42E−05	0.091606887
GOTERM_MF_DIRECT	GO:0018636	Phenanthrene 9,10-monooxygenase activity	3	3.75	7.42E−05	0.091606887
GOTERM_MF_DIRECT	GO:0004032	Alditol:NADP+ 1-oxidoreductase activity	3	3.75	2.58E−04	0.318095483

showed that upregulated IRGs were mainly involved in the immune response (BP, GO: 0006955), external side of plasma membrane (CC, GO: 0009897), and antigen binding (MF, GO: 0003823). The downregulated IRGs were mainly involved in the cellular response to jasmonic acid stimulus (BP, GO: 0071395), neuronal cell body (CC, GO: 0043025), and oxidoreductase activity, and in acting on NAD(P)H, quinone or similar compounds as acceptors (MF, GO: 0016655) (**Figures 3A-C,E; Table 2**). The KEGG pathway enrichment results in the upregulated IRGs were mainly involved in cytokine–cytokine receptor interactions, chemokine signaling pathways, and cell adhesion molecules (CAMs). However, the KEGG pathway enrichment results of downregulated IRGs were mainly involved in arachidonic acid metabolism, metabolic pathways, and tyrosine metabolism (**Figures 3D,F; Table 3**).

Development of a Prognostic Model for the Training Cohort

To generate a prognostic model for lung adenocarcinoma, univariate regression analysis was first performed to screen the key prognostic genes in the training cohort. Thereafter, 58 significantly differentially expressed IRGs correlated with prognosis were considered for LASSO regression analysis. Finally, three key IRGs (*CLEC17A*, *INHA*, and *XIRP1*) were selected to generate an immune prognostic model. The results of the multivariate Cox regression analysis are summarized in **Table 4**. The risk score was determined using the following formula:

[Expression level of *CLEC17A* × (−0.13549042)] + [Expression level of *INHA* × (0.01207179)] + [Expression level of *XIRP1* × (0.6263501)].

TABLE 3 | Top five KEGG pathway enrichment results.

Category	Term	Count	%	*p*-value	Genes	FDR
Upregulated IRGs						
KEGG_PATHWAY	Cytokine–cytokine receptor interaction	28	5.405405405	2.94E−13	CCL1, IL21R, CXCL9, TNFRSF8, CXCL6, CXCL11, IL7R, IL10, CXCL10, CCL23, CCL21, IL10RA, CSF2RB, IL1B, CSF1R, IL2RA, TNFRSF13B, CCL19, CCL18, TNFSF8, CCR8, CCL13, CCL14, TNFSF13B, CCR5, CCR4, CXCL13, CCR2	3.53E−10
KEGG_PATHWAY	Chemokine signaling pathway	19	3.667953668	3.51E−08	CCL1, PIK3CG, ITK, CXCL9, CCL19, CXCL6, CXCL11, CCL18, CXCL10, CCR8, DOCK2, CCL13, CCL23, CCL14, CCR5, CCL21, CXCL13, CCR4, CCR2	4.22E−05
KEGG_PATHWAY	Cell adhesion molecules (CAMs)	15	2.895752896	1.03E−06	PTPRC, CADM3, SELL, ICAM3, ITGAM, PDCD1LG2, HLA-DQA1, CD86, CD80, ICOS, CD22, CD4, CD226, SPN, CD28	0.00123743
KEGG_PATHWAY	B cell receptor signaling pathway	9	1.737451737	7.44E−05	PIK3CG, CD19, CR2, FCGR2B, CD22, PIK3AP1, CD79B, CD79A, BTK	0.089383945
KEGG_PATHWAY	Phagosome	12	2.316602317	2.37E−04	MRC1, MARCO, MSR1, FCGR2B, OLR1, FCGR2C, FCGR1A, CD209, TLR4, FCGR3A, ITGAM, HLA-DQA1	0.284714595
Downregulated IRGs						
KEGG_PATHWAY	Arachidonic acid metabolism	4	5	0.002057483	AKR1C3, GPX2, CBR1, PLA2G10	2.102810979
KEGG_PATHWAY	Metabolic pathways	13	16.25	0.002420062	ETNPPL, DDC, ODC1, PLA2G10, OGDHL, HAL, HGD, TAT, AKR1C3, CBR1, HMGCS2, ENO3, NAT8L	2.469211516
KEGG_PATHWAY	Tyrosine metabolism	3	3.75	0.009368241	DDC, HGD, TAT	9.255598588
KEGG_PATHWAY	Metabolism of xenobiotics by cytochrome P450	3	3.75	0.038441569	AKR1C2, CBR1, AKR1C1	33.26837318
KEGG_PATHWAY	Phenylalanine metabolism	2	2.5	0.069378576	DDC, TAT	52.38108893

TABLE 4 | Multivariate Cox regression analysis of key immune-related genes.

Gene	Coef	HR	HR.95L	HR.95H	*p*-value
CLEC17A	−0.13549042	0.192289385	0.071601478	0.516402855	0.001071204
INHA	0.01207179	1.141665832	1.046649718	1.245307623	0.002804616
XIRP1	0.6263501	2.024671234	1.219239069	3.362173761	0.006410729

Evaluation of the Prognostic Model in the Training Cohort

LASSO regression analysis was performed to construct and evaluate the prognostic model (**Figures 4A,B**). Patients were divided into high- and low-risk-score groups in accordance with the best separation of risk scores. The high-risk-score group had significantly worse OS than the low-risk-score group ($p < 0.0001$; **Figure 4C**). The area under the ROC curve for predicting the 1-, 3-, and 5-year survival of lung adenocarcinoma was 0.699, 0.631, and 0.669, respectively (**Figure 4D**).

Additionally, the risk curve indicated that the high-risk-score group had a higher mortality and worse prognosis than the low-risk-score group (cutoff value: 0.889; **Figure 4E**). Further analysis of the relationship between risk score and pathological stage revealed that patients with early-stage lung adenocarcinoma (stages 1 and 2) scored lower than those with advanced stage lung adenocarcinoma ($p = 0.043$; **Figure 4F**).

Univariate Cox analysis showed that pathological staging and risk score had statistical significance, while age and sex had no statistical significance (**Figure 4G**). However, multivariate Cox analysis showed that pathological stage (HR, 1.995; 95% CI, 1.113–3.574; $p = 0.020$) and risk score (HR, 1.120; 95% CI, 1.025–1.223; $p = 0.012$) were independent prognostic factors (**Figure 4H**).

GSEA of the Mechanism Underlying the Prognostic Differences Between the Two Groups

In this study, the possible molecular mechanisms of the prognosis difference between the two groups of patients were analyzed by GSEA analysis. The results showed that the GO and pathway enrichment in the high-risk-score group was mainly involved in metabolism-related pathways (**Figures 5A,C**). However, GO and pathway enrichment in the low-risk-score group was primarily focused on immunoregulation and immune cell activation (**Figures 5B,D**). The detailed GSEA results are described in **Table 5**.

Validation of the Prediction Model in the Testing Cohort

The Kaplan–Meier results showed that the high-risk group had worse OS than the low-risk group ($p < 0.0001$) (**Figure 6A**). The area under the ROC curve for predicting the 1-, 3-, and 5-year survival of lung adenocarcinoma was 0.725, 0.712, and 0.660, respectively (**Figure 6B**). Additionally, risk curve revealed that the high-risk-score group had a worse prognosis than the low-risk-score group (**Figure 6C**). These results were consistent with the results of the training set.

The Mechanism of Action of Hub IRGs in the TCGA Database

To further analyze the potential function of hub IRGs, our results were verified using the TCGA and GTEx databases. First, the mutation characteristics of these hub IRGs were analyzed among patients with lung adenocarcinoma. The mutation rates of these hub IRGs in patients with lung adenocarcinoma were 0.8, 1, and 2.6% (**Figure 7A**). Moreover, each hub gene had different mutation forms, including mutation, deletion, and amplification, in lung adenocarcinoma. For example, the mutation form of CLEC17A was mainly amplification, the mutation form of INHA was mainly amplification and missense mutation, while the mutation form of XIRP1 was mainly deep deletion and missense mutation (**Figure 7B**).

In addition, analysis of pathways in the GSCALite database revealed that CLEC17A is primarily involved in the activation of the epithelial–mesenchymal transition (EMT) and RAS pathways and cell cycle inhibition. INHA is primarily involved in the activation of the mTOR pathway and inhibition of the apoptosis pathway. XIRP1 was mainly involved in the activation of the apoptosis and the EMT pathways and inhibition of the DNA damage and the PI3K pathways (**Figures 7C,D**).

Finally, the TIMER database was used to analyze the correlation between hub IRGs and immune cells. The results showed that these key genes were significantly correlated with the infiltration of CD4+ T cells, CD8+ T cells, macrophages, B cells, and neutrophils. Assuming that a correlation coefficient >0.3 was considered a strong correlation, further analysis showed that CLEC17A was positively correlated with the infiltration of B cells and CD4+ T cells. However, INHA was negatively correlated with the infiltration of CD8+ T and dendritic cells. However, there was no strong correlation between XIRP1 and the infiltration of immune cells (**Figure 7E**). Moreover, the relationship between copy number variation (CNV) of hub IRGs and immune cell infiltration was further analyzed. The results showed that there were significant differences between the CNV of these hub IRGs and immune cell infiltration. Arm-level deletion of the CLEC17A gene was closely related to the infiltration of B cells, CD4+ T cells, macrophages, neutrophils, and dendritic cells. Arm-level gain of the INHA gene was closely related to the infiltration of CD4+ T cells. Arm-level deletion of the XIRP1 gene was closely related to the infiltration of CD4+ T cells and macrophages (**Figure 7F**).

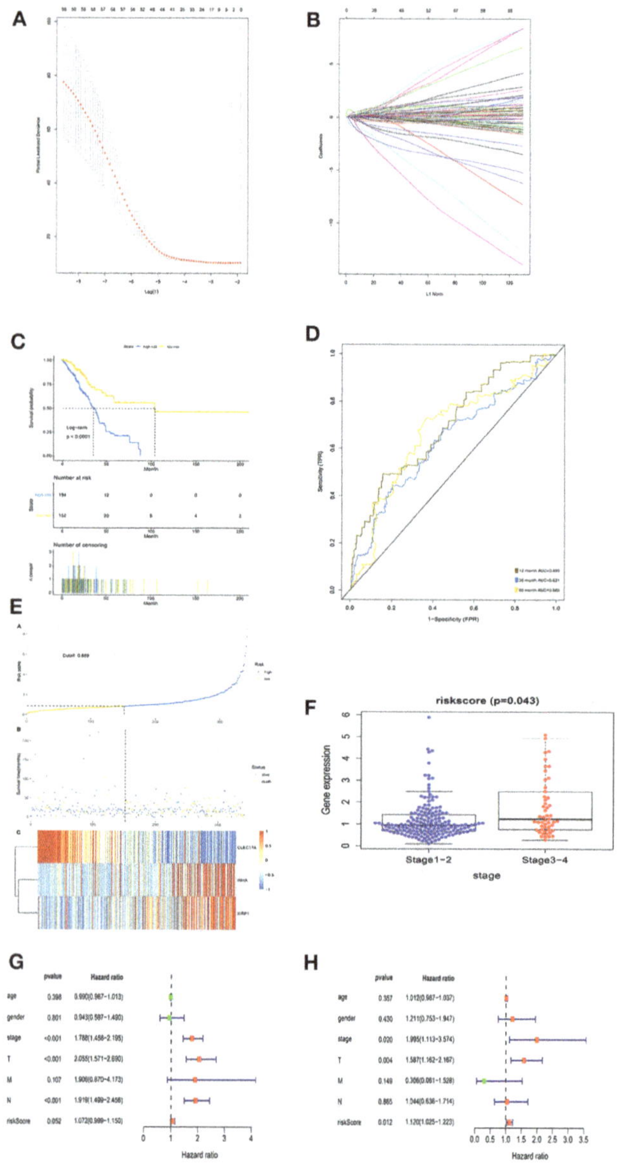

FIGURE 4 | LASSO regression analysis and identification of prognostic signatures in the training set. **(A)** Ten-fold cross-validation for turning parameter selection in the LASSO Cox regression model. **(B)** Coefficient profiles in the LASSO Cox regression model. **(C)** Survival curve of low- and high-risk groups stratified by immune-stromal score signature. **(D)** ROC analysis of the TCGA dataset for prognostic signature. **(E)** LASSO regression analysis of low- and high-risk groups. **(F)** Relationship between risk score and clinical stage. **(G)** The forest plot of the prognostic signature by univariate analysis. **(H)** The forest plot of the prognostic signature by multivariate Cox proportional regression analysis.

DISCUSSION

Tumor-infiltrating immune cells in the TME significantly contribute to the prognosis of lung adenocarcinoma. Therefore, it

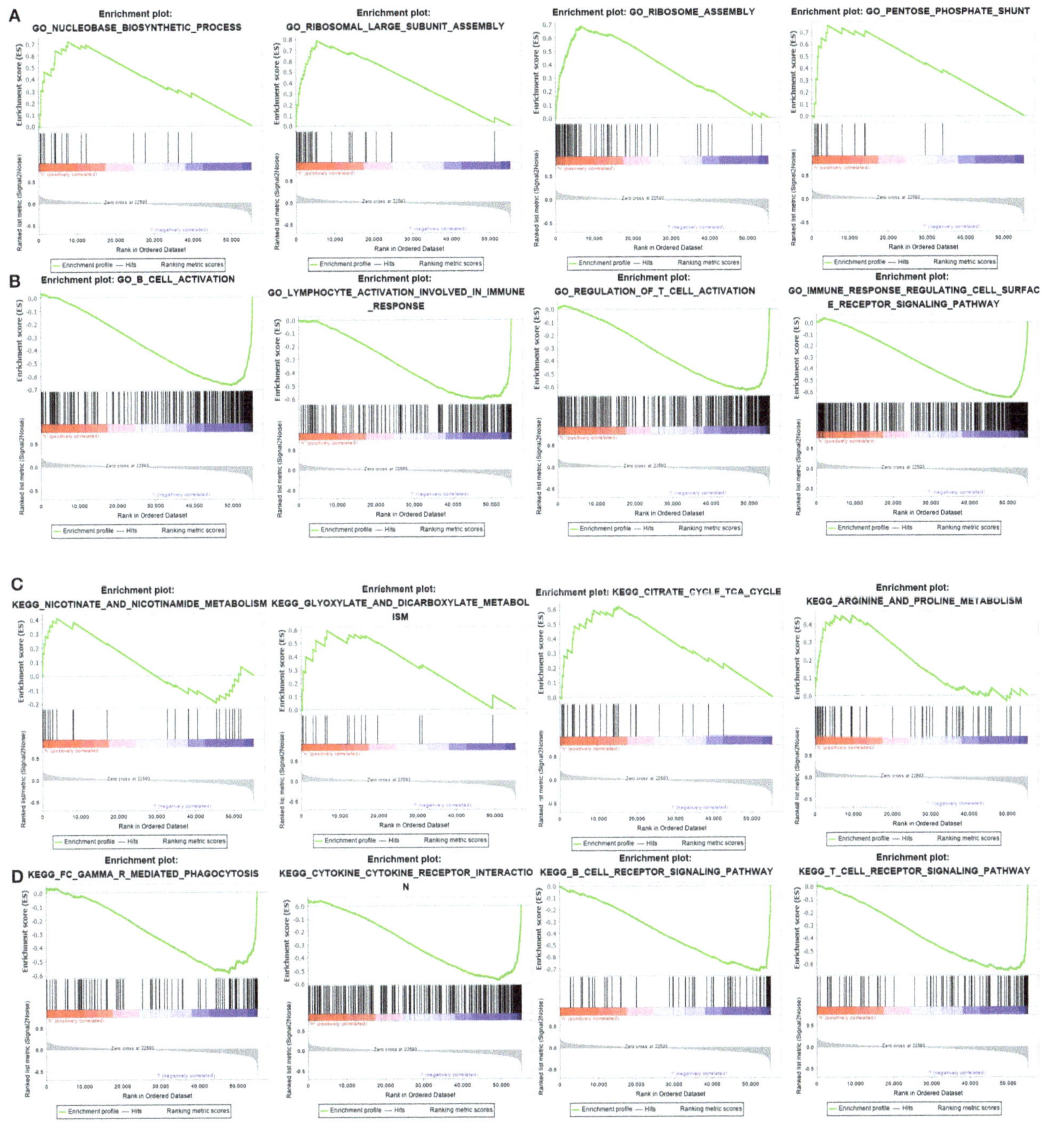

FIGURE 5 | GSEA analysis of differences in pathway enrichment in the training set. **(A,B)** GO terms in the high- and low-risk score groups. **(C,D)** KEGG pathway enrichment in the high- and low-risk score groups.

is essential to develop a TME-related immune prognostic model for appropriate clinical management of lung adenocarcinoma. Accordingly, the aim of this study was to develop a novel TME-related immune prognostic model for lung adenocarcinoma.

Although some studies have explored the prognostic value of TME-related IRGs in lung adenocarcinoma, certain key issues of these models remain to be resolved.

Yang et al. (18) used the CIBERSORT algorithm to analyze a TME-related prognostic immunity-based model for lung adenocarcinoma. This model was developed to evaluate the relative levels of the 22 immune cell phenotypes, primarily including B cells, T cells, macrophages, dendritic cells, plasma cells, natural killer cells, and mast cells. Moreover, this algorithm is primarily used to evaluate immune cells; however, it cannot be

TABLE 5 | Detailed results of gene set enrichment analysis.

NAME	ES	NES	NOM *p* value
GO Terms			
High score group			
GO_RIBOSOMAL_LARGE_SUBUNIT_ASSEMBLY	0.78643316	1.9444792	0.00203252
GO_PENTOSE_PHOSPHATE_SHUNT	0.7535411	1.8539398	0.008298756
GO_RIBOSOME_ASSEMBLY	0.68597955	1.8540714	0.016528925
GO_NUCLEOBASE_BIOSYNTHETIC_PROCESS	0.71662575	1.7974799	0.01980198
Low score group			
GO_B_CELL_ACTIVATION	−0.6719656	−2.3789294	0
GO_IMMUNE_RESPONSE_REGULATING_CELL_SURFACE_RECEPTOR_SIGNALING_PATHWAY	−0.654903	−2.3589978	0
GO_LYMPHOCYTE_ACTIVATION_INVOLVED_IN_IMMUNE_RESPONSE	−0.60444784	−2.3353372	0
GO_T_CELL_ACTIVATION	−0.6102059	−2.343195	0
KEGG Pathway Enrichment			
High score group			
KEGG_CITRATE_CYCLE_TCA_CYCLE	0.62047356	1.6142783	0.046184737
KEGG_GLYOXYLATE_AND_DICARBOXYLATE_METABOLISM	0.5940425	1.5761957	0.060194176
KEGG_ARGININE_AND_PROLINE_METABOLISM	0.45005503	1.4639851	0.055900622
KEGG_NICOTINATE_AND_NICOTINAMIDE_METABOLISM	0.4092993	1.3358487	0.115384616
Low score group			
KEGG_B_CELL_RECEPTOR_SIGNALING_PATHWAY	−0.72458243	−2.4734645	0
KEGG_T_CELL_RECEPTOR_SIGNALING_PATHWAY	−0.6531744	−2.3155243	0
KEGG_CYTOKINE_CYTOKINE_RECEPTOR_INTERACTION	−0.5735697	−2.178205	0.001968504
KEGG_FC_GAMMA_R_MEDIATED_PHAGOCYTOSIS	−0.5871511	−2.1173847	0

used to evaluate stromal cells in the TME. Yue et al. (19) used the ESTIMATE algorithm to investigate the TME-related immune prognostic characteristics of lung adenocarcinoma. However, they directly enumerated immune and stromal cells from their expression profiles of all genes expressed in lung adenocarcinoma and normal tissues. Moreover, differentially expressed IRGs were analyzed using Wilcoxon correlation analysis between tumor and normal tissue. However, some limitations are associated with the analysis of multi-dimensional tumor gene expression profiles through the Wilcoxon rank-sum test. These findings indicate that these TME-related prognostic immunity-based models have not been adequately evaluated. These issues can be resolved primarily by improving the algorithm of IRGs in the TME and to identify more specific TME-related IRGs for lung adenocarcinoma. Therefore, it is essential to develop a new TME-related immune prognostic model for lung adenocarcinoma.

To address these aforementioned limitations, in the present study, a new method was developed to identify differentially expressed IRGs. First, TME-related differentially expressed IRGs were identified exclusively from tumor samples by evaluating tumor-infiltrating immune cells and stromal cells via the ESTIMATE algorithm; this probably effectively reflected the TME-related IRGs in tumor tissue. Second, differentially expressed IRGs were analyzed on the basis of significant differences in OS between the high- and low-immune-score groups in terms of lung adenocarcinoma, rather than differences between lung adenocarcinoma and normal tissue using the Wilcoxon rank-sum test. The prognostic model, based on prognosis-associated differentially expressed genes, might more accurately predict the prognosis of lung adenocarcinoma. Finally, intersecting differentially expressed IRGs with significant prognostic characteristics in both immune and stromal scores were used for subsequent analysis. Both immune cells and stromal cells in each tumor sample were assessed, thus better reflecting the characteristics of the TME. Therefore, the TME-related immune prognostic model developed herein was different from those developed previously. In this study, we developed a more robust prognostic model of TME-related IRGs in lung adenocarcinoma.

Furthermore, this study shows that patients with lung adenocarcinoma and high immune scores had a better prognosis than those with low immune scores, which might be due to the involvement of upregulated IRGs in immune cell infiltration factors, such as cytokines and B cell immune pathways. Clinical studies have also shown that lung cancer patients with high immune infiltration of helper T cells have a better prognosis than those with low infiltration (20, 21). These findings were consistent with our results. Previous studies have suggested that IL-2 is involved in antitumor T cell infiltration, increasing the efficacy of immunotherapy (22). IL-33 also promotes myeloid-derived suppressor cells (MDSCs) and interferes with CD8+ T and natural killer (NK) cell infiltration (23). These studies have suggested that certain cytokines are involved in antitumor immune pathways, potentially elucidating the mechanisms associated with prognosis.

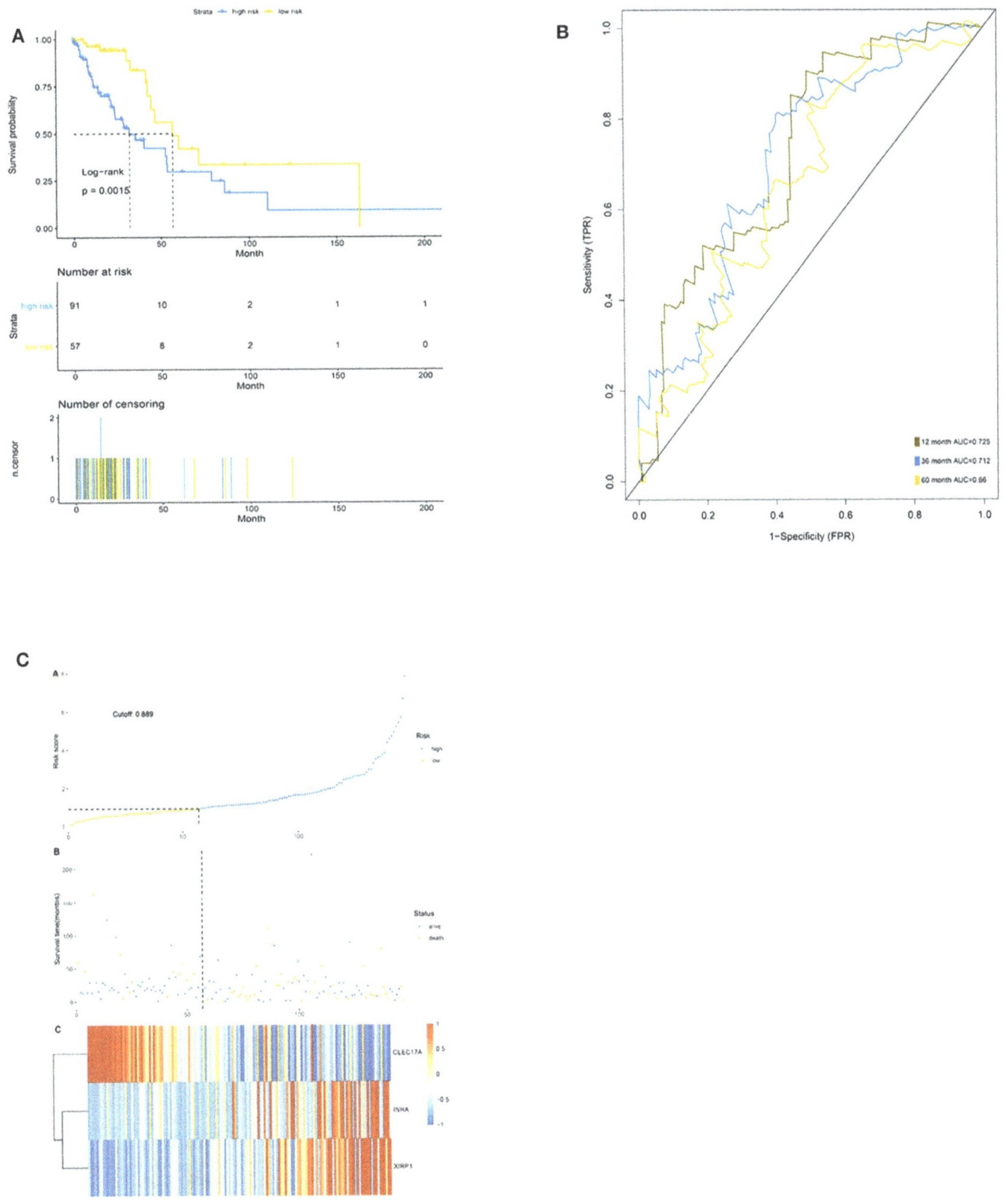

FIGURE 6 | Validation of the prediction features. **(A)** Survival curve of low- and high-risk groups stratified by immune-stromal score signature. **(B)** ROC analysis of the TCGA dataset for prognostic signature. **(C)** LASSO regression analysis of low- and high-risk groups.

Moreover, GSEA was performed to further investigate the potential mechanism underlying the differences in prognosis between the two groups. The present results indicate that the immunoregulation and immune cell activation pathways are potentially associated with a better prognosis. The underlying putative mechanism potentially involves the enrichment of B and T cell immune pathways. Furthermore, the infiltration of these immune cells is associated with an enhanced prognosis among patients with lung adenocarcinoma. Our results are concurrent with those of the aforementioned studies.

Furthermore, this study described the functional prediction of potential hub IRGs. An enhanced understanding of these potential hub genes is essential to elucidate their mechanisms of action in the TME in lung adenocarcinoma. The present results suggest that although these genes were prognosis-related IRGs, they harbored different mutations involved in different

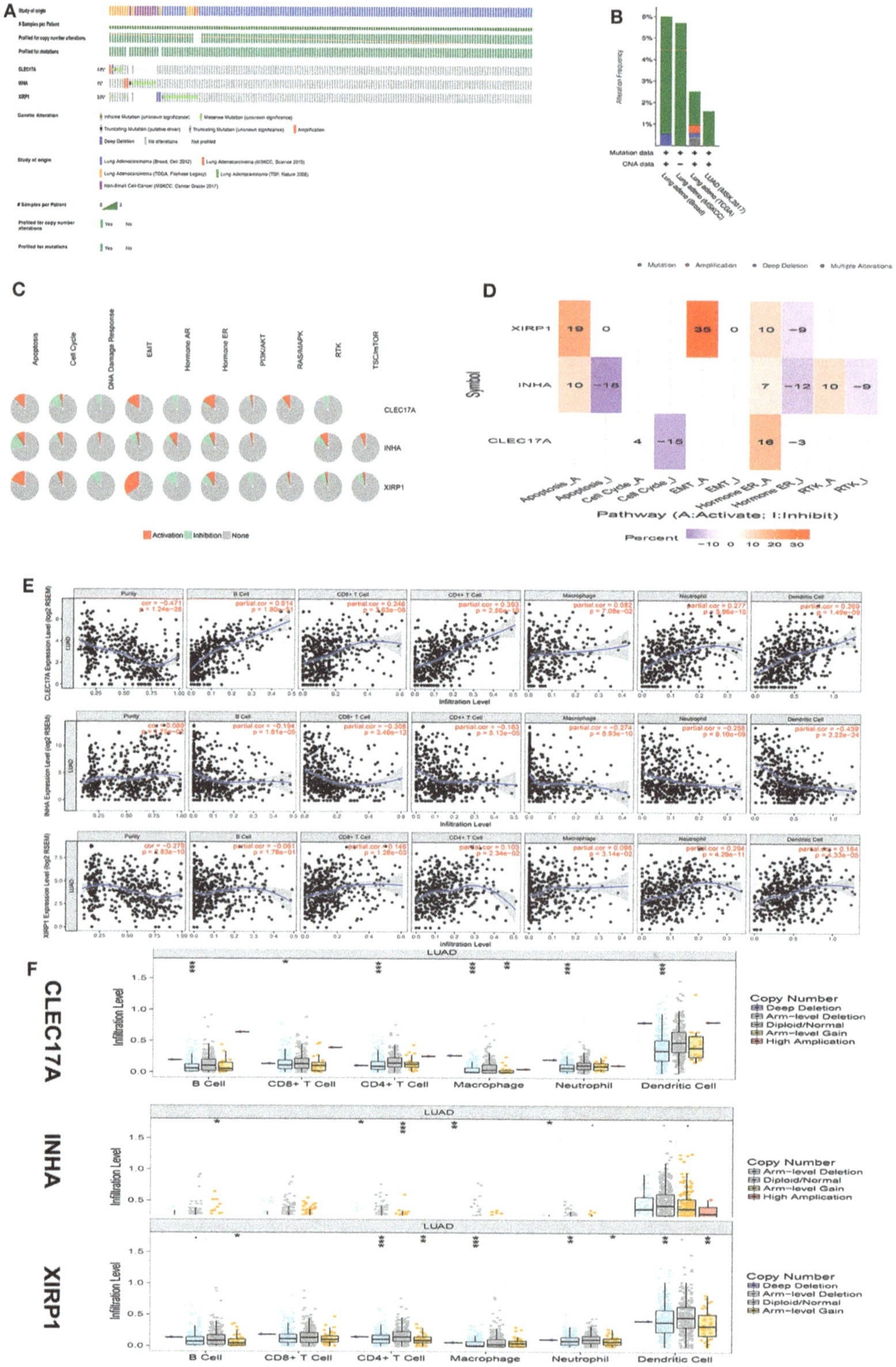

FIGURE 7 | Mechanism analysis of hub genes in the TCGA database. **(A)** Matrix heat map shows genomic alterations of hub genes in five lung datasets. **(B)** The alteration frequencies of hub genes across five studies on lung adenocarcinoma. **(C)** The pathways of hub genes were analyzed by the GSCALite tool. **(D)** Heatmap percentage of hub genes. **(E)** The correlation between the hub gene and immune cells was analyzed in the TIMER database. **(F)** The relationship between copy number variation (CNV) of hub genes and immune cell infiltration was further analyzed.

pathways in lung adenocarcinoma, indicating their potential involvement in different immunoregulatory pathways in lung adenocarcinoma. Further analysis of the function of these genes revealed that these hub genes and their CNVs were different. Moreover, the association between these hub genes and the infiltration of B cells, CD4+ T cells, CD8+ T cells, neutrophils, and other immune cells was also different. These results indicate that different CNVs of these hub genes warrant further differentiation to better understand the association between hub genes and immune cell infiltration. Based on the aforementioned results, our results indicate that *CLEC17A*, *INHA*, and *XIRP1* are potential novel biomarkers for the prognosis of lung adenocarcinoma.

CLEC17A is a human lectin found in lymph node B cells and is involved in a variety of biological processes, including cell adhesion, intercellular interactions, and pathogen recognition (24). Previous studies have shown that CLEC17A is related to the B cell receptor signaling pathway and plays an important role in the pathogenesis of chronic lymphocytic leukemia (25). The present results further indicate that CLEC17A is associated with immune cell infiltration in lung adenocarcinoma, concurrent with previous reports. XIRP1 is a striated muscle protein and belongs to the Xin actin-binding repeat-containing protein (XIRP) family. Previous studies have shown that the XIRP1 gene is related to hypertension and nervous system development (26, 27). The function of the gene has not been reported in tumors. However, our study showed that it was not only related to the TME in lung adenocarcinoma but is also related to the prognosis of lung adenocarcinoma. INHA encodes a member of the transforming growth factor-beta (TGF-beta) superfamily of proteins. The function of the gene has not been reported in lung cancer. Our results showed that INHA was a marker of poor prognosis in lung adenocarcinoma. The possible mechanism was that INHA was involved in tumor angiogenesis, leading to tumor metastasis and poor prognosis (28). Further studies are required to elucidate the roles of these hub genes in the TME in the pathogenesis of lung adenocarcinoma.

This study also had some limitations. First, this study only mined data in the TCGA database and did not combine GEO database analysis. However, in our study, patient data were segregated into training and testing cohorts. In addition, the results were verified and analyzed in comprehensive TCGA and GSCALite datasets. Second, the function of the hub gene in our study was analyzed based on the TCGA database, and the validation function of the hub gene needs to be further confirmed by basic experiments. Constructing an immune-related prognosis model was the focus of our research; hence, there was no basic experiment on hub prognostic genes. Third, our study only analyzed the correlation of differentially expressed IRGs with immune cell infiltration, thus lacking the correlation analysis of the expression of PDL1 and tumor mutational burden.

CONCLUSIONS

The robust TME-related immune prognostic model developed herein effectively predicted the prognosis of patients with lung adenocarcinoma, thus potentially guiding personalized treatment of lung adenocarcinoma in accordance with prognostic stratification. Further studies are required to elucidate the regulatory mechanisms of these IRGs in the TME and develop new treatment strategies.

AUTHOR CONTRIBUTIONS

XQ designed the study, analyzed the data, and drafted the paper. CQ critically revised it for important intellectual content. BQ and XK assisted in data acquisition and analysis. YH and WH revised the manuscript. All authors read and approved the final version of the manuscript.

ACKNOWLEDGMENTS

The authors would like to thank TCGA databases for the availability of the data.

SUPPLEMENTARY MATERIAL

Supplementary Table 1 | Immune-Stromal score of lung adenocarcinoma.

Supplementary Table 2 | Differential IRGs estimated by immune score.

Supplementary Table 3 | Differential IRGs estimated by stromal score.

Supplementary Table 4 | Intersection of differential IRGs.

REFERENCES

1. Romaszko AM, Doboszyńska A. Multiple primary lung cancer: a literature review. *Adv Clin Exp Med.* (2018) 27:725–30. doi: 10.17219/acem/68631
2. Schneider BJ, Ismaila N, Altorki N. Lung cancer surveillance after definitive Curative-Intent therapy: ASCO guideline summary. *JCO Oncol Pract.* (2020) 16:83–6. doi: 10.1200/JOP.19.00722
3. Singhi EK, Horn L, Sequist LV, Heymach J, Langer CJ. Advanced non-small cell lung cancer: sequencing agents in the EGFR-mutated/ALK-rearranged populations. *Am Soc Clin Oncol Educ Book.* (2019) 39:e187–e97. doi: 10.1200/EDBK_237821
4. Possidente L, Landriscina M, Patitucci G, Borgia L, Lalinga V, Vita G. ALK rearrangement in specific subtypes of lung adenocarcinoma: immunophenotypic and morphological features. *Med Oncol.* (2017) 34:76. doi: 10.1007/s12032-017-0936-z
5. Sgambato A, Casaluce F, Maione P, Gridelli C. Targeted therapies in non-small cell lung cancer: a focus on ALK/ROS1 tyrosine kinase inhibitors. *Expert Rev Anticancer Ther.* (2018) 18:71–80. doi: 10.1080/14737140.2018.1412260
6. Nasim F, Sabath BF, Eapen GA. Lung cancer. *Med Clin North Am.* (2019) 103:463–73. doi: 10.1016/j.mcna.2018.12.006
7. Woodard GA, Jones KD, Jablons DM. Lung cancer staging and prognosis. *Cancer Treat Res.* (2016) 170:47–75. doi: 10.1007/978-3-319-40389-2_3
8. Dafni U, Tsourti Z, Vervita K, Peters S. Immune checkpoint inhibitors, alone or in combination with chemotherapy, as first-line treatment for advanced non-small cell lung cancer. A systematic review and network meta-analysis. *Lung Cancer.* (2019) 134:127–40. doi: 10.1016/j.lungcan.2019.05.029

9. Varn FS, Tafe LJ, Amos CI, Cheng C. Computational immune profiling in lung adenocarcinoma reveals reproducible prognostic associations with implications for immunotherapy. *Oncoimmunology.* (2018) 7:e1431084. doi: 10.1080/2162402X.2018.1431084
10. Guo D, Wang M, Shen Z, Zhu J. A new immune signature for survival prediction and immune checkpoint molecules in lung adenocarcinoma. *J Transl Med.* (2020) 18:123. doi: 10.1186/s12967-020-02286-z
11. Song Q, Shang J, Yang Z, Zhang L, Zhang C, Chen J, et al. Identification of an immune signature predicting prognosis risk of patients in lung adenocarcinoma. *J Transl Med.* (2019) 17:70. doi: 10.1186/s12967-019-1824-4
12. Wood SL, Pernemalm M, Crosbie PA, Whetton AD. The role of the tumor-microenvironment in lung cancer-metastasis and its relationship to potential therapeutic targets. *Cancer Treat Rev.* (2014) 40:558–66. doi: 10.1016/j.ctrv.2013.10.001
13. Altorki NK, Markowitz GJ, Gao DC, Port JL, Saxena A, Stiles B, et al. The lung microenvironment: an important regulator of tumour growth and metastasis. *Nat Rev Cancer.* (2019) 19:9–31. doi: 10.1038/s41568-018-0081-9
14. Bonanno L, Zulato E, Pavan A, AttiliI, Pasello G, Conte P, et al. LKB1 and tumor metabolism: the interplay of immune and angiogenic microenvironment in lung cancer. *Int J Mol Sci.* (2019) 20:1874. doi: 10.3390/ijms20081874
15. Guo XY, ZhangYY, Liangtao Zheng LT, Zheng CH, Song JT, Zhang QM, et al. Global characterization of T cells in non-small-cell lung cancer by single-cell sequencing. *Nat Med.* (2018) 24:978–85. doi: 10.1038/s41591-018-0045-3
16. Stankovic B, Bjørhovde HA, Skarshaug R, Aamodt H, Frafjord A, Müller E, et al. Immune cell composition in human non-small cell lung cancer. *Front Immunol.* (2018) 9:3101. doi: 10.3389/fimmu.2018.03101
17. Jia D, Li SL, Li D, Xue HP, Yang D, Liu Y. Mining TCGA database for genes of prognostic value in glioblastoma microenvironment. *Aging (Albany NY).* (2018) 10:592–605. doi: 10.18632/aging.101415
18. Yang XD, Shi Y, Li M, Lu T, Xi JJ, Lin ZW, et al. Identification and validation of an immune cell infiltrating score predicting survival in patients with lung adenocarcinoma. *J Transl Med.* (2019) 17:217. doi: 10.1186/s12967-019-1964-6
19. Yue C, Ma H, Zhou Y. Identification of prognostic gene signature associated with microenvironment of lung adenocarcinoma. *Peer J.* (2019) 7:e8128. doi: 10.7717/peerj.8128
20. Liu X, Wu S, Yang Y, Zhao M, Zhu G, Hou Z. The prognostic landscape of tumor-infiltrating immune cell and immunomodulators in lung cancer. *Biomed Pharmacother.* (2017) 95:55–61. doi: 10.1016/j.biopha.2017.08.003
21. Sun J, Zhang Z, Bao S, Yan C, Hou P, Wu N, et al. Identification of tumor immune infiltration-associated lncRNAs for improving prognosis and immunotherapy response of patients with non-small cell lung cancer. *J Immunother Cancer.* (2020) 8:e000110. doi: 10.1136/jitc-2019-000110
22. Moynihan KD, Opel CF, Szeto GL, Tzeng A, Zhu EF, Engreitz JM, et al. Eradication of large established tumors in mice by combination immunotherapy that engages innate and adaptive immune responses. *Nat Med.* (2016) 22:1402–10. doi: 10.1038/nm.4200
23. Shen JX, Liu J, Zhang GJ. Interleukin-33 in malignancies: friends or foes? *Front Immunol.* (2018) 9:3051. doi: 10.3389/fimmu.2018.03051
24. Larsen FT, Bed'Hom B, Guldbrandtsen B, Dalgaard TS. Identification and tissue-expression profiling of novel chicken c-type lectin-like domain containing proteins as potential targets for carbohydrate-based vaccine strategies. *Mol Immunol.* (2019) 114:216–25. doi: 10.1016/j.molimm.2019.07.022
25. Johnston HE, Carter MJ, Larrayoz M, Clarke J, Garbis SD, Oscier D, et al. Proteomics profiling of CLL versus healthy B-cells identifies putative therapeutic targets and a subtype-independent signature of spliceosome dysregulation. *Mol Cell Proteomics.* (2018) 17:776–91. doi: 10.1074/mcp.RA117.000539
26. Ikawa T, Watanabe Y, Okuzaki D, Goto N, Okamura N, Yamanishi K, et al. A new approach to identifying hypertension-associated genes in the mesenteric artery of spontaneously hypertensive rats and stroke-prone spontaneously hypertensive rats. *J Hypertens.* (2019) 37:1644–56. doi: 10.1097/HJH.0000000000002083
27. Alazami AM, Patel N, Shamseldin HE, Anazi S, Al-Dosari MS, Alzahrani F, et al. Accelerating novel candidate gene discovery in neurogenetic disorders via whole-exome sequencing of prescreened multiplex consanguineous families. *Cell Rep.* (2015) 10:148–61. doi: 10.1016/j.celrep.2014.12.015
28. Singh P, Jenkins LM, Horst B, Alers V, Pradhan S, Kaur P, et al. Inhibin is a novel paracrine factor for tumor angiogenesis and metastasis. *Cancer Res.* (2018) 78:2978–89. doi: 10.1158/0008-5472.CAN-17-2316

2

Predicting EGFR and PD-L1 Status in NSCLC Patients using Multitask AI System based on CT Images

Chengdi Wang[1], Jiechao Ma[2], Jun Shao[1], Shu Zhang[2], Zhongnan Liu[2], Yizhou Yu[2,3] and Weimin Li[1]**

[1] Department of Respiratory and Critical Care Medicine, Med-X Center for Manufacturing, National Clinical Research Center for Geriatrics, Frontiers Science Center for Disease-related Molecular Network, West China Hospital, West China School of Medicine, Sichuan University, Chengdu, China, [2] AI Lab, Deepwise Healthcare, Beijing, China, [3] Faculty of Engineering, The University of Hong Kong, Hong Kong, Hong Kong SAR, China

***Correspondence:**
Weimin Li
weimi003@scu.edu.cn
Yizhou Yu
yizhouy@acm.org*

Background: Epidermal growth factor receptor (EGFR) genotyping and programmed death ligand-1 (PD-L1) expressions are of paramount importance for treatment guidelines such as the use of tyrosine kinase inhibitors (TKIs) and immune checkpoint inhibitors (ICIs) in lung cancer. Conventional identification of EGFR or PD-L1 status requires surgical or biopsied tumor specimens, which are obtained through invasive procedures associated with risk of morbidities and may be unavailable to access tissue samples. Here, we developed an artificial intelligence (AI) system that can predict EGFR and PD-L1 status in using non-invasive computed tomography (CT) images.

Methods: A multitask AI system including deep learning (DL) module, radiomics (RA) module, and joint (JO) module combining the DL, RA, and clinical features was developed, trained, and optimized with CT images to predict the EGFR and PD-L1 status. We used feature selectors and feature fusion methods to find the best model among combinations of module types. The models were evaluated using the areas under the receiver operating characteristic curves (AUCs).

Results: Our multitask AI system yielded promising performance for gene expression status, subtype classification, and joint prediction. The AUCs of DL module achieved 0.842 (95% CI, 0.825–0.855) in the EGFR mutated status and 0.805 (95% CI, 0.779–0.829) in the mutated-EGFR subtypes discrimination (19Del, L858R, other mutations). DL module also demonstrated the AUCs of 0.799 (95% CI, 0.762–0.854) in the PD-L1 expression status and 0.837 (95% CI, 0.775–0.911) in the positive-PD-L1 subtypes (PD-L1 tumor proportion score, 1%–49% and ≥50%). Furthermore, the JO module of our AI system performed well in the EGFR and PD-L1 joint cohort, with an AUC of 0.928 (95% CI, 0.909–0.946) for distinguishing EGFR mutated status and 0.905 (95% CI, 0.886–0.930) for discriminating PD-L1 expression status.

Conclusion: Our AI system has demonstrated the encouraging results for identifying gene status and further assessing the genotypes. Both clinical indicators and radiomics features showed a complementary role in prediction and provided accurate estimates to predict EGFR and PD-L1 status. Furthermore, this non-invasive, high-throughput, and interpretable AI system can be used as an assistive tool in conjunction with or in lieu of ancillary tests and extensive diagnostic workups to facilitate early intervention.

Keywords: EGFR, PD-L1, NSCLC, deep learning, computed tomography

INTRODUCTION

Lung cancer is the second most commonly diagnosed cancer and the leading cause of mortality tumor throughout the world (1, 2). In China, there are around 733,000 new cases of lung cancer annually, and with over 610,000 deaths due to lung cancer (3), accounting for 37% new cases and 39.2% death cases of the world, respectively (4). Approximately 85% of lung cancer patients were histologically identified as non-small cell lung cancer (NSCLC), of which comprises the most common subtype such as lung adenocarcinoma (LUAD) and lung squamous cell carcinoma (LUSC) (5). Targeted therapies, as represented by epidermal growth factor receptor (EGFR) tyrosine kinase inhibitors (TKIs), and immune checkpoint inhibitor (ICI) treatments targeted the programmed death-1 (PD-1) receptor on T cells, or the programmed death ligand-1 (PD-L1) expressed by tumor cells; these two treatment paradigms have significantly revolutionized cancer treatment and improved survival outcome for lung cancer. Identifying predictive biomarkers is therefore crucial for choosing individuals who are potentially suitable to therapy.

In the era of precision medicine, lung cancer treatment depended on the genetics. Patients with EGFR mutated lung adenocarcinoma could achieve a longer progression-free survival (PFS) from EGFR-TKIs than conventional chemotherapy (6–8). However, the medication and efficacy varied among NSCLC patients with EGFR 19Del, L858R, or other types of mutations (9, 10). Meanwhile, ICIs targeting PD-1 or PD-L1 offer promising paradigm to treatment in NSCLC with high PD-L1 expression. The first-line pembrolizumab monotherapy can enhance overall survival (OS) and PFS in lung cancer patients with PD-L1 tumor proportion score (TPS) ≥50% (11, 12). However, gene detection is determined by surgical or biopsied tissue-based assays at present, which has many limitations: difficulties in accessing suitable tumor tissues due to their extensive genetic heterogeneity; associated morbidities or tumor metastasis during the invasive biopsies; and different antibodies, multiple scoring criteria, and poor DNA quality resulting in high heterogeneity of results (13). What is more, gene mutations could change over the course and progression during whole therapy, making it impractical and challenging to obtain tumor biopsy during multiple times. However, molecular profiling of relative high costs is not routinely performed for every patient, especially in low-resource settings. Therefore, a non-invasive method for identifying the mutation status is urgently needed.

Radiological images reflect abundant information on the entire tumor in non-invasive way (14). Recent advances in machine learning have promoted the disease diagnosis based on computed tomography (CT) images. Conventional radiomics methods, which are tedious and time consuming, include image segmentation, feature extraction and selection, model building, and data analysis. The radiological characteristics are affected by manual segmentation and CT scan parameters, and repeated professional analysis by doctors is necessary (14). Advances in deep learning could overcome these problems and have demonstrated accurate, reliable, and reproducible performance on triage tasks for detecting the abnormalities and diagnosing the disease (15, 16). These proposed deep learning models and techniques have achieved a predictive performance in estimating malignancy risk in pulmonary nodules and diagnosing pneumonia quickly during the COVID-19 pandemic. Recent new and exciting developments in artificial intelligence (AI) have provided new potential opportunities to predict the EGFR mutation or PD-L1 expression status on the basis of CT images (17, 18). However, the small datasets and binary task limit its applicability in the routine clinical work. There still exists a considerable challenge to objectively evaluate the ability of the model to predict the gene mutation status and gene subtypes.

In the present study, we proposed an AI system to mine CT image information to predict EGFR mutation status and mutated subtype (i.e., 19Del and L858R) and investigate the PD-L1 expression level and positive PD-L1 subtypes (PD-L1 TPS, 1%–49% and ≥50%) and further simultaneously identify both EGFR and PD-L1 status, aiming to provide support for clinical decision-making.

MATERIALS AND METHODS

Patients Cohort and Data Collection

This study retrospectively included consecutive patients with NSCLC who visited West China Hospital of Sichuan University (Sichuan, China) from June 2019 and June 2021. The current study was performed in compliance with the Declaration of Helsinki and approved by the Institutional Review Board (IRB)/ Ethics Committee. Written informed consent was waived because the data used for system development were de-identified by removing personal information. Patients who meet the following inclusion criteria were collected into this study: (1) histologically verified primary NSCLC, (2) pathological analysis of tumor tissues with thorough EGFR or PD-L1 testing results, and (3) preoperative CT images. Patients were excluded if (1) clinical data such as age, sex, and stage were missing; (2) preoperative treatment was received; (3) the duration between CT examination and subsequent surgery exceeded 1 month; or (4) tumors <1cm in size and CT imaging artifact were found. Following the screening of exclusion criteria, we selected our primary cohort (n = 3,816) for model development. Furthermore, we created a subset of EGFR cohort (n = 3,629), PD-L1 cohort (n=873), and EGFR and PD-L1 joint cohort (n = 818) who underwent staining based on surgery or biopsy specimens and gene testing (EGFR, PD-L1 or both), with the goal of evaluating the performance of our models for three prediction tasks: gene mutation status, gene subtypes, and joint prediction.

EGFR gene status was determined to be mutated (including 19Del, L858R, and Others) and wild by amplification refractory mutation system-polymerase chain reaction (ARMS-PCR) or next-generation sequencing (NGS). PD-L1 expression status was identified as positive and negative according to PD-L1 TPS (≥1% vs. <1%; TPS is the percentage of tumor cells with membranous PD-L1 staining, with TPS ≥1% indicating positivity; TPS 1%-49% and ≥50% indicating low PD-L1+ and high PD-L1+, respectively) using SP142 antibody in immunohistochemical (IHC) assays performed on the Ventana Benchmark platform. After being reviewed by senior pathologists, these gene testing results were regarded as the gold criteria in the current study. The CT data utilized in this study came from a variety of suppliers (GE, Philips, Siemens United Imaging Health) to assess the resilience of our AI system in multiple clinical contexts. All CT scans had a resolution of 512 × 512, with slice spacing ranging from 0.625 to 5 mm in the axial direction. For the electronic health records (EHRs) data collection in our study, ideally, for a unique patient, his/her EHRs data should at least include basic information, i.e., age, sex, tumor stage, and smoking status, and radiology reports in line with international standards.

For multitask AI system, we collected multimodal data that comprised (a) deep learning features based on CT images, which consisted of a global texture feature and a tumor local texture feature; (b) radiomics features that extracted and analyzed a large number of advanced quantitative image features with high throughput; and (c) clinical features that included demographics, comorbidities, and clinical symptoms.

Data Pre-Processing

In this experiment, we obtained the training and testing cohorts from the EGFR/PD-L1 dataset by stratified and random sampling of patients at a ratio of 4:1. For the CT images, two groups of doctors were asked to delineate of the specific mask of the entire tumor. The tumor–mask pair was then fed into the radiomics model, which extracted radiomic characteristics, and the deep learning model, which extracted deep learning features. For deep learning feature analysis, a cubic region of interest (ROI) containing the entire tumor with surrounding information was supplied and retrieved local deep learning features by the local DL model, and the global DL model took the corresponding origin CT volume as input. Finally, as deep learning features, local deep feature and global deep feature were combined. Using pre-computed windowing information, all cubic ROI and origin CT volume pixels were normalized to 0–255, and all CT volumes were resized to the same size of 36 × 36 × 36 using third-order [illegible]line interpolation. To reduce overfitting, data augmentations [illegible] flip, random resizing cropping, random rotation, and random color jittering were used throughout the training phase. For the final model training and inference, a random crop of 32 × 32 × 32 would be employed.

Construction of AI System

We developed a deep-learning-based AI system for scalable gene prediction in patients. To summarize, our proposed AI system employed a modular pipeline method with four key components (**Figure 1**): deep learning module, radiomics module, clinical module, and feature fusion module. The following was a full description of the AI system.

For the deep learning module (**Figure 1B**), in order to pay more attention to contextual features (different lesion signs usually appear at the same time) and use these correlation lesion signs to improve the model's representation learning ability, this study proposed a novel dual-pathway deep learning network architecture that performs CT volume and tumor volume feature as local and global information, using the weighted-share backbone to capture the dependence between tumor detail information and the whole CT information in a large range. To be more specific, both the encoders of the framework (local and global) were composed of several 3D convolution and residual blocks, and the continuous multislice (tumor and full CT images) were used to form trainable 3D data patches, which were then fed as two branch inputs to realize multiscale local and global information extraction through progressive fusion, making full use of context texture information of 3D image space. In addition, due to the different roles of global feature and local feature in specific prediction, it was necessary to conduct corresponding modeling for different extracted features; therefore, we adopted an asymmetric non-local fusion layer to implicitly modeled the attentional mechanism. For each weight-sharing branch of the backbone, for 3D volumes, we applied a 3D ResNet-18 feature extractor and fine-tuned the parameters by the pre-trained model. As a consequence, transfer learning was employed to address the issue of insufficient training data by first learning the neural network's unique weights on the source data set. Because several gene mutations might co-exist or overlap on the same patient, a multilabel triage loss function with sigmoid active function was used instead of the standard multiclass classification loss.

The radiomics module (**Figure 1C**) retrieved and quantified a large number of characteristic data from tumor images and processed genetic and tumor information from more high-dimensional features that cannot be observed by the human naked eye to construct clinical features. The following pipeline steps were used to extract image radiomics features: (1) precise segmentation of suspected tumors, (2) extraction of large high-dimensional characteristics from suspected tumor area, and (3) filtered and reduced correlation features to prevent overfitting. To begin, 1,247 radiomics characteristics were extracted from each tumor–mask pair volume (segmented by the doctors). These characteristics included first-order (HU stats), shape, and texture properties.

The first-order feature depicted the intensity distribution of CT values in the volume of interest by common basic measures,

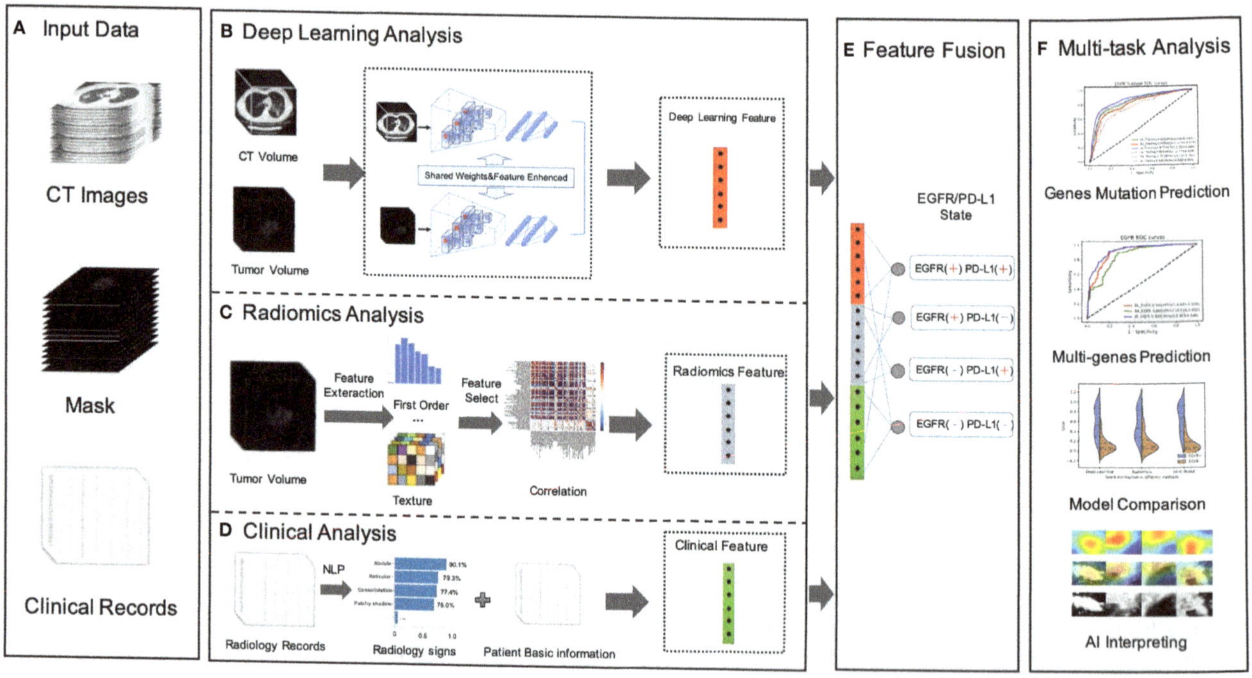

FIGURE 1 | Overall workflow in our study. **(A)** Data preparation stage included original CT image data, with manually labeled tumor images, NGS testing gene mutation status, gene mutation subtypes, radiology records, and patients' fundamental clinical indications. **(B)** A novel dual-pathway deep learning network architecture that performed CT volume and tumor volume feature extraction, named DL feature, using the trained backbone for gene prediction and further to fuse the extracted feature with another learnable pathway using an asymmetric non-local fusion module. **(C)** The pipeline of radiomics analysis model extracted radiomics features based on manually segmented contour of the tumor. **(D)** The clinical feature considered a full coverage of clinical information, including radiology signs that applied NLP techniques to extract structured labels from radiology reports. **(E)** The feature fusion utilized full connection to provide self-adaptation on the combination of deep learning features, radiomics features, and clinical features. **(F)** Validation of the proposed AI system.

such as mean, range, and standard deviation. The texture features were classified into five categories: (1) the gray-level co-occurrence matrix, (2) the gray-level difference matrix, (3) the gray-level run-length matrix, (4) the gray-level size-zone matrix, and (5) the gray-tone difference matrix in the neighborhood. Following that, for each feature in a specific tumor, we summarized and examined the distribution of the feature's values across nine filters and eight wavelet transformations in high dimensions. Then, the least absolute shrinkage and selection operator (LASSO) method was used on the feature set to eliminate the correlation radiomics characteristics with low variance (<0.8). Finally, around 100-dimensional features were selected as the most useful radiomics features in LASSO model.

The clinical module (**Figure 1D**) acquired structured abnormality symptoms and the patients' basic clinical information. Although CT imaging can provide some insight into the effectiveness of cancer immunotherapy, the clinical information of patients including age, sex, tumor staging, number, size, past recurrence, and medication status had all been linked to the efficacy of cancer immunotherapy. How to effectively combine imaging and clinical information to construct an individual prediction model remained another key problem. For the structured information, such as sex, we mainly used the one-hot strategy to convert category variables into a sparse vector space that machine learning algorithms can easily use. For the free-text reports, such as radiology record, we used the natural language processing (NLP) algorithm to perform free-text record analysis to predict patients' radiological abnormalities into a structured label vector format (binary vector of labels for the targeting abnormality). To create uniform length vectors, the raw free texts were first vectorized using a data vectorization process. The text classifier was then trained using supervised learning, which may be used to generate labels (e.g., radiological abnormalities) automatically. The text classifier was trained using pre-annotated text–label pairs. Then, these structured symptoms label vectors and structured patients' basic clinical information were merged into the combined vector as our clinical features.

The fusion module made use of the fully connectivity layer to provide self-adaptation based on a combination of deep learning (DL), radiomics (RA), and clinical (CL) features. Prior to the fusion action, both features were followed by a new conversion layer, specifically, a 512D-output full connection layer, which bridged the dimensional gap between the types of features and boosts the convergence of our feature fusion module. As a consequence, our model could jointly project these diverse features to an embedding feature space, allowing us to make better use of individual feature strength.

Statistical Analysis

The following measures were used to assess the performance of our classifiers: area under the receiver operating characteristic curve (AUC), accuracy, sensitivity, and specificity. The 95% confidence intervals (CIs) for the AUC were calculated through DeLong technique. The median and interquartile range (IQR) with a 95% CI were used to represent continuous variables. Independent sample t-test was used to assess the significance of mean age of EGFR mutant and EGFR genotyping patients. The same statistical analysis was performed for scores in the PD-L1 mutant group and the PPD-L1 negative (PD-L1-) and positive (low PD-L1+; high PD-L1+) groups. χ^2 test was used to evaluate the differences in sex and other symptoms in each cohort. The ANOVA test was used to determine whether there was a difference between the joint categories of genes mutant patients. All statistical tests were two-tailed, with statistical significance set at $P < 0.05$ considered as significant. Our implementation of the deep learning model used the Pytorch toolkit and Python 3.7.

RESULTS

Patient Characteristics of Enrolled Datasets

A total of 4,404 patients were initially identified who had been pathologically diagnosed with lung cancer and had undergone the molecular (EGFR or PD-L1) test (**Figure 2**). Following eligibility screening, this study included three cohorts of 3,816 eligible patients with consecutive chest CT images. The EGFR cohort (n = 3,629), PD-L1 cohort (n = 873), and EGFR and PD-L1 cohort (n = 818) were enrolled, divided into 80% training/internal validation and 20% testing sets, to develop and optimize our AI systems for differentiating positive EGFR mutation or PD-L1 expression status from negative ones. The sum of three cohorts were not equal to the number of total cohorts due to that molecular profiling of EGFR or PD-L1 was not routinely performed for every patient. Among the whole patients, the mean age was 59 years, and 2,067 (54.17%) patients were male. There were 2,067 (54.17%) never-smokers, 3,353 (87.87%) with no family history of cancer, and 2,937 (76.97%) LUAD patients. For tumor stage, patients with stages I, II, III, and IV were 1,136 (29.77%), 284 (7.44%), 742 (19.44%), and 1,475 (38.65%), respectively. There was no significant difference for age (p = 0.508), sex (p = 0.143), smoking status (p = 0.759), family history of cancer (p = 0.503), histopathology (p = 0.324), tumor stage (p = 0.497) among these three cohorts. Demographic and clinical characteristics of included dataset are depicted in **Table 1**.

Evaluation of Model Performance in Predicting EGFR Mutation Status

In this step, three models including deep learning (DL) model, radiomics (RA) model, and joint (JO) model combining the DL, RA, and CL features were trained and developed to distinguish the mutated EGFR from the wild EGFR patients and subsequently discriminate the mutated EGFR subtypes (19Del, L858R, and others). On the binary task of distinguishing mutated EGFR from wild ones, the AUCs of DL, RA, and JO models were 0.880 (95% CI, 0.871–0.892) and 0.842 (95% CI, 0.825–0.855), 0.838 (95% CI, 0.827–0.850) and 0.805 (95% CI, 0.789–0.827), and 0.919 (95% CI, 0.914-0.924) and 0.895 (95% CI, 0.883–0.907) in training and testing sets, separately (**Figure 3** and **Table 2**). Pertaining to three-way triage task discriminating the mutated EGFR subtypes, DL, RA, and JO models achieved the mean AUCs of 0.842 (95% CI, 0.828–0.855) and 0.805 (95% CI, 0.779–0.829), 0.809 (95% CI, 0.791–0.829) and 0.767 (95% CI, 0.735–0.791), and 0.873 (95% CI, 0.860–0.884) and 0.841 (95% CI, 0.818–0.864) in predicting 19Del, L858R, and other mutation status on the training and testing sets, respectively (**Figure 3** and **Table 2**). No matter which task, the proposed binary task and subtype classification, the performance of the joint model showed the best performance, and the combination of radiomics and clinical features contributed most to the EGFR prediction, which implied the associations and the complementarity of deep learning, radiomics, and clinical features.

Evaluation of Model Performance in Predicting PD-L1 Expression Status

The trained AI system was also evaluated on the PD-L1 cohort to distinguish the positive PD-L1-positive (PD-L1 TPS ≥1%) from the PD-L1-nagetive (PD-L1 TPS <1%) patients and subsequently discriminate the PD-L1-positive subtypes (low positive PD-L1, 1%–49%; high positive PD-L1, TPS ≥50%). On the binary task of distinguishing positive PD-L1 from negative PD-L1 ones, the AUCs of DL, RA, and JO models were 0.851 (95% CI, 0.833–0.872) and 0.799 (95% CI, 0.762–0.854), 0.819 (95% CI, 0.800–0.845) and 0.795 (95% CI, 0.748–0.843), 0.885 (95% CI, 0.867–0.905) and 0.867 (95% CI, 0.817–0.897) in training and testing sets, separately (**Figure 3** and **Table 2**). Pertaining to binary task classifying the positive-PD-L1 subtypes into low positive and high positive groups, DL, RA, and JO models achieved predictive performance with the AUCs of 0.911 (95% CI, 0.875–0.941) and 0.837 (95% CI, 0.775–0.911), 0.884 (95% CI, 0.841–0.917) and 0.836 (95% CI, 0.775–0.892), and 0.919 (95% CI, 0.889–0.942) and 0.864 (95% CI, 0.802–0.924) in the training and testing sets, respectively (**Figure 3** and **Table 3**). The performance of DL model outperformed RA models in both training and testing cohorts. What is more, JO model also performed superior than both DL and RA models. Both results confirmed that the JO model was sensitive to radiomics and clinical information and differentiating positive PD-L1 from negative PD-L1 with reasonable accuracy as a diagnostic tool.

Evaluation of Model Performance in Predicting Both EGFR and PD-L1 Expression Status

We next investigated the feasibility of assessing the multigenes mutation status. Three models also demonstrated the robust performance in the co-existing immunity cohort. In the multiple task in terms of four-way classification (multitask classifier) into EGFR(+)PD-L1(+), EGFR(+)PD-L1(−), EGFR(−)PD-L1(+), and EGFR(−)PD-L1(−) groups, DL, RA, and JO model achieved the

TABLE 1 | Clinical characteristics of patients used to measure EGFR mutation and PD-L1 expression status.

	Total (N = 3,816, %)	EGFR (N = 3,629, %)	PD-L1 (N = 873, %)	EGFR&PD-L1 (N = 818, %)	*p*-value
Age (years)	59.32	59.29	58.72	58.77	0.508
Sex, N(%)					0.143
Male	2,067(54.17)	1,955(53.87)	471(53.95)	449(54.89)	
Female	1,749(45.83)	1,674(46.13)	402(46.05)	369(45.11)	
Smoking status					0.759
Current or former	1,500(39.30)	1,413(38.94)	281(32.19)	257(31.42)	
Never	2,067(54.17)	1,981(54.59)	566(64.83)	543(66.38)	
Unknown	249(6.52)	235(6.47)	26(2.98)	18(2.2)	
Family history of cancer					0.503
Yes	248(6.50)	236(6.50)	69(7.90)	67(8.19)	
No	3,353(87.87)	3,188(87.85)	791(90.61)	745(91.08)	
Unknown	215(5.63)	205(5.65)	13(1.49)	6(0.73)	
Histopathology					0.324
LUAD	2,937(76.97)	2,787(76.80)	789(90.38)	743(90.83)	
LUSC	607(15.90)	592(16.31)	47(5.38)	42(5.13)	
Other	272(7.12)	250(6.89)	37(4.24)	33(4.03)	
Stage					0.497
I	1,136(29.77)	1,092(30.09)	354(40.55)	347(42.42)	
II	284(7.44)	272(7.50)	68(7.79)	63(7.7)	
III	742(19.44)	700(19.29)	160(18.33)	150(18.34)	
IV	1,475(38.65)	1,402(38.63)	260(29.78)	236(28.85)	
Unknown	179(4.69)	163(4.49)	31(3.55)	22(2.69)	
EGFR Mutation (%)					0.934
EGFR Wild	1,436(37.63)	1,436(39.57)	–	183(22.37)	
EGFR Mutant	2,193(57.47)	2,193(60.43)	–	635(77.63)	
PD-L1 Expression (%)					0.639
PD-L1-	562(64.38)	–	562(64.38)	539(65.89)	
PD-L1 +	311(35.62)	–	311(35.62)	279(34.11)	
Mutated EGFR Subtype (%)					0.367
19Del	919(24.08)	919(24.08)	–	–	
L858R	1,090(28.56)	1,090(30.04)	–	–	
Others	184(4.82)	184(5.07)	–	–	
Positive PD-L1 Expression (%)					0.215
≥50%	268(7.02)	–	268(30.70)	–	
1-49%	43(1.13)	–	43(4.93)	–	

EGFR, epidermal growth factor receptor; PD-L1, programmed death ligand-1; LUAD, lung adenocarcinoma; LUSC, lung squamous cell carcinoma.

AUCs of 0.906 (95% CI, 0.885–0.930) and 0.879 (95% CI, 0.854–0.906), 0.860 (95% CI, 0.816–0.902) and 0.856 (95% CI, 0.815–0.897), and 0.928 (95% CI, 0.909–0.946) and 0.905 (95% CI, 0.886–0.930) in the training and testing sets, respectively (**Figure 4**; **Table 4**). These results proved the potential of our joint model' ability to predict multigene events that may occur in at least two mutants on a single patient.

Deep Learning Model Interpretability

For each image, the attention of the model can be visualized for human interpretability and validation. High-resolution feature visualization provides an intuitive manner to understand the distribution of features used in this investigation. The aim of this section was to evaluate and validate the potential clinical application of the joint model of heatmaps as saliency models through CT volumes. In the attention map of the deep learning model through CAM, the dark color areas might be the tumor center, visualizing the attention regions located at the border of the lesion of a network to capture the discriminative information pertaining to the prediction results of distinct mutant categories (**Figure 5**). When the deep learning model predicts gene mutation status, it could simultaneously tell human experts which area draws the attention of the model. Additionally, the deep learning framework was based on pixel-level models, with the shallow layers of the model focused on textural information between pixels in CT images, such as horizontal and diagonal edges, while ignoring some general information about the tumor. On the contrary, as the network becomes deeper, more complicated characteristics, such as tumor semantics, were learned at the deep convolutional layer. Furthermore, the radiomics model concentrates primarily on some general tumor properties rather than on specific local low-dimensional tumor aspects. As a result, for a better understanding of the joint deep learning feature, we compared the model based only on deep learning feature and the joint model feature incorporating radiomics and clinical factors on the convolution filter.

DISCUSSION

Accurate and rapid quantification of EGFR mutation and PD-L1 expression status is of paramount importance in identifying of NSCLC patients more suitable for EGFR-TKI or ICI therapies,

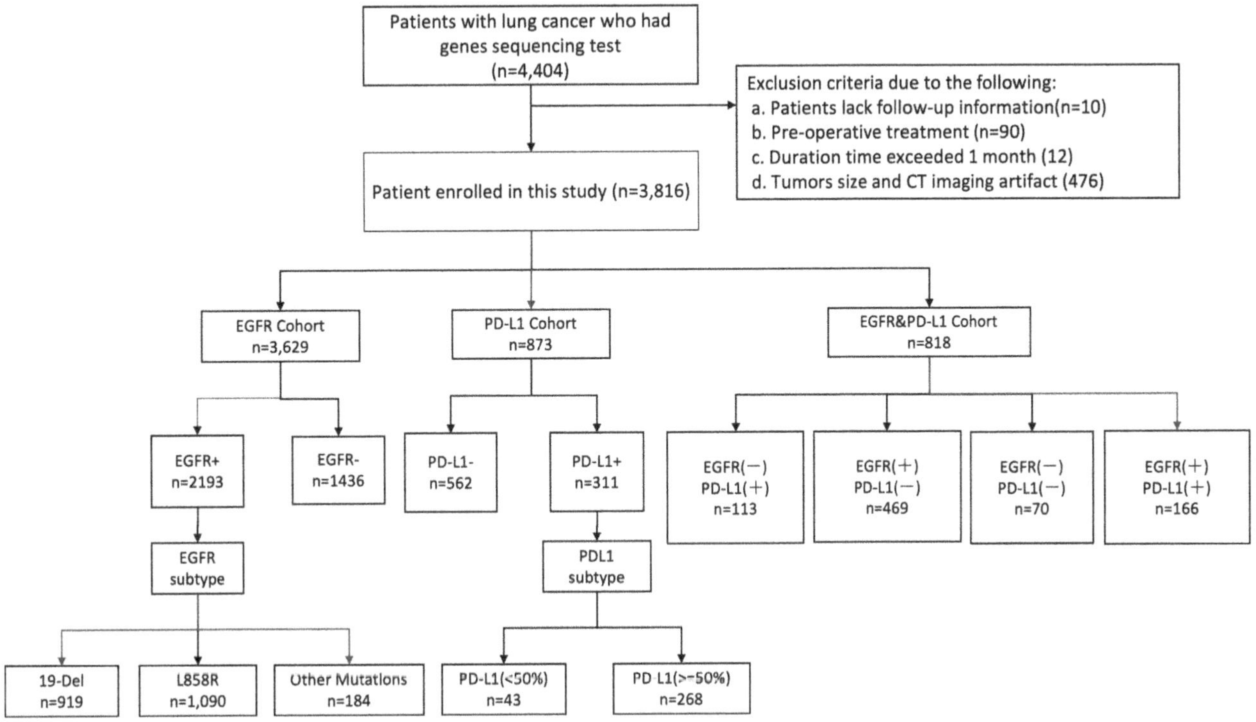

FIGURE 2 | Illustration of workflow in this study. Between June 2019 and June 2021, this study included primary cohort 3,816 consecutive patients with NSCLC who visited West China Hospital (Sichuan, China) for model development and validation. Additionally, we built a subset (EGFR cohort and PD-L1 cohort) for patients who underwent staining based on histological specimens and molecular test (EGFR, PD-L1), aiming to evaluate the performance of our models on predicting events gene mutation status and gene subtype. Cohort EGFR and PD-L1 was used to evaluate model performance in joint immunity prediction.

further guiding clinical decision-making. However, the dynamic change in proportion of cells expressing EGFR mutation or PD-L1 level and the invasive tissue/biopsy-based nature limit the applicability of EGFR or PD-L1 testing compared to image-based assays. Thus, there is a need for a non-invasive, accurate, reliable, and reproducible method to assess EGFR/PD-L1 status. In this study, we proposed a deep learning model using non-invasive chest CT images, which demonstrated the favorable performance to predict EGFR mutation/PD-L1 expression status and their subtypes for NSCLC patients.

According to the National Comprehensive Cancer Network (NCCN) Guidelines, multiple gene status especially EGFR and PD-L1 TPS should be known before deciding whether to use either targeted therapy or immunotherapy (19). However, gene detection posed a challenge, as suitable specimens were obtained through invasive procedure. These assessments were affected by heterogeneity of antibodies, platforms, and different clinicians. For example, the current study utilized SP142 antibody to score membrane-localized PD-L1 staining in tumor cells and tumor-infiltrating immune cells, which ignored cytoplasmic- or nuclei-located PD-L1. In addition, although the treatment strategy for NSCLC has rapidly evolved with the emergence of targeted therapy and immunotherapy, persistent drug responses remain limited to a subset of patients, such as the response rates of ICIs ranged from 14% to 20% in unselected patients (20, 21). Patients with PD-L1 level ≥50% would benefit from chemoimmunotherapy than single-agent immunotherapy (response rates of 60% and 40%, respectively) (11, 22, 23). The median PFS in patients with EGFR 19Del was longer than in patients with EGFR L858R treated with EGFR-TKI (10, 24). It was worth exploring the comprehensive method to assess precise gene status.

In clinical practice, CT scans are routinely available. Frontier studies combined radiological images and deep learning technology and have become trend in screening, diagnosis, gene prediction, and prognosis of lung cancer (15, 25, 26). Previous studies proposed deep learning models trained on CT images to predict high PD-L1 expression or EGFR mutated status of NSCLC (17, 18). Meanwhile, a deep-learning model based on radiology text reports was performed to estimate objective response of PD-1 blockade in NSCLC patients (27). However, these models only focused on binary tasks of gene status constructed on single-omics data, which were unsuitable for routine clinical work. Herein, we explored an approach with promising performance to predict gene mutation and further specific type based on large sample CT images and clinical features. This detailed molecular information including EGFR mutated (19Del, L858R, other) or wild; PD-L1 (≥50%) assists physician in accurate treatment. Additionally, several studies using deep learning inferred therapeutic effects of TKIs or ICIs in NSCLS patients (18, 28, 29). We would further update this

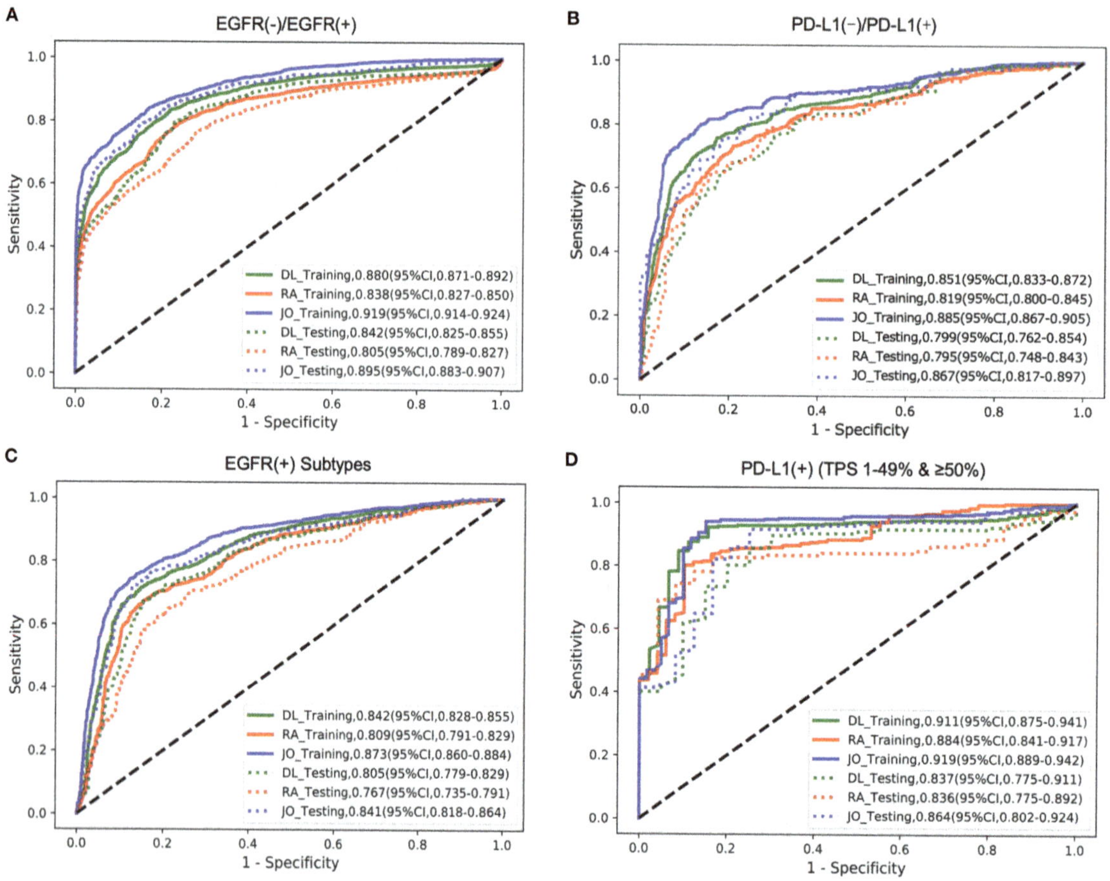

FIGURE 3 | The model performances in the prediction of two outcomes (EGFR cohort and PD-L1 cohort). The ROC curves for predicting **(A)** EGFR gene mutation status (mutant or wild); **(B)** PD-L1 status (positive or negative); **(C)** EGFR gene subtype mutations (19Del; L858R or Other); **(D)** PD-L1expression status (PD-L1 TPS 1%–49% or ≥50%). DL indicated that our image-based DL system used local tumor volume and global CT volume. RA indicated that our image-based radiomics model and the JO indicated that the joint model combined with the DL feature, radiomics feature, and clinical features. The solid line represents the performances on the training set, and the dotted line represents the effect on the test set.

TABLE 2 | Predictive performance of EGFR status and EGFR mutated subtypes using three methods in the training and testing cohorts.

Methods	Cohorts	AUC(95%CI)	Accuracy(%)	Sensitivity(%)	Specificity(%)
			EGDFR Mutation Status		
DL	Training	0.880(0.871-0.892)	0.805(0.797-0.815)	0.832(0.820-0.845)	0.783(0.769-0.798)
	Testing	0.842(0.825-0.855)	0.763(0.750-0.777)	0.797(0.777-0.818)	0.769(0.746-0.789)
Radiomics	Training	0.838(0.827-0.850)	0.769(0.758-0.779)	0.794(0.780-0.812)	0.760(0.743-0.771)
	Testing	0.805(0.789-0.827)	0.735(0.720-0.755)	0.768(0.748-0.793)	0.716(0.696-0.734)
Joint	Training	0.919(0.914-0.924)	0.840(0.831-0.850)	0.839(0.829-0.852)	0.831(0.820-0.844)
	Testing	0.895(0.883-0.907)	0.819(0.803-0.835)	0.791(0.765-0.816)	0.850(0.834-0.870)
			EGFR Subtypes		
DL	Training	0.842(0.828-0.855)	0.753(0.740-0.769)	0.716(0.696-0.739)	0.853(0.836-0.873)
	Testing	0.805(0.779-0.829)	0.732(0.707-0.755)	0.707(0.676-0.742)	0.815(0.787-0.849)
Radiomics	Training	0.809(0.791-0.829)	0.725(0.708-0.743)	0.672(0.647-0.702)	0.848(0.830-0.870)
	Testing	0.767(0.735-0.791)	0.697(0.663-0.728)	0.705(0.670-0.745)	0.742(0.712-0.773)
Joint	Training	0.873(0.860-0.884)	0.790(0.776-0.804)	0.758(0.739-0.778)	0.862(0.844-0.881)
	Testing	0.841(0.818-0.864)	0.767(0.746-0.790)	0.767(0.732-0.798)	0.827(0.803-0.858)

EGFR, epidermal growth factor receptor; PD-L1, programmed death ligand-1; DL model, deep learning model.

TABLE 3 | Predictive performance of PD-L1 status and PD-L1 expression using three methods in the training and testing cohorts.

Methods	Cohorts	AUC (95%CI)	Accuracy (%)	Sensitivity (%)	Specificity (%)
			PD-L1 Status		
DL	Training	0.851(0.833-0.872)	0.824(0.809-0.840)	0.758(0.729-0.791)	0.829(0.807-0.852)
	Testing	0.799(0.762-0.854)	0.770(0.727-0.800)	0.680(0.604-0.756)	0.793(0.746-0.839)
Radiomics	Training	0.819(0.800-0.845)	0.797(0.777-0.816)	0.732(0.688-0.775)	0.791(0.764-0.810)
	Testing	0.795(0.748-0.843)	0.759(0.717-0.797)	0.790(0.707-0.851)	0.716(0.659-0.769)
Joint	Training	0.885(0.867-0.905)	0.869(0.850-0.884)	0.801(0.768-0.842)	0.865(0.847-0.881)
	Testing	0.867(0.817-0.897)	0.808(0.771-0.846)	0.822(0.758-0.884)	0.752(0.714-0.810)
			Positive PD-L1 Expression with low and high PD-L1(+)		
DL	Training	0.911(0.875-0.941)	0.899(0.868-0.925)	0.924(0.894-0.943)	0.844(0.750-0.940)
	Testing	0.837(0.775-0.911)	0.868(0.820-0.910)	0.857(0.816-0.905)	0.750(0.611-0.933)
Radiomics	Training	0.884(0.841-0.917)	0.831(0.798-0.865)	0.802(0.764-0.837)	0.898(0.811-0.963)
	Testing	0.836(0.775-0.892)	0.796(0.745-0.854)	0.744(0.672-0.809)	0.917(0.810-1.000)
Joint	Training	0.919(0.889-0.942)	0.917(0.894-0.938)	0.941(0.918-0.960)	0.850(0.773-0.922)
	Testing	0.864(0.802-0.924)	0.884(0.845-0.934)	0.917(0.877-0.955)	0.750(0.636-0.875)

EGFR, epidermal growth factor receptor; PD-L1, programmed death ligand-1; DL model, deep learning model.

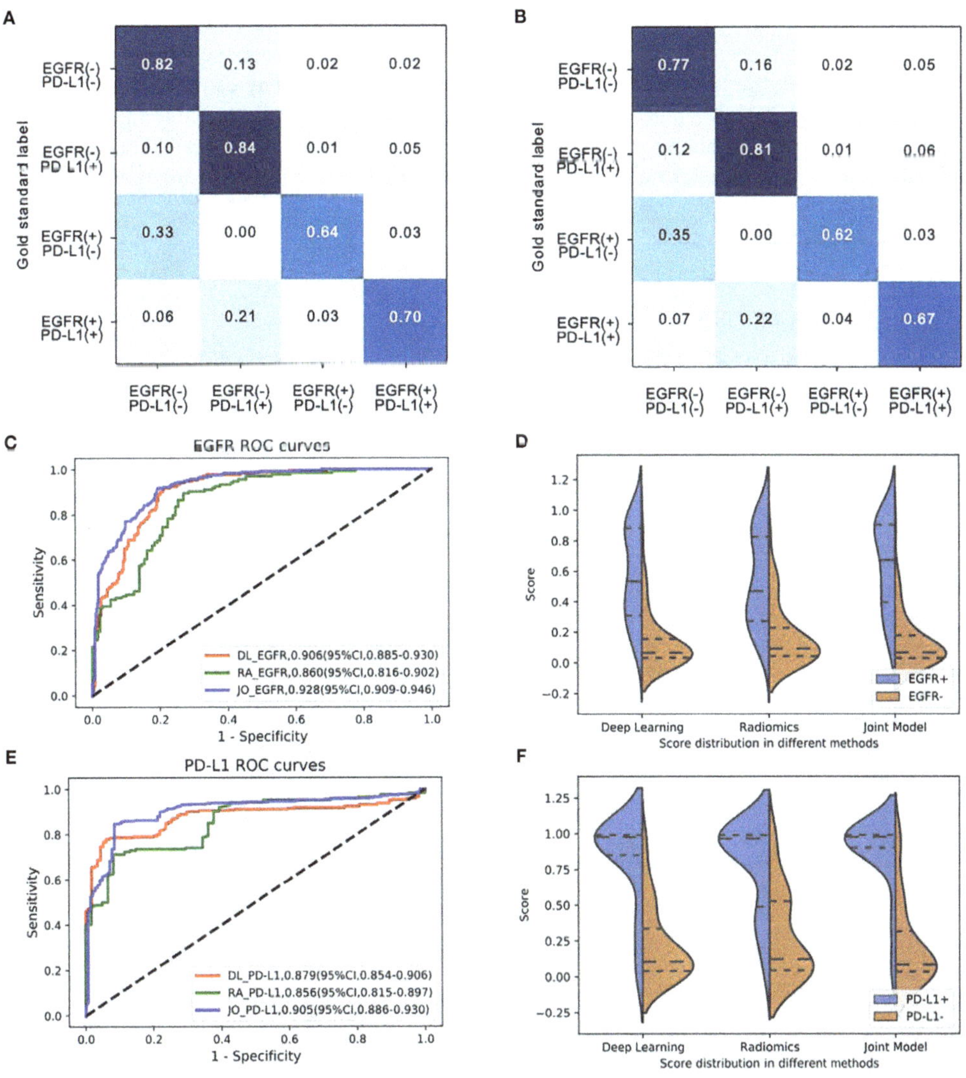

FIGURE 4 | The model performances in the prediction of joint-mutant genes (EGFR and PD-L1 cohort). Confusion matrix of **(A)** training set and **(B)** testing set indicated most errors occurred in the adjacent groups. **(C)** The ROC curves and **(D)** three model scores predicting EGFR mutation; **(E)** the ROC curves and **(F)** three model scores predicting PD-L1 expression status.

TABLE 4 | Predictive performance of EGFR and PD-L1 status performance using three methods in the joint cohort.

Methods	Categories	AUC (95% CI)	Accuracy (%)	Sensitivity (%)	Specificity (&)
			EGFR&PD-L1 Status		
DL	EGFR	0.906(0.885-0.930)	0.767(0.735-0.798)	0.920(0.884-0.954)	0.787(0.748-0.827)
	PD-L1	0.879(0.854-0.906)	0.793(0.762-0.819)	0.781(0.742-0.819)	0.939(0.904-0.969)
Radiomics	EGFR	0.860(0.816-0.902)	0.659(0.617-0.705)	0.896(0.856-0.944)	0.731(0.664-0.801)
	PD-L1	0.856(0.815-0.897)	0.719(0.677-0.766)	0.713(0.661-0.763)	0.918(0.864-0.972)
Joint	EGFR	0.928(0.909-0.946)	0.831(0.807-0.856)	0.917(0.883-0.941)	0.807(0.771-0.846)
	PD-L1	0.905(0.886-0.930)	0.848(0.825-0.874)	0.847(0.818-0.879)	0.915(0.876-0.951)

EGFR, epidermal growth factor receptor; PD-L1, programmed death ligand-1; DL model, deep learning model.

multitask AI system to predict the clinical outcomes of treatment more accurately.

In terms of algorithm, radiomics and deep learning features were integrated to mine CT image features. In addition, clinical features were integrated to try to build a prediction model with superior performance, which was more in line with routine clinical work. Not surprisingly, the performance of the integrated model was better than the deep learning model and radiomics model. This also reflected the trend of characteristic fusion. Although our AI system performed well in this aspect, it failed well short of the gold standard set by laboratory studies. To increase prediction accuracy, our AI system, for example, would benefit from other source data kinds. For example, clinical or laboratory information (such as blood biochemical analysis) might be incorporated as an additional information source to our joint AI system.

Our study has some limitations. First, this was a single-center study, and the predictive value of our model still needs to be validated in other medical centers. Second, this was a retrospective study. NSCLC patients may take multiple genes detection during treatment, which may cause some selection biases. Finally, this research only focused on EGFR and PD-L1. More extensive data would be collected to support additional mutation of NSCLC, such as ALK, ROS1, and KRAS mutation in the future.

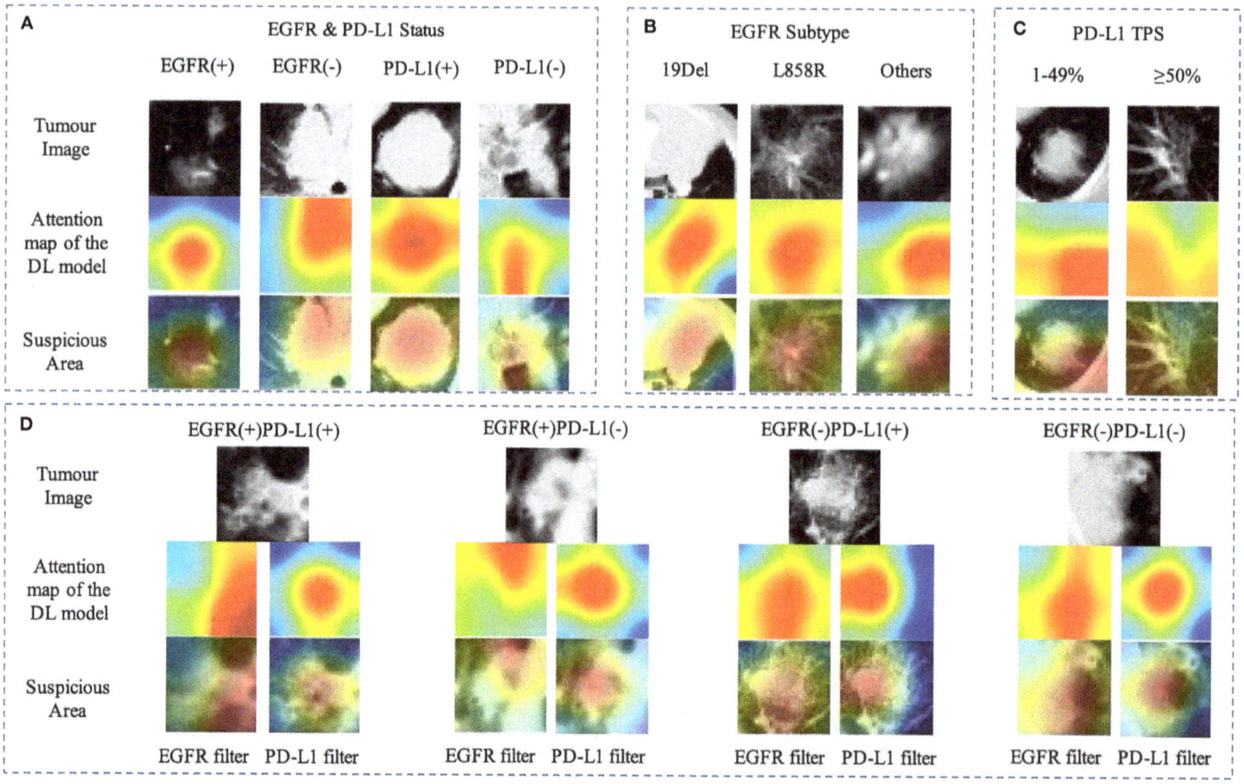

FIGURE 5 | Heatmap of characteristics that contributed to the prediction of gene mutation **(A)** EGFR and PD-L1 status; **(B)** EGFR subtype (19Del, L858R, or other); **(C)** PD-L1expression status (PD-L1 TPS, 1%–49% or ≥50%); **(D)** EGFR mutation combined with PD-L1 status using different filters. The first row showed the origin tumor image in the 3D volume; the second and third rows visualize the attention regions of a network for distinct mutant categories.

In conclusion, this study demonstrated an AI system's value in assisting medical professionals provide a non-invasive and easy-to-use method to identify the expression status of common genes EGFR and PD-L1 through CT images, which may serve as a predictive biomarker for guiding the target therapy and immunotherapy in NSCLC patients. Future refinement and improvement will expand its use into predicting other common genes mutation in larger and prospective trials.

AUTHOR CONTRIBUTIONS

WL and YY were involved in the study design. CW, JM, and JS were involved in the organization of the entire project, data analysis with a clinical perspective, and manuscript writing. CW and JS collected the imaging and clinical data. JM, SZ, and ZL were involved in the establishment of the algorithm. All authors contributed to the article and approved the submitted version.

REFERENCES

1. Sung H, Ferlay J, Siegel RL, Laversanne M, Soerjomataram I, Jemal A, et al. Global Cancer Statistics 2020: Globocan Estimates of Incidence and Mortality Worldwide for 36 Cancers in 185 Countries. *CA Cancer J Clin* (2021) 71 (3):209–49. doi: 10.3322/caac.21660
2. Wang C, Wu Y, Shao J, Liu D, Li W. Clinicopathological Variables Influencing Overall Survival, Recurrence and Post-Recurrence Survival in Resected Stage I Non-Small-Cell Lung Cancer. *BMC Cancer* (2020) 20(1):150. doi: 10.1186/s12885-020-6621-1
3. Chen W, Zheng R, Baade PD, Zhang S, Zeng H, Bray F, et al. Cancer Statistics in China, 2015. *CA Cancer J Clin* (2016) 66(2):115–32. doi: 10.3322/caac.21338
4. Shi JF, Wang L, Wu N, Li JL, Hui ZG, Liu SM, et al. Clinical Characteristics and Medical Service Utilization of Lung Cancer in China, 2005-2014: Overall Design and Results From a Multicenter Retrospective Epidemiologic Survey. *Lung Cancer* (2019) 128:91–100. doi: 10.1016/j.lungcan.2018.11.031
5. Herbst RS, Morgensztern D, Boshoff C. The Biology and Management of Non-Small Cell Lung Cancer. *Nature* (2018) 553(7689):446–54. doi: 10.1038/nature25183
6. Ramalingam SS, Vansteenkiste J, Planchard D, Cho BC, Gray JE, Ohe Y, et al. Overall Survival With Osimertinib in Untreated, EGFR-Mutated Advanced NSCLC. *N Engl J Med* (2020) 382(1):41–50. doi: 10.1056/NEJMoa1913662
7. Tang W, Li X, Xie X, Sun X, Liu J, Zhang J, et al. EGFR Inhibitors as Adjuvant Therapy for Resected Non-Small Cell Lung Cancer Harboring EGFR Mutations. *Lung Cancer* (2019) 136:6–14. doi: 10.1016/j.lungcan.2019.08.001
8. Mitsudomi T, Morita S, Yatabe Y, Negoro S, Okamoto I, Tsurutani J, et al. Gefitinib Versus Cisplatin Plus Docetaxel in Patients With Non-Small-Cell Lung Cancer Harbouring Mutations of the Epidermal Growth Factor Receptor (Wjtog3405): An Open Label, Randomised Phase 3 Trial. *Lancet Oncol* (2010) 11(2):121–8. doi: 10.1016/s1470-2045(09)70364-x
9. Gieszer B, Megyesfalvi Z, Dulai V, Papay J, Kovalszky I, Timar J, et al. EGFR Variant Allele Frequency Predicts EGFR-TKI Efficacy in Lung Adenocarcinoma: A Multicenter Study. *Transl Lung Cancer Res* (2021) 10 (2):662–74. doi: 10.21037/tlcr-20-814
10. Liu X, Hong L, Nilsson M, Hubert SM, Wu S, Rinsurongkawong W, et al. Concurrent Use of Aspirin With Osimertinib Is Associated With Improved Survival in Advanced EGFR-Mutant Non-Small Cell Lung Cancer. *Lung Cancer* (2020) 149:33–40. doi: 10.1016/j.lungcan.2020.08.023
11. Mok TSK, Wu YL, Kudaba I, Kowalski DM, Cho BC, Turna HZ, et al. Pembrolizumab Versus Chemotherapy for Previously Untreated, PD-L1-Expressing, Locally Advanced or Metastatic Non-Small-Cell Lung Cancer (Keynote-042): A Randomised, Open-Label, Controlled, Phase 3 Trial. *Lancet* (2019) 393(10183):1819–30. doi: 10.1016/s0140-6736(18)32409-7
12. Brody R, Zhang Y, Ballas M, Siddiqui MK, Gupta P, Barker C, et al. PD-L1 Expression in Advanced NSCLC: Insights Into Risk Stratification and Treatment Selection From a Systematic Literature Review. *Lung Cancer* (2017) 112:200–15. doi: 10.1016/j.lungcan.2017.08.005
13. Büttner R, Gosney JR, Skov BG, Adam J, Motoi N, Bloom KJ, et al. Programmed Death-Ligand 1 Immunohistochemistry Testing: A Review of Analytical Assays and Clinical Implementation in Non-Small-Cell Lung Cancer. *J Clin Oncol* (2017) 35(34):3867–76. doi: 10.1200/jco.2017.74.7642
14. Zhou Y, Xu X, Song L, Wang C, Guo J, Yi Z, et al. The Application of Artificial Intelligence and Radiomics in Lung Cancer. *Precis Clin Med* (2020) 3(3):214–27. doi: 10.1093/pcmedi/pbaa028
15. Ardila D, Kiraly AP, Bharadwaj S, Choi B, Reicher JJ, Peng L, et al. End-To-End Lung Cancer Screening With Three-Dimensional Deep Learning on Low-Dose Chest Computed Tomography. *Nat Med* (2019) 25(6):954–61. doi: 10.1038/s41591-019-0447-x
16. Zhang K, Liu X, Shen J, Li Z, Sang Y, Wu X, et al. Clinically Applicable Ai System for Accurate Diagnosis, Quantitative Measurements, and Prognosis of Covid-19 Pneumonia Using Computed Tomography. *Cell* (2020) 181 (6):1423–33.e11. doi: 10.1016/j.cell.2020.04.045
17. Wang S, Shi J, Ye Z, Dong D, Yu D, Zhou M, et al. Predicting EGFR Mutation Status in Lung Adenocarcinoma on Computed Tomography Image Using Deep Learning. *Eur Respir J* (2019) 53(3):1800986. doi: 10.1183/13993003.00986-2018
18. Tian P, He B, Mu W, Liu K, Liu L, Zeng H, et al. Assessing PD-L1 Expression in Non-Small Cell Lung Cancer and Predicting Responses to Immune Checkpoint Inhibitors Using Deep Learning on Computed Tomography Images. *Theranostics* (2021) 11(5):2098–107. doi: 10.7150/thno.48027
19. Ettinger DS, Wood DE, Aisner DL, Akerley W, Bauman JR, Bharat A, et al. NCCN Guidelines Insights: Non-Small Cell Lung Cancer, Version 2.2021. *J Natl Compr Canc Netw* (2021) 19(3):254–66. doi: 10.6004/jnccn.2021.0013
20. Chen DS, Mellman I. Elements of Cancer Immunity and the Cancer-Immune Set Point. *Nature* (2017) 541(7637):321–30. doi: 10.1038/nature21349
21. Xia L, Liu Y, Wang Y. PD-1/PD-L1 Blockade Therapy in Advanced Non-Small-Cell Lung Cancer: Current Status and Future Directions. *Oncologist* (2019) 24(Suppl 1):s31–s41. doi: 10.1634/theoncologist.2019-IO-S1-s05
22. Reck M, Rodríguez-Abreu D, Robinson AG, Hui R, Csőszi T, Fülöp A, et al. Pembrolizumab Versus Chemotherapy for PD-L1-Positive Non-Small-Cell Lung Cancer. *N Engl J Med* (2016) 375(19):1823–33. doi: 10.1056/NEJMoa1606774
23. Herbst RS, Giaccone G, de Marinis F, Reinmuth N, Vergnenegre A, Barrios CH, et al. Atezolizumab for First-Line Treatment of PD-L1-Selected. *N Engl J Med* (2020) 383(14):1328–39. doi: 10.1056/NEJMoa1917346
24. Wu YL, Cheng Y, Zhou X, Lee KH, Nakagawa K, Niho S, et al. Dacomitinib Versus Gefitinib as First-Line Treatment for Patients With EGFR-Mutation-Positive Non-Small-Cell Lung Cancer (ARCHER 1050): A Randomised, Open-Label, Phase 3 Trial. *Lancet Oncol* (2017) 18(11):1454–66. doi: 10.1016/s1470-2045(17)30608-3
25. Lu MT, Raghu VK, Mayrhofer T, Aerts H, Hoffmann U. Deep Learning Using Chest Radiographs to Identify High-Risk Smokers for Lung Cancer Screening Computed Tomography: Development and Validation of a Prediction Model. *Ann Intern Med* (2020) 173(9):704–13. doi: 10.7326/m20-1868
26. Wang C, Shao J, Lv J, Cao Y, Zhu C, Li J, et al. Deep Learning for Predicting Subtype Classification and Survival of Lung Adenocarcinoma on Computed Tomography. *Transl Oncol* (2021) 14(8):101141. doi: 10.1016/j.tranon.2021.101141
27. Arbour KC, Luu AT, Luo J, Rizvi H, Plodkowski AJ, Sakhi M, et al. Deep Learning to Estimate RECIST in Patients With NSCLC Treated With PD-1 Blockade. *Cancer Discov* (2021) 11(1):59–67. doi: 10.1158/2159-8290.Cd-20-0419
28. Mu W, Jiang L, Zhang J, Shi Y, Gray JE, Tunali I, et al. Non-Invasive Decision Support for NSCLC Treatment Using PET/CT Radiomics. *Nat Commun* (2020) 11(1):5228. doi: 10.1038/s41467-020-19116-x
29. Mu W, Jiang L, Shi Y, Tunali I, Gray JE, Katsoulakis E, et al. Non-Invasive Measurement of PD-L1 Status and Prediction of Immunotherapy Response Using Deep Learning of PET/CT Images. *J Immunother Cancer* (2021) 9(6): e002118. doi: 10.1136/jitc-2020-002118

3

Harmonization of Molecular Testing for Non-Small Cell Lung Cancer: Emphasis on PD-L1

Evgeny N. Imyanitov[1,2], *Alexandr O. Ivantsov*[1,2] *and Ilya V. Tsimafeyeu*[3*]

[1] *Department of Tumor Growth Biology, N.N. Petrov Institute of Oncology, St. Petersburg, Russia,* [2] *Department of Clinical Genetics, St.-Petersburg Pediatric Medical University, Saint Petersburg, Russia,* [3] *Institute of Oncology, Hadassah Moscow, Moscow, Russia*

Correspondence:
Ilya V. Tsimafeyeu
tsimafeyeu@gmail.com

Comprehensive molecular testing plays a critical role in the choice of treatment for non-small lung cell cancer (NSCLC). The analysis of druggable alterations in EGFR, BRAF, MET, KRAS, ALK, ROS1, RET and NTRK1/2/3 genes is more or less standardized and can be achieved using a single diagnostic platform, e.g., next generation sequencing (NGS) or polymerase chain reaction (PCR). In contrast to above targets, PD-L1 testing requires the use of immunohistochemistry (IHC). There are multiple PD-L1 IHC assays, which utilize distinct antibodies and detection systems. These PD-L1 tests are tailored to distinct drugs, often rely on different thresholds and scoring guidelines, and are characterized by incomplete inter-laboratory and inter-observer reproducibility. Several studies evaluated the performance of PD-L1 RNA expression tests, as PCR-based RNA analysis is compatible with other NSCLC molecular testing platforms, can be performed in a semi-automated manner, and has a potential for proper standardization. These investigations revealed a correlation between PD-L1 protein and RNA expression; however, there were NSCLCs demonstrating decent amounts of PD-L1 transcript in the absence of PD-L1 IHC staining. Clinical studies are required to evaluate, which of the two PD-L1 testing approaches, i.e., RNA or protein expression measurement, has a better predictive value.

Keywords: non-small cell lung cancer, molecular testing, PD-L1, PCR, review

While only a decade ago the laboratory diagnosis of non-small cell lung cancer (NSCLC) required mainly conventional morphological analysis, the process of examination of NSCLC tissues is getting increasingly complex nowadays, thanks to the invention of new targeted drugs. EGFR tyrosine kinase inhibitors (TKIs) were the first to trigger the molecular profiling of lung cancer, as they demonstrated high response rates in tumors with EGFR exon 19 and 21 drug-sensitizing mutations. Subsequent advances were based on the discovery of ALK and ROS1 rearrangements, which also turned to be linked to the pronounced tumor sensitivity to corresponding TKIs. Interestingly, the development of gefitinib, erlotinib and crizotinib actually preceded the identification of their genuine molecular targets, so the incorporation of these drugs into the NSCLC management was somehow attributed to some chance discoveries. This is in stark contrast with the history of the invention of inhibitors of the mutated BRAF, which is clearly an output of a pre-planned research, starting from the systematic search for kinase activating mutations and eventually resulting in the intentional development of specific antagonists of the BRAF V600E protein. There is a multitude of new NSCLC drug targets, e.g., NTRK1-3 and RET gene fusions, MET exon 14 skipping mutations, KRAS G12C substitutions, etc. In addition, administration of several inhibitors of immune checkpoints involves testing for PD-L1 expression (1–3).

NSCLC diagnostic pipeline includes a spectrum of molecular assays which usually rely on distinct laboratory platforms. The analysis of EGFR, BRAF, and KRAS mutations usually requires allele-specific PCR and/or gene sequencing. The detection of ALK, ROS, RET, and NTRK1-3 rearrangements may be based on the immunohistochemistry (IHC) guided detection of the overexpression of the kinase portion of the corresponding protein or on the break-apart FISH assay (3). The methodology of MET testing remains to be standardized (4). PD-L1 expression analysis is apparently the most complicated assay for the time being. There are several approved antibodies for the PD-L1 status evaluation. These antibodies are tailored to particular diagnostic platforms, linked to the use of distinct therapeutic modulators of the PD-L1/PD1 pathway, have different scoring guidelines and utilize varying thresholds between "positive" and "negative" samples. The detailed listing of PD-L1 antibodies, detection systems, associated therapeutic compounds and staining patterns is provided in several reviews (5–7). Most importantly, while the majority of clinical trials involving PD-L1/PD1 pathway inhibitors generally demonstrate an association between PD-L1 expression and clinical benefit from the drug, there is a great variability across the NSCLC studies with regard to medical applicability of observed findings (**Table 1**).

Many NSCLCs are diagnosed as a metastatic disease, therefore tumor tissue material is represented by a single tiny biopsy sample. These samples must be divided for mutational analysis (PCR, sequencing) and visualization-based tests (IHC, FISH). There is a great need for a "one-for-all" approach, which would allow for a comprehensive NSCLC examination performed on a single platform. Next generation sequencing (NGS) provides a viable diagnostic opportunity, as it is capable of detecting all relevant genetic alterations within a single run. At the present time, NGS has significant limitations, such as relatively high cost, need for significant turn-around time, and requirement for sophisticated equipment (3, 26, 27). Furthermore, NGS is not yet fully compatible with a high-precision analysis of gene expression. There are ongoing efforts to utilize PCR for all types of NSCLC molecular analysis. These assays include simultaneous isolation of DNA and RNA in a single tube, synthesis of complementary DNA (cDNA) on the RNA template, conventional analysis of mutations and the test for 5′/3′-end unbalanced expression of rearranged kinases. The latter approach allows for identification of all druggable gene fusions irrespective of the translocation variant (28). PCR analysis is relatively non-expensive and is more flexible for the incorporation of new predictive tests, as exemplified by the development of the assay for detection of MET exon 14 skipping mutations (4).

While many NSCLC tests can be performed by a number of interchangeable approaches, PD-L1 analysis remains restricted to IHC technology. Use of IHC scoring is time-consuming and may be a subject of significant interobserver variability (5–7). Explicit analysis of the comparability of the existing IHC assays has been recently published by Koomen et al. (29). PD-L1 IHC comparative studies generally demonstrate acceptable results with regard to assays' interchangeability, inter-observer variability, and inter-laboratory agreement. However, it is necessary to keep in mind that the pathologists involved in research activities and scientific publishing are likely to have somewhat better standards of the laboratory practice, so the real-world inconsistencies in the IHC performance may be substantially higher when compared to pre-planned investigations. In addition, while the numerical comparisons of PD-L1 scores show good correlation, there is an alarming rate of discordance when clinically accepted thresholds are utilized (29). Consider a situation in which one pathologist determines the proportion of PD-L1 tumor cells slightly below 1%, while another pathologist determines this proportion to be slightly over 1%. When formal correlation coefficients for continuous numerical variables are calculated, these two results will be considered concordant; however, in clinical practice this difference may critically affect the access to immune therapy, as PD-L1 score of 1% is a commonly accepted threshold for consideration of immune therapies in several clinical scenarios.

Measurement of RNA expression of the gene of interest can offer advantages over IHC. In particular, PCR-based RNA expression analysis offers better reproducibility, as it evaluates not the quantity of the gene-specific transcript *per se*, but the ratio between the RNA messages of the gene-target and gene-referee. Furthermore, PCR tests are usually performed in a semi-automated manner, so they are less labor-consuming as compared to morphology-based analyses (30–32). However, RNA testing has several limitations. First, gene transcription is not always an equivalent of gene translation, as the production and decay of gene-specific RNAs and proteins involves different layers of regulation. Second, IHC analysis is capable to assess intracellular localization of the protein, while RNA assays evaluate only the bulk amount of gene product. Third, some analytical solutions, such as PD-L1 IHC assays, offer individual scoring for various cell types, for example, tumor cells and immune cells (6, 7). This advantage is not compatible with currently established PCR procedures. Several studies attempted to investigate in parallel the expression of PD-L1 on the level of RNA and protein in cell cultures and tumor tissues. These small-scale studies provided generally encouraging results indicating that the correlation between PD-L1 RNA and protein level does exist (30–36).

Recently published CLOVER study represents the first systematic attempt to evaluate the feasibility of PCR-based PD-L1 testing in comparison with IHC (37). The authors analyzed 437 NSCLC samples by three PD-L1 IHC assays (Ventana SP142, Ventana SP263, Dako 22C3) and by the laboratory-developed real-time PCR test for PD-L1 RNA expression. In agreement with other investigations, the CLOVER study showed significant concordance between the SP263 and the 22C3 IHC, while the SP142 produced lower rate of PD-L1 positive tumors. Indeed, the Blueprint Phase 1 study, which included 39 lung tumors stained with four different antibodies, showed that SP263 and 22C3 assays demonstrated similar IHC patterns in the majority of cases, while SP142 stained fewer number of tumor cells with generally lower intensity (38). The Blueprint Phase 2 study

TABLE 1 | Selected clinical studies on immune checkpoint inhibitors, which evaluated associations between clinical outcomes and the level of PD-L1 expression analysis.

References	Brief description of the study	Survival	Predictive role of PD-L1
Pembrolizumab (IHC: 22C3)			
Herbst et al. (8) (KEYNOTE-010)	Assessment of long-term outcomes of pembrolizumab vs. docetaxel monotherapy in previously treated NSCLC with PD-L1 expression in >/=1% tumor cells	OS PD-L1 1-49%: pembrolizumab: 11.8 months; docetaxel: 8.4 months PD-L1 >/=50%: pembrolizumab: 16.9 months; docetaxel: 8.2 months	Dramatic improvement of OS for pembrolizumab in patients with PD-L1 expression in >/=50% tumor cells; moderate improvement of OS in patients with PD-L1 expression score 1–49%
Gadgeel et al. (9) (KEYNOTE-189)	First-line therapy, non-squamous NSCLC: pembrolizumab or placebo plus pemetrexed and platinum	OS PD-L1 <1%: pembrolizumab plus chemotherapy: 17.2 months; pembrolizumab plus placebo: 10.2 months PD-L1 1-49%: pembrolizumab plus chemotherapy: 21.8 months; pembrolizumab plus placebo: 12.1 months PD-L1 >/=50%: pembrolizumab plus chemotherapy: not reached; pembrolizumab plus placebo: 10.1 months PFS PD-L1 <1%: pembrolizumab plus chemotherapy: 6.2 months; pembrolizumab plus placebo: 5.1 months PD-L1 1-49%: pembrolizumab plus chemotherapy: 9.2 months; pembrolizumab plus placebo: 4.9 months PD-L1 >/=50%: pembrolizumab plus chemotherapy: 11.1 months; pembrolizumab plus placebo: 4.8 months	Pembrolizumab plus chemotherapy outperformed pembrolizumab plus placebo regardless of the PD-L1 status, however the magnitude of the effect was higher in tumors with high PD-L1 expression
Garon et al. (10) (KEYNOTE-001)	Assessment of long-term outcomes of pembrolizumab monotherapy in treatment-naïve and previously treated patients	OS in treatment-naïve patients: PD-L1 <1%: not evaluated (low number of patients) PD-L1 1–49%: 19.5 months PD-L1 >/=50%: 35.4 months OS in previously treated patients: PD-L1 <1%: 8.6 months PD-L1 1–49%: 8.5 months PD-L1 >/=50%: 15.4 months	Pembrolizumab treatment was associated with improved OS in patients with PD-L1 expression in >/=50% tumor cells
Mok et al. (11) (KEYNOTE-042)	First-line therapy: pembrolizumab vs. chemotherapy for NSCLC with PD-L1 expression in >/=1% tumor cells	OS: PD-L1 >/=1%: pembrolizumab: 16.7 months; chemotherapy: 12.1 months PD-L1 >/=20%: pembrolizumab: 17.7 months; chemotherapy: 13.0 months PD-L1 >/=50%: pembrolizumab: 20.0 months; chemotherapy: 12.2 months PFS: PD-L1 >/=1%: pembrolizumab: 5.4 months; chemotherapy: 6.5 months PD-L1 >/=20%: pembrolizumab: 6.2 months; chemotherapy: 6.6 months PD-L1 >/=50%: pembrolizumab: 7.1 months; chemotherapy: 6.4 months	Improvement of OS for pembrolizumab was observed both for PD-L1 >/=50% and >/=1% expression thresholds, however the magnitude of the effect was greater for the high expressors
Paz-Ares et al. (12) (KEYNOTE-407)	First-line therapy, squamous NSCLC: pembrolizumab or placebo plus chemotherapy	OS: PD-L1 <1%: pembrolizumab plus chemotherapy: 15.9 months; pembrolizumab plus placebo: 10.2 months PD-L1 1–49%: pembrolizumab plus chemotherapy: 14.0 months; pembrolizumab plus placebo: 11.6 months PD-L1 >/=50%: pembrolizumab plus chemotherapy: not reached; pembrolizumab plus placebo: not reached PFS: PD-L1 <1%: pembrolizumab plus chemotherapy: 6.3 months; pembrolizumab plus placebo: 5.3 months PD-L1 1–49%: pembrolizumab plus chemotherapy: 7.5 months; pembrolizumab plus placebo: 5.2 months PD-L1 >/=50%: pembrolizumab plus chemotherapy: 8.0 months; pembrolizumab plus placebo: 4.2 months	Pembrolizumab plus chemotherapy outperformed pembrolizumab plus placebo regardless of the PD-L1 status

(Continued)

TABLE 1 | Continued

References	Brief description of the study	Survival	Predictive role of PD-L1
Nivolumab (IHC: 28-8)			
Hellmann et al. (13) (CHECKMATE 227)	First-line therapy: nivolumab plus ipilimumab vs. nivolumab alone vs. chemotherapy for NSCLC with PD-L1 expression in >/=1% tumor cells; nivolumab plus ipilimumab vs. nivolumab plus chemotherapy vs. chemotherapy for NSCLC with PD-L1 expression in <1% tumor cells	OS: PD-L1 <1%: nivolumab plus ipilimumab: 17.2 months; nivolumab plus chemotherapy: 15.2 months; chemotherapy: 12.2 months PD-L1 >/=1%: nivolumab plus ipilimumab: 17.1 months; nivolumab alone: 15.7 months; chemotherapy: 14.9 months PD-L1 >/=50%: nivolumab plus ipilimumab: 21.2 months; nivolumab alone: 18.1 months; chemotherapy: 14.0 months PFS: PD-L1 <1%: nivolumab plus ipilimumab: 5.1 months; nivolumab alone: 5.6 months; chemotherapy: 4.7 months PD-L1 >/=1%: nivolumab plus ipilimumab: 5.1 months; nivolumab alone: 4.2 months; chemotherapy: 5.6 months PD-L1 >/=50%: nivolumab plus ipilimumab: 6.7 months; nivolumab alone: 5.6 months; chemotherapy: 5.6 months	Nivolumab plus ipilimumab outperformed chemotherapy regardless of the PD-L1 status, however the difference was more pronounced in patients with PD-L1 expression in >/=50% tumor cells
Ready et al. (14) (CHECKMATE 568)	First-line therapy: nivolumab plus ipilimumab	PFS: PD-L1 <1%: 2.8 months PD-L1 >/=1%: 6.8 months PD-L1 >/=50%: 6.8 months	PD-L1 expression was associated with higher rate of objective responses and longer PFS
Carbone et al. (15) (CHECKMATE 026)	First-line therapy: nivolumab vs. chemotherapy for NSCLC with PD-L1 expression in >/=1% tumor cells	OS: PD-L1 >/=1%: nivolumab: 13.7 months; chemotherapy: 13.8 months PD-L1 >/=5%: nivolumab: 14.4 months; chemotherapy: 13.2 months PD-L1 >/=50%: nivolumab: 15.9 months; chemotherapy: 13.9 months PFS: PD-L1 >/=1%: nivolumab: 4.2 months; chemotherapy: 5.8 months PD-L1 >/=5%: nivolumab: 4.2 months; chemotherapy: 5.9 months PD-L1 >/=50%: nivolumab: 5.4 months; chemotherapy: 5.8 months	No predictive value for PD-L1 expression
Borghaei et al. (16) (CHECKMATE 057)	Nivolumab vs. docetaxel monotherapy in previously treated patients with non-squamous NSCLC	OS: PD-L1 <1%: nivolumab: 10.5 months; docetaxel: 10.1 months PD-L1 >/=1%: nivolumab: 17.7 months; docetaxel: 9.0 months PD-L1 >/=5%: nivolumab: 19.4 months; docetaxel: 8.1 months PD-L1 >/=10%: nivolumab: 19.9 months; docetaxel: 8.0 months PFS: PD-L1 <1%: nivolumab: 2.1 months; docetaxel: 3.6 months PD-L1 >/=1%: nivolumab: 4.2 months; docetaxel: 4.5 months PD-L1 >/=5%: nivolumab: 5.0 months; docetaxel: 3.8 months PD-L1 >/=10%: nivolumab: 5.0 months; docetaxel: 3.7 months	Nivolumab outperformed docetaxel only in patients with PD-L1 expression in >/=1% tumor cells
Brahmer et al. (17) (CHECKMATE 017)	Nivolumab vs. docetaxel monotherapy in previously treated patients with squamous NSCLC	OS: PD-L1 <1%: nivolumab: 8.7 months; docetaxel: 5.9 months PD-L1 >/=1%: nivolumab: 9.3 months; docetaxel: 7.2 months PD-L1 >/=5%: nivolumab: 10.0 months; docetaxel: 6.4 months PD-L1 >/=10%: nivolumab: 11.0 months; docetaxel: 7.1 months	No predictive role of the PD-L1 status

(Continued)

TABLE 1 | Continued

References	Brief description of the study	Survival	Predictive role of PD-L1
		PFS: PD-L1 <1%: nivolumab: 3.1 months; docetaxel: 3.0 months PD-L1 >/=1%: nivolumab: 3.3 months; docetaxel: 2.8 months PD-L1 >/=5%: nivolumab: 4.8 months; docetaxel: 3.1 months PD-L1 >/=10%: nivolumab: 3.7 months; docetaxel: 3.3 months	
Atezolizumab (IHC: SP142)			
Socinski et al. (18) (IMpower 150)	First-line therapy: atezolizumab plus carboplatin plus paclitaxel (ACP) vs. bevacizumab plus carboplatin plus paclitaxel (BCP) vs. atezolizumab plus BCP (ABCP) for non-squamous NSCLC	ABCP vs. BCP comparison, PFS: TC3 or IC3: 12.6 months vs. 6.8 months TC1/2/3 or IC1/2/3: 11.0 months vs. 6.8 months TC1/2 or IC1/2: 8.3 months vs. 6.6 months TC0/1/2 and IC0/1/2: 8.0 months vs. 6.8 months TC0 and IC0: 7.1 months vs. 6.9 months	Addition of atezolizumab to carboplatin, paclitaxel and bevacizumab improved PFS regardless of the PD-L1 status, however the magnitude of the effect was higher for tumors with high PD-L1 expression
Rittmeyer et al. (19) (OAK)	Atezolizumab vs. docetaxel monotherapy in previously treated NSCLC patients	OS: TC3 or IC3: 20.5 months vs. 8.9 months TC2/3 or IC2/3: 16.3 months vs. 10.8 months TC1/2/3 or IC1/2/3: 15.7 months vs. 10.3 months TC0 and IC0: 12.6 months vs. 8.9 months	Atezolizumab outperformed docetaxel regardless of the PD-L1 status, however the magnitude of the effect was higher for tumors with high PD-L1 expression
Fehrenbacher et al. (20) (POPLAR)	Atezolizumab vs. docetaxel monotherapy in previously treated NSCLC patients	OS: TC3 or IC3: 15.5 months vs. 11.1 months TC2/3 or IC2/3: 15.1 months vs. 7.4 months TC1/2/3 or IC1/2/3: 15.5 months vs. 9.2 months TC0 and IC0: 9.7 months vs. 9.7 months	Atezolizumab outperformed docetaxel only in patients with PD-L1 expression in >/=1% tumor cells or >/=1% tumor-infiltrating immune cells
Avelumab: (IHC: 73-10)			
Barlesi et al. (21) (JAVELIN Lung 200)	Avelumab vs. docetaxel monotherapy in previously treated NSCLC patients	OS: PD-L1 >/=1%: avelumab: 11.4 months; docetaxel: 10.3 months PD-L1 >/=50%: avelumab: 13.6 months; docetaxel: 9.2 months PD-L1 >/=80%: avelumab: 17.1 months; docetaxel: 9.3 months	Improved outcomes for avelumab were observed only in patients with high PD-L1 expression
Gulley et al. (22) (JAVELIN Solid Tumor)	Avelumab in previously treated NSCLC patients	OS: PD-L1 <1% tumor cells: 4.6 months PD-L1 >/=1% tumor cells: 8.9 months PD-L1 >/=5% tumor cells: 10.6 months PD-L1 >/=25% tumor cells: 8.4 months PD-L1 </=10% immune cells in hot-spots: 8.5 months PD-L1 >/=10% immune cells in hot-spots: 8.9 months PFS: PD-L1 <1% tumor cells: 5.9 weeks PD-L1 >/=1% tumor cells: 12.0 weeks PD-L1 >/=5% tumor cells: 11.9 weeks PD-L1 >/=25% tumor cells: 11.9 weeks PD-L1 </=10% immune cells in hot-spots: 11.3 weeks PD-L1 >/=10% immune cells in hot-spots: 8.4 weeks	Improved outcomes for avelumab were observed when PD-L1 expression in >/=1% tumor cells was used as a threshold
Durvalumab (IHC: SP263)			
Rizvi et al. (23) (MYSTIC)	First-line therapy: durvalumab with or without tremelimumab vs. standard chemotherapy	OS: PD-L1 <1%: durvalumab plus tremelimumab: 11.9 months; durvalumab alone: 10.1 months; chemotherapy: 10.3 months PD-L1 >/=1%: durvalumab plus tremelimumab: 10.9 months; durvalumab alone: 14.6 months; chemotherapy: 12.3 months PD-L1 25–49%: durvalumab plus tremelimumab: 10.5 months; durvalumab alone: 11.1 months; chemotherapy: 13.3 months PD-L1 >/=50%: durvalumab plus tremelimumab: 15.2 months; durvalumab alone: 18.3 months; chemotherapy: 12.7 months	Improved outcomes for durvalumab were observed only in patients with high PD-L1 expression

(Continued)

TABLE 1 | Continued

References	Brief description of the study	Survival	Predictive role of PD-L1
Paz-Ares et al. (24) (PACIFIC)	Durvalumab vs. placebo after chemoradiotherapy in unresectable stage III NSCLC	OS: PD-L1 <1%: durvalumab 33.1 months; placebo: 45.6 months PD-L1 1–24%: durvalumab 43.3 months; placebo: 30.5 months PD-L1 >/=25%: durvalumab: not reached; placebo: 21.1 months PFS: PD-L1 <1%: durvalumab 10.7 months; placebo: 5.6 months PD-L1 1–24%: durvalumab: not reached; placebo: 9.0 months PD-L1 >/=25%: durvalumab 17.8 months; placebo: 3.7 months	Improved PFS for durvalumab was observed across all subgroups; improved OS for durvalumab was seen for patients with PD-L1 expression in >/=1% tumor cells
Garassino et al. (25) (ATLANTIC)	Durvalumab as a third-line or later treatment in NSCLC patients	OS: Cohort EGFR+/ALK+: PD-L1 <25%: 9.9 months PD-L1 >/=25%: 13.3 months Cohort EGFR-/ALK-: PD-L1 <25%: 9.3 months PD-L1 >/=25%: 10.9 months Cohort PD-L1>/=90%: not reached PFS: Cohort EGFR+/ALK+: PD-L1 <25%: 1.9 months PD-L1 >/=25%: 1.9 months Cohort EGFR-/ALK-: PD-L1 <25%: 1.9 months PD-L1 >/=25%: 3.3 months Cohort PD-L1>/=90%: 2.4 months	PD-L1 expression was associated with improved outcomes

OS, overall survival; PFS, progression-free survival; IHC, immunohistochemistry; TC, tumor cells; IC, immune cells; the details for TC and IC scoring are explained in (20).

essentially replicated these results using a "real-world" series of 81 lung cancer specimens (39). The CLOVER study compared the performance of PCR-based PD-L1 expression measurement against conventional IHC assays. Strikingly, negative PCR tests appeared to be a reliable predictor for the lack of PD-L1 expression as determined by immunohistochemistry. This is an expected observation, given that the PCR is considered to be an ultrasensitive method for detection of biological molecules; so if the gene product cannot be detected by PCR it is unlikely to be seen by other methods. However, positive predictive value of PCR was low, as many PD-L1 RNA expressing tumors turned out to be PD-L1-negative by IHC analysis.

The results of the CLOVER study may potentially be relevant to already existing PCR diagnostic pipelines. It is relatively easy to add one more gene-specific assay to established PCR procedures, so if PCR is indeed helpful to identify PD-L1 non-expressors, its use may avoid unnecessary IHC tests. The reliability of this approach remains to be determined in subsequent studies. Overall, the CLOVER investigation calls for further efforts related to the harmonization of PD-L1 testing. Contrary to many studies, the CLOVER considered PD-L1 RNA measurement as a categorical variable by grouping tumors as "positive" and "negative" (37). It is essential to consider RNA expression as a continuous variable. Furthermore, the estimation of meaningful thresholds requires tedious consideration of various clinical and laboratory endpoints. The CLOVER study utilized a conditional threshold for the PCR test and did not adjust its value; so the additional efforts are needed to define the categories of PD-L1 expressors using biologically or clinically relevant criteria. Most importantly, the CLOVER investigation used IHC tests as a comparator for PCR assays. Ideally, studies of this type should consider treatment outcomes instead of surrogate markers; this is particularly true for PD-L1 testing, given that many PD-L1/PD1 targeted drugs show activity irrespective of the results of PD-L1 analysis (6, 7).

The instances of discordant results of PD-L1 expression measurement deserve a more systematic investigation on a case-by-case basis, given that the outcome of PD-L1 testing may dramatically influence clinical treatment decisions. There are examples of surprising discordance, when the same specimen is strongly positive by one antibody but clearly negative by another IHC assay (38, 39). Several factors may contribute to these discrepancies. Human error may be one of the factors when large series of tumors are analyzed. The Blueprint project revealed that the inter-observer variability may play a role in the interpretation of the results of PD-L1 staining (38). PD-L1 IHC assays calculate only the proportion of stained cells, while the intensity of the staining is not considered; therefore, the cut-off point between weak and absent staining may be defined differently. Intratumoral heterogeneity of PD-L1 expression may also contribute to these discrepancies, given that even serial sections may differ from each other with regard to the percentage of stained cells. The process of industrial development of distinct PD-L1 antibodies by definition involves distinct protein epitopes and distinct animals, so the individual antibody clones may differ in their ability to recognize various PD-L1 isoforms. The incorporation of the RNA testing adds complexity to this issue. It is not impossible that some tumor specimens lose their ability to interact with diagnostic antibodies during the archiving process; these samples may retain detectable PD-L1 RNA expression but show PD-L1 negativity by IHC.

There is a growing enthusiasm towards the use of PCR-based expression assays as a substitute or complement for IHC analysis. For example, Oncotype Dx breast cancer panel includes estrogen receptor, progesterone receptor and HER2 measurement to aid conventional IHC testing (40). Some studies demonstrate that Ki-67 RNA-based expression analysis has non-inferior or even better clinical performance as compared to conventional IHC tests (41, 42). There are several reported PCR-based biomarkers, which could assist the administration of immune checkpoint inhibitors (18, 43). It is highly likely that PD-L1 testing will undergo significant modification in a very near future.

AUTHOR CONTRIBUTIONS

All authors listed have made a substantial, direct and intellectual contribution to the work, and approved it for publication.

REFERENCES

1. Canon J, Rex K, Saiki AY, Mohr C, Cooke K, Bagal D, et al. The clinical KRAS (G12C) inhibitor AMG 510 drives anti-tumour immunity. *Nature.* (2019) 575:217–23. doi: 10.1038/s41586-019-1694-1
2. Halliday PR, Blakely CM, Bivona TG. Emerging targeted therapies for the treatment of non-small cell lung cancer. *Curr Oncol Rep.* (2019) 21:21. doi: 10.1007/s11912-019-0770-x
3. Sokolenko AP, Imyanitov EN. Molecular diagnostics in clinical oncology. *Front Mol Biosci.* (2018) 5:76. doi: 10.3389/fmolb.2018.00076
4. Mitiushkina NV, Kholmatov MM, Tiurin VI, Romanko AA, Yatsuk OS, Sokolova TN, et al. Comparative analysis of expression of mutant and wild-type alleles is essential for reliable PCR-based detection of MET exon 14 skipping. *Biochimie.* (2019) 165:267–74. doi: 10.1016/j.biochi.2019.08.014
5. Cottrell TR, Taube JM. PD-L1 and emerging biomarkers in immune checkpoint blockade therapy. *Cancer J.* (2018) 24:41–6. doi: 10.1097/PPO.0000000000000301
6. Camidge DR, Doebele RC, Kerr KM. Comparing and contrasting predictive biomarkers for immunotherapy and targeted therapy of NSCLC. *Nat Rev Clin Oncol.* (2019) 16:341–55. doi: 10.1038/s41571-019-0173-9
7. Pirker R. Biomarkers for immune checkpoint inhibitors in advanced nonsmall cell lung cancer. *Curr Opin Oncol.* (2019) 31:24–8. doi: 10.1097/CCO.0000000000000496
8. Herbst RS, Garon EB, Kim DW, Cho BC, Perez-Gracia JL, Han JY, et al. Long-term outcomes and retreatment among patients with previously treated, programmed death-ligand 1-positive, advanced non–small-cell lung cancer in the KEYNOTE-010 study. *J Clin Oncol.* (2020) 38:1580–90. doi: 10.1200/JCO.19.02446
9. Gadgeel S, Rodríguez-Abreu D, Speranza G, Esteban E, Felip E, Dómine M, et al. Updated analysis from KEYNOTE-189: pembrolizumab or placebo plus pemetrexed and platinum for previously untreated metastatic nonsquamous non-small-cell lung cancer. *J Clin Oncol.* (2020) 38:1505–17. doi: 10.1200/JCO.19.03136
10. Garon EB, Hellmann MD, Rizvi NA, Carcereny E, Leighl NB, Ahn MJ, et al. Five-year overall survival for patients with advanced non–small-cell lung cancer treated with pembrolizumab: results from the phase I KEYNOTE-001 study. *J Clin Oncol.* (2019) 37:2518–27. doi: 10.1200/JCO.19.00934
11. Mok TSK, Wu YL, Kudaba I, Kowalski DM, Cho BC, Turna HZ, et al. Pembrolizumab versus chemotherapy for previously untreated, PD-L1-expressing, locally advanced or metastatic non-small-cell lung cancer (KEYNOTE-042): a randomised, open-label, controlled, phase 3 trial. *Lancet.* (2019) 393:1819–30. doi: 10.1016/S0140-6736(18)32409-7
12. Paz-Ares L, Luft A, Vicente D, Tafreshi A, Gümüş M, Mazières J, et al. Pembrolizumab plus chemotherapy for squamous non-small-cell lung cancer. *N Engl J Med.* (2018) 379:2040–51. doi: 10.1056/NEJMoa1810865
13. Hellmann MD, Paz-Ares L, Bernabe Caro R, Zurawski B, Kim SW, Carcereny Costa E, et al. Nivolumab plus ipilimumab in advanced non-small-cell lung cancer. *N Engl J Med.* (2019) 381:2020–31. doi: 10.1056/NEJMoa1910231
14. Ready N, Hellmann MD, Awad MM, Otterson GA, Gutierrez M, Gainor JF, et al. First-line nivolumab plus ipilimumab in advanced non-small-cell lung cancer (CheckMate 568): outcomes by programmed death ligand 1 and tumor mutational burden as biomarkers. *J Clin Oncol.* (2019) 37:992–1000. doi: 10.1200/JCO.18.01042
15. Carbone DP, Reck M, Paz-Ares L, Creelan B, Horn L, Steins M, et al. First-line nivolumab in stage IV or recurrent non-small-cell lung cancer. *N Engl J Med.* (2017) 376:2415–26. doi: 10.1056/NEJMoa1613493
16. Borghaei H, Paz-Ares L, Horn L, Spigel DR, Steins M, Ready NE, et al. Nivolumab versus docetaxel in advanced nonsquamous non-small-cell lung cancer. *N Engl J Med.* (2015) 373:1627–39. doi: 10.1056/NEJMoa1507643
17. Brahmer J, Reckamp KL, Baas P, Crinò L, Eberhardt WE, Poddubskaya E, et al. Nivolumab versus docetaxel in advanced squamous-cell non-small-cell lung cancer. *N Engl J Med.* (2015) 373:123–35. doi: 10.1056/NEJMoa1504627
18. Socinski MA, Jotte RM, Cappuzzo F, Orlandi F, Stroyakovskiy D, Nogami N, et al. Atezolizumab for first-line treatment of metastatic nonsquamous NSCLC. *N Engl J Med.* (2018) 378:2288–301. doi: 10.1056/NEJMoa1716948
19. Rittmeyer A, Barlesi F, Waterkamp D, Park K, Ciardiello F, von Pawel J, et al. Atezolizumab versus docetaxel in patients with previously treated non-small-cell lung cancer (OAK): a phase 3, open-label, multicentre randomised controlled trial. *Lancet.* (2017) 389:255–65. doi: 10.1016/S0140-6736(16)32517-X
20. Fehrenbacher L, Spira A, Ballinger M, Kowanetz M, Vansteenkiste J, Mazieres J, et al. Atezolizumab versus docetaxel for patients with previously treated non-small-cell lung cancer (POPLAR): a multicentre, open-label, phase 2 randomised controlled trial. *Lancet.* (2016) 387:1837–46. doi: 10.1016/S0140-6736(16)00587-0
21. Barlesi F, Vansteenkiste J, Spigel D, Ishii H, Garassino M, de Marinis F, et al. Avelumab versus docetaxel in patients with platinum-treated advanced non-small-cell lung cancer (JAVELIN lung 200): an open-label, randomised, phase 3 study. *Lancet Oncol.* (2018) 19:1468–79. doi: 10.1016/S1470-2045(18)30673-9
22. Gulley JL, Rajan A, Spigel DR, Iannotti N, Chandler J, Wong DJL, et al. Avelumab for patients with previously treated metastatic or recurrent non-small-cell lung cancer (JAVELIN solid tumor): dose-expansion cohort of a multicentre, open-label, phase 1b trial. *Lancet Oncol.* (2017) 18:599–610. doi: 10.1016/S1470-2045(17)30240-1
23. Rizvi NA, Cho BC, Reinmuth N, Lee KH, Luft A, Ahn MJ, et al. Durvalumab with or without tremelimumab vs standard chemotherapy in first-line treatment of metastatic non-small cell lung cancer: the MYSTIC phase 3 randomized clinical trial. *JAMA Oncol.* (2020) 6:661–74. doi: 10.1001/jamaoncol.2020.0237
24. Paz-Ares L, Spira A, Raben D, Planchard D, Cho BC, Özgüroglu M, et al. Outcomes with durvalumab by tumour PD-L1 expression in unresectable, stage III non-small-cell lung cancer in the PACIFIC trial. *Ann Oncol.* (2020) 31:798–806. doi: 10.1016/j.annonc.2020.03.287
25. Garassino MC, Cho BC, Kim JH, Mazières J, Vansteenkiste J, Lena H, et al. Durvalumab as third-line or later treatment for advanced non-small-cell lung cancer (ATLANTIC): an open-label, single-arm, phase 2 study. *Lancet Oncol* (2018) 19:521–36. doi: 10.1016/S1470-2045(18)30144-X

26. Garinet S, Laurent-Puig P, Blons H, Oudart JB. Current and future molecular testing in NSCLC, what can we expect from new sequencing technologies? *J ClinMed.* (2018) 7:E144. doi: 10.3390/jcm7060144
27. Morganti S, Tarantino P, Ferraro E, D'Amico P, Duso BA, Curigliano G. Next Generation sequencing (NGS): a revolutionary technology in pharmacogenomics and personalized medicine in cancer. *Adv Exp Med Biol.* (2019) 1168:9–30. doi: 10.1007/978-3-030-24100-1_2
28. Iyevleva AG, Raskin GA, Tiurin VI, Sokolenko AP, Mitiushkina NV, Aleksakhina SN, et al. Novel ALK fusion partners in lung cancer. *Cancer Lett.* (2015) 362:116–21. doi: 10.1016/j.canlet.2015.03.028
29. Koomen BM, Badrising SK, van den Heuvel MM, Willems SM. Comparability of PD-L1 immunohistochemistry assays for non-small-cell lung cancer: a systematic review. *Histopathology.* (2020) 76:793–802. doi: 10.1111/his.14040
30. Vannitamby A, Hendry S, Makadia T, Danks J, Slavin J, Irving L, et al. A novel approach to detect programed death ligand 1 (PD-L1) status and multiple tumor mutations using a single non-small-cell lung cancer (NSCLC) bronchoscopy specimen. *J Mol Diagn.* (2019) 21:186–97. doi: 10.1016/j.jmoldx.2018.10.001
31. Vannitamby A, Hendry S, Irving L, Steinfort D, Bozinovski S. Novel multiplex droplet digital PCR assay for scoring PD-L1 in non-small cell lung cancer biopsy specimens. *Lung Cancer.* (2019) 134:233–7. doi: 10.1016/j.lungcan.2019.06.029
32. Brüggemann C, Kirchberger MC, Goldinger SM, Weide B, Konrad A, Erdmann M, et al. Predictive value of PD-L1 based on mRNA level in the treatment of stage IV melanoma with ipilimumab. *J Cancer Res Clin Oncol.* (2017) 143:1977–84. doi: 10.1007/s00432-017-2450-2
33. Shimoji M, Shimizu S, Sato K, Suda K, Kobayashi Y, Tomizawa K, et al. Clinical and pathologic features of lung cancer expressing programmed cell death ligand 1 (PD-L1). *Lung Cancer.* (2016) 98:69–75. doi: 10.1016/j.lungcan.2016.04.021
34. Le Goux C, Damotte D, Vacher S, Sibony M, Delongchamps NB, Schnitzler A, Terris B, et al. Correlation between messenger RNA expression and protein expression of immune checkpoint-associated molecules in bladder urothelial carcinoma: a retrospective study. *Urol Oncol.* (2017) 35:257–63. doi: 10.1016/j.urolonc.2017.01.014
35. Chen S, Crabill GA, Pritchard TS, McMiller TL, Wei P, Pardoll DM, et al. Mechanisms regulating PD-L1 expression on tumor and immune cells. *J Immunother Cancer.* (2019) 7:305. doi: 10.1186/s40425-019-0770-2
36. Gullo I, Oliveira P, Athelogou M, Gonçalves G, Pinto ML, Carvalho J, et al New insights into the inflamed tumor immune microenvironment of gastric cancer with lymphoid stroma: from morphology and digital analysis to gene expression. *Gastric Cancer.* (2019) 22:77–90. doi: 10.1007/s10120-018-0836-8
37. Tsimafeyeu I, Imyanitov E, Zavalishina L, Raskin G, Povilaitite P, Savelov N, et al. Agreement between PDL1 immunohistochemistry assays and polymerase chain reaction in non-small cell lung cancer: CLOVER comparison study. *Sci Rep.* (2020) 10:3928. doi: 10.1038/s41598-020-60950-2
38. Hirsch FR, McElhinny A, Stanforth D, Ranger-Moore J, Jansson M, Kulangara K, et al. PD-L1 immunohistochemistry assays for lung cancer: results from phase 1 of the blueprint PD-L1 IHC assay comparison project. *J Thorac Oncol.* (2017) 12:208–22. doi: 10.1016/j.jtho.2016.11.2228
39. Tsao MS, Kerr KM, Kockx M, Beasley MB, Borczuk AC, Botling J, et al. PD-L1 Immunohistochemistry comparability study in real-life clinical samples: results of blueprint phase 2 project. *J Thorac Oncol.* (2018) 13:1302–11. doi: 10.1016/j.jtho.2018.05.013
40. McVeigh TP, Kerin MJ. Clinical use of the oncotype DX genomic test to guide treatment decisions for patients with invasive breast cancer. *Breast Cancer.* (2017) 9:393–400. doi: 10.2147/BCTT.S109847
41. Yamamoto S, Ibusuki M, Yamamoto Y, Fu P, Fujiwara S, Murakami K, et al. Clinical relevance of Ki67 gene expression analysis using formalin-fixed paraffin-embedded breast cancer specimens. *Breast Cancer.* (2013) 20:262–70. doi: 10.1007/s12282-012-0332-7
42. Gao W, Wu J, Chen X, Lin L, Fei X, Shen K, et al. Clinical validation of Ki-67 by quantitative reverse transcription-polymerase chain reaction (RT-PCR) in HR+/HER2- early breast cancer. *J Cancer.* (2019) 10:1110–6. doi: 10.7150/jca.29337
43. Paré L, Pascual T, Seguí E, Teixidó C, Gonzalez-Cao M, Galván P, et al. Association between PD1 mRNA and response to anti-PD1 monotherapy across multiple cancertypes. *Ann Oncol.* (2018) 29:2121–8. doi: 10.1093/annonc/mdy335

4

Co-Occurring Alteration of NOTCH and DDR Pathways Serves as Novel Predictor to Efficacious Immunotherapy in NSCLC

Zhimin Zhang[1†], Yanyan Gu[2†], Xiaona Su[3†], Jing Bai[4†], Wei Guan[3], Jungang Ma[3], Jia Luo[3], Juan He[3], Bicheng Zhang[1], Mingying Geng[3], Xuefeng Xia[4], Yanfang Guan[4], Cheng Shen[5] and Chuan Chen[3*]*

[1] *Cancer Center, Renmin Hospital of Wuhan University, Wuhan, China,* [2] *Department of Nutrition, Changzheng Hospital, Second Military Medical University, Shanghai, China,* [3] *Cancer Center, Daping Hospital, Army Medical University (Third Military Medical University), Chongqing, China,* [4] *Geneplus-Beijing Institute, Beijing, China,* [5] *Department of Thoracic Surgery, Daping Hospital, Army Medical University (Third Military Medical University), Chongqing, China*

***Correspondence:**
Cheng Shen
sc941@sina.com
Chuan Chen
sinkriver@126.com

[†]*These authors have contributed equally to this work*

Although immune checkpoint inhibitors (ICIs) have shown remarkable benefit for treatment of advanced non-small lung cancer (NSCLC), only a minority of patients can achieve durable responses and the most patients produce an ultra-rapid progressive disease. Here, we collected the availably published datasets and mined the determinants of response to immunotherapy on pathway levels. One hundred six NSCLC patients treated with immunotherapy were combined from Rizvi et al. and Hellman et al. studies (whole exon sequencing). Two independent validation datasets consisted of the MSKCC cohort (targeted sequencing) and data by Anagnostou and colleagues (whole exon sequencing). The Cancer Genome Atlas (TCGA) somatic mutation and gene expression data were applied to explore the immunobiology features. In the first combined cohort, we detected NOTCH pathway altered in 71% patients with durable clinical benefit (DCB) while only 36% among no durable benefit (NDB) ($p = 0.005$). Compared to NDB group, co-occurrence of NOTCH and at least two DDR (co-DDR) pathway was discovered in DCB group and contributed to a prolonged progression-free survival (PFS) [22.1 *vs* 3.6 months, $p < 0.0001$, HR, 0.34, 95% confidence interval (CI), 0.2–0.59]. In two independent datasets, co-occurrence of NOTCH+/co-DDR+ was also validated to be a better immunotherapy efficacy [Cohort 2: 13 *vs* 6 months, $p = 0.034$, HR, 0.55, 95% CI, 0.31–0.96; Cohort 3: 21 *vs* 11 months, $p = 0.067$, HR, 0.45, 95% CI, 0.18–1.1]. By analyzing TCGA cohort, we found patients with coexisting NOTCH+/co-DDR+ pathway had a higher TMB, more infiltration of CD4+T cells. Overall, co-occurrence of NOTCH and co-DDR pathway reflect a better immunotherapy efficacy in advanced NSCLC. This genomic predictor show promise in stratifying patients that suit for immunotherapy for future clinical practice.

Keywords: NOTCH pathway, DDR pathway, co-occurring mutations, immunotherapy, predictive biomarker, non-small cell lung cancer

INTRODUCTION

Immune checkpoint inhibitors (ICIs) has shown remarkable benefit for treatment of advanced non-small lung cancer (NSCLC) (1, 2). Nevertheless, only a limited patient population can generate durable responses after immunotherapy, while the majority of patients undergo inferior survival (3, 4). Therefore, there is an urgent need to stratify the patients who will benefit from ICIs.

A plethora of studies have shown biomarkers for predicting response to immunotherapy. The most heavily studied biomarker was programmed death-ligand 1 (PD-L1) expression correlated to efficacious immunotherapy (5–8), but subsequent trials proven a sizeable proportion of patients still achieve durable responses with PD-L1 negative (2, 9). Furthermore, some genomic markers have been reported for predicting the response to ICI, including tumor mutation burden (TMB) (10, 11), tumor neoantigen burden (TNB) (12, 13), and DNA repair alterations (14–16). Meanwhile, several studies explored the alterations on pathway level that correlates to ICI. Zhang et al. found NOTCH signaling related to better ICI efficacy (17). Wang et al. revealed co-mutations in DNA damage response (DDR) pathways could serve as predictors of response to ICB (18).

Due to the interactions and dependencies among different pathways, we supposed single pathway was not high enough to reflect the response of ICI. Therefore, we focused on the co-occurrent pathways to predict the superior survival outcomes after immunotherapy. Availably published datasets were collected from four studies. The first cohort was combined by data from Rizvi et al. and Hellman et al., which was used to identify the co-occurrent pathways correlated to ICI (15, 19). We further validated the co-occurrent pathways correlated to better efficacy after immunotherapy in two independent datasets (data from Anagnostou et al. and the MSKCC cohort) (20, 21). Using the somatic mutation and gene expression data from TCGA, we explored the immunobiology features about the co-occurrent pathway.

MATERIALS AND METHODS

Datasets Used

We collected four publicly available datasets treated with immunotherapy (**Supplementary Table 1**). Thirty-four NSCLC patients sequenced by WES were downloaded from Rizvi et al. Another 75 patients with WES data were derived from Hellman et al. studies. Data from the two studies were merged as the first combined cohort. After excluding three patients lack of efficacy information, data from 106 patients was obtained. The second cohort was from Anagnostou et al., including 89 NSCLC patients treated with ICIs. Two patients were excluded because of lacking definitive response evaluation. For the third cohort, MSKCC cohort was downloaded from cBioPortal (http://www.cbioportal.org/study/summary?id=tmb_mskcc_2018). We also acquired the genome mutation from 1026 NSCLC patients and transcriptome expression data from 59 advanced NSCLC patients in TCGA.

Pathway Alterations

Genes involved in 10 oncogenic signaling pathways and eight DDR pathways were listed in **Supplementary Table 2**. The 10 canonical oncogenic signaling pathways were downloaded from (22) and included: cell cycle, Hippo signaling, Myc signaling, Notch signaling, oxidative stress response/Nrf2, PI-3-Kinase signaling, receptor-tyrosine kinase (RTK)/RAS/MAP-Kinase signaling, TGFb signaling, p53 and b-catenin/Wnt signaling. Eight DDR pathways analyzed were: mismatch repair (MMR); base excision repair (BER); check point factors (CPF); Fanconi anemia (FA); homologous recombination repair (HRR); nucleotide excision repair (NER); non-homologous end-joining (NHEJ); and DNA translesion synthesis (TLS) (23). We defined pathway alteration as at least one gene in this pathway mutated. Co-DDR was defined as two or more DDR pathway altered. Co-occurring alteration of NOTCH and DDR pathway was referred as NOTCH+/co-DDR+.

Immune Infiltration Analysis

SsGSEA was utilized to calculate the enrichment scores (ES) of immune cell types in the tumor microenvironment (24). Gene signatures of 28 immune cell types were downloaded from previous study (25). Tumors were further subclassified into different immune groups using the Euclidean distance and "ward.D" clustering. The expression levels of genes were first z-score normalized across all patients. Then we calculated the mean z-scores for each group and ranked in descending order. Based on the pre-ranked GSEA method, for each immune cell signature, we defined the q-value <10% and NES >0 as the enrichment, while the q-value <10% and NES <0 as the depletion.

Statistical Analyses

We performed univariable and multivariable Cox regression analyses to identify potential predictors of survival. Survival curves were estimated with the Kaplan-Meier product-limit method and compared by log-rank test. Comparisons of TMB, TNB, and expression levels between different groups were used with the Wilcoxon rank-sum test or t test. Enrichment analysis of gene function was calculated by GSEA with Benjamini-Hochberg correction for multiple hypothesis testing ($q < 0.05$). All statistical analyses were performed in the R statistical environment version 3.6.2.

RESULTS

Pathway Alterations in NSCLC Treated With Immunotherapy

We collected WES data from 106 NSCLC patients treated with immunotherapy derived from published data as the discovery cohort (15, 19). Of these patients, 51 (48.1%) achieved durable clinical benefit and 55 (51.9%) had no response to the immunotherapy. The clinical features and efficacy outcomes were summarized in **Table 1**. To unravel the determinants of response to immunotherapy on pathway levels, we mapped all mutated genes to 10 oncogenic signaling pathways and eight DDR pathways (**Supplementary Table 2, Figure 1**). A tumor sample was considered as altered in a given pathway if one or more genes in this pathway contained non-synonymous mutations. Data from 99 patients succeeded to map to pathways that were further analyzed. The most frequently altered pathway was RTK/RAS in both DCB and NDB group (80 *vs* 82%), followed by HIPPO pathway (65% in DCB *vs* 52% in NDB). Notably, 71% patients with DCB had alteration in NOTCH pathway while only 36% in NDB group (p = 0.005). This was consistent with previous study that NOTCH signaling correlated with better ICI efficacy (17). More DDR-related pathways were altered in DCB. Co-mutations in DDR

TABLE 1 | Clinical characteristics of discovery cohort.

	Total	DCB	NDB	P-value
Histology				
Squamous	87 (82.1%)	44 (86.3%)	43 (78.2%)	0.32
Non-squamous	19 (17.9%)	7 (13.7%)	12 (21.8%)	
Sex				
Female	54 (50.9%)	26 (51.0%)	28 (50.9%)	1
Male	52 (49.1%)	25 (49.0%)	27 (49.1%)	
Smoking Status				
Current/Former	85 (80.2%)	43 (84.3%)	42 (76.4%)	0.34
Never	21 (19.8%)	8 (15.7%)	13 (23.6%)	
PD L1 expression				
Strong	18 (17.0%)	14 (27.5%)	4 (7.3%)	0.045
Weak	48 (45.3%)	21 (41.2%)	27 (49.1%)	
Negative	31 (29.2%)	12 (23.5%)	19 (34.5%)	
Unknown	9 (8.5%)	4 (7.84%)	5 (9.1%)	
Best Overall Response				
CR/PR	34 (32.1%)	34 (66.7%)	0 (0.0%)	<0.001
PD/NE	36 (34.0%)	0 (0.0%)	36 (65.5%)	
SD	36 (34.0%)	17 (33.3%)	19 (34.5%)	
Treatment				
PD-1 blockade	31 (29.2%)	14 (27.5s%)	17 (30.9%)	0.83
PD-1 plus CTLA-4 blockade	75 (70.8%)	37 (72.5%)	38 (69.1%)	

CR, complete response; CTLA-4, cytotoxic T-cell lymphocyte-4; DCB, durable clinical benefit; NDB, no durable benefit; NE, not evaluable; PD, progressive disease; PD-1, programmed cell death-1; PR, partial response; SD, stable disease.

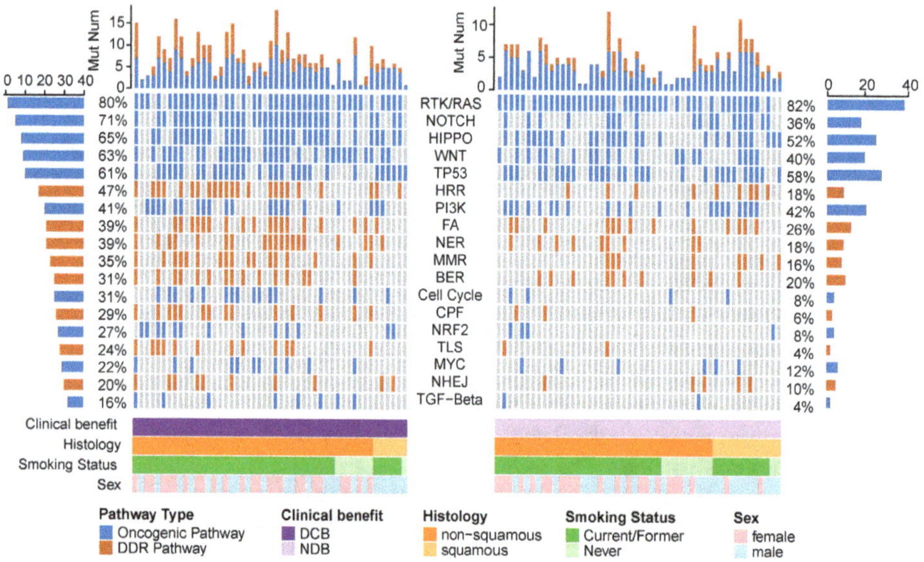

FIGURE 1 | Pathway alterations in NSCLC with or without efficacious immunotherapy. Stacked plot showed the number of mutated pathway (histogram, top). Clinical characters are listed at the bottom of the figure. The prevalence of mutated pathways was calculated at left (in DCB group) and right (in NDB group). Orange represents the oncogenic pathway and blue stands for the DDR pathway.

pathways (hereafter referred as co-DDR) have been reported to a better clinical benefit to ICI by Wang et al. (18), we also detected a higher prevalence of co-DDR pathway alteration in DCB group (69.3 *vs* 30%, p = 0.0002). Taken together, alterations on pathway level can reflect the divergent response in immunotherapy.

Identification of NOTCH Co-occurring Pathways to Distinguish ICI Efficacy

Given that single pathway fails to adequately reveal the response of ICI, we applied a co-occurrence strategy to investigate how the NOTCH co-occurring pathways impacted the ICI efficacy. Comparing to NDB group, we identified the HIPPO and/or co-DDR pathway co-occurring with NOTCH pathway, which displayed a better clinical benefit (**Figure 2A**). After testing in univariate and multivariate cox regression for progressive free survival (PFS), only co-occurrence of NOTCH and co-DDR pathway proved to be an independently protective factor for PFS (**Figure 2B**, **Supplementary Figure 1**). Thus, 99 patients were further stratified into two groups according to the co-occurrent alteration of NOTCH and co-DDR pathways (hereafter referred as NOTCH+/co-DDR+). Altered genes for each pathway of NOCTH+/co-DDR+ were shown in **Supplementary Figure 2**. We defined the patients with NOTCH+/co-DDR+ as "GoodBenefit" (37 patients) and others were "BadBenefit" (62 patients). Patients grouped as "GoodBenefit" showed a longer PFS (22.1 *vs* 3.6 months, p < 0.0001, **Figure 2C**). Notably, co-occurrence of NOTCH+/co-DDR+ showed more prolonged PFS than single pathway (alteration either in NOTCH or co-DDR pathway) (**Supplementary Figure 3A**). In the NOTCH+/co-DDR+ group, we also detected higher tumor mutation burden (TMB, **Figure 2D**), higher tumor neoantigen burden (TNB, **Figure 2E**), more durable clinical benefit (p < 0.001, **Figure 2F**), and more improved objective response (p < 0.001, **Figure 2G**). These

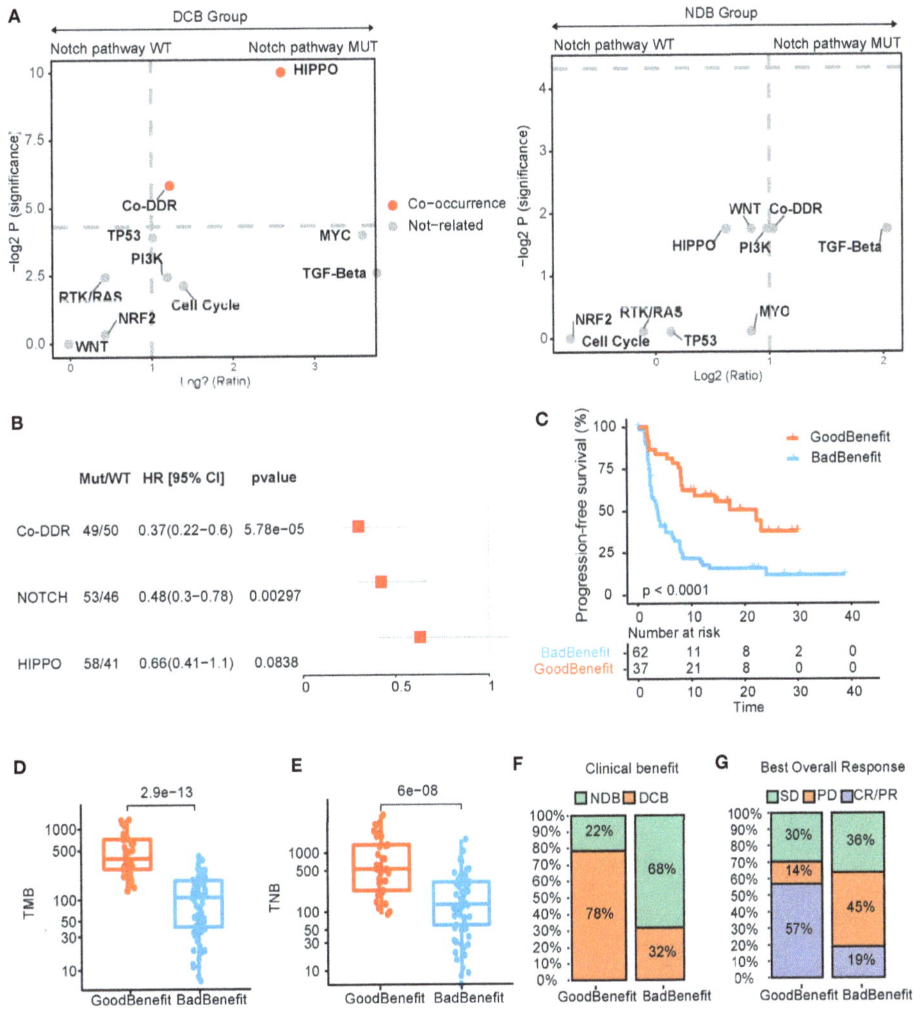

FIGURE 2 | NOTCH co-occurring pathways that contributed to ICI efficacy. **(A)** log2 (odds ratio) and -log2 (p value) for enrichment of altered pathways co-occurred with and without NOTCH pathway. **(B)** Forest plot displaying univariate cox regression analyses for PFS of individually considered pathway. **(C)** Kaplan-Meier survival curves for PFS comparing "GoodBenefit" *versus* "BadBenefit." **(D, E)** Boxplot of TMB **(D)** and TNB **(E)** in "GoodBenefit" *versus* "BadBenefit." **(F, G)** Percentage of patients with clinical benefit evaluation **(F)** and objective response **(G)**.

results were also observed when we stratified patients into the following three groups: CoPath (NOTCH+/co-DDR+) *versus* SinglePath (alterations in NOTCH or at least two DDR pathway) *versus* wild type (**Supplementary Figures 3B–E**). In summary, we identified NOTCH co-occurring with co-DDR pathways reflecting a better immunotherapy efficacy.

Independent Validation of the Model in Two Cohorts

To evaluate whether the co-occurrence of NOTCH+/co-DDR+ could serve as a potential predictor of immunotherapy efficacy, we crossed-validated our findings using two independent cohorts who received ICI therapies.

One validated dataset was from Anagnostou and colleagues (20), 87 NSCLC patients with definitive response evaluation were obtained. Using our stratification criteria, 26 patients were grouped into "GoodBenefit," where 61 were classified as "BadBenefit." Utilizing the univariate cox regression for PFS, "GoodBenefit" group showed a decreased risk of PFS (**Figure 3A**). Comparing to the group of "BadBenefit," patients with co-existing pathways had longer PFS (13 *vs* 6 months, p = 0.034, HR, 0.55, 95% CI, 0.31–0.96) (**Figure 3B**). As expected, the TMB was

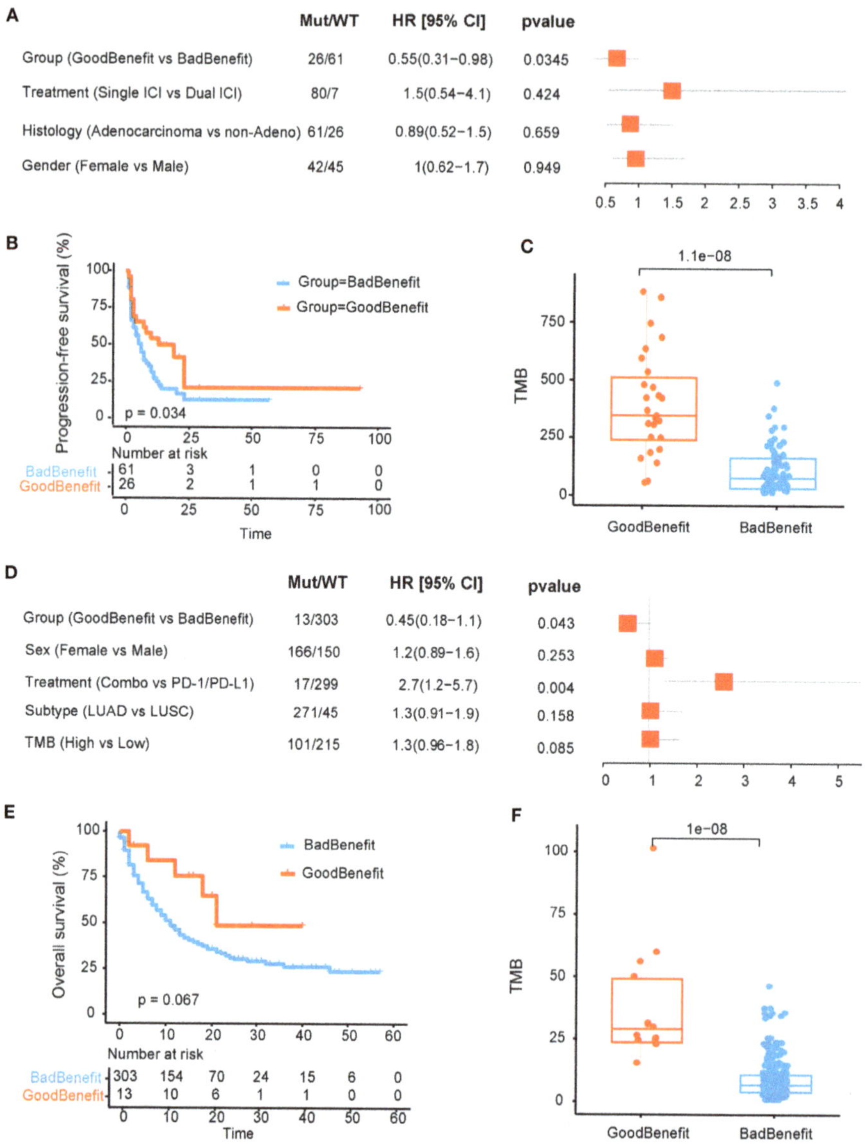

FIGURE 3 | Validation of NOTCH/co-DDR co-occurring pathways to ICI efficacy in Anagnostou et al. cohort **(A–C)** and MSKCC cohort **(D–F)**. **(A)** Forest plot displaying univariate cox regression analyses for PFS of individually considered pathway for Anagnostou et al. dataset. **(B)** Kaplan-Meier survival curves for PFS comparing "GoodBenefit" *versus* "BadBenefit." **(C)** Boxplot of TMB in "GoodBenefit" *versus* "BadBenefit." **(D)** Forest plot displaying univariate cox regression analyses for OS of individually considered pathway for MSKCC data. **(E)** Kaplan-Meier survival curves for OS comparing "GoodBenefit" *versus* "BadBenefit." **(F)** Boxplot of TMB in "GoodBenefit" *versus* "BadBenefit."

significantly higher in "GoodBenefit" group than "BadBenefit" group (**Figure 3C**). When Comparing among the three groups (NOTCH+/co-DDR+ *versus* NOTCH or co-DDR occurrence *versus* Wildtype), co-occurrence of NOTCH/co-DDR also exhibited superior survival outcomes and the highest TMB (**Supplementary Figures 4A, B**).

For another independent cohort from MSKCC, 1,661 patients received immunotherapy by targeted sequencing, we retained the 316 NSCLC tissue [271 lung adenocarcinoma (LUAD) and 45 Lung squamous cell carcinoma (LUSC)] for further analyses (21). Co-occurrence of NOTCH+/co-DDR+ was found act as a protective factor (**Figure 3D**). Overall survival in co-occurrence group was prolonged, although did not reached the statistical significance (21 *vs* 11 months, p = 0.067, HR, 0.45, 95% CI, 0.181.1, **Figure 3E**). We speculated the limited genes from panel may underestimate the pathway alteration. In this cohort, targeted capture panel comprised of 341 and 410 genes, respectively, covering 10 oncogenic pathways and seven DDR pathways without TLS pathway. In addition, the TMB was significantly higher in "GoodBenefit" group (**Figure 3F**). When compared among the three groups, the co-occurrent group still performed improved OS prognostication and higher TMB (**Supplementary Figures 4C, D**).

Genomic Characteristics of NOTCH/co-DDR Co-occurrence in TCGA Cohort

We next explored the genomic characteristics in TCGA cohort according to our stratification criterion. One thousand twenty-six NSCLC WES data and clinical features were downloaded. All mutated genes were mapped to 18 canonical pathways. TMB in "GoodBenefit" group was significantly higher than "BadBenefit" group regardless of stage (**Supplementary Figure 5A**). Considering the predictor of NOTCH+/co-DDR+ was trained based on advanced NSCLC and without EGFR mutation. We filtered out the patients with early stage and EGFR alteration. Ultimately, 120 advanced NSCLC patients retained; 39.2% (47) patients were classified as "GoodBenefit" group while 60.8% (73) as "BadBenefit" group. This ratio of potential efficiency coincided with previous reports on NSCLC patients beneficial of ICIs delivery (26–29). In order to exclude NOTCH+/co-DDR+ as a potential prognostic factor, we performed the survival analyses in TCGA cohort treated with standard treatment. No significant difference of overall survival was detected between GoodBenefit *versus* BadBenefit group or among three groups (**Figure 4A, Supplementary Figure 5B**). This result demonstrated co-occurrent NOTCH+/co-DDR+ was not a prognostic factor *per se*, but can serve as predictor in condition of immunotherapy. Recent studies have shown the TMB was a predictor of the pathological response to immune checkpoint inhibitors treatment in advanced lung cancer patients, we next checked the TMB distribution in our groups. Comparing to wildtype, higher TMB was observed in "GoodBenefit" group (**Figure 4B**). In details, the TMB was significantly higher in co-occurrence group than those harbored single pathway (either NOCTH or co-DDR alteration) and wildtype (neither NOTCH nor co-DDR alteration) (**Supplementary Figure 5C**).

Immunobiology Features of NOTCH/co-DDR Co-occurrence

To further explore the immunobiology features of NOTCH+/co-DDR+ co-occurrence, we obtained 59 of 120 patients from TCGA whose RNA-seq data were available. The single sample gene set enrichment analysis (ssGSEA) method was employed to deconvolute the relative abundance of each immune cell type. By unsupervised clustering, we classified the 59 NSCLC into three clusters [immune-high (n = 27), immune-intermediate (n = 15), and immune-low (n = 17), **Figure 5A**]. Patients with NOTCH+/co-DDR+ co-occurrence had no preference to specific immune group (immune-high 14/27 *vs* immune-intermediate 3/15 *vs* immune-low 6/17, p = 0.12). Of note, CD4+ T cell were enriched in NOTCH+/co-DDR+ group (**Figure 5B**). We also found Interleukin 4 (IL-4), a quintessential T helper type 2 (Th2) cytokine produced by CD4+ T cells, expressed lower in "GoodBenefit" group (**Figure 5C**). TNFRSF18 was up-regulated in "GoodBenefit" group (**Figure 5C**), playing a role in promoting T effector cell activity by inducing proliferation and supporting survival in T cells, while also suppressing Treg activity (30). Another Tumor necrosis factor superfamily, TNFSF15 was downregulated in "GoodBenefit" group. TNFSF15 has been reported being an inhibitor of endothelial cell growth (31). Functional enrichment analyses revealed "GoodBenefit" group up-

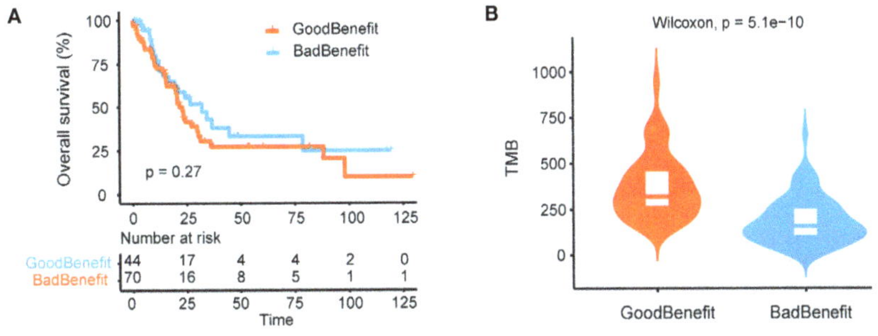

FIGURE 4 | Genomic characteristics of NOTCH/co-DDR co-occurring pathways in TCGA cohort. **(A)** Kaplan-Meier survival curves for OS comparing "GoodBenefit" *versus* "BadBenefit." **(B)** Violin plot of TMB between "GoodBenefit" *versus* "BadBenefit."

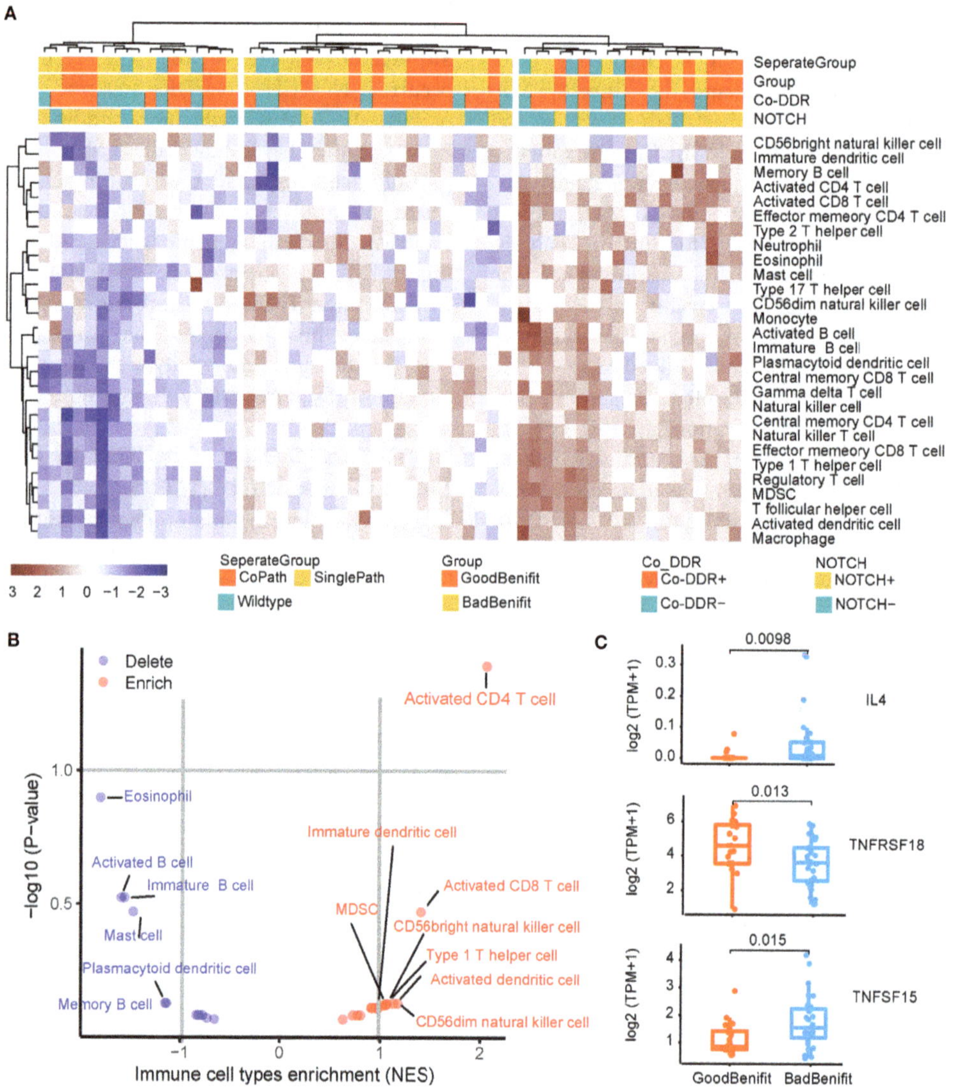

FIGURE 5 | Immunobiology features of NOTCH/co-DDR co-occurrence. **(A)** Heatmap of immune infiltration in each patient. **(B)** Volcano plots for the enrichment (red) and depletion (blue) of immune cell types for GoodBenefit and BadBenefit. The expression levels of genes were first z-score normalized across all patients. Then we calculated the mean z-scores for each group and ranked in descending order. Based on the pre-ranked GSEA method, for each immune cell signature, we defined the q-value <10% and NES >0 as the enrichment, while the q-value <10% and NES <0 as the depletion. Immune cells with absolute NES greater than 1 were shown. **(C)** Normalized express of immune-related genes between Goodbenefit *versus* Badbenefit.

regulated growth factor receptor pathway, down-regulated DNA repair pathways and immune response pathways, this tumor context may contribute to the clinical benefit of ICI (**Supplementary Figure 6**).

DISCUSSION

In this study, we demonstrated the co-occurrence of NOTCH and co-DDR pathways can predict the superior survival outcomes after immunotherapy in advanced NSCLC. This phenomenon was first identified in one combined cohort and validated across another two independent cohorts. All the data we analyzed was performed WES, except one validated cohort from MSKCC (targeted sequencing). Using WES data was an advantage because it can cover enough genes of the pathway, overcoming the deficiency of targeted sequencing. To the best of our knowledge, this is the first report focusing on co-occurrence event on pathway level to explore the determinants of response to ICIs.

To explore whether there were dominant gene mutations in the co-occurring pathway, we depicted the co-occurring event on gene level involved in NOTCH and DDR pathways (**Supplementary Figure 1**). It can be observed that more alterations occurred in DCB group than NDB group. However, the overall mutation incidence on gene level was quite low. The most frequently mutated genes in

NOTCH pathway were NOTCH1 (7%), NOTCH2 (7%), and JAG2 (7%). Meanwhile, low mutation rates of genes were observed in DDR pathway. Taken together, our data suggested that different genes converging to the co-occurring pathways effect the immunotherapy effect, rather than the specific gene of co-occurrence drives.

Although a single pathway of NOTCH or co-DDR has been reported as a predictor to ICI, we revealed co-occurrent NOTCH+/co-DDR+ pathway preferred in DCB and was more predictive to patients beneficial of ICIs delivery. In the first combined cohort, patients carrying co-mutations in NOTCH and co-DDR pathways had significantly longer PFS as compared to the SinglePath (alterations in NOTCH or at least two DDR pathway) or wild type, and the TMB was gradually decreasing. As for the validation dataset of cohort 2, we also observed the longer PFS in CoPath group than SinglePath, but there was no significant different in SinglePath *versus* Wild type. Thus, we speculated alteration in single pathway of NOTCH or co-DDR was incomplete correlate of immunotherapy.

Patients carrying alterations of NOTCH+/co-DDR+ pathway associated with increased TMB, TNB, and more infiltration of CD4+ T cell. Previous study has revealed that alterations in co-DDR pathway appeared to higher TMB and TNB (18). Since a higher mutation and neoantigen load could induce T cell-mediated antitumor response (32), we speculated that alterations in co-DDR contributed to more mutation and neoepitope, and further increased the likelihood of recognition by T cell. NOTCH signaling pathway has been reported as a pivotal role in regulating T cell modulation, differentiation, and activation (33, 34). In addition, previous study also reported NOTCH can control the fate of various T cell types, including Th1, Th2, and the regulatory T cells (35). In our result, we found co-occurrence of NOTCH/co-DDR tended to infiltrate more CD4+ T cell, but down-regulated the cytokine of Th2, suggesting more CD4 T cell that not secrete Th2 exist in NOTCH/co-DDR group. Moreover, recent studies have shown that NOTCH signaling is required for optimal T-cell-mediated anti-tumor immunity (36). Collectively, one potential explanation may be alteration of co-DDR pathway cause more mutations producing immunogenic neoantigens that are recognized and targeted by T cells and NOTCH pathway mediate more infiltration of CD4+ T cells and enhance effector T-cell activity. However, the underlying mechanism of co-ordination between NOTCH and co-DDR pathways and how these pathways shape together the microenvironment suit for immunotherapy should be further investigated in the future. Expanded data and more experiments are warranted to reveal the mechanism on how these pathways cross-talk to determine a better response to immunotherapy.

In conclusion, preliminary data from three cohorts showed evidence that co-mutations in NOTCH and co-DDR pathways indicated better immunotherapy efficacy. This genomic marker provided a new dimension to predict the superior survival outcomes in response to immunotherapy.

AUTHOR CONTRIBUTIONS

CC, CS, and ZZ conceived and designed the present study. ZZ, YYG, XS, and JB contributed equally to this work. ZZ and CC wrote the manuscript. ZZ, YYG, and XS collected and interpreted data. JB and WG performed the data analysis. JM, JL, and XX gave material support. JH, BZ, and YFG helped in improving the language and correcting grammar mistakes. All authors contributed to the article and approved the submitted version.

REFERENCES

1. Reck M, Rodríguez-Abreu D, Robinson AG, Hui R, Csőszi T, Fülöp A, et al. Pembrolizumab Versus Chemotherapy for Pd-L1–Positive Non–Small-Cell Lung Cancer. *N Engl J Med* (2016) 375:1823–33. doi: 10.1056/NEJMoa 1606774
2. Socinski MA, Jotte RM, Federico C, Francisco O, Daniil S, Naoyuki N, et al. Atezolizumab for First-Line Treatment of Metastatic Nonsquamous Nsclc. *N Engl J Med* (2018) 378:Nejmoa1716948–1716948. doi: 10.1056/NEJMoa1716948
3. Camidge DR, Doebele RC, Kerr KM. Comparing and Contrasting Predictive Biomarkers for Immunotherapy and Targeted Therapy of Nsclc. *Nat Rev Clin Oncol* (2019) 16:341–55. doi: 10.1038/s41571-019-0173-9
4. Gibney GT, Weiner LM, Atkins MB. Predictive Biomarkers for Checkpoint Inhibitor-Based Immunotherapy. *Lancet Oncol* (2016) 17:E542–542e551. doi: 10.1016/S1470-2045(16)30406-5
5. Garon EB, Rizvi NA, Hui R, Leighl N, Gandhi L. Pembrolizumab for the Treatment of Non–Small-Cell Lung Cancer. *N Engl J Med* (2015) 372:2018–28. doi: 10.1056/NEJMoa1501824
6. Chae YK, Pan A, Davis AA, Raparia K, Mohindra NA, Matsangou M, et al. Biomarkers for Pd-1/Pd-L1 Blockade Therapy In Non-Small-Cell Lung Cancer: Is Pd-L1 Expression a Good Marker for Patient Selection. *Clin Lung Cancer* (2016) 17:350–61. doi: 10.1016/J.Cllc.2016.03.011
7. Tumeh PC, Harview CL, Yearley JH, Shintaku IP, Taylor EJ, Robert L, et al. Pd-1 Blockade Induces Responses by Inhibiting Adaptive Immune Resistance. *Nature* (2014) 515:568–71. doi: 10.1038/Nature13954
8. Anagnostou V, Forde PM, White JR, Niknafs N, Hruban C, Naidoo J, et al. Dynamics of Tumor and Immune Responses During Immune Checkpoint Blockade in Non-Small Cell Lung Cancer. *Cancer Res* (2019) 79:1214–25. doi: 10.1158/0008-5472.Can-18-1127
9. Motzer RJ, Rini BI, Mcdermott DF, Redman BG, Kuzel TM, Harrison MR, et al. Nivolumab for Metastatic Renal Cell Carcinoma: Results of a Randomized Phase Ii Trial. *J Clin Oncol* (2014) 33:1430–7. doi: 10.1200/JCO.2014.59.0703
10. Hellmann MD, Callahan MK, Awad MM, Calvo E, Ascierto PA, Atmaca A, et al. Tumor Mutational Burden and Efficacy of Nivolumab Monotherapy and in Combination With Ipilimumab in Small-Cell Lung Cancer. *Cancer Cell* (2018) 33:853–61.e4. doi: 10.1016/j.ccell.2019.01.011
11. Carbone DP, Reck M, Paz-Ares L, Creelan B, Horn L, Steins M, et al. First-Line Nivolumab in Stage Iv or Recurrent Non-Small-Cell Lung Cancer. *N Engl J Med* (2017) 376:2415–26. doi: 10.1056/Nejmoa1613493
12. Van Allen EM, Miao D, Schilling B, Shukla SA, Blank C, Zimmer L, et al. Genomic Correlates of Response to Ctla-4 Blockade in Metastatic Melanoma. *Science* (2015) 350:207–11. doi: 10.1126/science.aad0095
13. Gubin MM, Zhang X, Schuster H, Caron E, Ward JP, Noguchi T, et al. Checkpoint Blockade Cancer Immunotherapy Targets Tumour-Specific Mutant Antigens. *Nature* (2014) 515:577–81. doi: 10.1038/Nature13988
14. Finn OJ. Cancer immunology. *Cancer Immunol* (2008) 358:2704–15. doi: 10.1056/NEJMra072739
15. Rizvi NA, Hellmann MD, Snyder A, Kvistborg P, Makarov V, Havel JJ, et al. Mutational Landscape Determines Sensitivity to Pd-1 Blockade in Non-Small Cell Lung Cancer. *Science* (2015) 348:124–8. doi: 10.1126/science.aaa1348

16. Bhangoo MS, Boasberg P, Mehta P, Elvin JA, Ali SM, Wu W, et al. Tumor Mutational Burden Guides Therapy in a Treatment Refractory Pole-Mutant Uterine Carcinosarcoma. *Oncologist* (2018) 23:518. doi: 10.1634/theoncologist.2017-0342
17. Zhang K, Hong X, Song Z, Xu Y, Liu L. IIdentification of Deleterious NOTCH Mutation as Novel Predictor to Efficacious Immunotherapy in NSCLC. *Clin Cancer Res* (2020) 26:3649–661. doi: 10.1158/1078-0432.CCR-19-3976
18. Wang Z, Zhao J, Wang G, Zhang F, Zhang Z, Zhang F, et al. Comutations in Dna Damage Response Pathways Serve as Potential Biomarkers for Immune Checkpoint Blockade. *Cancer Res* (2018) 78:6486–96. doi: 10.1158/0008-5472.Can-18-1814
19. Hellmann MD, Nathanson T, Rizvi H, Creelan BC, Sanchez-Vega F, Ahuja A, et al. Genomic Features of Response to Combination Immunotherapy in Patients With Advanced Non-Small-Cell Lung Cancer. *Cancer Cell* (2018) 33:843–52.e4. doi: 10.1016/j.ccell.2018.03.018
20. Anagnostou V, Niknafs N, Marrone K, Bruhm DC, White JR, Naidoo J, et al. Multimodal Genomic Features Predict Outcome of Immune Checkpoint Blockade in Non-Small-Cell Lung Cancer. *Nat Cancer* (2020) 1:99–111. doi: 10.1038/s43018-019-0008-8
21. Samstein RM, Lee C, Shoushtari AN, Hellmann MD, Shen R, Janjigian YY, et al. Tumor Mutational Load Predicts Survival After Immunotherapy Across Multiple Cancer Types. *Nat Genet* (2019) 51:202–6. doi: 10.1038/s41588-018-0312-8
22. Sanchez-Vega F, Mina M, Armenia J, Chatila WK, Luna A, La KC, et al. Oncogenic Signaling Pathways in the Cancer Genome Atlas. *Cell* (2018) 173:321–37.E10. doi: 10.1016/J.Cell.2018.03.035
23. Scarbrough PM, Weber RP, Iversen ES, Brhane Y, Amos CI, Kraft P, et al. a Cross-Cancer Genetic Association Analysis of the Dna Repair and Dna Damage Signaling Pathways for Lung, Ovary, Prostate, Breast, and Colorectal Cancer. *Cancer Epidemiol Biomarkers Prev* (2016) 25:193–200. doi: 10.1158/1055-9965.EPI-15-0649
24. Hnzelmann S, Castelo R, Guinney J. Gsva: Gene Set Variation Analysis for Microarray and Rna-Seq Data. *BMC Bioinformatics* (2013) 14:7–7. doi: 10.1186/1471-2105-14-7
25. Charoentong P, Finotello F, Angelova M, Mayer C, Efremova M, Rieder D, et al. Pan-Cancer Immunogenomic Analyses Reveal Genotype-Immunophenotype Relationships and Predictors of Response to Checkpoint Blockade. *Cell Rep* (2017) 18:248–62. doi: 10.1016/j.celrep.2016.12.019
26. Barlesi F, Vansteenkiste J, Spigel D, Ishii H, Garassino M, De Marinis F, et al. Avelumab versus docetaxel in patients with platinum-treated advanced non-small-cell lung cancer (JAVELIN Lung 200): An open-label, randomised, phase 3 study. *Lancet Oncol* (2018) 19:1468–79. doi: 10.1016/S1470-2045(18)30673-9
27. Borghaei H, Paz-Ares L, Horn L, Spigel DR, Steins M, Ready NE, et al. Nivolumab Versus Docetaxel in Advanced Nonsquamous Non–Small-Cell Lung Cancer. *N Engl J Med* (2015) 373:1627–39. doi: 10.1056/NEJMoa1507643
28. Garassino MC, Cho B, Kim J, Mazières J, Vansteenkiste J, Lena H, et al. Durvalumab as Third-Line or Later Treatment for Advanced Non-Small-Cell Lung Cancer (Atlantic): an Open-Label, Single-Arm, Phase 2 Study. *Lancet Oncol* (2018) 19:521–36. doi: 10.1016/S1470-2045(18)30144-X
29. Herbst RS, Baas P, Kim D, Felip E, Pérez-Gracia JL, Han J, et al. Pembrolizumab Versus Docetaxel for Previously Treated, Pd-L1-Positive, Advanced Non-Small-Cell Lung Cancer (Keynote-010): a Randomised Controlled Trial. *Lancet* (2016) 387:1540–50. doi: 10.1016/S0140-6736(15)01281-7
30. Mahoney KM, Rennert PD, Freeman GJ. Combination Cancer Immunotherapy and New Immunomodulatory Targets. *Nat Rev Drug Discov* (2015) 14:561–84. doi: 10.1038/nrd4591
31. Yu J, Tian S, Metheny-Barlow L, Chew LJ, Hayes AJ, Pan H, et al. Modulation of Endothelial Cell Growth Arrest and Apoptosis by Vascular Endothelial Growth Inhibitor. *Circ Res* (2001) 89:1161–7. doi: 10.1161/hh2401.101909
32. Keenan TE, Burke KP, Van Allen EM. Genomic Correlates of Response to Immune Checkpoint Blockade. *Nat Med* (2019) 25:1. doi: 10.1038/s41591-019-0382-x
33. Laky K, Fowlkes BJ. Notch Signaling in Cd4 and Cd8 T Cell Development. *Curr Opin Immunol* (2008) 20:197–202. doi: 10.1016/J.Coi.2008.03.004
34. Janghorban M, Xin L, Rosen JM, Zhang XH. Notch Signaling as a Regulator of the Tumor Immune Response: to Target or Not to Target. *Front Immunol* (2018) 9:1649:1649. doi: 10.3389/Fimmu.2018.01649
35. Luo X, Xu L, Li Y, Tan H. Notch Pathway Plays a Novel and Critical Role in Regulating Responses of T and Antigen-Presenting Cells in Agvhd. *Front Immunol* (2017) 33:169–81. doi: 10.1007/s10565-016-9364-7
36. Kelliher MA, Roderick JE. NOTCH Signaling in T-Cell-Mediated Anti-Tumor Immunity and T-Cell-Based Immunotherapies. *Front Immunol* (2018) 9:1718 doi: 10.3389/fimmu.2018.01718

5

Obesity, Sarcopenia and Outcomes in Non-Small Cell Lung Cancer Patients Treated with Immune Checkpoint Inhibitors and Tyrosine Kinase Inhibitors

Karam Khaddour[1,2], Sandra L. Gomez-Perez[3], Nikita Jain[1], Jyoti D. Patel[4] and Yanis Boumber[4,5]*

[1] Department of Medicine, Rosalind Franklin University of Medicine and Science, McHenry, IL, United States, [2] Department of Medicine, Division of Hematology and Oncology, University of Illinois at Chicago, Chicago, IL, United States, [3] Department of Clinical Nutrition, Rush University Medical Center, Chicago, IL, United States, [4] Division of Hematology/Oncology, Feinberg School of Medicine, Northwestern University, Robert H. Lurie Comprehensive Cancer Center, Chicago, IL, United States, [5] Institute of Fundamental Medicine and Biology, Kazan Federal University, Kazan, Russia

***Correspondence:**
Karam Khaddour
Karam.khaddour@gmail.com

Body composition refers to the proportional content of body fat mass and lean body mass that can lead to a continuum of different phenotypes ranging from cachectic/sarcopenic state to obesity. The heterogenetic phenotypes of body composition can contribute to formation of some cancer types and can sometimes lead to disparate outcomes. Both of these extremes of the spectrum exist in patients with non-small cell lung carcinoma (NSCLC). The discovery of new pathways that drive tumorigenesis contributing to cancer progression and resistance have expanded our understanding of cancer biology leading to development of new targeted therapies including tyrosine kinase inhibitors (TKI) and immune checkpoint inhibitors (ICI) that have changed the landscape of NSCLC treatment. However, in the new era of precision medicine, the impact of body composition phenotypes on treatment outcomes and survival is now being elucidated. In this review, we will discuss the emerging evidence of a link between body composition and outcomes in patients with NSCLC treated with TKI and ICI. We will also discuss suggested mechanisms by which body composition can impact tumor behavior and anti-tumor immunological response.

Keywords: non-small cell lung cancer, body composition, obesity, sarcopenia, tyrosine kinase inhibitor, immune checkpoint inhibitor, overall survival

---

Abbreviations: ALK, anaplastic lymphoma kinase gene; BMI, body mass index; CI, confidence interval; cm, centimeter; CT, computed tomography; CTLA-4, cytotoxic associated lymphocyte antigen-4; DEXA, dual-energy x-ray absorptiometry; EGFR, epidermal growth factor receptor; HR, hazard ratio; HU, Hounsfield unit; IARC, international agency for research on cancer; ICI, immune checkpoint inhibitor; IL-6, interleukin-6; IL-10, interleukin-10; IL-15, interleukin-15; IMAC, Intermuscular adipose content; irAEs, immune related adverse events; kg, kilogram; L3, third lumbar; m, meter; NA, not available; NK, natural killer; NR, not reached; PD-1, programmed death 1; PD-L1, programmed death-ligand-1; PFS, progression free survival; PMI, psoas muscle index; N, number; NSCLC, non-small cell lung cancer; ORR, objective response rate; OS, overall survival; SMI, skeletal muscle index; SCFM, sub-cutaneous fat mass; STAT3, signal transduction and activator of transcription 3; TGF-β, transforming growth factor-β; TKI, tyrosine kinase inhibitor; Treg, T-regulatory; TTF, time to treatment failure; VSR, visceral to subcutaneous adipose tissue area ratio; WHO, world health organization.

INTRODUCTION

Body composition refers to the proportional distribution of different body mass contents amongst various compartments including adipose tissue and lean body mass. The most clinically distinct body phenotypes are obesity and sarcopenia. Obesity plays a significant role in tumorigenesis. It is believed that some cancers develop in obese individuals because of the chronic meta-inflammation associated with obesity in which an abundance of hormones and cytokines can potentiate epithelial cell proliferation and cancer formation (1). The link between obesity and cancer development in multiple tumor types has long been recognized in multiple epidemiological studies including a landmark report by the International Agency for Research on Cancer (IARC) showing an increased incidence of several solid and hematological malignancies in obese patients compared to the general population (2). Interestingly, this link is weak in the case of lung cancer (2).

In addition to its role in cancer development, obesity has now emerged as a prognostic factor that may predict cancer mortality (3–5). Obesity can be associated with either inferior or superior outcomes, depending on the cancer type. For example, systematic reviews and meta-analyses of population-based follow-up studies of obese patients with non-metastatic prostate and breast cancer across all clinical stages found a higher mortality in obese compared to normal weight patients regardless of treatment modality (4, 5). Surprisingly, obese and overweight patients with lung cancer seem to have better survival rates compared to normal weight subjects with a relative risk (RR) of 0.78 (95% CI: 0.75–0.82) in overweight and 0.79 (95% CI: 0.73–0.86) in obese patients respectively, however, this only applies to smokers (3). Moreover, a more recent Chinese study confirmed a strong inverse relationship between body mass index (BMI) and lung cancer mortality, which was again seen primarily in smokers (6).

The favorable effect of obesity on mortality in patients with non-small cell lung cancer (NSCLC) which is the most common type of lung cancer has been demonstrated in patients with local and metastatic disease who received different treatment modalities including surgery, radiation, and chemotherapy (7, 8). For example, Yang et al. demonstrated that obesity was associated with longer survival in lung cancer patients (N= 14,751) which was consistent among all stages (local, regional and distant) (7) Furthermore, a large retrospective study showed a trend for better survival in obese patients with NSCLC treated with combination doublet chemotherapies (N= 2,585) (9).

The other clinically distinct phenotype of body composition is sarcopenia which is defined by severe reduction of lean body mass and wasting of skeletal muscle. Sarcopenia has been identified as an independent prognostic factor for mortality in some cancer types including NSCLC (10, 11). In addition, a distinct overlap syndrome of increased adipose tissue (obesity) and loss of lean body mass (sarcopenia) has been recognized as an important factor contributing to worse prognosis in some cancers including NSCLC (12). These effects of obesity on mortality and worse prognosis in the presence of sarcopenia in cancer patients have generated an unprecedented interest in the field of oncology to study the interconnection between body composition phenotypes and cancer behavior including NSCLC (which will be the focus of this review) in an attempt to solve this conundrum. What adds to the importance of analyzing this association is that lung cancer has the highest prevalence, annual incidence and mortality rates worldwide compared to all cancer types in men and women (13). Likewise, body composition phenotypes such as obesity and sarcopenia are prevalent in lung cancer patients. As an example, up to 43% of patients with NSCLC cancer can develop sarcopenia and cachectic syndrome (14) and approximately about half of NSCLC patients are considered to have a BMI >25 mg/m^2 (considered overweight or obese) (15).

Recently, there has been a revolution in our understanding of lung cancer biology with the detection of driver mutations such as epidermal growth factor receptor (EGFR) mutation as well as the exploration of the role of immune system dysfunction in cancer progression (16–18). These discoveries have transformed the outcomes of advanced lung cancer with the development of tyrosine kinase inhibitors (TKI) targeting driver mutations such as EGFR directed TKIs and immune checkpoint inhibitors (ICI) which unleash the host immune system against tumor cells (19–24). This recent development of therapeutics in NSCLC was accompanied by a huge effort to identify patients who benefit the most from these medications given that a significant proportion of patients do not respond (25). Given the established link between different body composition and outcomes in NSCLC that was outlined by prior research, it was plausible for researchers to analyze whether different body phenotypes could be a predictive factor for response and outcomes with novel therapies.

With an evolving landscape of treatment options in advanced and metastatic lung cancer, it is imperative to further understand if body composition phenotypes can predict response and outcomes to these new classes of medications and whether there is a mechanistic effect of proportionate body components and tumor microenvironment. In this review, we first introduce the common approaches used in clinical research to estimate body composition including obesity and sarcopenia. Next, we discuss the available evidence of a biological crosstalk between different body composition phenotypes and tumor microenvironment in NSCLC. Lastly, we highlight the available studies conducted to analyze the implications of body composition phenotypes on survival outcomes in patients with NSCLC who were treated with either EGFR TKI or ICI; we also provide our recommendations on the conceptual utility of incorporating body composition calculations into prospective trials.

DISCUSSION

Methods Used To Estimate Body Composition in Patients With Non-Small Cell Lung Cancer

Many measures have been used in recent and ongoing research investigating the effect of body composition phenotypes on cancer outcomes including NSCLC. The most conventional and easiest method of estimating body composition to identify obesity is through calculation of BMI which is defined by weight divided by the square of body height [kg/m^2]. Based on the world health organization (WHO) classification, individuals can be divided into six groups to estimate the degree of obesity (**Table 1**) (26, 27). However, the complexity and heterogeneity of body composition and nutritional status might not be reflected accurately with the use of BMI alone due to its low sensitivity as indicted by discrepancies between BMI and central obesity (15, 28). In addition, calculation of BMI does not offer an accurate depiction of lean body mass which, when reduced, is considered an independent prognostic factor for high mortality in patients with NSCLC (10, 11). It has also been recognized that a subset of obese patients (defined by BMI > 30 kg/m^2) are considered to be metabolically healthy whereby they are considered to have a favorable distribution of fat mass with a normal inflammatory profile which potentially reduces the risk incurred by diseases related to obesity such as cancer and cardiovascular disease (29). Moreover, the calculation of BMI cannot distinguish between different patterns of body fat distribution (subcutaneous versus visceral) which could lead to multiple heterogeneous obesity phenotypes that could be associated with different biology and are not accurately reflected by BMI (30). Lastly, definition of obesity based on WHO classification can vary depending on ethnicity (26). This has led to the utilization of other indicators and calculations of adipose tissue content to study their relationship with outcomes in NSCLC patients such as visceral fat mass, subcutaneous fat mass, visceral to subcutaneous ratio, and fat mass index among others (31).

The measurement of sarcopenia is based on calculation of skeletal muscle index (SMI) (32, 33). Calculation of SMI is defined as total cross-sectional skeletal muscle mass (cm^2) normalized by height (m^2). Skeletal muscle mass also referred to as skeletal muscle area is derived from the total skeletal muscle mass of the eight abdominal muscles (psoas, erector spinae, quadratus lumborum, transversus abdominis, latissimus dorsi, external, and internal obliques, and rectus abdominis) measured by surface area (cm^2) at the third lumbar (L3) landmark using a single cross-sectional computed tomography (CT) image (32, 34). The L3 landmark is visible in CT scan protocols routinely performed for diagnostic and monitoring reasons in most cancer populations: abdomen (T10-L4), chest- abdomen (T1-L4), or chest-abdomen-pelvis (T1-L5). The use of a single CT image for regional body composition analysis at L3 has been described and validated in great detail in several seminal papers (32, 34, 35). The most valuable feature of this L3 landmark is that it is linearly related to whole-body fat free mass, appendicular skeletal muscle mass and whole-body fat mass as measured by dual-energy x-ray absorptiometry (DXA) in non-cancer and cancer populations (34). In brief, the CT scanner differentiates between adipose, skeletal muscle, and other compartments like bone based on specific attenuation thresholds according to the CT unit of measurement, the Hounsfield unit (HU) scale (e.g., skeletal muscle attenuation threshold is -29 to 150 HU). Cross-sectional tissue surface areas (cm^2) are semi-automatically determined by a medical imaging software such as SliceOmatic v 5.0 (Tomovision Montreal, Quebec, Canada) based on HU tissue-specific thresholds (34, 35) (**Figure 1**). Then, tissue boundaries are manually corrected as needed by a trained investigator following the semi-automatic analysis. Cutoff points for sarcopenia using the L3 SMI according to ethnicity, gender and BMI (sarcopenic obesity) have been validated with adverse cancer-related outcomes in several studies (32, 33).

TABLE 1 | World health organization classification of obesity based on body mass index.

Body Mass Index (BMI) (kg/m^2)*	Definition
<18.5	Underweight
18.5 – 24.9	Normal weight
25.0 – 29.9	Overweight (Pre-obesity)
30.0 – 34.9	Obesity class 1
35.0 – 39.9	Obesity class 2
≥40	Obesity class 3

BMI cut off points used to define obesity can vary depending on ethnicity (26).

Sarcopenic obesity is defined as low skeletal muscle mass (i.e., sarcopenia) according to a SMI cut-off such as <38.5 cm^2/m^2 for women and <52.4 cm^2/m^2 for men in the context of a BMI > 30 kg/m^2 as published by Prado et al. (32). Similarly, sarcopenia and sarcopenic obesity can also be determined using BMI and SMI specific cut-offs for men (SMI < 43 cm^2/m^2 for underweight and normal weight men, SMI < 53 cm^2/m^2 for overweight and obese men) and for women (<41 cm^2/m^2 across all BMI categories) as published by Martin et al. (33). Although the Martin et al. and Prado et al. SMI cut-off values have been used extensively by other investigators, there is currently no consensus on CT-derived SMI reference cut-off values to identify sarcopenia or sarcopenic obesity in healthy and clinical populations and is an active area of research. In addition, the L3 landmark may not be ideal for assessing SMI in patients with lung cancer, including NSCLC, who often only undergo chest CT scans (i.e., L3 vertebral landmark often not visible, T1-L1). Several research studies have examined alternative chest CT scan landmarks including lumber one (L1) and two (L2) and have provided potential SMI cut-offs for sarcopenia in healthy and in lung cancer populations, however these landmarks have not been adequately tested or validated particularly in large racially diverse cancer populations (35–38). Thus, identifying an appropriate and valid single vertebral landmark from a chest CT scan and derivation of specific cut-offs at these newer landmarks to identify sarcopenia also remains an emerging area of research.

Various researchers have used single muscle groups to determine sarcopenia such as the psoas muscle index (PMI) also usually at the L3 region (39) (see **Figure 1**). The major advantage of using a single muscle group is the speed by which this analysis can be conducted in comparison to having to capture all the muscle groups at this landmark. A major criticism for the use of single muscle groups is that it does not correlate with total lumbar skeletal muscle area and thus not representative of the entirety of the lumbar muscle groups and more importantly appears to be a poor indicator of clinical

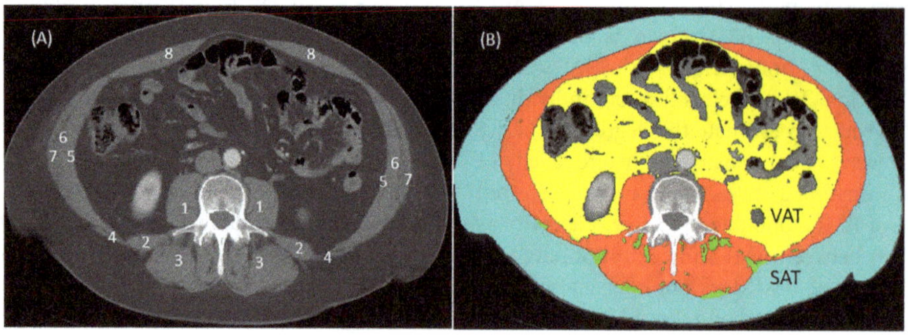

FIGURE 1 | Computed tomography (CT) image at third lumbar (L3) before **(A)** and after **(B)** analysis using sliceOmatic software (Tomovision, Montreal, Quebec, Canada). In the image without coloring **(A)**, individual muscle groups are represented by numbers and these are: 1 = psoas; 2 = quadratus lumborum; 3 = erector spinae; 4 = latissimus dorsi; 5 = transversus abdominis; 6 = internal obliques; 7 = external obliques; 8 = rectus abdominis. In the image with coloring **(B)**, analysis is based on Hounsfield unit thresholds for each tissue: skeletal muscles (red) -29 to 150 HU; subcutaneous adipose tissue (SAT) in teal and intermuscular adipose tissue (IMAT) in green -30 to -190 HU; visceral adipose tissue (VAT) in yellow -50 to -150 HU; air in black -1,000 HU; bone (L3 vertebra) 400 to 4,000 HU). Skeletal muscle index (SMI) is calculated from the total surface area (cm^2) of skeletal muscles (in red, image **(B)** normalized (divided) for height (m^2). For example, the total L3 skeletal muscle (in red, image **(B)** for this image is 166 cm^2 assuming that this person is female with a height of 164 cm or 2.68 m^2 the SMI for this person = 166 cm^2/2.68 m^2 or 61.4 cm^2/m^2. Using the Prado et al. (32) cut off of SMI < 38 cm^2/m^2 for women, this individual would not have sarcopenia. Some researchers use single muscle groups such as the psoas muscles (1 in image **(A)** normalized for height to determine sarcopenia. Although using single muscle groups to determine sarcopenia is debatable, only the surface area for both psoas muscles (1 in image **(A)** would be used to calculate psoas muscle index (PMI). Thus, PMI = psoas muscle surface areas (cm^2) divided by height (m^2).

outcomes in cancer populations (40, 41). Given these limitations, the use of PMI is less favorable than the well-established and validated technique using total lumbar skeletal muscle area for the calculation of SMI as previously described.

The importance of identifying sarcopenia comes from the fact that it has high prevalence across all BMI subtypes as well as having a detrimental prognostic effect on patients with NSCLC (42, 43).

As previously mentioned, an overlap syndrome of sarcopenia and obesity (sarcopenic obesity) has been identified and associated with adverse clinical implications in different cancer types, including NSCLC. For example, an observational study of patients with NSCLC who were treated with chemotherapy found that patients with sarcopenic obesity had shorter overall survival (OS) compared to obese patients without sarcopenia (44). The variable methodologies used to estimate body composition from obesity to sarcopenia and their effect on cancer progression and outcomes pose a challenge on how to compare and derive conclusions from studies in NSCLC. Nevertheless, the effort to analyze the effect of different elements of body composition and outcomes in NSCLC is of much importance, as each phenotype could have distinct biological implications on the host and the tumor.

What Is the Effect of Obesity on Non-Small Cell Lung Cancer and Anti-Tumor Immune Response?

Obesity is considered a protective factor in both early stage and advanced NSCLC patients who are treated with surgery or chemotherapy (7, 45). This effect can be explained partially by the fact that obese patients who receive chemotherapy tend to develop less medication related toxicities leading to lower discontinuation rates of cancer treatment (46). However, the biological landscape associated with obesity seems to be more complex and is believed to play a role in cancer behavior and progression. As an example, some hormonal factors in obese patients such as leptin plasma levels can affect prognosis in NSCLC, as low leptin levels correlate with shortened OS (47). Inversely, adiponectin, which is another hormone secreted from the adipose tissue has been suggested as a factor contributing to tumor progression in NSCLC, but biological mechanisms explaining the action of this hormone are not well understood (48). Different body composition phenotypes in obese patients and their variable hormonal and inflammatory profiles have led to distinguishing obesity as "metabolically unhealthy obesity" versus "metabolically healthy obesity" whereby patients can have a high BMI consistent with obesity definition but have a favorable fat distribution with decreased systemic inflammation leading to low disease morbidity (29).

The biological and immunological aspects of the inverse relationship between obesity and prognosis in NSCLC, termed "obesity paradox" can be explained through several mechanisms (49). Obesity can lead to exhaustion of T-cells resulting in increased tumor growth and it can upregulate programmed death-1 (PD-1) expression on CD8+ T-cells in tumor mice models (50). PD-1 receptors are checkpoint protein receptors present on immune cells that when bound to their respective ligand receptor can decrease anti-tumor efficacy of the host immune system against tumor cells (51). Although, the mechanism by which obesity can increase PD-1 expression has not been fully elucidated, increased levels of leptin secreted from adipose tissues has been suggested to boost cascade signaling indirectly through signal transduction and activator of transcription 3 (STAT3) which leads to upregulation of PD-1 receptors on T-cells (**Figure 2**). This can, in part, explain the improved response rates and survival noted in patients with

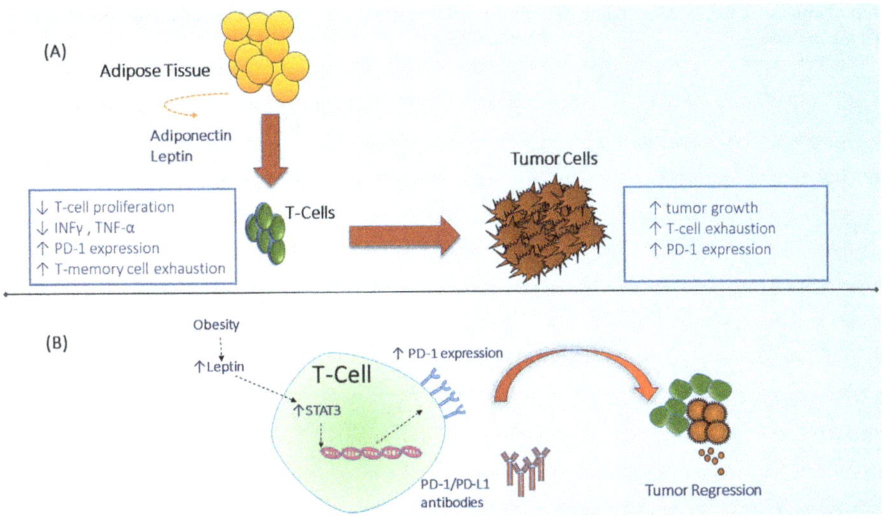

FIGURE 2 | Obesity effect on immune system function and anti-tumor mechanisms. **(A)** Adipose cells in the fat tissue secrete different adipokines including adiponectine and leptin that can alter immune system function by suppressing T-cell proliferation, decreasing INF-y, TNF-a, and increasing T-cell memory dysfunction which in turn can lead to enhanced tumor escape from immune surveillance leading to tumor growth and progression (48). Obesity related tumors can as well be associated with increased expression of checkpoint proteins which have a negative regulatory effect on immune cell proliferation (50). **(B)** The mechanism by which obesity can interact with immune checkpoint receptors in the tumor microenvironment is believed to be through increased secretion of leptin which in turn increases PD-1 expression on CD8+ T-cells through STAT3 signaling (50). Increased expression of PD-1 receptors can lead to enhanced response to immune checkpoint monoclonal antibodies and immune cells mediated tumor regression (50).

obesity across different tumor types who are treated with ICI including PD-1/PD-L1 (programmed death ligand-1) inhibitors that target the interaction of these checkpoint receptors (52–54). Moreover, obesity can modulate other T-cell subsets such as T-regulatory (Treg) cells which function as immunosuppressant cells and when down regulated in obese patients, they can reduce production of interleukin-10 (IL-10) which leads to exacerbation of the chronic inflammatory state (55). Similarly, Treg cells have been found in the tumor microenvironment of NSCLC and lead to an inhibitory effect on effector T-cell proliferation (56). Therefore, the effect of obesity on Treg cells can play a role in modulating Treg response in NSCLC although this has not been studied yet. Another type of immune cell that is important in obesity and NSCLC are the Natural Killer (NK) cells which are responsible for innate immunity and anti-cancer function. NK cells have been shown to be impaired in patients with obesity (57). Likewise, NSCLC patients can lack the cytotoxic effect of NK cells and have defective granulation leading to decreased innate anti-tumor response (57–59). Finally, obesity can affect the balance between macrophage subtypes (M1- M2) favoring the M1 subtype (pro-inflammatory cells) over M2 (immunosuppressive and pro-tumorigenic) (60). An increase in M2 macrophages can lead to increased host immunosuppression and more aggressive tumor behavior which could theoretically explain the improved outcome profile noted in patients with NSCLC who are obese (61) (**Table 2**). This collective evidence suggests an alteration of anti-tumor immune function and the favorable outcomes in obese patients with NSCLC which can partially explain the improved outcomes noted recently with the use of ICI since this class of medications primarily affects the T-cell but also has been found to have partial mechanisms of action through other immune cells such as NK cells and macrophages (65, 66).

What is the Effect of Sarcopenia on Non-Small Cell Lung Cancer and Anti-Tumor Immune Response?

Sarcopenia is usually considered to be a consequence of the changes accompanying malignancy such as malnutrition and alterations in the hormonal milieu including the surge of cytokines due to the presence of the tumor (67). However, the presence of sarcopenia which is manifested by reduced lean body mass including decreased skeletal muscle mass is believed to influence host immune system leading to immune senescence (68). Hence, sarcopenia can have a deleterious effect on the anti-tumor response mediated by the immune system. Also, altered cytokines levels such as elevated IL-6 and decreased IL-15 can affect immune cell function. For example, skeletal muscle cells are essential producers of IL-15 which have a positive effect on NK cell expansion, proliferation and cytotoxic effects (63, 64, 69). As such, subclasses of NK cells express PD-1 receptors and their downregulation in sarcopenia can partially explain the decreased response and worse outcomes in NSCLC patients treated with ICI (70, 71) (**Figure 3**). It should be noted that although the role of NK cells in prognosis of NSCLC patients has been suggested, the mechanism behind their role in the tumor microenvironment in lung cancer is still not well-defined (75). Similarly, it has been found that in IL-15 deficient mice models there is a reduction in the presence of CD8+ which suggests that lack of IL-15 can lead to less targetable cytotoxic T-cells by ICI (62, 76). In addition, the levels of IL-6 are increased in sarcopenic patients which can

TABLE 2 | Immune cell modulation in obesity, sarcopenia and non-small cell lung cancer.

Immune Cell Type	Modulation of immune cells, cytokines in Obesity	Modulation of immune cells, cytokines in Sarcopenia	Modulation of immune cells, cytokines in NSCLC	Reference
T-Cell				
CD8+	↑ CD8+/CD4+ ratio ↑ expression of PD-1 on CD8+	↓IL-15 ↓CD8+	↑ PD-1 expression on CD8+	50, 62
Treg	Dysregulated Treg ↓IL-10 ↑ Immunosuppression ↑ Inflammation	NA	↑ Treg (immunosuppression) ↑ CTLA-4	55, 56
NK Cells	↓ Cytotoxic NK cells	↓ IL-15 ↓ NK cell activity	↓NK Degranulation ↓ Lytic activity	55–59, 63 64
Macrophage	↓ M2 Macrophages (pro-tumorigenic)	NA	Some NSCLC ↑ M2 Macrophages which leads to immune suppression	60, 61

CTLA-4, cytotoxic lymphocyte associated antigen-4; IL-10, interleukin-10; IL-15, interleukin-15; NA, not available; NK, natural killer cells; NSCLC, non-small cell lung cancer; PD-1, programmed death-1; Treg, T- regulatory cells.

contribute to tumor growth and alters the function of immune cells including T-cell subsets (77). The possible role the pleiotropic effect of IL-6 on the immune system has tempted researchers to study the effect of targeting this proinflammatory pathway in combination with PD-1 blockade and preclinical results have shown a synergistic effect on T-cell trafficking and antitumor immunity (78). Likewise, the levels of transforming growth factor-β (TGF-β) are altered in association with sarcopenia and have been found to have a negative effect on the regulation of immune system leading to T-cell exhaustion and dysfunctional NK cells (72–74) (**Table 2**). This cumulative interconnection between sarcopenia and immune dysregulation has also been examined as in obesity to determine whether lower lean body mass impacts the response and prognosis in patients with NSCLC.

The evidence of an existing molecular and pathological relationships between different components of body composition and improved outcomes in obese and non-sarcopenic patients has been described in several retrospective studies and meta-analyses (39, 79, 80). In the following sections, we will summarize the current evidence of the impact of body composition phenotypes and cancer-related outcomes in patients with NSCLC treated with TKI-EGFR or ICI.

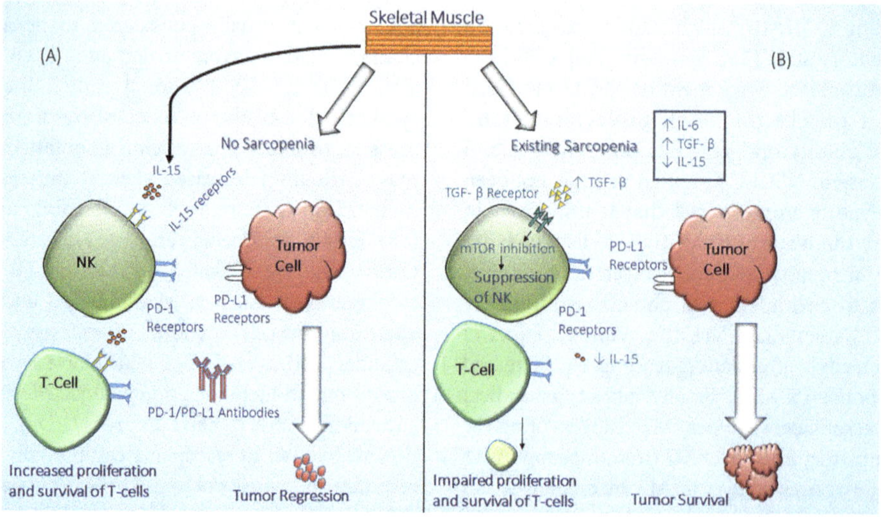

FIGURE 3 | Effect of sarcopenia on immune system function and anti-tumor mechanisms. **(A)** in individuals without skeletal muscle wasting (no sarcopenia), there is sufficient production and secretion of IL-15 by skeletal muscle cells which in turn can bind to IL-15 receptors on the natural killer (NK) cell surface and T-cells leading to enhanced functional natural killer cell and proliferation and maintenance of T-cells including CD8+ T-cells against tumor (69). **(B)** In the presence of significant muscle wasting (sarcopenia), there is decreased production and secretion of IL-15 by skeletal muscle cells (69), as well as an increased chronic inflammatory status in the body associated with high levels of IL-6 and TGF-β (72–74). The latter can lead to NK suppression through mTOR inhibition leading to dysfunctional NK cell which cannot effectively eliminate malignant cells (63, 64, 75). Decreased IL-15 production can lead as well to impaired maintenance, proliferation, and survival of T-cells which are considered potential targets for immune checkpoint inhibitors.

Tyrosine Kinase Inhibitors, Body Composition, and Outcomes in Non-Small Cell Lung Cancer

Targeted therapy has changed the landscape of the management and prognosis in NSCLC. Targetable alterations in NSCLC include mutations in the epidermal growth factor receptor (EGFR) (accounting for up to 15% NSCLC in Europe and United States, and up to 45% in Southeast Asia) (81, 82), translocation in the anaplastic lymphoma kinase gene (ALK) (accounting for approximately 5% of cases), with a lower frequency of other mutations (ROS1, BRAF, NTRAK, and HER2) (83). Most of the phase 3 randomized controlled trials testing tyrosine kinase inhibitors (TKI) that led to approval of these targeted therapies in patients with NSCLC did not conduct subgroup analyses according to body composition (19, 20, 84). However, evidence suggests that body composition can affect outcomes in patients with NSCLC who harbor EGFR mutation and are treated with EGFR TKIs (85). A retrospective study of 630 patients with metastatic EGFR-mutant NSCLC who received either gefitinib or erlotinib (as first or later line therapy) found a relationship between higher BMI and improved progression free survival (PFS) in patients with BMI $\geq$ 25 kg/m^2 compared to BMI < 18.5 kg/m^2 (15.6 months versus 8.5 months, respectively) and OS (28.8 months versus 26.7 months, respectively) (85). Multivariate analysis in this study showed BMI as an independent risk factor in terms of PFS and OS (85). Another study used body weight (kg) to estimate PFS and OS in patients with stage IV NSCLC who were treated with gefitinib (cut off point 53 kg) (N = 138) and found a trend towards improved PFS and OS in patients with higher body weight (> 53 kg), however, it was statistically non-significant (86). Lin et al. examined the impact of weight loss prior to starting gefitinib (defined as loss of more than 5% of body weight in a 3 months period before diagnosis) on objective response rate (ORR), PFS and OS. This retrospective analysis included 75 patients and found no difference in ORR but improved PFS in patients with weight loss <5% compared to patients >5% of weight loss (12.4 months versus 7.6 months; hazard ratio [HR] 0.356, 95% confidence interval [CI] 0.212–0.596, p <0.001). This study also reported an improved OS in patients with <5% weight loss compared to those with >5% weight loss (28.5 months vs. 20.7 months, respectively; HR 0.408, 95% CI 0.215–0.776, p = 0.006) (87). In contrast, another study in patients with NSCLC who received osimertinib (N= 47) did not show any significant relationship between BMI, PFS, and OS (88). The only study that examined the association of both measures (sarcopenia and BMI) with outcomes in patients with NSCLC and EGFR mutation was a retrospective study of 167 patients who received gefitinib, erlotinib, or afatinib as a first or later line therapy (89). This study showed a BMI < 18.5 kg/m^2 to be an independent prognostic factor for worse PFS (HR 1.70 [1.03–2.81], p= 0.04) and OS (HR 1.72 [1.11–2.67], p = 0.02). However, sarcopenia defined by measurements of psoas muscle index (PMI), intermuscular adipose tissue content (IMAC), and visceral to subcutaneous adipose tissue area ratio (VSR) failed to show any effect on different outcomes (89).

Previous discrepancies in the findings of different studies challenge the theory of the effect of body composition on outcomes when NSCLC is treated with EGFR TKI. However, most studies were retrospective and observational in nature and included small sample sizes which could have undermined the relationship between body composition and efficacy of TKIs. The lack of a proposed mechanism supporting a link between body composition and signaling pathways using targetable mutations such as in EGFR mutations poses a question on whether body composition should be examined further as a marker of treatment response in this patient population. However, given the impact of body composition as an independent prognostic factor in NSCLC that have already been established with surgery and chemotherapy and its relationship with altered outcomes in patients treated with different modalities supports the need for further investigation examining these associations. Future studies examining the link between body composition and cancer-related outcomes should consider including the following parameters: better patient selection (i.e., appropriate inclusion and exclusion criteria), larger sample sizes, inclusion of newer medications like osimertinib, as well as accounting for confounding factors such as performance status and metastatic sites (90, 91).

Immune Checkpoint Inhibitors, Body Composition, and Outcomes in Non-Small Cell Lung Cancer

The discovery of immune checkpoint molecules has revolutionized our understanding of tumor biology and resistance mechanisms (92, 93). Immune checkpoints are receptor proteins that are expressed by various immune cells that when bound to their ligands lead to suppression of effector immune cell function (94). Some inhibitory checkpoints can be related to decreased anti-tumor effect against malignant cells which usually use checkpoint ligation to escape immune surveillance (17–19). The two first targetable checkpoint receptors in tumor microenvironment discovered were cytotoxic associated lymphocyte antigen-4 (CTLA-4) and programmed death-1 (PD-1) (92, 93). Their discovery led to the development of monoclonal antibodies directed against checkpoint receptors which entered the clinical realm in NSCLC and changed the standard of care after demonstrating improved PFS and OS as first or later line therapy (21–24, 95, 96). However, not all patients retain a good response to these medications with only some patients deriving benefits with a sustained response. This has led to an effort to discover and develop predictive biomarkers to identify appropriate patient selection. Many biomarkers have emerged as predictor markers such as programmed death- ligand 1 expression (PD-L1), tumor mutational burden, and lymphocyte infiltration in tumor bed (97–99). However, adoption of these biomarkers as a conventional method to predict response and survival can be challenging given the lack of standardized definition and methodology used to quantify some of these biomarkers. Thus, the utilization of simpler available patient characteristics such as gender or body habitus seemed plausible to understand if there is any association with response to immune checkpoint inhibitors (ICI) (98–100).

The prognostic implication of body composition and survival in cancer patients has long been established in different tumor types regardless of stage or treatment approach (33, 101, 102). This concept was later adopted by researchers to examine body composition as a predictive rather than a prognostic marker for response to ICI. Perhaps the earliest link between body composition and survival when using ICI was established in melanoma patients. The work by Daly et al. demonstrated that loss of muscle mass (sarcopenia) can be associated with worse OS in melanoma patients treated with CTLA-4 inhibitors (103). This was followed by other studies that corroborated the findings as a proof of concept and were soon tested in different malignancies including NSCLC (53, 79, 104). There are two different approaches that were used to study the association between body composition and survival. The first was considering the effect of adipose tissue and obesity on survival in patients treated with ICI; while the other approach used skeletal muscle indices as a surrogate for sarcopenia. The feasibility of using such indicators to understand the interconnection was convenient given the simple methodology used to obtain these variables and soon led to several observational and comparative retrospective studies that are summarized in **Table 3** (31, 39, 52, 105–113). The findings from retrospective studies seem to be consistent with a trend towards improved PFS and OS in patients with NSCLC treated with PD-1/PD-L1 inhibitors and have been verified with meta-analyses (79, 114). Both high BMI (overweight and obese) and normal SMI (absence of sarcopenia) were associated with improved survival. It should be noted that different cut points were used to identify overweight, obese and sarcopenic patients as these indicators have different established cut points depending on variable factors such as ethnicity and health status (cancer versus no cancer) (26, 33). The use of predictive biomarkers combined with body composition status has proved a stronger correlation than using body composition alone in predicting improved PFS and OS in NSCLC patients treated with ICI in a recent large retrospective study (52). In this important paper, stronger OS/PFS benefit was observed in overweight and obese patients with PD-L1 positive tumors (defined by PD-L1 expression of > 5% of tumor cells or tumor infiltrating immune cells) compared to normal weight patients, which implies that in NSCLC, PD-L1 expressed by either tumor cells or by immune cells is critical for OS prediction in obese patients, and obesity is secondary to PD-L1 tumor status (52). Interestingly, evidence suggests that occurrence of immune related adverse events (irAEs) of any grade in different cancer types is higher in overweight and obese patients, while irAEs themselves are associated with improved PFS and OS (114, 115). Therefore, in analyzing the effect of obesity/sarcopenia on survival in NSCLC patients treated with ICI, future studies should consider analyzing the effect of body composition in different subpopulations such as patients with PD-L1 positive tumors, high tumor mutational burden, and also occurrence of irAEs. Limitations that can hinder the robustness of the previously mentioned findings in **Table 3** include the retrospective nature of the studies and small sample sizes which are both prone to sampling error and inability to detect a significant difference in specific sub-groups (such as high PD-L1 expression, irAEs).

How to Implement Body Composition Phenotypes in Designing Future Clinical Trials for Patients With Advanced Non-Small Cell Lung Cancer?

Current effort in the management of NSCLC is focused on targeting pathways involved in immune surveillance against tumor cells as well as developing novel drugs against resistant mutations that emerge after exposure to specific targeted therapy. Alongside this effort, it appears to be important to further identify subpopulations who will derive the best benefit. Given the emerging evidence of a crosstalk between different body compositions and cancer biology it will be important to incorporate subgroup analysis in prospective clinical trials when testing current available medication or novel therapies in NSCLC. This would help determine if body composition phenotypes could serve as predictive indicators for the implemented therapies or whether they serve as prognostic factors in NSCLC.

Another area of interest for future research is the changing landscape of cytokine production in obese and sarcopenic NSCLC patient categories and their effect on cancer biology and whether supplementary targeting of specific inflammatory or cytokine pathways could augment the response to immunotherapy. For instance, administration of IL-15 which has been shown to boost anti-tumor immunity *in vitro* (116). Lastly, it would be intriguing to analyze life style modification such as modulation of nutritional status and exercise or medical interventions to stabilize components of body composition such as lean body mass or adipose tissue and their effect on body composition balance and the outcomes in NSCLC when treated with ICI and other novel therapies. The impact of exercise in improving outcomes has already been established although no focus was put on weight changes as a response to therapy (117). Another example, is the use of anamorelin a ghrelin receptor agonist which maintains lean body mass and has been tested previously for the treatment of cachexia-sarcopenia syndrome in NSCLC (118).

CONCLUSION

In conclusion, the study of body composition as a predictive marker in NSCLC patients treated with novel immune and targeted therapies is an area of compelling interest. Future studies should focus on incorporating subgroup analysis in large prospective trials to better analyze this association. Given that in several studies, obesity plays predictive role among smokers or primarily in PD-L1 positive NSCLC tumors, further studies focusing on BMI among these subsets are warranted. Inclusion of newer promising biomarkers such as

TABLE 3 | Studies on effect of body composition on tumor response and survival in patients with stage IV non-small cell lung cancer treated with immune checkpoint inhibitors.

Publication	Sample Size	Male, %	Number of PD-L1 Positive Patients	Immune Checkpoint Inhibitor	Surrogate for Body Composition	Cut-off for Surrogate	End Point	Results*	P-Value
Kichenadasse et al. (52)	1434	890 (62)	938 **	Atezolizumab	BMI	Per WHO Class	OS	Obesity vs. normal weight. HR 0.64 [CI 95%, 0.51-0.81]	P < 0.001
							PFS	Overweight and obese vs. normal weight HR 0.88 [CI 95%, 0.78-0.99]	P = 0.03
Cortellini et al. (105)	976 total with 635 NSCLC cases	663 (67.9)	NA	Pembrolizumab, Nivolumab, Atezolizumab	BMI	Overweight/ obese >= 25 vs. non-overweight <25	ORR	41.3 % vs 20.9%	P < 0.0001
							TTF	9.3 [95% CI: 8.1-11.6] vs 3.6 [95% CI: 3.2 - 4.1] months HR= 0.51 [95% CI: 0.44 – 0.60]	P < 0.0001
							PFS	11.7 [95% CI: 9.4 – 15] vs 3.7 [95% CI: 3.2 – 4.1] months HR= 0.46 [95%CI: 0.39 – 0.54]	P < 0.0001
							OS	26.6 [95% CI: 21.4 – 36.8] vs 6.6 [95% CI: 5.8 – 8.5] months HR= 0.33 [95%CI: 0.28 – 0.41]	P < 0.0001
Ichihara et al. (106)	Cohort 1: 84	68 (80.9)	84 ***	Pembrolizumab	BMI	22	ORR	(evaluated in 74 pts.) 0% complete response 44.6% -partial response, 32.4%- stable disease, 23%- progressive disease	
							PFS	7.3 vs. 4.7 months (HR): 0.94; 95 % CI: 0.53–1.65	P = 0.84
							OS	NR vs. 17 months HR: 0.67; 95 % CI: 0.32–1.40	P = 0.29
	Cohort 2: 429	338 (78.7)	45	Pembrolizumab, Nivolumab, Atezolizumab			ORR	(evaluated 403 pts.) 1.5% complete response, 23.3% partial response, 36.2% stable disease, 3% progressive disease	
							PFS	3.7 vs 2.8 months HR: 0.79; 95 % CI: 0.64–0.98	P = 0.036
							OS	15.4 vs 13.5 months HR: 0.73; 95 % CI: 0.57–0.95	P = 0.021
							High PDL-1 and High BMI vs Low PDL-1 and Low BMI	PFS: 17 vs 3.5 months OS: NR vs 16.1 months	P = 0.007 P = 0.031
Magri et al. (107)	46	28 (60.87)	NA	Nivolumab	Weight loss	Weight loss > 5% prior to therapy vs weight loss <5%	OS	2 vs 10 months	P = 0.0076
Popinat et al. (31)	55	41 (75)	13 ****	Nivolumab	SCFM	5 kg/m^2	1-year OS	HR: 0.75	P = 0.006
Minami et al. (108)	74	48 (64.8)	28 *****	Nivolumab, Pembrolizumab, Atezolizumab	BMI,	BMI cutoff point 18.5 Higher BMI vs lower BMI	OS	15.8 vs. 3.3 months HR = 1.83 (0.79 - 4.21)	P < 0.01
							PFS	No significant difference	-
					IMAC	Men: 0.358 Women: 0.229	OS	Low IMAC favorable for OS (HR 0.43, 95% CI 0.18 - 0.998)	P = 0.0496
							PFS	No significant difference	-

(Continued)

TABLE 3 | Continued

Publication	Sample Size	Male, %	Number of PD-L1 Positive Patients	Immune Checkpoint Inhibitor	Surrogate for Body Composition	Cut-off for Surrogate	End Point	Results*	P-Value
Shiroyama et al. (39)	42	26 (61.9)	NA	Nivolumab, Pembrolizumab	PMI Sarcopenia vs non-sarcopenia	Male: 6.36 cm^2/m^2 Female: 3.92 cm2/m2	PFS Overall response rate	2.1 vs 6.8 months 9.1 % vs. 40%	P= 0.004 P = 0.025
Nishioka et al. (109)	38	26 (68.4)	16 ****	Nivolumab, Pembrolizumab	Psoas Muscle Major Area change Sarcopenia vs non-sarcopenia	Change of equal or more than 10%	ORR PFS	0 % versus 41% 47 vs. 204 days [CI 23-76] vs [CI 59-NA]	P = 0.0154 P = 0.00186
Katayama et al. (110)	35	24 (68.6)	22****	Pembrolizumab, Nivolumab, Atezolizumab	BMI	>20	PFS OS	HR 0.43 [CI 95%, 0.19-0.95] No significant findings	P = 0.036 -
Tsukagoshi etr al. (111)	30	23 (76.7)	NA	Nivolumab	SMI	Male: 6.36 cm2/m2. Female 3.92 cm2/m2	PFS OS Partial response	7.5 vs 2.8 months 25 vs. 10 months 35.3% vs 0%	P = 0.008 P = 0.03 P = n/a
Roch et al. (112)	142	93 (65.5)	56 *** This cut off was only for those with pembrolizumab as first line	Pembrolizumab, Nivolumab	SMI Sarcopenia vs no-sarcopenia	Male: 52.4 cm^2/m^2 Female: 38.5 cm2/m2	PFS OS	2.3 vs 4.1 months 7.6 vs. 12.6 months	P = 0.56 P = 0.08
					Evolving Sarcopenia	(SMI) loss of ≥ 5%. Similar to definition of cachexia	PFS OS	2.3 vs 5.1 months 11.2 vs 15.2 months	P = 0.04 P = 0.07
Takada et al. (113)	103	84 (81.6)	25***	Nivolumab, pembrolizumab	SMI Low SMI vs. high SMI	Male: 25.63 cm2/m2 Female: 21.73 cm2/ m2	PFS OS	HR 1.6 [CI 95%, 1.02- 2.50] HR 2.04 [CI 95%, 1.14- 3.63	P = 0.0399 P = 0.0155
					BMI (univariate analysis)	Male: 21.9 Female 19.8	PFS OS RR	Not significant HR 1.20 (0.78–1.86) HR 1.88 (1.09–3.27) No effect of SMI or BMI on response rate	P = 0.4047 P = 0.0243 P = 0.0117

** Results reported comparing the higher than cut point group to the lower than cut point group; results are reported as either median PFS, OS or hazard ratios with confidence intervals.*

*** PD-L1 positivity identified by ≥5%*

**** PD-L1 positivity identified by ≥ 50%*

***** PD-L1 >1%*

****** Tumor proportion score > 1%*

Results are reported across different tumor types of which the majority were non-small cell lung cancer.

BMI, body mass index; CI, confidence interval; HR, hazard ratio; IMAC, Intermuscular adipose content; NA, not available; NR, not reached; PD-L1, programmed death-ligand-1; PFS, progression free survival; PMI, psoas muscle index; NSCLC, non-small cell lung cancer; ORR, objective response rate; OS, overall survival; SMI, skeletal muscle index; SCFM, sub-cutaneous fat mass; TTF, time to treatment failure; WHO, world health organization.

type of EGFR mutations, PD-L1 expression and tumor mutational burden (TMB) in combination with body composition seems plausible. Unifying the definitions and cut points of different surrogate indicators of obesity or sarcopenia can be challenging but would improve our understanding of the effect of obesity and sarcopenia on survival in non-small cell lung cancer patients in the era of precision medicine.

AUTHOR CONTRIBUTIONS

KK conceptualized the idea of the manuscript with supervision from YB. KK performed literature search and wrote the manuscript in consultation with YB. KK provided **Figures 2, 3** and constructed **Tables 1–3**. SG-P wrote the section *Methods Used in Estimating Body Composition* and provided **Figure 1**. NJ verified the information mentioned in the manuscript and contributed to **Tables 2, 3**. JP and YB supervised the project. All authors contributed to the article and approved the submitted version.

REFERENCES

1. Himber C, Delphan M, Scherer D, Bowers LW, Hursting S, Ulrich CM. Signals from the adipose microenvironment and the obesity-cancer link: a systematic review. *Cancer Prev Res (Phila)* (2017) 10(9):494–506. doi: 10.1158/1940-6207.CAPR-16-0322
2. Lauby-Secretan B, Scoccianti C, Loomis D, Grosse Y, Bianchini F, Straif K, et al. Body Fatness and Cancer-Viewpoint of the IARC Working Group. *N Engl J Med* (2016) 375(8):794–8. doi: 10.1056/NEJMsr1606602
3. Calle EE, Rodriguez C, Walker-Thurmond K, Thun MJ. Overweight, obesity, and mortality from cancer in a prospectively studied cohort of U.S. adults. *N Engl J Med* (2003) 348:1625–38. doi: 10.1056/NEJMoa021423
4. Cao Y, Ma J. Body mass index, prostate cancer-specific mortality, and biochemical recurrence: a systematic review and meta-analysis. *Cancer Prev Res (Phila)* (2011) 4(4):486–501. doi: 10.1158/1940-6207.CAPR-10-0229
5. Chan DS, Vieira AR, Aune D, Bandera EV, Greenwood DC, McTiernan A, et al. Body mass index and survival in women with breast cancer—systematic literature review and meta-analysis of 82 follow-up studies. *Ann Oncol* (2014) 25:1901–14. doi: 10.1093/annonc/mdu042
6. Yang L, Yang G, Zhou M, Smith M, Ge H, Boreham J, et al. Body mass index and mortality from lung cancer in smokers and nonsmokers: a nationally representative prospective study of 220,000 men in China. *Int J Cancer* (2009) 125(9):2136–43. doi: 10.1002/ijc.24527
7. Yang R, Cheung MC, Pedroso FE, Byrne MM, Koniaris LG, Zimmers TA. Obesity and weight loss at presentation of lung cancer are associated with opposite effects on survival. *J Surg Res* (2011) 170:e75–83. doi: 10.1016/j.jss.2011.04.061
8. Ferguson MK, Im HK, Watson S, Johnson E, Wigfield CH, Vigneswaran WT. Association of body mass index and outcomes after major lung resection. *Eur J Cardiothorac Surg* (2014) 45(4):e94–9; discussion e99. doi: 10.1093/ejcts/ezu008
9. Dahlberg SE, Schiller JH, Bonomi PB, Sandler AB, Brahmer JR, Ramalingam SS, et al. Body mass index and its association with clinical outcomes for advanced non-small-cell lung cancer patients enrolled on Eastern Cooperative Oncology Group clinical trials. *J Thorac Oncol* (2013) 8 (9):1121–7. doi: 10.1097/JTO.0b013e31829cf942
10. Jeong SM, Lee DH, Giovannucci EL. Predicted lean body mass, fat mass and risk of lung cancer: prospective US cohort study. *Eur J Epidemiol* (2019) 34 (12):1151–60. doi: 10.1007/s10654-019-00587-2
11. Buentzel J, Heinz J, Bleckmann A, Bauer C, Röver C, Bohnenberger H, et al. Sarcopenia as Prognostic Factor in Lung Cancer Patients: A Systematic Review and Meta-analysis. *Anticancer Res* (2019) 39(9):4603–12. doi: 10.21873/anticanres.13640
12. Suzuki Y, Okamoto T, Fujishita T, Katsura M, Akamine T, Takamori S, et al. Clinical implications of sarcopenia in patients undergoing complete resection for early non-small cell lung cancer. *Lung Cancer* (2016) 101:92–7. doi: 10.1016/j.lungcan.2016.08.007
13. Bray F, Ferlay J, Soerjomataram I, Siegel RL, Torre LA, Jemal A. Global cancer statistics 2018: GLOBOCAN estimates of incidence and mortality worldwide for 36 cancers in 185 countries. *CA Cancer J Clin* (2018) 68 (6):394–424. doi: 10.3322/caac.21492
14. Yang M, Shen Y, Tan L, Li W. Prognostic Value of Sarcopenia in Lung Cancer: A Systematic Review and Meta-analysis. *Chest* (2019) 156(1):101–11. doi: 10.1016/j.chest.2019.04.115
15. Yu D, Zheng W, Johansson M, Lan Q, Park Y, White E, et al. Overall and Central Obesity and Risk of Lung Cancer: A Pooled Analysis. *J Natl Cancer Inst* (2018) 110(8):831–42. doi: 10.1093/jnci/djx286
16. Walunas TL, Lenschow DJ, Bakker CY, Linsley PS, Freeman GJ, Green JM, et al. CTLA-4 can function as a negative regulator of T cell activation. *Immunity* (1994) 1(5):405–13. doi: 10.1016/1074-7613(94)90071-x
17. Freeman GJ, Long AJ, Iwai Y, Bourque K, Chernova T, Nishimura H, et al. Engagement of the PD-1 immunoinhibitory receptor by a novel B7 family member leads to negative regulation of lymphocyte activation. *J Exp Med* (2000) 192(7):1027–34. doi: 10.1084/jem.192.7.1027
18. Waterhouse P, Penninger JM, Timms E, Wakeham A, Shahinian A, Lee KP, et al. Lymphoproliferative disorders with early lethality in mice deficient in Ctla-4. *Science* (1995) 270(5238):985–8. doi: 10.1126/science.270.5238.985
19. Cappuzzo F, Ciuleanu T, Stelmakh L, Cicenas S, Szczésna A, Juhász E, et al. Erlotinib as maintenance treatment in advanced non-small-cell lung cancer: a multicentre, randomised, placebo-controlled phase 3 study. *Lancet Oncol* (2010) 11:521–29. doi: 10.1016/S1470-2045(10)70112-1
20. Fukuoka M, Wu YL, Thongprasert S, Sunpaweravong P, Leong SS, Sriuranpong V, et al. Biomarker analyses and final overall survival results from a phase III, randomized, open-label, first-line study of gefitinib versus carboplatin/paclitaxel in clinically selected patients with advanced non-small-cell lung cancer in Asia (IPASS). *J Clin Oncol* (2011) 29(21):2866–74. doi: 10.1200/JCO.2010.33.4235
21. Herbst RS, Baas P, Kim DW, Felip E, Perez-Gracia JL, Han JY, et al. Pembrolizumab versus docetaxel for previously treated, PD-L1-positive, advanced non-small-cell lung cancer (KEYNOTE-010): a randomised controlled trial. *Lancet* (2016) 387(10027):1540–50. doi: 10.1016/S0140-6736(15)01281-7
22. Rittmeyer A, Barlesi F, Waterkamp D, Park K, Ciardiello F, von Pawel J, et al. Atezolizumab versus docetaxel in patients with previously treated non-small-cell lung cancer (OAK): a phase 3, open-label, multicentre randomised controlled trial. *Lancet* (2017) 389(10066):255–65. doi: 10.1016/S0140-6736 (16)32517-X
23. Borghaei H, Paz-Ares L, Horn L, Spigel DR, Steins M, Ready NE, et al. Nivolumab versus Docetaxel in Advanced Nonsquamous Non-Small-Cell Lung Cancer. *N Engl J Med* (2015) 373(17):1627–39. doi: 10.1056/NEJMoa1507643

24. Brahmer J, Reckamp KL, Baas P, Crinò L, Eberhardt WE, Poddubskaya E, et al. Nivolumab versus Docetaxel in Advanced Squamous-Cell Non-Small-Cell Lung Cancer. *N Engl J Med* (2015) 373(2):123–35. doi: 10.1056/NEJMoa1504627
25. Haslam A, Gill J, Prasad V. Estimation of the Percentage of US Patients With Cancer Who Are Eligible for Immune Checkpoint Inhibitor Drugs. *JAMA Netw Open* (2020) 3(3):e200423. doi: 10.1001/jamanetworkopen.2020.0423
26. Razak F, Anand SS, Shannon H, Vuksan V, Davis B, Jacobs R, et al. Defining obesity cut points in a multiethnic population. *Circulation* (2007) 115 (16):2111–8. doi: 10.1161/CIRCULATIONAHA.106.635011
27. Organization WHO. *Obesity: Preventing and Managing the Global Epidemic.* World Health Organization (2000).
28. Romero-Corral A, Somers VK, Sierra-Johnson J, Thomas RJ, Collazo-Clavell ML, Korinek J, et al. Accuracy of body mass index in diagnosing obesity in the adult general population. *Int J Obes (Lond)* (2008) 32(6):959–66. doi: 10.1038/ijo.2008.11
29. Kovarik M, Hronek M, Zadak Z. Clinically relevant determinants of body composition, function and nutritional status as mortality predictors in lung cancer patients. *Lung Cancer* (2014) 84(1):1–6. doi: 10.1016/j.lungcan.2014.01.020
30. Shimizu H, Shimomura Y, Hayashi R, Ohtani K, Sato N, Futawatari T, et al. Serum leptin concentration is associated with total body fat mass, but not abdominal fat distribution. *Int J Obes Relat Metab Disord* (1997) 21(7):536–41. doi: 10.1038/sj.ijo.0800437
31. Popinat G, Cousse S, Goldfarb L, Becker S, Gardin I, Salaün M, et al. Sub-cutaneous Fat Mass measured on multislice computed tomography of pretreatment PET/CT is a prognostic factor of stage IV non-small cell lung cancer treated by nivolumab. *Oncoimmunology* (2019) 8(5):e1580128. doi: 10.1080/2162402X.2019.1580128
32. Prado CM, Lieffers JR, McCargar LJ, Reiman T, Sawyer MB, Martin L, et al. Prevalence and clinical implications of sarcopenic obesity in patients with solid tumours of the respiratory and gastrointestinal tracts: a population-based study. *Lancet Oncol* (2008) 9(7):629–35. doi: 10.1016/S1470-2045(08) 70153-0
33. Martin L, Birdsell L, MacDonald N, Reiman T, Clandinin MT, McCargar LJ, et al. Cancer Cachexia in the Age of Obesity: Skeletal Muscle Depletion Is a Powerful Prognostic Factor, Independent of Body Mass Index. *J Clin Oncol* (2013) 31:1539–47. doi: 10.1200/JCO.2012.45.2722
34. Mourtzakis M, Prado CM, Lieffers JR, Reiman T, McCargar LJ, Baracos VE. A practical and precise approach to quantification of body composition in cancer patients using computed tomography images acquired during routine care. *Appl Physiol Nutr Metab* (2008) 33(5):997–1006. doi: 10.1139/H08-075
35. Shen W, Punyanitya M, Wang Z, Gallagher D, St-Onge MP, Albu J, et al. Total body skeletal muscle and adipose tissue volumes: estimation from a single abdominal cross-sectional image. *J Appl Physiol (1985)* (2004) 97 (6):2333–8. doi: 10.1152/japplphysiol.00744.2004
36. Derstine BA, Holcombe SA, Ross BE, Wang NC, Su GL, Wang SC. Skeletal muscle cutoff values for sarcopenia diagnosis using T10 to L5 measurements in a healthy US population. *Sci Rep* (2018) 8(1):11369. doi: 10.1038/s41598-018-29825-5
37. Kim EY, Kim YS, Park I, Ahn HK, Cho EK, Jeong YM, et al. Evaluation of sarcopenia in small-cell lung cancer patients by routine chest CT. *Support Care Cancer* (2016) 24(11):4721–6. doi: 10.1007/s00520-016-3321-0
38. Recio-Boiles A, Galeas JN, Goldwasser B, Sanchez K, Man LMW, Gentzler RD, et al. Enhancing evaluation of sarcopenia in patients with non-small cell lung cancer (NSCLC) by assessing skeletal muscle index (SMI) at the first lumbar (L1) level on routine chest computed tomography (CT). *Support Care Cancer* (2018) 26(7):2353–9. doi: 10.1007/s00520-018-4051-2
39. Shiroyama T, Nagatomo I, Koyama S, Hirata H, Nishida S, Miyake K, et al. Impact of sarcopenia in patients with advanced non-small cell lung cancer treated with PD-1 inhibitors: A preliminary retrospective study. *Sci Rep* (2019) 9(1):2447. doi: 10.1038/s41598-019-39120-6
40. Baracos VE. Psoas as a sentinel muscle for sarcopenia: a flawed premise. *J Cachexia Sarcopenia Muscle* (2017) 8(4):527–8. doi: 10.1002/jcsm.12221
41. Rutten IJG, Ubachs J, Kruitwagen RFPM, Beets-Tan RGH, Olde Damink SWM, Van Gorp T. Psoas muscle area is not representative of total skeletal muscle area in the assessment of sarcopenia in ovarian cancer. *J Cachexia Sarcopenia Muscle* (2017) 8(4):630–8. doi: 10.1002/jcsm.12180
42. Baracos VE, Reiman T, Mourtzakis M, Gioulbasanis I, Antoun S. Body composition in patients with non-small cell lung cancer: a contemporary view of cancer cachexia with the use of computed tomography image analysis. *Am J Clin Nutr* (2010) 91(4):1133S–7S. doi: 10.3945/ajcn.2010.28608C
43. Shachar SS, Williams GR, Muss HB, Nishijima TF. Prognostic value of sarcopenia in adults with solid tumours: A meta-analysis and systematic review. *Eur J Cancer* (2016) 57:58–67. doi: 10.1016/j.ejca.2015.12.030
44. Gonzalez MC, Pastore CA, Orlandi SP, Heymsfield SB. Obesity paradox in cancer: new insights provided by body composition. *Am J Clin Nutr* (2014) 99(5):999–1005. doi: 10.3945/ajcn.113.071399
45. Lam VK, Bentzen SM, Mohindra P, Nichols EM, Bhooshan N, Vyfhuis M, et al. Obesity is associated with long-term improved survival in definitively treated locally advanced non-small cell lung cancer (NSCLC). *Lung Cancer* (2017) 104:52–7. doi: 10.1016/j.lungcan.2016.11.017
46. Kashiwabara K, Yamane H, Tanaka H. Toxicity and prognosis in overweight and obese women with lung cancer receiving carboplatin-paclitaxel doublet chemotherapy. *Cancer Invest* (2013) 31(4):251–7. doi: 10.3109/07357907.2013.784778
47. Kerenidi T, Lada M, Tsaroucha A, Georgoulias P, Mystridou P. Gourgoulianis KI. Clinical significance of serum adipokines levels in lung cancer. *Med Oncol* (2013) 30:507. doi: 10.1007/s12032-013-0507-x
48. Boura P, Loukides S, Grapsa D, Achimastos A, Syrigos K. The diverse roles of adiponectine in non-small-cell lung cancer: current data and future prespectives. *Future Oncol* (2015) 11:2193–203. doi: 10.2217/fon.15.96
49. Zhang X, Liu Y, Shao H, Zheng X. Obesity paradox in lung cancer prognosis: evolving biological insights and clinical implications. *J Thoracic Oncol* (2017) 12(10):1478–88. doi: 10.1016/j.jtho.2017.07.022
50. Wang Z, Aguilar EG, Luna JI, Dunai C, Khuat LT, Le CT, et al. Paradoxical effects of obesity on T cell function during tumor progression and PD-1 checkpoint blockade. *Nat Med* (2019) 25(1):141–51. doi: 10.1038/s41591-018-0221-5
51. Weber J. Immune checkpoint proteins: a new therapeutic paradigm for cancer–preclinical background: CTLA-4 and PD-1 blockade. *Semin Oncol* (2010) 37(5):430–9. doi: 10.1053/j.seminoncol.2010.09.005
52. Kichenadasse G, Miners JO, Mangoni AA, Rowland A, Hopkins AM, Sorich MJ. Association between body mass index and overall survival with immune checkpoint inhibitor therapy for advanced non–small cell lung cancer. *JAMA Oncol* (2019) 6(4):512–8. doi: 10.1001/jamaoncol.2019.5241
53. McQuade JL, Daniel CR, Hess KR, Mak C, Wang DY, Rai RR, et al. Association of body-mass index and outcomes in patients with metastatic melanoma treated with targeted therapy, immunotherapy, or chemotherapy: a retrospective, multicohort analysis. *Lancet Oncol* (2018) 19(3):310–22. doi: 10.1016/S1470-2045(18)30078-0
54. De Giorgi U, Procopio G, Giannarelli D, Sabbatini R, Bearz A, Buti S, et al. Association of Systemic Inflammation Index and Body Mass Index with Survival in Patients with Renal Cell Cancer Treated with Nivolumab. *Clin Cancer Res* (2019) 25(13):3839–46. doi: 10.1158/1078-0432.CCR-18-3661
55. Han JM, Patterson SJ, Speck M, Ehses JA, Levings MK. Insulin inhibits IL-10-mediated regulatory T cell function: implications for obesity. *J Immunol* (2014) 192(2):623–9. doi: 10.4049/jimmunol.1302181
56. Woo EY, Yeh H, Chu CS, Schlienger K, Carroll RG, Riley JL, et al. Cutting edge: Regulatory T cells from lung cancer patients directly inhibit autologous T cell proliferation. *J Immunol* (2002) 168(9):4272–6. doi: 10.4049/jimmunol.168.9.4272
57. Bahr I, Jahn J, Zipprich A, Pahlow I, Spielmann J, Kielstein H. Impaired natural killer cell subset phenotypes in human obesity. *Immunol Res* (2018) 66:234–44. doi: 10.1007/s12026-018-8989-4
58. Carrega P, Morandi B, Costa R, Frumento G, Forte G, Altavilla G, et al. Natural killer cells infiltrating human nonsmall-cell lung cancer are enriched in CD56 bright CD16(-) cells and display an impaired capability to kill tumor cells. *Cancer* (2008) 112(4):863–75. doi: 10.1002/cncr.23239
59. Platonova S, Cherfils-Vicini J, Damotte D, Crozet L, Vieillard V, Validire P, et al. Profound coordinated alterations of intratumoral NK cell phenotype and function in lung carcinoma. *Cancer Res* (2011) 71(16):5412–22. doi: 10.1158/0008-5472.CAN-10-4179
60. Kraakman MJ, Murphy AJ, Jandeleit-Dahm K, Kammoun HL. Macrophage polarization in obesity and type 2 diabetes: weighing down our understanding of macrophage function? *Front Immunol* (2014) 5:470. doi: 10.3389/fimmu.2014.00470

61. Dai F, Liu L, Che G, Yu N, Pu Q, Zhang S, et al. The number and microlocalization of tumor-associated immune cells are associated with patient's survival time in non-small cell lung cancer. *BMC Cancer* (2010) 10:220. doi: 10.1186/1471-2407-10-220
62. Kennedy MK, Glaccum M, Brown SN, Butz EA, Viney JL, Embers M. Reversible defects in natural killer and memory CD8 t cell lineages in interleukin 15-deficient mice. *J Exp Med* (2000) 191(5):771–80. doi: 10.1084/jem.191.5.771
63. Carson WE, Giri JG, Lindemann MJ, Linett ML, Ahdieh M, Paxton R, et al. Interleukin (IL) 15 is a novel cytokine that activates human natural killer cells via components of the IL-2 receptor. *J Exp Med* (1994) 180(4):1395–403. doi: 10.1084/jem.180.4.1395
64. Van den Bergh J, Willemen Y, Lion E, Van Acker H, De Reu H, Anguille S, et al. Transpresentation of interleukin-15 by IL-15/IL-15Rα mRNA-engineered human dendritic cells boosts antitumoral natural killer cell activity. *Oncotarget* (2015) 6(42):44123–33. doi: 10.18632/oncotarget.6536
65. Dong W, Wu X, Ma S, Wang Y, Nalin AP, Zhu Z, et al. The Mechanism of Anti-PD-L1 Antibody Efficacy against PD-L1-Negative Tumors Identifies NK Cells Expressing PD-L1 as a Cytolytic Effector. *Cancer Discov* (2019) 9 (10):1422–37. doi: 10.1158/2159-8290.CD-18-1259
66. Xiong H, Mittman S, Rodriguez R, Moskalenko M, Pacheco-Sanchez P, Yang Y, et al. Anti-PD-L1 Treatment Results in Functional Remodeling of the Macrophage Compartment. *Cancer Res* (2019) 79(7):1493–506. doi: 10.1158/0008-5472.CAN-18-3208
67. Argilés JM, Busquets S, Felipe A, López-Soriano FJ. Molecular mechanisms involved in muscle wasting in cancer and ageing: cachexia versus sarcopenia. *Int J Biochem Cell Biol* (2005) 37(5):1084–104. doi: 10.1016/j.biocel.2004.10.003
68. Nelke C, Dziewas R, Minnerup J, Meuth SG, Ruck T. Skeletal muscle as potential central link between sarcopenia and immune senescence. *EBioMedicine* (2019) 49:381–8. doi: 10.1016/j.ebiom.2019.10.034
69. Nielsen AR, Mounier R, Plomgaard P, Mortensen OH, Penkowa M, Speerschneider T, et al. Expression of interleukin-15 in human skeletal muscle effect of exercise and muscle fibre type composition. *J Physiol* (2007) 584(Pt 1):305–12. doi: 10.1113/jphysiol.2007.139618
70. Moretta L, Bottino C, Pende D, Vitale M, Mingari MC, Moretta A. Different checkpoints in human NK-cell activation. *Trends Immunol* (2004) 25 (12):670–6. doi: 10.1016/j.it.2004.09.008
71. Chiossone L, Vivier E. Immune checkpoints on innate lymphoid cells. *J Exp Med* (2017) 214(6):1561–3. doi: 10.1084/jem.20170763
72. Burks TN, Cohn RD. Role of TGF-β signaling in inherited and acquired myopathies. *Skelet Muscle* (2011) 1(1):19. doi: 10.1186/2044-5040-1-19
73. Mariathasan S, Turley SJ, Nickles D, Castiglioni A, Yuen K, Wang Y, et al. TGFβ attenuates tumour response to PD-L1 blockade by contributing to exclusion of T cells. *Nature* (2018) 554(7693):544–8. doi: 10.1038/nature25501
74. Viel S, Marçais A, Guimaraes FS, Loftus R, Rabilloud J, Grau M, et al. TGF-β inhibits the activation and functions of NK cells by repressing the mTOR pathway. *Sci Signal* (2016) 9(415):ra19. doi: 10.1126/scisignal.aad1884
75. Carrega P, Ferlazzo G. Natural Killers Are Made Not Born: How to Exploit NK Cells in Lung Malignancies. *Front Immunol* (2017) 8:277. doi: 10.3389/fimmu.2017.00277
76. Conlon KC, Lugli E, Welles HC, Rosenberg SA, Fojo AT, Morris JC, et al. Redistribution, hyperproliferation, activation of natural killer cells and CD8 T cells, and cytokine production during first-in-human clinical trial of recombinant human interleukin-15 in patients with cancer. *J Clin Oncol* (2015) 33(1):74–82. doi: 10.1200/JCO.2014.57.3329
77. Maggio M, Guralnik JM, Longo DL, Ferrucci L. Interleukin-6 in aging and chronic disease: a magnificent pathway. *J Gerontol A Biol Sci Med Sci* (2006) 61(6):575–84. doi: 10.1093/gerona/61.6.575
78. Tsukamoto H, Fujieda K, Miyashita A, Fukushima S, Ikeda T, Kubo Y, et al. Combined Blockade of IL6 and PD-1/PD-L1 Signaling Abrogates Mutual Regulation of Their Immunosuppressive Effects in the Tumor Microenvironment. *Cancer Res* (2018) 78(17):5011–22. doi: 10.1158/0008-5472.CAN-18-0118
79. Xu H, Cao D, He A, Ge W. The prognostic role of obesity is independent of sex in cancer patients treated with immune checkpoint inhibitors: A pooled analysis of 4090 cancer patients. *Int Immunopharmacol* (2019) 74:105745. doi: 10.1016/j.intimp.2019.105745
80. Cortellini A, Verna L, Porzio G, Bozzetti F, Palumbo P, Masciocchi C, et al. Predictive value of skeletal muscle mass for immunotherapy with nivolumab in non-small cell lung cancer patients: A "hypothesis-generator" preliminary report. *Thorac Cancer* (2019) 10(2):347–51. doi: 10.1111/1759-7714.12965
81. Kawaguchi T, Koh Y, Ando M, Ito N, Takeo S, Adachi H, et al. Prospective Analysis of Oncogenic Driver Mutations and Environmental Factors: Japan Molecular Epidemiology for Lung Cancer Study. *J Clin Oncol* (2016) 34 (19):2247–57. doi: 10.1200/JCO.2015.64.2322
82. Han B, Tjulandin S, Hagiwara K, Normanno N, Wulandari L, Laktionov K, et al. EGFR mutation prevalence in Asia-Pacific and Russian patients with advanced NSCLC of adenocarcinoma and non-adenocarcinoma histology: The IGNITE study. *Lung Cancer* (2017) 113:37–44. doi: 10.1016/j.lungcan.2017.08.021
83. Chia PL, Mitchell P, Dobrovic A, John T. Prevalence and natural history of ALK positive non-small-cell lung cancer and the clinical impact of targeted therapy with ALK inhibitors. *Clin Epidemiol* (2014) 6:423–32. doi: 10.2147/CLEP.S69718
84. Ding Z, Chen Y, Hong Y, Fu Y, Tong L, Li Q, et al. Obesity has an impact on the efficacy of EGFR-TKI in nonsmall cell lung cancer patients harboring EGFR mutation: A real-world study. *Ann Oncol* (2019) 30(suppl_2):ii38–68. doi: 10.1093/annonc/mdz063
85. Park S, Park S, Lee SH, Suh B, Keam B, Kim TM, et al. Nutritional status in the era of target therapy: poor nutrition is a prognostic factor in non-small cell lung cancer with activating epidermal growth factor receptor mutations. *Korean J Intern Med* (2016) 31(6):1140–9. doi: 10.3904/kjim.2015.062
86. Imai H, Kuwako T, Kaira K, Masuda T, Miura Y, Seki K, et al. Evaluation of gefitinib efficacy according to body mass index, body surface area, and body weight in patients with EGFR-mutated advanced non-small cell lung cancer. *Cancer Chemother Pharmacol* (2017) 79(3):497–505. doi: 10.1007/s00280-016-3232-2
87. Lin L, Zhao J, Hu J, Huang F, Han J, He Y, et al. Impact of Weight Loss at Presentation on Survival in Epidermal Growth Factor Receptor Tyrosine Kinase Inhibitors (EGFR-TKI) Sensitive Mutant Advanced Non-small Cell Lung Cancer (NSCLC) Treated with First-line EGFR-TKI. *J Cancer* (2018) 9 (3):528–34. doi: 10.7150/jca.22378
88. Ono T, Igawa S, Ozawa T, Kasajima M, Ishihara M, Hiyoshi Y, et al. Evaluation of osimertinib efficacy according to body surface area and body mass index in patients with non-small cell lung cancer harboring an EGFR mutation: A prospective observational study. *Thorac Cancer* (2019) 10 (4):880–9. doi: 10.1111/1759-7714.13018
89. Minami S, Ihara S, Nishimatsu K, Komuta K. Low Body Mass Index Is an Independent Prognostic Factor in Patients With Non-Small Cell Lung Cancer Treated With Epidermal Growth Factor Receptor Tyrosine Kinase Inhibitor. *World J Oncol* (2019) 10(6):187–98. doi: 10.14740/wjon1244
90. Kawaguchi T, Takada M, Kubo A, Matsumura A, Fukai S, Tamura A, et al. Performance status and smoking status are independent favorable prognostic factors for survival in non-small cell lung cancer: a comprehensive analysis of 26,957 patients with NSCLC. *J Thorac Oncol* (2010) 5(5):620–30. doi: 10.1097/JTO.0b013e3181d2dcd9
91. Tamura T, Kurishima K, Nakazawa K, Kagohashi K, Ishikawa H, Satoh H, et al. Specific organ metastases and survival in metastatic non-small-cell lung cancer. *Mol Clin Oncol* (2015) 3(1):217–21. doi: 10.3892/mco.2014.410
92. Brunet JF, Denizot F, Luciani MF, Roux-Dosseto M, Suzan M, Mattei MG, et al. A new member of the immunoglobulin superfamily–CTLA-4. *Nature* (1987) 328(6127):267–70. doi: 10.1038/328267a0
93. Agata Y, Kawasaki A, Nishimura H, Ishida Y, Tsubata T, Yagita H, et al. Expression of the PD-1 antigen on the surface of stimulated mouse T and B lymphocytes. *Int Immunol* (1996) 8(5):765–72. doi: 10.1093/intimm/8.5.765
94. Azoury SC, Straughan DM, Shukla V. Immune Checkpoint Inhibitors for Cancer Therapy: Clinical Efficacy and Safety. *Curr Cancer Drug Targ* (2015) 15(6):452–62. doi: 10.2174/156800961506150805145120
95. Reck M, Rodríguez-Abreu D, Robinson AG, Hui R, Csőszi T, Fülöp A, et al. Pembrolizumab versus Chemotherapy for PD-L1-Positive Non-Small-Cell Lung Cancer. *N Engl J Med* (2016) 375(19):1823–33. doi: 10.1056/NEJMoa1606774

96. Gandhi L, Rodríguez-Abreu D, Gadgeel S, Esteban E, Felip E, De Angelis F, et al. Pembrolizumab plus Chemotherapy in Metastatic Non-Small-Cell Lung Cancer. *N Engl J Med* (2018) 378(22):2078–92. doi: 10.1056/NEJMoa1801005
97. Arora S, Velichinskii R, Lesh RW, Ali U, Kubiak M, Bansal P, et al. Existing and Emerging Biomarkers for Immune Checkpoint Immunotherapy in Solid Tumors. *Adv Ther* (2019) 36(10):2638–78. doi: 10.1007/s12325-019-01051-z
98. Willis C, Fiander M, Tran D, Korytowsky B, Thomas JM, Calderon F, et al. Tumor mutational burden in lung cancer: a systematic literature review. *Oncotarget* (2019) 10(61):6604–22. doi: 10.18632/oncotarget.27287
99. Brambilla E, Le Teuff G, Marguet S, Lantuejoul S, Dunant A, Graziano S, et al. Prognostic Effect of Tumor Lymphocytic Infiltration in Resectable Non-Small-Cell Lung Cancer. *J Clin Oncol* (2016) 34(11):1223–30. doi: 10.1200/JCO.2015.63.0970
100. Conforti F, Pala L, Bagnardi V, De Pas T, Martinetti M, Viale G, et al. Cancer immunotherapy efficacy and patients' sex: a systematic review and meta-analysis. *Lancet Oncol* (2018) 19(6):737–46. doi: 10.1016/S1470-2045(18) 30261-4
101. Antoun S, Lanoy E, Iacovelli R, Albiges-Sauvin L, Loriot Y, Merad-Taoufik M, et al. Skeletal muscle density predicts prognosis in patients with metastatic renal cell carcinoma treated with targeted therapies. *Cancer* (2013) 119(18):3377–84. doi: 10.1002/cncr.28218
102. Sabel MS, Lee J, Cai S, Englesbe MJ, Holcombe S, Wang S. Sarcopenia as a prognostic factor among patients with stage III melanoma. *Ann Surg Oncol* (2011) 18(13):3579–85. doi: 10.1245/s10434-011-1976-9
103. Daly LE, Power DG, O'Reilly á, Donnellan P, Cushen SJ, O'Sullivan K, et al. The impact of body composition parameters on ipilimumab toxicity and survival in patients with metastatic melanoma. *Br J Cancer* (2017) 116 (3):310–7. doi: 10.1038/bjc.2016.431
104. Richtig G, Hoeller C, Wolf M, Wolf I, Rainer BM, Schulter G, et al. Body mass index may predict the response to ipilimumab in metastatic melanoma: An observational multi-centre study. *PLoS One* (2018) 13(10):e0204729. doi: 10.1371/journal.pone.0204729
105. Cortellini A, Bersanelli M, Buti S, Cannita K, Santini D, Perrone F, et al. A multicenter study of body mass index in cancer patients treated with anti-PD-1/ PD-L1 immune checkpoint inhibitors: when overweight becomes favorable. *J Immuno Ther Cancer* (2019) 7(1):57. doi: 10.1186/s40425-019-0527-y.
106. Ichihara E, Harada D, Inoue K, Sato K, Hosokawa S, Kishino D, et al. The impact of body mass index on the efficacy of anti-PD-1/PD-L1 antibodies in patients with non-small cell lung cancer. *Lung Cancer* (2020) 139:140–5. doi: 10.1016/j.lungcan.2019.11.011
107. Magri V, Gottfried T, Di Segni M, Urban D, Peled M, Daher S, et al. Correlation of body composition by computerized tomography and metabolic parameters with survival of nivolumab-treated lung cancer patients. *Cancer Manag Res* (2019) 11:8201–7. doi: 10.2147/CMAR.S210958
108. Minami S, Ihara S, Tanaka T, Komuta K. Sarcopenia and Visceral Adiposity Did Not Affect Efficacy of Immune-Checkpoint Inhibitor Monotherapy for Pretreated Patients With Advanced Non-Small Cell Lung Cancer. *World J Oncol* (2020) 11(1):9–22. doi: 10.14740/wjon1225
109. Nishioka N, Uchino J, Hirai S, Katayama Y, Yoshimura A, Okura N, et al. Association of Sarcopenia with and Efficacy of Anti-PD-1/PD-L1 Therapy in Non-Small-Cell Lung Cancer. *J Clin Med* (2019) 8(4):450. doi: 10.3390/ jcm8040450
110. Katayama Y, Shimamoto T, Yamada T, Takeda T, Yamada T, Shiotsu S, et al. Retrospective Efficacy Analysis of Immune Checkpoint Inhibitor Rechallenge in Patients with Non-Small Cell Lung Cancer. *J Clin Med* (2019) 9(1):102. doi: 10.3390/jcm9010102
111. Tsukagoshi M, Yokobori T, Yajima T, Maeno T, Shimizu K, Mogi A, et al. Skeletal muscle mass predicts the outcome of nivolumab treatment for non-small cell lung cancer. *Med (Baltimore)* (2020) 99(7):e19059. doi: 10.1097/ MD.0000000000019059
112. Roch B, Coffy A, Jean-Baptiste S, Palaysi E, Daures JP, Pujol JL, et al. Cachexia - sarcopenia as a determinant of disease control rate and survival in non-small lung cancer patients receiving immune-checkpoint inhibitors. *Lung Cancer* (2020) 143:19–26. doi: 10.1016/j.lungcan.2020.03.003
113. Takada K, Yoneshima Y, Tanaka K, Okamoto I, Shimokawa M, Wakasu S, et al. Clinical impact of skeletal muscle area in patients with non-small cell lung cancer treated with anti-PD-1 inhibitors. *J Cancer Res Clin Oncol* (2020) 146(5):1217–25. doi: 10.1007/s00432-020-03146-5
114. Zhou X, Yao Z, Yang H, Liang N, Zhang X, Zhang F. Are immune-related adverse events associated with the efficacy of immune checkpoint inhibitors in patients with cancer? A systematic review and meta-analysis. *BMC Med* (2020) 18(1):87. doi: 10.1186/s12916-020-01549-2
115. Cortellini A, Bersanelli M, Santini D, Buti S, Tiseo M, Cannita K, et al. Another side of the association between body mass index (BMI) and clinical outcomes of cancer patients receiving programmed cell death protein-1 (PD-1)/ Programmed cell death-ligand 1 (PD-L1) checkpoint inhibitors: A multicentre analysis of immune-related adverse events. *Eur J Cancer* (2020) 128:17–26. doi: 10.1016/j.ejca.2019.12.031
116. Berger A, Colpitts SJ, Seabrook MSS, Furlonger CL, Bendix MB, Moreau JM, et al. Interleukin-15 in cancer immunotherapy: IL-15 receptor complex versus soluble IL-15 in a cancer cell-delivered murine leukemia model. *J Immunother Cancer* (2019) 7(1):355. doi: 10.1186/s40425-019-0777-8
117. Peddle-McIntyre CJ, Singh F, Thomas R, Newton RU, Galvão DA, Cavalheri V. Exercise training for advanced lung cancer. *Cochrane Database Syst Rev* (2019) 2(2):CD012685. doi: 10.1002/14651858.CD012685.pub2
118. Zhang H, Garcia JM. Anamorelin hydrochloride for the treatment of cancer-anorexia-cachexia in NSCLC. *Expert Opin Pharmacother* (2015) 16(8):1245–53. doi: 10.1517/14656566.2015.1041500

6

Pan-Cancer Analysis of IGF-1 and IGF-1R as Potential Prognostic Biomarkers and Immunotherapy Targets

Yinqi Zhang[1,2†], Chengqi Gao[3†], Fei Cao[2,3†], Ying Wu[2,3†], Shuanggang Chen[4], Xue Han[2,3], Jingqin Mo[1], Zhiyu Qiu[2,3], Weijun Fan[2,3], Penghui Zhou[3] and Lujun Shen[2,3*]*

[1] Zhongshan School of Medicine, Sun Yat-Sen University, Guangzhou, China, [2] Department of Minimally Invasive Interventional Therapy, Sun Yat-Sen University Cancer Center, Guangzhou, China, [3] State Key Laboratory of Oncology in South China, Collaborative Innovation Center of Cancer Medicine, Sun Yat-Sen University, Guangzhou, China, [4] Department of Oncology, Yuebei People's Hospital, Shantou University Medical College, Shaoguan, China

***Correspondence:**
Lujun Shen
shenlj@sysucc.org.cn
Penghui Zhou
zhouph@sysucc.org.cn

†These authors have contributed equally to this work

Aim: Insulin-like growth factor-1 receptor (IGF-1R) is one of the main members of the tyrosine protein kinase receptor family. This receptor binds insulin-like growth factor-1 (IGF-1) with a high affinity. IGF-1 is a member of a family of proteins involved in mediating growth and development. However, the correlations of IGF-1 and IGF-1R to prognosis and tumor-infiltrating lymphocytes in different cancers remain unclear.

Method: This research comprehensively analyzed the expression pattern of IGF-1 and IGF-1R and the influence of IGF-1 and IGF-1R on clinical significance in prognosis prediction among 33 types of malignancies using The Cancer Genome Atlas (TCGA) and the Cancer Cell Line Encyclopedia (CCLE) databases. The correlation between IGF-1, IGF-1R, and cancer immunity was explored.

Results: IGF-1 and IGF-1R displayed inconsistent gene expression levels among diverse cancer cell lines. Typically, high expression level of IGF-1 and IGF-1R was detected in most malignant tumors. High expression of IGF-1 was closely bound up with the unfavorable overall survival (OS) for patients in BLCA, CHOL, and LAML upon Cox and Kaplan-Meier analyses. While high expression of IGF-1R was closely bound up with the unfavorable overall survival (OS) for patients in BLCA, LIHC, and LUAD. Furthermore, high expression level of IGF-1 and IGF-1R were closely connected with high degrees of tumor infiltrates, including CD4+ T cell, dendritic cells, and macrophages. In addition, we found that IGF-1 was commonly positively correlated with the expression of gene markers including LAIR1, ICOS, CD40LG, CTLA4, CD48, CD28, CD200R1, HAVCR2, and CD86.

Whereas, IGF-1R was commonly positively correlated with the expression of gene markers including NRP1 and CD276. More importantly, IGF-1 and IGF-1R expression were correlated with tumor mutation burden (TMB), microsatellite instability (MSI), mismatch repair (MMR), and DNA methyltransferase (DNMT) of different types of cancers.

Conclusions: The impact of high IGF-1 and IGF-1R on prognosis and immune infiltrates differs across cancer types. Anti-IGF-1R therapy may inhibit tumor growth and contribute to immunotherapy in LIHC and KIRC.

Keywords: pan-cancer, IGF-1, IGF-1R, prognostic biomarker, immunity

INTRODUCTION

Insulin-like growth factor 1 receptor (IGF-1R), one of the main members of tyrosine protein kinase receptor family, plays an important role in maintaining the malignant phenotype and tumor anti-apoptosis. Insulin-like growth factor-1 (IGF-1), ligand of IGF-1R, is a kind of growth hormone mainly synthesized in liver. Population studies provide substantial direct and circumstantial evidence that cancer risk and cancer prognosis are influenced by IGF-1 and insulin levels (1). The overexpression of IGF-1 and its receptor IGF-1R have been implicated in carcinogenesis and are also considered risk factors for the progression of diverse human cancers (2–4). On the other hand, studies have proved that anti-IGF-1R monoclonal antibody has potential therapeutic value in diverse cancers (5–7). Researchers have also found that the differentiation of *ex vivo*-expanded CD34+ cells through manipulation of RAS/MAPK, IGF-1R, and TGF-β signaling pathways is an efficient approach for generating functional NK cells that can be used for cancer immunotherapy (8). However, the correlations of IGF-1 and IGF-1R to prognosis and tumor-infiltrating lymphocytes in different cancers remain unclear. Since cancer is a leading cause of death worldwide, and the low efficacy of many existing therapies is a major clinical challenge, it is essential to understand the prognostic and immunological impact of IGF-1 and IGF-1R among cancer types comprehensively in order to develop novel immunotherapies.

Molecular-level pan-cancer analyses have provided insights into the common features and heterogeneity of various human malignancies. Since the establishment of The Cancer Genome Atlas based on various human cancer samples and normal tissues at epigenomic, genomic, proteomic, and transcriptomic levels, diverse cancer samples are offered so that deeper pan-cancer analysis could be conducted (9). Therefore, we conducted a pan-cancer analysis taking advantage of its large datasets. The analysis aimed to (a) describe the expression of IGF-1 and IGF-1R among different cancer types; (b) assess the prognostic values of IGF-1 and IGF-1R among varied tumors; and (c) evaluate the associations between IGF-1/IGF-1R and tumor immunity features including intratumoral immune infiltrates, checkpoint markers, tumor mutation burden (TMB), and microsatellite instability (MSI), which have been identified as biomarkers for predicting response to immune checkpoint inhibitor treatment (10).

METHODS

Patient Datasets and Processing

The Cancer Genome Atlas (TCGA), a milestone of the cancer genomics project, characterizes thousands of primary cancer samples and matched adjacent noncarcinoma samples from 33 types of cancers. In this study, the TCGA level 3 RNA sequencing processed data and the corresponding clinical annotations were acquired using the UCSC cancer genome browser (https://tcga.xenahubs.net, accessed May 2020). The Cancer Cell Line Encyclopedia (CCLE) public project is established through the comprehensive characterization of tremendous human tumor models at both genetic and pharmacological levels (https://portals.broadinstitute.org/ccle). To examine the differential gene expression in cancers at a larger a scale, the CCLE database containing the RNA-sequencing datasets for over 1,000 cell lines (https://portals.broadinstitute.org/ccle) was used in this study. The approval from the Ethics Committee was exempted as only the open-access data were used.

IGF-1/IGF-1R Differential Expression and Survival-Associated Cancers

To compare the gene expression levels between cancer and adjacent noncarcinoma samples, data regarding the gene expression profiles of IGF-1/IGF-1R were extracted from the 33 cancer types in TCGA to from an expression matrix. It is thereafter merged with corresponding clinical information by patient ID. Univariate Cox model was applied in calculating the associations between gene expression levels and patient survival among 33 cancer types, and a difference of $p < 0.05$ for IGF-1 and IGF-1R in a specific cancer indicated statistical significance. The survival-associated forest plot is also made. Moreover, the Kaplan-Meier (KM) analysis by log-rank test was conducted to compare the overall survival (OS) and disease-specific survival (DSS) for TCGA cancer patients stratified based on the median gene expression level of IGF-1/IGF-1R.

IGF-1/IGF-1R and Tumor Immune Microenvironment

The tumor-infiltrating immunocyte levels among different types of cancers were estimated by Tumor Immune Estimation Resource (TIMER, https://cistrome.shinyapps.io/timer/) (11) and CIBERSORT (12) based on related gene expression data, through deconvolution statistical method. The relationships between each immune infiltrate among 33 cancer types and IGF-1/IGF-1R expression were analyzed.

Estimation of STromal and Immune cells in MAlignant Tumor tissues using Expression data (ESTIMATE) is used to predict tumor purity and the infiltrating stromal cells/ immunocytes in tumor tissue based on gene expression profiles (13). The ESTIMATE algorithm produces three scores based on the gene set enrichment analysis (GSEA) of single samples, including stromal score, which determines stromal cells in tumor tissues and immune score, which stands for the immunocyte infiltration level in tumor tissues. In this study, ESTIMATE algorithm is used to estimate the stromal and immune scores in tumor tissues according to corresponding transcriptional data and calculated the correlations of these scores with the expression of IGF-1/IGF-1R.

The relationships between the expression level of IGF-1/IGF-1R and the gene markers in tumor infiltrating immunocytes selected with reference to previous research were further conducted (14, 15). Correlation analysis was conducted to generate the estimated statistical significance and Spearman's correlation coefficient. The somatic mutation data of all TCGA patients were downloaded (https://tcga.xenahubs.net) in order to calculate TMB scores and MSI scores and explore the correlation of IGF1/IGF-1R with MMR genes and DNMT.

Gene Set Enrichment Analysis

GSEA were performed on IGF-1 and IGF-1R to understand the interrelated biological functions and pathways of IGF-1/IGF-1R. The molecular signature Database (MSigDB) H (hallmark gene sets) collection of chemical and genetic perturbations and KEGG subsets of canonical pathways and cancer modules were employed, and the analysis was completed on Sangerbox (http://sangerbox.com/). Normalized enrichment scores (NES) were used to show GSEA results, accounting for the size and degree to which a gene set is overrepresented at the top or bottom of the ranked list of genes (nominal p-value <0.05 and FDR ≤ 0.25). Bioconductor (http://bioconductor.org/) and R software (http:///www.r-project.org/) were used to visualize the enrichment maps of results.

Statistical Analysis

In the present work, the clinical survival types, including OS and disease-specific survival (DSS), were selected for analysis. Generally, OS is deemed as the duration from the date of diagnosis to the date of death due to any course, DSS is considered disease progression or death due to the disease.

Wilcox log rank test was adopted to determine the presence or absence of a markedly increased sum of gene expression z-scores in cancer tissues compared with adjacent normal tissues. Meanwhile, Kruskal-Wallis test was employed to compare the difference in the expression of IGF-1 and IGF-1R. Survival was analyzed by the KM curves, log-rank test, and the Cox proportional hazard regression model. Spearman' test was utilized for correlation analysis. The R language (version 3.6.0; R Foundation) was used for all analyses. A two-sided difference of $p < 0.05$ indicated statistical significance.

RESULTS

Pan-Cancer Expression Landscape of IGF-1 and IGF-1R

Comparison of expression of IGF-1/IGF-1R between normal and tumor samples across TCGA cancer types and the combined datasets based on integrated database of GTEx and TCGA datasets were conducted and shown in **Figure 1**. Consistent high expression level of IGF-1 could be seen in normal tissues than most types of tumor based on both comparisons, and significant decreased expression of IGF-1 could be seen in tumor samples including ACC, BLCA, BRCA, CESC, CHOL, COAD, ESCA, LAML. LGG, LIHC, LUAD, OV, PRAD, READ, SKCM, STAD, TGCT, THCA, UCEC, and UCS based on the integrated database. Whereas, high expression level of IGF-1R could be seen in most types of tumors than normal tissue based on both comparisons, and significant increased expression of IGF-1R could be seen in tumor samples including BRCA, CHOL, COAD, ESCA, GBM, HNSC, LAML, LGG, LIHC, LUAD, LUSC, PAAD, PRAD, SKCM, STAD, TGCT, and THCA based on the integrated database. Patients with different tumor stage and gender did not differ in the expression of IGF-1/IGF-1R in tumor samples.

Correlation of IGF-1/IGF-1R Expression Level and Overall Survival of Cancer Patients

Figures 2 and **3** summarized the results of OS analyses of IGF-1 and IGF-1R expression across the 33 cancer types. In univariate analysis, high expression of IGF-1 in tumor samples correlates with unfavorable prognosis in BLCA (HR = 1.09, p = 0.0012), CHOL (HR = 1.27, p = 0.0011) and LAML (HR = 3.88, p = 0.018); whereas, high expression of IGF-1 correlates with favorable prognosis in SARC (HR = 0.93, p = 0.00063) (**Figures 2A–D**). Cox regression model confirmed the prognostic impact of IGF-1 in BLCA (p = 4.4e–0.6), CHOL (p = 3.8e–0.2), LAML (p = 7.8e–0.3), and SARC (p = 4.2e–0.2) with the same trend (**Figure 2E**). On the other hand, high expression of IGF-1R in tumor samples correlates with unfavorable prognosis in BLCA (HR = 1.01, p = 0.045), LIHC (HR = 1.06, p = 0.013), and LUAD (HR = 1.01, p = 0.024); whereas, high expression of IGF-1R correlates with favorable prognosis in KIRC (HR = 0.97, p < 0.0001) and LAML (HR = 0.98, p = 0.0011) (**Figures 3A–E**). Cox regression model confirmed the prognostic impact of IGF-1R in BLCA (p = 4.0e–0.2), LIHC (p = 1.3e–0.2), LUAD (p = 2.7e–0.2), KIRC (p = 9.3e–0.8), and LAML (p = 3.2e –0.2) with the same trend (**Figure 3F**).

Correlation of IGF-1/IGF-1R Expression Level and Immune Infiltrates

Systemic analysis of immune infiltrates in different cancer types could be conducted by using a deconvolution statistical approach to infer tumor-infiltrating lymphocyte (TIL) counts based on gene expression data thanks to TIMER (https://cistrome.shinyapps.io/timer/). In this study, we analyzed the impact of IGF-1 and IGF-1R on the abundance of six immune infiltrates in cancers that harbor prognostic value, which are B cells, CD4+

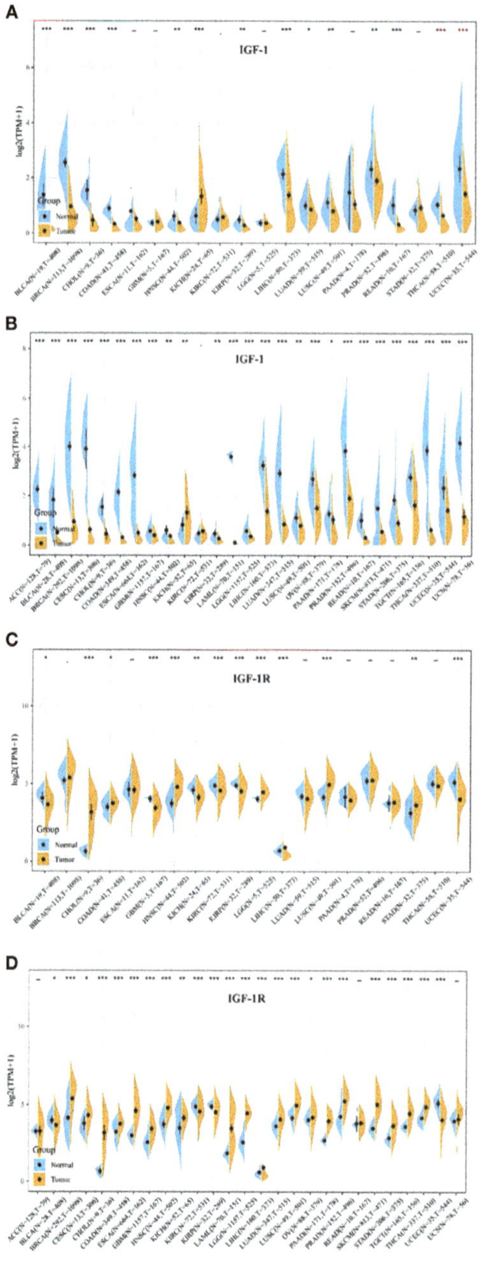

FIGURE 1 | IGF-1/IGF-1R expression levels in different types of human cancers. The expression levels of IGF-1 between tumor and normal tissues were compared in 20 cancer types based on the TCGA database **(A)** and 27 cancer types based on the integrated database from TCGA and GTEx datasets **(B)**. The expression levels of IGF-1R between tumor and normal tissues were compared in 20 cancer types based on the TCGA database **(C)** and 27 cancer types based on the integrated database from TCGA and GTEx datasets **(D)**. Consistent high expression level of IGF-1 could be seen in normal tissues than most types of tumor based on both comparisons, and significant decreased expression of IGF-1 could be seen in tumor samples including ACC, BLCA, BRCA, CESC, CHOL, COAD, ESCA, LAML, LGG, LIHC, LUAD, OV, PRAD, READ, SKCM, STAD, TGCT, THCA, UCEC, and UCS based on the integrated database. Consistent high expression level of IGF-1R could be seen in most types of tumor than normal tissue based on the both comparisons, and significant increased expression of IGF-1R could be seen in tumor samples including BRCA, CHOL, COAD, ESCA, GBM, HNSC, LAML, LGG, LIHC, LUAD, LUSC, PAAD, PRAD, SKCM, STAD, TGCT, and THCA based on the integrated database. "*, **, ***" means $p < 0.05$, $p < 0.01$ and $p < 0.001$, respectively.

cells, CD8+ cells, dendritic cells, macrophages, and neutrophils. The correlation between the expression of IGF-1/IGF-1R and the immune infiltration levels across diverse cancer types is derived from TIMER. As for IGF-1, three of the most significant associations were BLCA (**Figure 4A**), BRCA (**Figure 4B**), and CHOL (**Figure 4C**). While for IGF-1R, three of the most significant associations were BLCA (**Figure 4D**), LIHC (**Figure 4E**), and PRAD (**Figure 4F**). TIMER showed that both

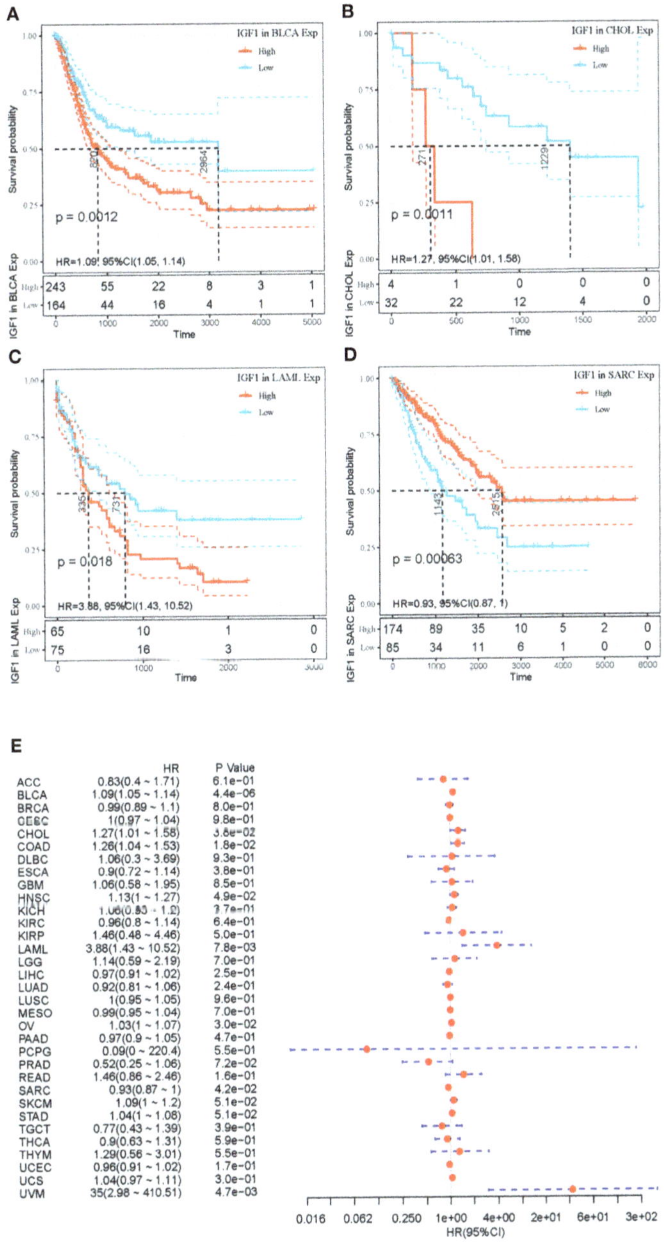

FIGURE 2 | Selected Kaplan-Meier plots and forest plot comparing the high and low expressions of IGF-1 on overall survival across different cancers. **(A–C)** Kaplan-Meier method showed high expression of IGF-1 correlated with unfavorable prognosis in BLCA, CHOL, and LAML. **(D)** Kaplan-Meier method showed high expression of IGF-1 correlated with favorable prognosis in SARC. **(E)** Forest plot displaying the impact of high expression of IGF-1 on OS across 33 cancer types using Cox regression model. Confidence level is shown in dashed lines.

IGF-1 and IGF-1R are positively correlated with the abundance of CD4+ T cell, dendritic cells, and macrophages.

The ESTIMATE method is developed to calculate the immune and stromal scores of cancer tissues. By adopting the ESTIMATE method, we calculated the immune, stromal scores, respectively. As for IGF-1, three of the most significant correlation according to stromal scores were found in ESCA, GBM, and LGG (**Figures 5A–C**), while three of the most significant correlation according to immune scores were found in GBM, LGG, and LUSC (**Figures 5D–F**). As for IGF-1R, three of the most significant correlation according to stromal scores were found in LIHC, LGG, and COAD (**Figures 5G–I**), while three of the most significant correlation according to immune scores were found in BRCA, KIRC, and LUAD (**Figures 5J–L**).

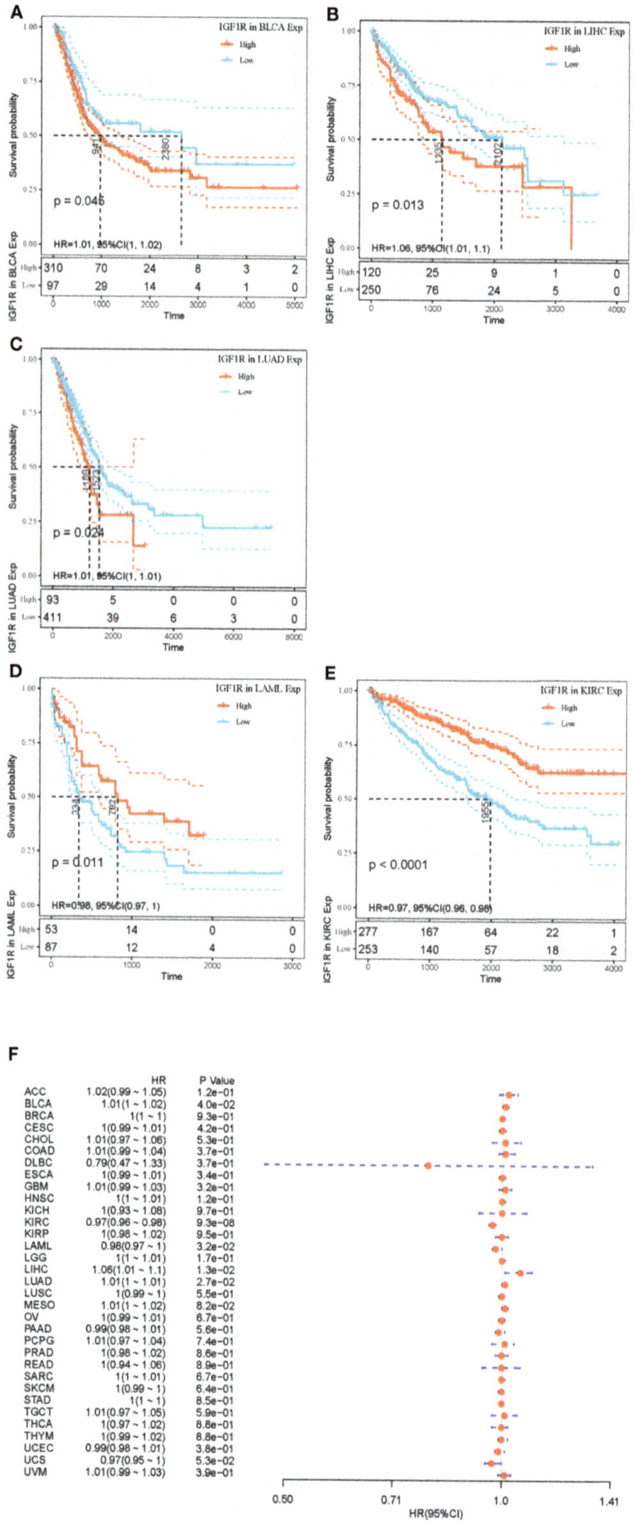

FIGURE 3 | Selected Kaplan-Meier plots and forest plot comparing the high and low expressions of IGF-1R on overall survival across different cancers. **(A–C)** Kaplan-Meier method showed high expression of IGF-1R correlated with unfavorable prognosis in BLCA, LIHC, and LUAD. **(D, E)** Kaplan-Meier method showed high expression of IGF-1R correlated with favorable prognosis in LAML and KIRC. **(F)** Forest plot displaying the impact of high expression of IGF-1R on OS across 33 cancer types using Cox regression model.

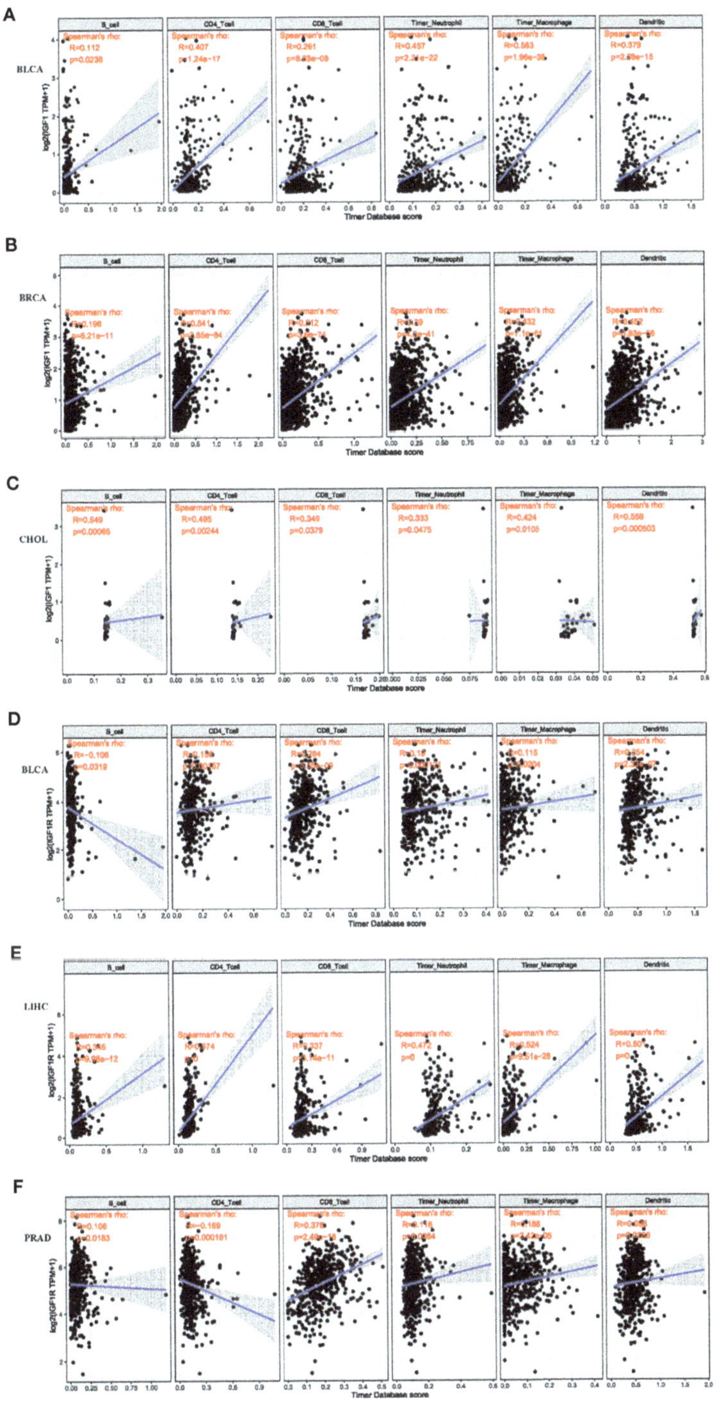

FIGURE 4 | Correlation of IGF-1 expression level with immune infiltration level in BLCA, BRCA, and CHOL. Correlation of IGF-1R expression level with immune infiltration level in BLCA, LIHC, and PRAD. **(A–C)** IGF-1 expression is significantly positively correlated with CD4+ T cell, dendritic cell, and macrophage infiltration in BLCA, BRCA, and CHOL. **(D–F)** IGF-1R expression is significantly positively correlated with CD4+ T cell, dendritic cell, and macrophage infiltration in BLCA, LIHC, and PRAD.

Correlation Analysis on Checkpoint Gene Markers

To further explored the potential mechanism of immune inhibition of IGF-1/IGF-1R signaling, the associations of IGF-1/IGF-1R expressions with multiple checkpoint markers were compared across different cancer types (**Figure 6**). Generally, IGF-1 expression positively correlates with the expression of LAIR1, ICOS, CD40LG, CTLA4, CD48, CD28, CD200R1,

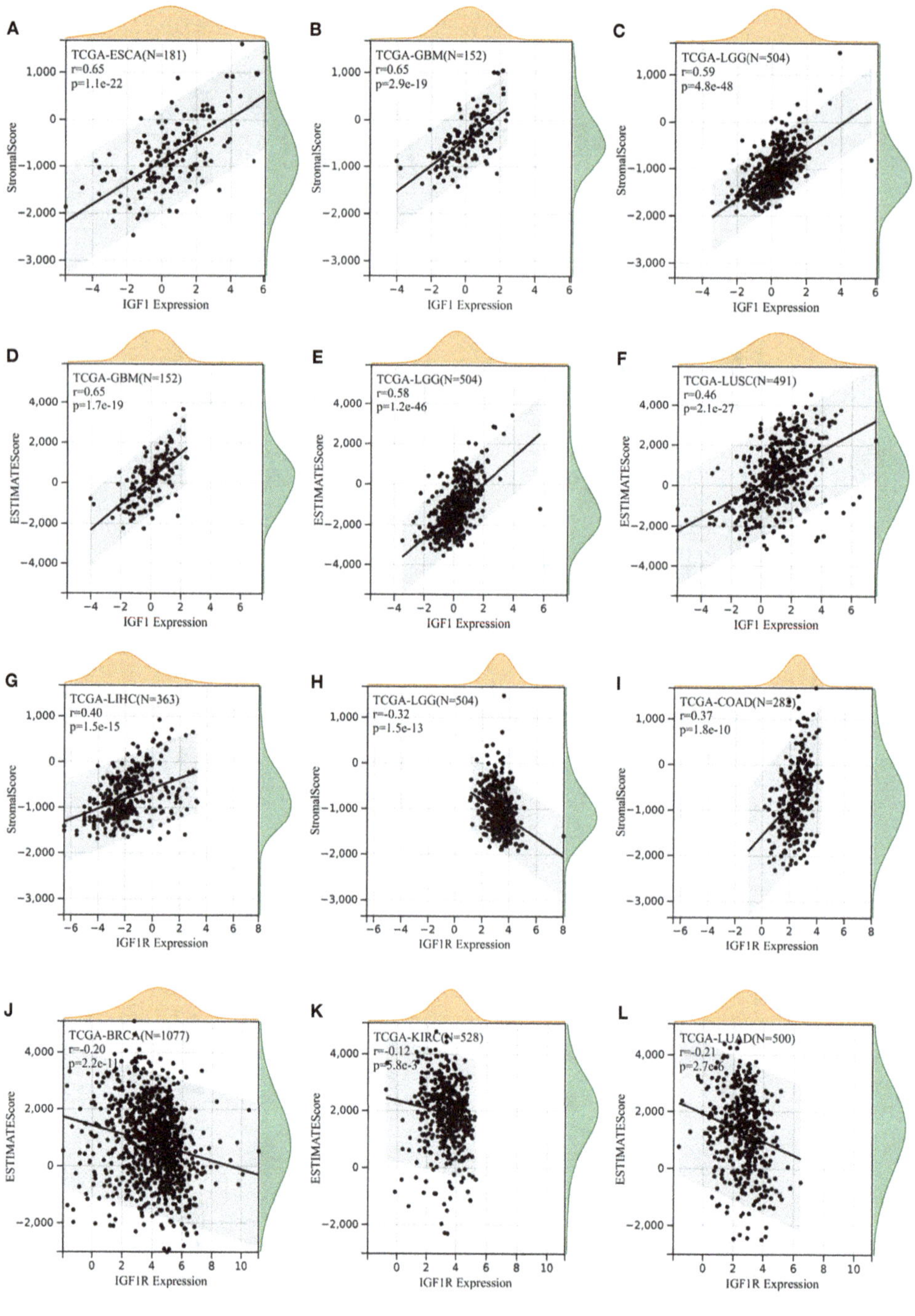

FIGURE 5 | Correlation of IGF-1/IGF-1R expression with estimate score. **(A–C)** IGF-1 expression significantly correlated with stromal scores in esophageal carcinoma (ESCA), glioblastoma multiforme (GBM), and lower-grade glioma (LGG). **(D–F)** IGF-1 expression significantly correlated with immune scores in glioblastoma multiforme (GBM), lower-grade glioma (LGG), and lung squamous cell carcinoma (LUSC). **(G–I)** IGF-1R expression significantly correlated with stromal scores in liver hepatocellular carcinoma (LIHC), lower-grade glioma (LGG), and lung squamous cell carcinoma (LUSC). **(J–L)** IGF-1R expression significantly correlated with immune scores in breast invasive carcinoma (BRCA), kidney renal clear cell carcinoma (KIRC), and lung adenocarcinoma (LUAD).

HAVCR2, and CD86 in the majority of 33 cancer types (**Figure 6A**). On the other hand, IGF-1R expression positively correlates with the expression of NRP1 and CD276 in the majority of 33 cancer types (**Figure 6B**).

Correlation Analysis on TMB, MSI, MMR, and DNMT

Tumor mutational burden (TMB) is a quantifiable biomarker which is used to reflect the number of mutations contained in malignancies.

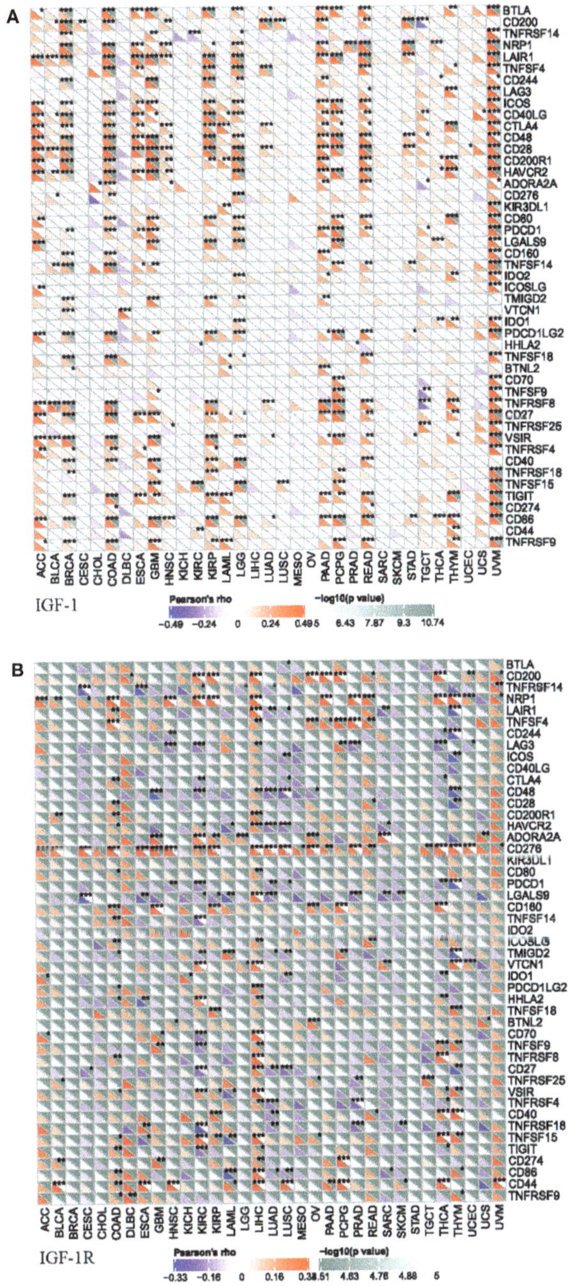

FIGURE 6 | Correlation of IGF-1 **(A)** and IGF-1R **(B)** expressions with expression of immune checkpoint genes across 33 cancer types. "*, **, ***" means significant correlation $p < 0.05$, $p < 0.01$ and $p < 0.001$, respectively.

Microsatellite instability (MSI) refers to the occurrence of new microsatellite alleles due to the insertion or deletion of duplicate units and cause changes in the length of a microsatellite compared with normal tissue. The association of TMB/MSI with IGF-1/IGF-1R expression was evaluated. Expression of IGF-1 positively correlated with TMB in THYM, CHOL, LAML, LIHC, and OV while negatively correlated with the TMB in BLCA, BRCA, CESC, COAD, DLBC, ESCA, GBM, HNSC, KICH, KIRC, KIRP, LGG, LUAD, LUSC, MESO, PAAD, PCPG, PRAD, READ, SARC, STAD, TGCT, THCA, UCEC, UCS, and UVMP (**Figure 7A**). Expression of IGF-1R positively correlated with TMB in GBM, HNSC, KICH, LAML, LGG, MESO, SKCM, and THYM while negatively correlated with TMB in BLCA, BRCA, CESC, COAD, ESCA, KIRC, KIRP, LIHC, OV, PAAD, PRAD, READ, STAD, TGCT, THCA, UCEC, UCS, and UVM (**Figure 7B**). The correlations of IGF-1/IGF-1R with MSI are shown in **Figures 7C, D**.

The correlation analysis between MMR genes (MLH1, MSH2, MSH6, PMS2, EPCAM) and IGF-1/IGF-1R expression was further

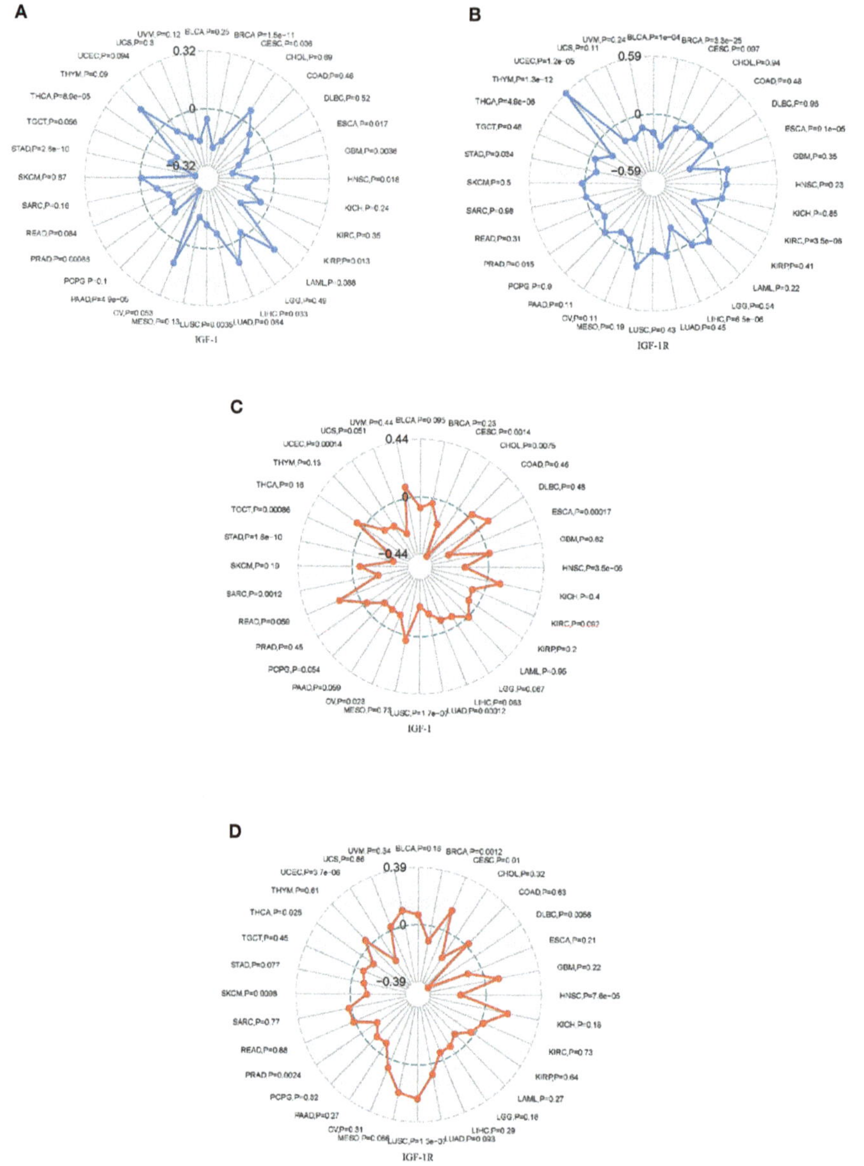

FIGURE 7 | Radar map plotting the correlation of tumor mutation burden (TMB) **(A)** and microsatellite instability (MSI) **(B)** with IGF-1 expression across 33 cancer types. Radar map plotting the correlation of tumor mutation burden (TMB) **(C)** and microsatellite instability (MSI) **(D)** with IGF-1R expression across 33 cancer types.

performed. IGF-1 expression was correlated with at least one MMR genes in BRCA, COAD, HNSC, LIHC, PAAD, STAD, and TGCT (**Supplementary Figure S1**). IGF-1R expression was correlated with at least one MMR genes in almost all of the 33 cancer types except for BRCA, STAD, and UCS (**Supplementary Figure S2**). Moreover, the correlation analysis between DNMT (DNMT1, DNMT2, DNMT3A, and DNMT3B) and IGF-1/IGF-1R expression was also conducted. The result is as shown in **Supplementary Figures S3** and **S4**.

Functional Analysis by Gene Set Enrichment Analysis

The biological role of IGF-1 and IGF-1R were illustrated through GSEA. The pan-cancer functional KEGG and HALLMARK terms of IGF-1/IGF-1R are shown in **Figure 8**, respectively. Generally, the top 3 negatively enriched KEGG terms in high IGF-1 subgroups were hematopoietic cell lineage, cytokine cytokine receptor interaction, and B-cell receptor signaling pathway (**Figure 8A**), and the top positively enriched KEGG terms were glutathione metabolism, pentose phosphate pathway, fructose and mannose metabolism, and base excision repair (**Figure 8B**). The top 3 negatively enriched HALLMARK terms in high IGF-1 subgroups were epithelial mesenchymal transition, KRAS upsignaling, and allograft rejection (**Figure 8C**), and the top positively enriched HALLMARK terms were MYC targets V2, reactive oxygen species pathway, oxidative phosphorylation, and DNA repair (**Figure 8D**). As for IGF-1R, the top 3 negatively enriched KEGG terms were WNT signaling pathway,

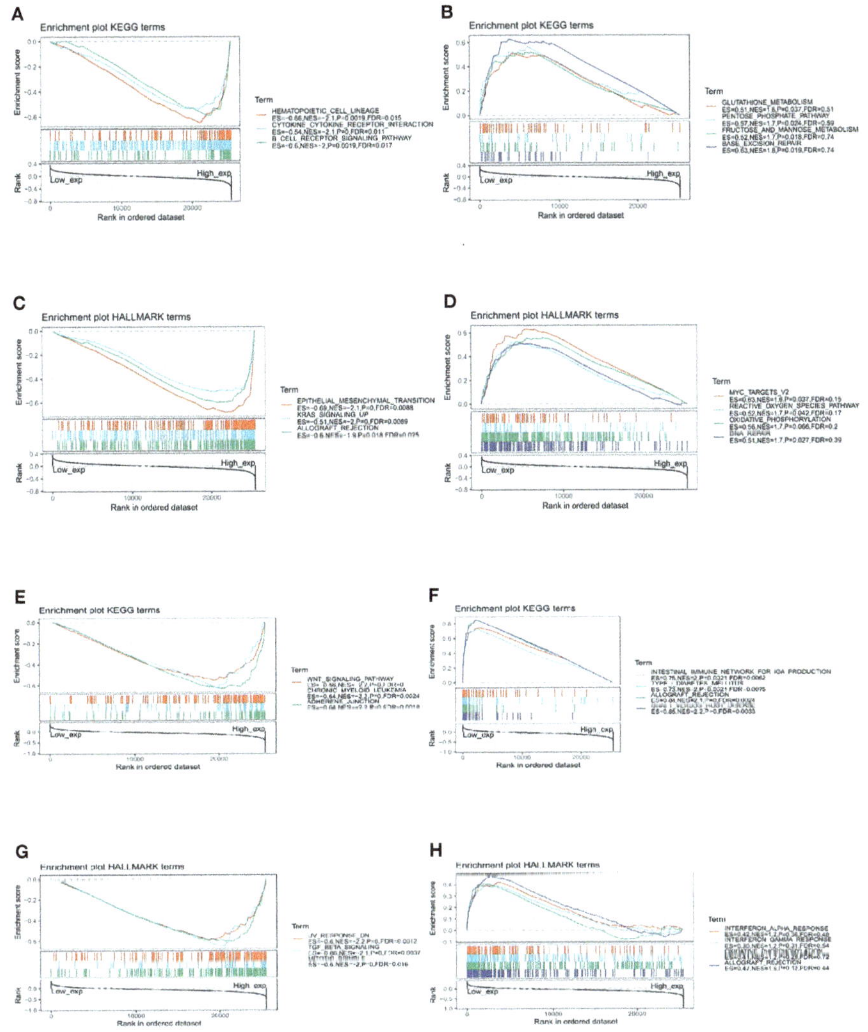

FIGURE 8 | Functional Enrichment of KEGG and HALLMARK terms on IGF-1 and IGF-1R through GSEA. The top 3 negatively and positively enriched KEGG terms on IGF-1 are displayed in **(A, B)**, respectively. The top 3 negatively and positively enriched KEGG terms on IGF-1 are displayed in **(C, D)**, respectively. The top 3 negatively and positively enriched KEGG terms on IGF-1R are displayed in **(E, F)**, respectively. The top 3 negatively and positively enriched KEGG terms on IGF-1R are displayed in **(G, H)**, respectively.

chronic myeloid leukemia, and adherens junction (**Figure 8E**), and the top positively enriched KEGG terms were intestinal immune network for IgA production, type I diabetes mellitus, allograft rejection, and graft-versus-host disease (**Figure 8F**). The top 3 negatively enriched HALLMARK terms in high IGF-1R subgroups were UV response DN, TGF beta signaling, and mitotic spindle (**Figure 8G**), and the top positively enriched HALLMARK terms were interferon alpha response, interferon gamma response, oxidative phosphorylation, and allograft rejection (**Figure 8H**).

DISCUSSION

The present work illustrated a comprehensive workflow for pan-cancer analysis and thoroughly investigated the role of IGF-1 and IGF-1R in cancers. The prognostic impact of IGF-1 and IGF-1R expression among different cancer types was reported. It was found that most cancer types showed a higher IGF-1/IGF-1R alteration frequency and the expression of IGF-1 and IGF-1R served as the prognostic factor in some cancer types, including BLCA and LAML upon both Cox and KM survival analyses. However, the relationship between IGF-1/IGF-1R overexpression and tumor immunity was still unclear. Secondly, though IGF-1 and IGF-1R share the same signaling pathway, whether they have different prognostic and immunologic values in different types of cancer needs further investigation. Moreover, the relationship between IGF1/IGF1R expression and tumor prognoses, such as TMB, MSI, MMR, and DNMT, which can predict the efficacy of immunotherapy, remains unclear. Base on this, our bioinformatics analysis studied the IGF-1/IGF-1R expression-associated KEGG terms and HALLMARK pathways.

Our study showed that IGF-1 and IGF-1R harbor distinct prognostic values among different cancer types. The low expression of IGF-1 served as a favorable prognostic factor in some cancer types, including BLCA, CHOL, LAML, and UVM; whereas in SARC, high expression of IGF-1 served as a favorable prognostic factor. On the other hand, high expression of IGF-1R served as a significant prognostic factor in such cancer types including KIRC and LAML; whereas in BLCA, LIHC, and LUAD, low expression of IGF-1R served as a favorable prognostic factor. Previous study has proven that the epithelial-mesenchymal transition (EMT) process of gastric cancer cells could be induced by IGF-1 through the IGF-1R/STAT3 signaling pathway so that cancer cells would achieve metastasis (16). It has also been found that in liver cancer, IGF-1 promotes the invasion and metastasis of liver cancer cells by inhibiting the degradation of cathepsin B (17). Wu et al. proved that the increasing secretion of IGF-1 and CCL20 promotes brain metastasis of lung cancer cells by polarizing microglia and suppressing innate immune function (18). Studies done by Somri-Gannam et al. provide evidence that IGF-1R axis inhibition could be a therapeutic strategy for ovarian cancer by restoring dendritic cell (DC)-mediated antitumor immunity (19). Therefore, the distinct prognostic value of changeable IGF-1/IGF-1R expression across different cancers may result from its synthetic effect of immune suppressive activity and tumor suppressive activity in each cancer type. The distinct prognostic value of IGF-1 and IGF-1R expression may give rise to some new researches and questions for discussion. Both IGF-1 and IGF-1R are positively correlated with the abundance of CD4+ T cell, dendritic cells, and macrophages. Cellular infiltration of CD4+ T cell, dendritic cells, and macrophages would lead to immunosuppressive tumor microenvironment and cause unfavorable prognosis. The expression of IGF-1 is positively correlated with the expression of most immune checkpoint genes in UVM. The expression of IGF-1R is positively correlated with the expression of CD276 in most cancer types, and since CD276 is related to immunosuppression, this may explain why the increased expression of IGF-1R in tumor has an impact on the prognosis.

The expressions of IGF-1 and IGF-1R were correlated with TMB and MSI in some cancer types. TMB could impact the patient response to immune checkpoint inhibitors through affecting the generation possibility of immunogenic peptide (20). MSI is a vital index to predict tumor genesis and development (21). The NCCN guidelines have recommended MSI testing for all rectum adenocarcinoma (READ) subtypes, and the READ mortality can be reduced by the early detection of MSI (22). FDA has approved the use of Keytruda for the treatment of MSI-H solid tumors. As a result, TMB and MSI can serve as the predicting factors for efficacy. The expressions of IGF-1/IGF-1R share negative correlation with TMB and MSI in most cancer types, which means high expression of IGF-1/IGF-1R indicates immunosuppression. Our findings provide clues on the correlation between IGF-1/IGF-1R expression and cancer immunity and suggest that it could be a potential predictive maker of the efficacy of immunotherapy. Our study systematically compared the immune effects of IGF-1 and IGF1-R, which is conducive to localize the target molecules more accurately. A series of drugs targeting IGF-1/IGF1-R in the treatment of cancer are in clinical trials. The associated results may be released in the next 5 years.

Our study has several limitations. First, the result of our study should be interpreted with caution since checkpoint inhibitor treatment has not been analyzed in our study. Second, the result of our study lacks external validation in other public datasets. We need clinical specimens from our center for further verification. Only the gene expression level was analyzed in this study; we may conduct a more comprehensive analysis from the perspective of single and multiple omics. More efforts are needed to undermine the value of IGF-1/IGF-1R as a potential target of immunotherapy.

To conclude, our comprehensive pan-cancer analysis has characterized IGF-1/IGF-1R expression in different cancer cell lines and tissues. According to our results, IGF-1 and IGF-1R can serve as a valuable prognostic biomarker in some cancer types. They are also related to cancer immunity and could be potential predictive maker of the efficacy of immunotherapy, which may help develop the new targeted treatment.

AUTHOR CONTRIBUTIONS

LS and PZ designed and implemented the study design. YZ, CG, FC, YW, and SC participated in data analysis. XH, JM, ZQ, and WF managed and advised on the project. YZ, CG, FC, and YW wrote the paper. All authors contributed to the article and approved the submitted version.

SUPPLEMENTARY MATERIAL

Supplementary Figure 1 | Correlations of IGF-1 expression with MMR genes.

Supplementary Figure 2 | Correlations of IGF-1R expression with MMR genes.

Supplementary Figure 3 | Correlations of IGF-1 expression with DNMT.

Supplementary Figure 4 | Correlations of IGF-1R expression with DNMT.

REFERENCES

1. Pollak M. Insulin and Insulin-Like Growth Factor Signalling in Neoplasia. *Nat Rev Cancer* (2008) 8(12):915–28. doi: 10.1038/nrc2536
2. Majchrzak-Baczmańska D, Malinowski A. Does IGF-1 Play a Role in the Biology of Endometrial Cancer? *Ginekologia Polska* (2016) 87(8):598–604. doi: 10.5603/gp.2016.0052
3. Majchrzak-Baczmańska D, Malinowski A, Głowacka E, Wilczyński M. Does IGF-1 Play a Role in the Biology of Ovarian Cancer? *Ginekologia Polska* (2018) 89(1):13–9. doi: 10.5603/GP.a2018.0003
4. Li Y, Liu Q, He H, Luo W. The Possible Role of Insulin-Like Growth Factor-1 in Osteosarcoma. *Curr Problems Cancer* (2019) 43(3):228–35. doi: 10.1016/j.currproblcancer.2018.08.008

5. Ma H, Zhang T, Shen H, Cao H, Du J. The Adverse Events Profile of Anti-IGF-1R Monoclonal Antibodies in Cancer Therapy. *Br J Clin Pharmacol* (2014) 77(6):917 28. doi: 10.1111/bcp.12228
6. Wang W, Zhang Y, Lv M, Feng J, Peng H, Geng J, et al. Anti-IGF-1R Monoclonal Antibody Inhibits the Carcinogenicity Activity of Acquired Trastuzumab-Resistant SKOV3. *J Ovarian Res* (2014) 7:103. doi: 10.1186/s13048-014-0103-5
7. Lu H, Jiang Z. Advances in Antibody Therapeutics Targeting Small-Cell Lung Cancer. *Adv Clin Exp Med Off Organ Wroclaw Med Univ* (2018) 27(9):1317–23. doi: 10.17219/acem/70159
8. Shokouhifar A, Anani Sarab G, Yazdanifar M, Fereidouni M, Nouri M, Ebrahimi M. Overcoming the UCB HSCs -Derived NK Cells Dysfunction Through Harnessing RAS/MAPK, IGF-1R and TGF-β Signaling Pathways. *Cancer Cell Int* (2021) 21(1):298. doi: 10.1186/s12935-021-01983-z
9. Tomczak K, Czerwińska P, Wiznerowicz M. The Cancer Genome Atlas (TCGA): An Immeasurable Source of Knowledge. *Contemp Oncol (Poznan Poland)* (2015) 19:A68–77. doi: 10.5114/wo.2014.47136
10. Rizzo A, Ricci A, Brandi G. PD-L1, TMB, MSI, and Other Predictors of Response to Immune Checkpoint Inhibitors in Biliary Tract Cancer. *Cancers* (2021) 13(3). doi: 10.3390/cancers13030558
11. Li T, Fan J, Wang B, Traugh N, Chen Q, Liu J, et al. TIMER: A Web Server for Comprehensive Analysis of Tumor-Infiltrating Immune Cells. *Cancer Res* (2017) 77(21):e108–e10. doi: 10.1158/0008-5472.can-17-0307
12. Newman A, Steen C, Liu C, Gentles A, Chaudhuri A, Scherer F, et al. Determining Cell Type Abundance and Expression From Bulk Tissues With Digital Cytometry. *Nat Biotechnol* (2019) 37(7):773–82. doi: 10.1038/s41587-019-0114-2
13. Becht E, Giraldo N, Lacroix L, Buttard B, Elarouci N, Petitprez F, et al. Estimating the Population Abundance of Tissue-Infiltrating Immune and Stromal Cell Populations Using Gene Expression. *Genome Biol* (2016) 17 (1):218. doi: 10.1186/s13059-016-1070-5
14. Cristescu R, Mogg R, Ayers M, Albright A, Murphy E, Yearley J, et al. Pan-Tumor Genomic Biomarkers for PD-1 Checkpoint Blockade-Based Immunotherapy. *Sci (New York NY)* (2018) 362(6411). doi: 10.1126/science.aar3593
15. Pan J, Zhou H, Cooper L, Huang J, Zhu S, Zhao X, et al. LAYN Is a Prognostic Biomarker and Correlated With Immune Infiltrates in Gastric and Colon Cancers. *Front Immunol* (2019) 10:6. doi: 10.3389/fimmu.2019.00006
16. Xu L, Zhou R, Yuan L, Wang S, Li X, Ma H, et al. IGF1/IGF1R/STAT3 Signaling-Inducible IFITM2 Promotes Gastric Cancer Growth and Metastasis. *Cancer Lett* (2017) 393:76–85. doi: 10.1016/j.canlet.2017.02.014
17. Lei T, Ling X. IGF-1 Promotes the Growth and Metastasis of Hepatocellular Carcinoma *via* the Inhibition of Proteasome-Mediated Cathepsin B Degradation. *World J Gastroenterol* (2015) 21(35):10137–49. doi: 10.3748/wjg.v21.i35.10137
18. Wu S, Xing F, Sharma S, Wu K, Tyagi A, Liu Y, et al. Nicotine Promotes Brain Metastasis by Polarizing Microglia and Suppressing Innate Immune Function. *J Exp Med* (2020) 217(8). doi: 10.1084/jem.20191131
19. Somri-Gannam L, Meisel-Sharon S, Hantisteanu S, Groisman G, Limonad O, Hallak M, et al. IGF1R Axis Inhibition Restores Dendritic Cell Antitumor Response in Ovarian Cancer. *Trans Oncol* (2020) 13(8):100790. doi: 10.1016/j.tranon.2020.100790
20. Chan T, Yarchoan M, Jaffee E, Swanton C, Quezada S, Stenzinger A, et al. Development of Tumor Mutation Burden as an Immunotherapy Biomarker: Utility for the Oncology Clinic. *Ann Oncol Off J Eur Soc Med Oncol* (2019) 30 (1):44–56. doi: 10.1093/annonc/mdy495
21. Chang L, Chang M, Chang H, Chang F. Microsatellite Instability: A Predictive Biomarker for Cancer Immunotherapy. *Appl Immunohistochem Mol Morphol AIMM* (2018) 26(2):e15–21. doi: 10.1097/pai.0000000000000575
22. Ganesh K, Stadler Z, Cercek A, Mendelsohn R, Shia J, Segal N, et al. Immunotherapy in Colorectal Cancer: Rationale, Challenges and Potential. *Nat Rev Gastroenterol Hepatol* (2019) 16(6):361–75. doi: 10.1038/s41575-019-0126-x

7

Imperfect Predictors for Lung Cancer Immunotherapy—A Field for Further Research

Kamila Wojas-Krawczyk[1*] *and Tomasz Kubiatowski*[2]

[1] *Department of Pneumonology, Oncology and Allergology, Medical University of Lublin, Lublin, Poland,* [2] *Department of Clinical Oncology, Saint John of Dukla Oncology Centre of the Lublin Region, Lublin, Poland*

Correspondence:
Kamila Wojas-Krawczyk
kamilawojas@wp.pl

The armamentarium for lung cancer immunotherapy has been strengthened using two groups of monoclonal antibodies: 1) anti-PD-1 antibodies, including pembrolizumab and nivolumab, which block the programmed death 1 receptor on the lymphocyte surface, resulting in increasing activity of these cells, and 2) anti-PD-L1 antibodies, including atezolizumab, durvalumab, and avelumab, which block the ligand for the PD-1 molecule on tumor cells and on tumor-infiltrating immune cells. The effectiveness of both groups of antibodies has been proven in many clinical trials, which translates into positive immunotherapeutic registrations for cancer patients. Regarding the predictive factor, PD-L1 expression on cancer cells is the only biomarker validated in prospective clinical trials used for qualification to immunotherapy in advanced non-small cell lung cancer (NSCLC) patients. However, it is not an ideal one. Unfortunately, no clinical benefits could be noted in patients with high PD-L1 expression on tumor cells against the effectiveness of immunotherapy that may be observed in patients without PD-L1 expression. Furthermore, the mechanism of antitumor immune response is extremely complex, multistage, and depends on many factors. Cancer cells could be recognized by the immune system, provided tumor-specific antigen presentation, and these arise as a result of somatic mutations in tumor cells. Based on novel immunotherapy registration, high tumor mutation burden (TMB) has become an important predictive factor. The intensity of lymphocyte infiltration in tumor tissue may be another predictive factor. The effectiveness of anti-PD-L1 immunotherapy is observed in patients with high expression of genes associated with the effector function of T lymphocytes (i.e., their ability to produce IFN-gamma). This does not end the list of potential factors that become useful in qualification of cancer patients for immunotherapy. There remains a need to search for new and perfect predictive factors for immunotherapy.

Keywords: predictive factors, PD-L1, PD-1, immunotherapy, non-small cell lung cancer

INTRODUCTION

The immune system is a key player in the efficient monitoring and destruction of cancer cells (1). Let us follow briefly how it works. The immune response cycle begins with the recognition of tumor antigens by antigen-presenting cells and presents them to T lymphocytes in the lymph nodes. Activated cytotoxic T lymphocytes (CTLs) migrate to peripheral tissues, actively seeking the antigen (2, 3). At the site of recognition, the intracellular cytotoxic proteins are released from the CTLs, and together with the nonspecific mechanisms provided by macrophages or NK cells, the cancer cells are eliminated (1–4). Why does this system fail in some cases? It seems that the reasons lie both on the side of insufficient immune system activation and the growing tumor tissue (2, 4). First, the immune checkpoints expressed on immune system cells [CTLA-4 on T regulatory cells, PD-1 on T lymphocytes, PD-L1 on tumor-infiltrating immune cells (IC), e.g., macrophages] play a crucial role in maintaining a balance between immune system overactivation and extinguishing its action (5, 6). Whereas tumor cells (TC) that expressed the PD-L1 molecule could very effectively block the activity of PD-1-positive T lymphocytes. Keeping this in mind, how could we suppress the inhibiting activity of cancer cells and restore the cytotoxic activity of T lymphocytes? It is time for immunotherapy.

From the moment that Professor James Allison and Professor Tasuko Honjo discovered the checkpoint molecules, the next step was to create specific monoclonal antibodies that, by blocking these molecules, restore immune system activity (7, 8). Since this moment, immunotherapy with immunological checkpoint inhibitors (ICIs) has revolutionized cancer treatment, especially for patients without actionable driver mutations (8, 9). In 2016, the American Society of Clinical Oncology named immunotherapy as a top cancer advance of the year.

In the field of lung cancer immunotherapy, two groups of ICIs are widely used. Anti-PD-1 antibodies include pembrolizumab and nivolumab and block the PD-1 receptor on the lymphocyte surface. Anti-PD-L1 antibodies include atezolizumab, durvalumab, and avelumab and block the ligand for the PD-1 molecule on TC and on tumor-infiltrating IC (8–11). Now, one of the most important questions tormenting oncologists is how to choose patients with lung cancer who will benefit the most from immunotherapy? The solution to this problem is to choose the right and most sensitive biomarker (12, 13). At present, the only validated biomarker with a qualification for cancer patients for ICIs is the percentage of TC and/or IC with PD-L1 expression (12–14). Moreover, tumor mutational burden (TMB) and microsatellite instability assay also have a predictive value in qualification for immunotherapy (14–16). However, one should remember the availability of tissue material from cancer patients. What should we do if we cannot collect the cancer cells, or if the tumor is heterogeneous and we only have a small biopsy of tumor tissue? Does the determination of selected markers in the blood serum or plasma of cancer patients give reliable results and indicate those who should be treated with ICIs? Should we make every effort to reobtain tissue material?

In this article, we focus on the advantages and disadvantages of all biomarkers that are approved or were tested in clinical trials and that could be used in qualification of cancer patients for immunotherapy.

BIOMARKERS RELATED TO TUMOR TISSUE

PD-L1 Expression

Immunohistochemical (IHC) testing for PD-L1 expression has become standard in the diagnosis of predictive factors in lung cancer (15–17). IHC is a relatively simple technique that is not related to any major problems. In many prospective trials, the efficacy of ICIs over standard chemotherapy as first-line therapy is demonstrated in patients with TC positive for PD-L1 (15–17). The KEYNOTE-024 study led to pembrolizumab registration in patients with metastatic non-small cell lung cancer (NSCLC) with expression of PD-L1 on ≥50% of TC (18). In this study, a significant increase in overall survival (OS) was observed in patients receiving pembrolizumab compared to patients treated with chemotherapy (18).

Moreover, based on the risk–benefit profile depicted in the KEYNOTE-042 study, pembrolizumab monotherapy can be extended by FDA registration (but not by the European Medicines Agency registration) as first-line therapy to patients with locally advanced or metastatic NSCLC without sensitizing *EGFR* or *ALK* alterations and with low PD-L1 expression (≥1%) as determined by an FDA-approved test (19).

However, advanced NSCLC patients, regardless of PD-L1 expression on TC, benefited from first-line combination therapy with platinum-based chemotherapy and pembrolizumab (KEYNOTE-189 and KEYNOTE-407 studies) (18–21). Regarding 2nd-line treatment, significantly longer survival was observed in locally advanced or advanced NSCLC patients receiving nivolumab (CheckMate-017 and CheckMate-057 studies) or atezolizumab (OAK study) compared with docetaxel regardless of PD-L1 expression although it should be noted that greater benefits were observed in patients with higher percentages of TC with PD-L1 expression (22–24). Pembrolizumab in the 2nd-line treatment could be used in patients with ≥1% of TC with PD-L1 expression (KEYNOTE-010 study) (25, 26). It should be mentioned that significant clinical efficacy of maintenance durvalumab therapy was observed in locally advanced NSCLC patients who received concurrent chemoradiotherapy (PACIFIC trial) (27, 28). In this study, patients were enrolled regardless of PD-L1 expression, but *post hoc* subgroup analysis of progression-free survival (PFS) and OS showed significant clinical benefits from durvalumab therapy when PD-L1 expression was present on ≥1% of TC (27). Recently, the FDA approved three new therapeutic strategies for first-line therapy in metastatic NSCLC patients: atezolizumab in patients with ≥50% of TC with PD-L1 expression (Impower-110 study); combination therapy with nivolumab and ipilimumab in patients with ≥1% of PD-L1 positive TC (CheckMate-227 study); and combination therapy with nivolumab, ipilimumab, and chemotherapy in patients regardless of PD-L1 expression on TC (CheckMate-9LA study) (29–33).

Additionally, an important issue regarding the benefit from immunotherapy in PD-L1 negative patients was raised in the CheckMate 227 trial (30, 34). In the subset of PD-L1 negative tumors, a significantly stronger survival benefit was observed in patients treated with nivolumab plus ipilimumab compared with chemotherapy. However, direct comparison of OS in PD-L1 negative tumors between combined immunotherapy and chemo-immunotherapy was not performed; a higher response rate for chemo-immunotherapy rather than for the nivolumab plus ipilimumab combination (38% *vs.* 27%) was observed. Based on that, we could speculate that immunotherapy combination and chemo-immunotherapy regimens demonstrated similar efficacy in PD-L1 negative patients (30, 34).

The abovementioned important clinical trials that resulted in immunotherapy registration clearly indicate that PD-L1 expression was an important factor for stratifying patients to receive ICIs and to obtain clinical efficacy (14–16, 35). However, it is surprising that different therapies used in different lines are registered in patients with different PD-L1 status on TC. It should be considered whether PD-L1 expression is an ideal biomarker or whether is it associated with ambiguity and controversy. Among the many unsolved questions concerning PD-L1 expression, the following aspect should be mentioned: 1) use of different cutoff levels for the percentage of PD-L1 positive TC for different ICIs; 2) differences in testing platforms; 3) the heterogeneous expression of this molecule through the tumor; its dependence on the histological type of TC; and the history of treatment (chemotherapy and radiotherapy could change PD-L1 expression on TC).

The scoring system for PD-L1 expression is varied for each immunotherapeutic. There were two categories in clinical trials with pembrolizumab: ≥50% of TC with PD-L1 expression is considered sufficient although <50% was insufficient for qualification for first-line therapy (18, 21). Pembrolizumab could be administered as second-line therapy if PD-L1 expression was observed on ≥1% of TC and in the first line with low PD-L1 expression (≥1%) but only in the United States (18, 19, 21, 35). Unlike this, nivolumab and atezolizumab could be ordered irrespective of PD-L1 expression on TC in second-line therapy (22–24, 31). However, in clinical studies with nivolumab in the second line, patients were stratified for PD-L1 expression into 4 groups: <1%, ≥1%, ≥5%, and ≥10% of PD-L1 positive TC. An even more complex scale was adopted in the OAK study. The efficacy of atezolizumab was assessed in 4 groups based on the PD-L1 expression on TC and tumor-infiltrating IC. Percentages of PD-L1-expressing TC were as follows: TC3 ≥50%, TC2 ≥5% and <50%, TC1 ≥1% and <5%, and TC0 <1% and percentage of tumor area infiltration by IC were as follows: IC3 ≥10%, IC2 ≥5% and <10%, IC1 ≥1% and <5%, and IC0 <1% (24). In the PACIFIC trial, ≥25% and ≥1% of TC with PD-L1 expression was used for assessment of durvalumab therapy efficacy; however, clinical benefits were observed irrespective of PD-L1 expression (27, 28). One should also remember that effectiveness of different treatment lines is also associated with various methods of qualification for treatment based on PD-L1 expression assessment.

As was mentioned, testing for PD-L1 expression by the IHC technique is considered to be a standard in predictive factor diagnosis. Unfortunately, each clinical trial with different immunotherapeutics used different anti-PD-L1 antibody clones and a different commercially available platform for testing. Trials with nivolumab used a 28-8 antibody clone, studies with pembrolizumab used a 22C3 clone, studies with atezolizumab used a 142 clone, and trials with durvalumab used an SP263 clone. The epitopes for anti-PD-L1 binding are in the extracellular domain for 28-8 and 22C3 antibody clones, and those for SP142 and SP263 are in the cytoplasmic domain (12, 21–24, 33, 35, 36).

In previous years, two large studies concerning the specificity and sensitivity of all the anti-PD-L1 antibody clones were conducted (Blueprint-1 and Blueprint-2) (35, 37, 38). In both studies, three companion assays—with 22C3 (used for pembrolizumab), 28-2 (used for nivolumab), and SP263 (used for durvalumab) antibody clones—achieved comparable specificity and sensitivity. Clone SP142, used for atezolizumab, was found to be less sensitive (37–39).

A quite complicated situation was resolved in 2015. The FDA approved the IHC 22C3 pharmDx assay as a companion diagnostic for the identification of NSCLC patients for pembrolizumab therapy (11, 12, 18). Moreover, in 2017, an IHC assay using the SP263 antibody clone, previously used for PD-L1 testing in clinical trials with durvalumab, received the CE mark for its use in PD-L1 testing during qualification for pembrolizumab immunotherapy. Therefore, PD-L1 expression is no longer required to be tested with the 22C3 antibody although this test is still approved for diagnosis (14–16).

The last problem associated with PD-L1 diagnosis is the heterogeneity of its expression within the tumor and its variability observed between primary and metastatic sites (14, 15, 40). Mansfield and colleagues examined paired primary lung tumor tissue and metastatic brain tissue and demonstrated that many of the brain metastases significantly lacked PD-L1 expression even when it was present in the primary lung cancer specimens (40).

During qualification of NSCLC patients for ICI treatment, all the limitations related to PD-L1 expression assessment described above as well as the spatial and temporal heterogeneity of the tumor microenvironment should be kept in mind.

Tumor Mutational Burden

Cancer cells can be recognized by the immune system if there are tumor-specific antigens on their surface, and these arise as a result of somatic mutations in TC (14–16, 41, 42). During TC transformation, their genetic materials are very unstable, and gene reparation does not always occur properly. The total number of mutations within a tumor genome counted per coding area of a tumor genome is defined as the TMB (39). A higher number of somatic mutations causes an increased number of neoantigens, which translates into increased immunogenicity of such tissues (39). Cancer tissues with high TMB are thought to be more sensitive to immunological checkpoint inhibitors. Therefore, TMB could be a potential important biomarker in qualification to ICI therapy. Indeed, it has been used in numerous clinical studies (39, 41, 42).

The first studies that indicated its predictive value related to second-line therapy were clinical trials with atezolizumab (24, 31, 33). The OAK and POPLAR studies assessed TMB in patients' blood and used a different cutoff level for TMB: 10, 16, and 20 mutations (mut) per megabase (Mb). Both studies reported a positive correlation between the number of mutations and OS as well as PFS of patients treated with atezolizumab. Moreover, both studies used the same platform for TMB assessment (Foundation One) (24, 31, 33, 35, 36).

The CheckMate-227 study is extremely important for the use of TMB as a predictive marker. In this study, combination therapy with ipilimumab and nivolumab was administered in first-line settings for chemotherapy-naive stage IV or recurrent NSCLC patients (32, 43, 44). The cutoff level for TMB was estimated at 10 mut/Mb. A significantly higher OS (18.3 months) was observed for high TMB patients (≥10 mut/Mb) when compared with patients (12.7 months) with low TMB (<10 mut/Mb). Furthermore, the significant efficacy of immunotherapy observed in patients with high TMB was irrespective of PD-L1 expression on tumor cells. The benefit of combination immunotherapy was observed even in patients with high TMB and <1% of TC with PD-L1 expression (32, 43, 44).

This biomarker could serve as a more sensitive predictor of immunotherapy benefit than PD L1 expression on TC. However, it does not happen because, as a biomarker, TMB has some strong limitations (44–46). First, different clinical studies used various cutoff levels for defining TMB, ranging from 10 to 15 mut/Mb in tissue and from 6 to even 20 mut/Mb in plasma-derived, cell-free DNA (44, 47). In some studies, the cutoff scale was two points and in others 3 points and some of the studies defined TMB as high, medium, or low. In this regard, there is no standard definition of TMB that could be used to determine the level of mutations in further studies. However, the CheckMate 568 study used combination therapy (nivolumab and ipilimumab in untreated advanced NSCLC patients) and demonstrated that there was no evidence of increased immunotherapy efficacy in patients with very high TMB (≥15 mut/Mb) compared to patients with high TMB (≥10 mut/Mb) (43).

Second, different platforms were used for TMB estimation and various genetic techniques, including whole genome sequencing (WGS), whole exome sequencing (WES), or comprehensive genomic sequencing (CGS). Some panels require parallel sequencing of a paired normal specimen to exclude germline variants from analysis; others remove germline variants from tumor sequencing results (39, 45, 46). A harmonization study of TMB determination in NSCLC samples using three different commercially available sequencing methods was conducted by Garido-Martin and colleagues. They suggested that wider sequencing for more accurate TMB assessment is needed to reduced misclassification (48).

Ultimately, different materials were tested from NSCLC patients: tissue biopsies or peripheral blood. It should be noted that, in both peripheral blood and tumor tissue, the percentage of results that could not be analyzed was relatively high (32, 47). In the CheckMate 227 study, which used tissue materials and the Foundation One CDx assay, the rejection rate was estimated at 47% of analyzed specimens (32). This suggests that, for reliable TMB testing, particularly good quality material is required. These facts translated into FDA registration of nivolumab in combination with ipilimumab in advanced NSCLC patients based on the results of the CheckMate 227 study. This combination therapy can be administered as first-line therapy in patients with ≥1% of TC expressing PD-L1. TMB in these patients does not need to be evaluated (11, 32, 39, 43).

Taken together, TMB has a notably great potential as a predictive biomarker. Indeed, further standardization of methods used in TMB assessment and systematic evaluation of TMB across different sequencing platforms should be undertaken before it is fully incorporated into clinics.

Immunoprofile and Gene Expression Signature of Tumor Tissue

Studies carried out in many different cancers have proven that the presence of IC, especially tumor infiltrating T lymphocytes (TILs) in the tumor tissue, is associated with higher benefits from immunotherapy (14–16, 49, 50). These observations are widely described in patients with breast cancer or melanoma (49, 50). Moreover, using data regarding ICI effectiveness in various malignancies, it has been indicated that tumors have three immunoprofiles based on their immune system activation: 1) "hot" tumors, which are strongly infiltrated by T lymphocytes and with many inflammatory signals; 2) "cold" tumors, which have scant IC infiltration or inflammatory signs; and 3) tumors with immune exclusion, in which immune cells are at the periphery or within the stromal tissue (49–51).

Are similar divisions of cancerous tissue described in NSCLC, and even more interestingly, has analysis of the immune system in cancerous tissue ever been used as a predictor for ICI efficacy?

In the case of lung cancer, it seems that a clear division into three types of tumor tissue has never been used prospectively as an ICI predictor in clinical trials. Rather, the immune gene signature profile, particularly those associated with IC activation (e.g., INF-γ signaling), instead of immunological examination, is correlated with immunotherapy outcome (14, 15, 31). In the POPLAR trial, in which the efficacy of atezolizumab was compared with docetaxel in a second-line setting, retrospective analysis showed that significant improvement in patient survival was associated with a high expression of the interferon-γ gene and genes associated with the T-effector activation (defined by *CD8A*, *GZMA*, *GZMB*, *IFN-γ*, *EOMES*, *CXCL9*, *CXCL10*, and *TBX21* gene expression) (31). All these genes had high co-expression in tested tumor specimens, which have been previously associated with activated T cells, immune cytolytic activity, and interferon-γ expression (31). It is obvious that tissue with high expression of these mentioned genes meets the criteria for a "hot, inflamed tumor," but it was based on genetic, not immunological, examination. The "hot" tumors are associated with denser PD-1-positive T lymphocytes infiltration with a preexisting primed immune response, and they are more likely to respond to an anti-PD-1 or anti-PD-L1 blockade used as monotherapy (31, 49).

Are these relationships also observed when we use a combination of immunotherapy, which seems to have a great importance for the future? In the IMpower 150 study, among patients with no PD-L1 expression on TC, with low expression of the genes responsible for T-effector activation, and with liver metastases, a significantly longer median PFS was observed in the group of patients receiving combination therapy (atezolizumab, bevacizumab, chemotherapy) than in patients receiving only bevacizumab with platinum doublets (33). However, when tissue samples were qualified as "inflamed," more benefits from combination therapy were observed in patients carrying "hot" tumors.

The greater efficacy of immunotherapy in patients with "inflamed" than in patients with "non-inflamed" tumors seems to be well documented in the literature (50, 51). What about the tumor, where the preexisting immune response is located at the invasive tumor margin? Lung cancer trials are rather scarce on this observation. However, it seems, based on melanoma trials, that tumor regression after therapeutic PD-1 blockade requires tumor infiltration by CD8-positive cells (50). Pretreatment samples obtained from melanoma patients who later responded to pembrolizumab therapy showed a higher number of CD8-positive, PD-1-positive, and PD-L1-expressing cells at the invasive tumor margin and inside tumors (52).

Currently, none of anti-PD-1 or anti-PD-L1 antibodies could be administered based on the immunological status of the tumor tissue (11, 12). However, immunological analysis or estimation of the gene expression profile in cancer tissue could be considered to be a reliable biomarker in the prospective qualification for immunotherapy. What should be chosen for the future direction? Immunological analysis of the existing immune response in cancer tissue could be added into the basic pathomorphological diagnosis. This is a relatively quick and inexpensive technique, but it requires several serially cut tissue specimens. Molecular analysis of cancerous tissue evaluated by gene expression could be carried out simultaneously in one tissue fragment, but it requires a specific molecular platform as a microarray. However, for both these methods, a bright future is ahead, and expanding the benefits from immunotherapy based on profiling of immune and genetic characteristic of tumors is possible, but prospective validation is still needed.

Genetics Biomarkers

Very recent studies indicate that some genetic abnormalities could be considered as predictive biomarkers for immunotherapy. *STK11/LKB1*-inactivating mutations have been significantly linked to a primary resistance to PD-1 inhibitors (53). Patients harboring the *STK11* mutation had a significantly lower expression of PD-L1 molecules on TC and higher TMB score and no clinical benefits were observed when they received immune checkpoint inhibitors with a median survival of only 6 months. Moreover, the presence of this mutation strongly correlated with the low immune cell infiltration within the tumor tissue (53). That indicates that an *STK11*-positive tumor could be defined as the cold type, which directly translates into poor immunogenicity. Quite often the *STK11* mutation significantly coexists with the *KRAS* and *KEAP1* mutations in cancer patients. The kelch-like ECH-associated protein 1 (Keap1)-nuclear factor erythroid 2-related factor 2 (Nrf2) intracellular pathway is defined as a factor regulating genes related to the cellular protective response as well as to resisting the action of chemotherapy drugs (54, 55). Malfunctioning of *Nrf2* and *Keap1* genes has been observed in lung cancer, and it is possible that they are associated with tumor progression, cytoprotection, and poor prognosis. However, clinical implementation of Nrf2 inhibitors in patients with advanced NSCLC may be a useful therapeutic approach for patients harboring *KEAP1-NRF2* mutations, increasing the chance for clinical response (54, 55).

In the context of genetic markers, their determinations seem to be of great importance in predicting resistance to immunotherapy. T cell–mediated cytotoxicity could be deregulated by mutations in genes involved in chromatin remodeling pathways. The mutations in the *SWI/SNF* (SWItch/sucrose nonfermentable) complex as well as in the *PBAF* complex (PBRM1, ARID2, and BRD7) regulate the chromatin opening for the IFN pathway in TC, resulting in an increased resistance to lymphocyte cytotoxicity. This resistance can be reversed by *PBRM1* as well as *ARID1A* gene inactivation (56).

BIOMARKERS RELATED TO PERIPHERAL BLOOD

One could imagine an ideal situation in which biomarker determinations for ICI qualification is performed in a material as easily accessible as peripheral blood. This is already established for patients progressing on EGFR tyrosine kinase inhibitors when the presence of the Thr790Met mutation in the *EGFR* gene is examined in peripheral blood for osimertinib qualification (57, 58). Is there any chance that biomarkers tested in peripheral blood would indicate a group of patients benefiting more from immunotherapy? To date, most published analysis of peripheral blood biomarkers has been tested retrospectively (12–14). However, it seems that they have a lot of information about the activity of the immune system in cancer patients.

PERIPHERAL BLOOD SOLUBLE BIOMARKERS

The most investigated serum soluble biomarker is blood tumor mutational burden (bTMB), estimated by commercial platforms (e.g., the FoundationOne CDx assay) in cell-free DNA (not in peripheral blood circulating cancer cells) (59, 60). The most recognizable studies that determined bTMB were POPLAR, OAK, and CheckMate 227 (24, 31, 32). Gandara et al. described a novel, technically robust, blood-based assay to measure bTMB based on hybridization-capture methodology, which is distinct from tissue-based approaches (47). First, they showed positive correlation between blood and tissue TMB in advanced NSCLC patients treated with second- or third-line immunotherapy included in the POPLAR trial. The cutoff points for bTMB that significantly correlated with outcomes of patients treated with atezolizumab were confirmed in the OAK study (24, 31, 47). They found that significantly longer PFS in atezolizumab-treated patients was associated with higher bTMB, and the definition of high TMB was estimated as ≥16 mut/Mb (24, 31, 47). Both studies have undoubtedly shown that bTMB could be a predictive biomarker for ICI qualification. Notwithstanding patients with bTMB ≥16 mut/Mb showed benefits from combination immunotherapy (tremelimumab plus durvalumab) in the MYSTIC clinical trial. In addition, patients with TMB ≥10 mut/Mb in tissue usually had TMB ≥16 mut/Mb in their blood serum (61, 62). The MYSTIC trial was a negative study in which the clinical benefit of combination therapy over chemotherapy was not demonstrated, but this study allowed a prospective determination of the TMB ≥10 mut/Mb cutoff threshold for the CheckMate 227 study.

PERIPHERAL BLOOD–SOLUBLE PD-1 AND PD-L1

The soluble form of PD-L1 (sPD-L1) is usually undetectable in the plasma of healthy people (63). However, detection of sPD-L1 is associated with a poor prognosis in various cancers. Moreover, a high level of sPD-L1 is associated with systemic inflammation and with activation of a nonspecific immune response (63). Taken together, this factor could be considered a predictive marker for immunotherapy qualification. So far, only one study has looked at the use of sPD-L1 as a prognostic factor in NSCLC patients. Interestingly, in the group of EGFR-mutated NSCLC patients, the increased level of sPD-L1 during erlotinib therapy was associated with a better prognosis. It is remarkably interesting because it is obviously known that patients with driving mutations do not receive benefits from immunotherapy (63). Meyo MT et al. showed the potential predictive role of soluble sPD-1 and sPD-L1 expression examination in metastatic NSCLC patients receiving nivolumab therapy (63). After two cycles of nivolumab therapy, increased sPD-1 levels, compared with the baseline value, independently correlated with longer PFS (adjusted HR=3.32; p=0.013) and OS (adjusted HR=0.33; p=0.006), and this relation was not seen when analyzing other soluble biomarkers (e.g., sCD40L, sCD44, or VEGFA). The authors proposed that composite biomarker analysis using sPD-1 and sPD-L1 could predict nivolumab efficacy (63). Zhang J et al. determined the expression of circulating PD-L1 in samples taken from 109 advanced NSCLC and 65 healthy patients (64). The results were analyzed with the association between clinicopathologic features and prognosis. First, Zhang J et al. showed higher PD-L1 expression in advanced NSCLC patients compared with the healthy controls (p<0.001). Moreover, high PD-L1 expression was positively correlated with shorter OS compared with low expression (18.7 vs. 26.8 months, p < 0.001). The presented results may give hope for the future use of sPD-1 or sPD-L1 determinations as prognostic factors (64). Moreover, the high levels of these molecules were related to intense inflammation and unspecific immune response activation, which is also considered to be a positive factor from immunotherapy benefits.

PLASMA-CIRCULATING TUMOR DNA AND PD-L1-CARRIED EXOSOMES

When we discuss the determination of predictive factors in a patient's blood serum, do not forget about the possibility of examining plasma-circulating tumor DNA (ctDNA). Ricciuti B et al. showed that assessment of plasma ctDNA would enable early detection of response to immunotherapy in NSCLC patients even before radiological examinations (65). Advanced NSCLC patients treated with first-line pembrolizumab +/- platinum doublet chemotherapy were enrolled in this study, and plasma samples were collected prior to starting therapy and serially during treatment. ctDNA was analyzed by NGS using targeted amplification of hot spots (65). Ricciuti B et al. showed that median PFS (mPFS) and median OS (mOS) were significantly longer among patients with low ctDNA levels tested at baseline compared with those with an increase in ctDNA (mPFS: 13.7 vs. 3.4 months, HR:0.20, P < 0.01; mOS: 32.8 vs. 14.7 months, HR:0.06, P < 0.01) (65). Similarly, Jia N et al., in a study of metastatic colorectal cancer patients treated with a first-line chemotherapy regimen, showed that changes in ctDNA determined by various techniques may have a strong predictive value for the assessment of patients' responses (66). Taken together, these results suggest that rapid changes in ctDNA could be applied as an early pharmacodynamic biomarker of response or resistance to immunotherapies (65, 66). Unfortunately, today it seems that the potential related to ctDNA examination is not fully utilized in the clinic.

The presence of exosomes that carry PD-L1 molecules on their surface may be another predictive factor of response to anti-PD-1 or anti-PD-L1 antibody therapy (67, 68). Exosomes, which are extracellular vehicles, are produced by cancer cells and released into the tumor microenvironment. In malignant melanoma patients, the high level of PD-L1-carried exosomes positively correlated with IFN-γ and indicated a high-level stimulation of an adaptive response in the early course of the disease (67, 68). Studies reported by Chen G et al. indicated that the level of PD-L1-carried exosomes could be a predictive factor that stratifies patients qualified for immunotherapy into two groups: responders with a high level of PD-L1-carried exosomes and nonresponders with a low level of these molecules (69). However, there are two important issues that should be kept in mind. First, there are methodological difficulties in examining the level of exosomes. At present, this test is not performed as a routine predictive factor but as research used for scientific purposes. Second, we should consider whether patients with high levels of PD-L1-carried exosomes should be treated with anti-PD-L1 or anti-PD-1 monoclonal antibodies or with antibodies specifically blocking PD-L1 exosomes or with combination therapy that can lock both of these points. These questions need to be answered in the future.

PERIPHERAL BLOOD CELLULAR BIOMARKERS

We should consider the use of conventional signs of inflammation tested in peripheral blood, such as LDH, C-reactive protein, or IL-6 concentration. Current data indicate only retrospective analysis of inflammatory-associated factors in NSCLC patients who received immunotherapy (12–15).

The simple analysis of selected peripheral blood parameters provides basic but particularly important information about the patients' immune system status. However, it is problematic to talk about predictive factors based on simple blood testing. This testing could be a great source of information about rapid progression during ICI therapy (70). For instance, the neutrophil-to-lymphocyte ratio (NLR), which could be simply calculated from a complete blood testing report, attracted a lot of interest regarding detection of rapid progression during ICI treatment (71, 72). The studies conducted in the tumor microenvironment of different solid cancers demonstrated that increased neutrophil infiltration should be considered as a factor promoting tumor progression (70–72). The NLR has also been studied in NSCLC patients. Takeda and colleagues reported that NLR could distinguish between nonresponders and responders to nivolumab therapy at an early stage of treatment, which is crucial for rapid progression diagnosis (73). The results show that low NLR (<5) after 4 weeks of nivolumab administration was significantly associated with higher median PFS compared to patients with NLR≥5. Takeda et al. indicate that the expression of these markers fluctuates dramatically during treatment; therefore, repeated evaluation is essential (73). Liu J and colleagues explored the systemic immune-inflammation index (SII), which combines NLR and platelet-to-lymphocyte ratio (PLR) (74). SII is a novel inflammatory marker, and it is considered to be an independent risk factor for the development of solid cancer. Low SII, NLR, and PLR were significantly associated with higher median PFS for metastatic NSCLC patients treated with nivolumab as second- or third-line treatment (74).

A literature review shows that more effort is made to retrospectively assess baseline peripheral blood biomarkers and associate them with clinical outcomes in NSCLC patients treated with immunotherapy (71, 72). Tanizaki and colleagues evaluated the relationship between survival and peripheral blood parameters measured before nivolumab initiation, including absolute neutrophil count (ANC), absolute lymphocyte count (ALC), absolute monocyte count, absolute eosinophil count (AEC), serum C-reactive protein, and lactate dehydrogenase concentrations (70). Low ANC, high ALC, and high AEC were significantly and independently associated with both higher mPFS and mOS in multivariable analysis. Additionally, the patients with only one positive predictive factor had a significantly worse outcome than those with two or three factors. All patients with ≥50% PD-L1 expression on TC had at least two favorable factors (70). This may suggest that high PD-L1 expression on TC influences systemic inflammation parameters, and combined analysis of those parameters could better predict response to ICI therapy. Unfortunately, the studies have been conducted on a small group of patients, and future validation is still necessary.

Some studies report that clinical benefits could be predicted based on regulatory T cell examination in patients with melanoma (75). Moreover, a high percentage of myeloid-derived stem cells (MDSCs) in peripheral blood was negatively correlated with the clinical benefit for ipilimumab-treated patients (75). Regrettably, those examinations are of very marginal importance.

CONCLUSION

Unquestionably, the effectiveness of immunotherapy has been proven in many clinical studies and documented by numerous registration approaches. Nevertheless, the issue that still raises some concerns is the use of appropriate biomarkers for qualification of cancer patients to immunotherapy. The presented work summarizes the most important information about biomarkers that could be used in the clinic. All this information is summarized in **Table 1**, but be aware of the following points. First, NSCLC patients should always be qualified for immunotherapy in regard to the registration summary of each immunotherapeutic based on the predictive factors that are dedicated to them. Currently, expression of the PD-L1 molecule on TC for immunotherapy of advanced NSCLC patients is the only predictive factor validated in prospective clinical trials. However, recently, new immunotherapeutic registrations are based on TMB as a predictive factor although this has not been validated as deeply as PD-L1 expression.

Based on the clinical trials conducted so far, we could conclude that one perfect predictive biomarker does not exist, and during qualifying cancer patients for immunotherapy, at least two biomarkers should be taken into account. One should remember that the immune system is a complex network of intercellular interactions, and it is difficult to talk about a single factor that determines its activity. Unfortunately, it seems that we will never achieve the situation that occurs for molecularly targeted therapy, in which one driving mutation affects treatment effectiveness. In addition, the situation with biomarkers could be more complicated when new immunotherapies targeting the remaining negative immune control points, anti-TIGIT or anti-TIM-3, are introduced in the clinic.

TABLE 1 | Summary of the most important advantages or disadvantages of the described biomarkers used in qualification of NSCLC patients to immunotherapy.

Biomarkers related to tumor tissue	
PD-L1 expression on tumor cells or tumor-infiltrating-immune cells	• only validated biomarker in many prospective trials • positivity for PD-L1 expression was defined using different values of PD-L positive tumor cells percentage • evaluation of percentage of tumor area infiltrated with immune cells expressing PD-L1 is extremely difficult and useless • expression was tested with different platforms • tumor tissue could demonstrate heterogenicity for PD-L1 expression • PD-L1 expression could depend on the histological type of tumor cells and patients' history of treatment
Tumor mutational burden	• proven to be a valuable factor in combination therapy regardless of PD-L1 expression • various cutoff levels for defining TMB level • different platforms were used for TMB estimation • different samples were tested for TMB with high rejection rate related to tumor samples
Immunoprofile of tumor tissue	• has never been used in prospective trials with ICI therapy • immunological analysis could be added into the basic pathomorphological diagnosis • relatively quick and inexpensive technique • requires several serially cut tissue specimens
Gene expression signature	• interferon-γ gene signature retrospectively demonstrated predictive value for ICIs therapy • molecular analysis could be carried out simultaneously in one tissue specimen • required specific molecular platform
Mutations in immunotherapy-resistance genes: *STK11*, *KEAP1*	• estimated by NGS technique or single-gene testing • significantly associated with poorer OS • lacks prospective validation in clinical trials
Biomarkers related to peripheral blood	
Peripheral blood-soluble biomarkers	
Blood TMB	• positive correlation between blood and tissue TMB was shown • determined in the most easily accessible blood samples • has never been used prospectively as an ICI therapy predictor
Soluble PD-1, PD-L1	• increase level at baseline correlated with ICI benefit • used as additional research • used only as retrospective factors
ctDNA and PD-L1-carried exosomes	• rapid changes in ctDNA as an early pharmacodynamic biomarker of response or resistance to ICIs • used as additional research • used only as retrospective factors
Inflammation parameters tested in blood analysis: LDH, C-reactive protein, IL-6 plasma, or serum concentration	• no impact on ICI effectiveness • used as additional research • usually in scientific research
Peripheral blood cellular biomarkers	
Neutrophil-to-lymphocyte ratio (NLR)	• simple analysis performed during completed blood testing • could be a great source of information about the rapid progression during ICI therapy • it fluctuates dramatically during treatment; repeated evaluation is essential
Systemic inflammation parameters: absolute neutrophil count (ANC), absolute lymphocyte count (ALC), absolute monocyte count, absolute eosinophil count (AEC)	• has never been used prospectively as a ICI predictor • significantly and independently associated with PFS and OS • systemic inflammation parameters combined with PD-L1 expression could better predict response for ICIs therapy

Second, we do not dismiss the possibility of using knowledge about additional biomarkers. We should also remember that many biomarkers that have not been registered so far can greatly facilitate monitoring of immunotherapy effectiveness. They are imperfect indeed but still could be important to prevent rapid tumor progression or for identification of the site effects of immunotherapy.

AUTHOR CONTRIBUTIONS

KW-K—literature review, preparing the manuscript, editing the manuscript TK—literature review, preparing the manuscript. All authors contributed to the article and approved the submitted version.

REFERENCES

1. Nicholson LD. The immune system. *Essays Biochem* (2016) 60(3):275–301. doi: 10.1042/EBC20160017
2. Dunn GP, Bruce AT, Ikeda H, LJ O, Schreiber RD. Cancer immunoediting: from immunosurveillance to tumor escape. *Nat Immunol* (2002) 3(11):991–98. doi: 10.1038/ni1102-991
3. Chen DS, Mellman I. Oncology meets immunology: the cancer-immunity cycle. *Immunity* (2013) 39(1):1–10. doi: 10.1016/j.immuni.2013.07.012
4. Chen DS, Mellman I. Elements of cancer immunity and the cancer-immune set point. *Nature* (2017) 18;541(7637):321–30. doi: 10.1038/nature21349
5. Brunner-Weinzierl MC, Rudd CE. CTLA-4 and PD-1 control of T-cell motility and migration: implications for tumor immunotherapy. *Front Immunol* (2018) 9:2737. doi: 10.3389/fimmu.2018.02737. eCollection 2018.
6. Buchbinder EI, Desai A. CTLA-4 and PD-1 pathways: similarities, differences, and implications of their inhibition. *Am J Clin Oncol* (2016) 39(1):98–106. doi: 10.1097/COC.0000000000000239
7. The Scientist. (2018). Available at: https://www.the-scientist.com/news-opinion/james-allison-and-tasuku-honjo-win-nobel-prize-64879 (Accessed May 26, 2020).
8. Valecha GK, Vennepureddy A, Ibrahim U, Safa F, Samra B, Atallah JP. Anti-PD-1/PD-L1 antibodies in non-small cell lung cancer: the era of immunotherapy. *Expert Rev Anticancer Ther* (2017) 17(1):47–59. doi: 10.1080/14737140.2017.1259574
9. Lee HT, Lee SH, Heo YS. Molecular interactions of antibody drugs targeting PD-1, PD-L1, and CTLA-4 in immuno-oncology. *Molecules* (2019) 26;24 (6):1190. doi: 10.3390/molecules24061190
10. Chen R, Tao Y, Xu X, Shan L, Jiang H, Yin Q, et al. The efficacy and safety of nivolumab, pembrolizumab, and atezolizumab in treatment of advanced non-small cell lung cancer. *Discov Med* (2018) 26(143):155–66.
11. Hargadon KM, Johnson CE, Williams CJ. Immune checkpoint blockade therapy for cancer: An overview of FDA-approved immune checkpoint inhibitors. *Int Immunopharmacol* (2018) 62:29–39. doi: 10.1016/j.intimp.2018.06.001
12. Bodor JN, Boumber Y, Borghaei H. Biomarkers for immune checkpoint inhibition in non-small cell lung cancer (NSCLC). *Cancer* (2020) 126(2):260–70. doi: 10.1002/cncr.32468
13. Cyriac G, Gandhi L. Emerging biomarkers for immune checkpoint inhibition in lung cancer. *Semin Cancer Biol* (2018) 52(Pt 2):269–77. doi: 10.1016/j.semcancer.2018.05.006
14. Gibney GT, Weiner LM, Atkins MB. Predictive biomarkers for checkpoint inhibitor-based immunotherapy. *Lancet Oncol* (2016) 17(12):e542–2. doi: 10.1016/S1470-2045(16)30406-5
15. Spencer KR, Wang J, Silk AW, Ganesan S, Kaufman HL, Mehnert JM. Biomarkers for immunotherapy: current developments and challenges. *Am Soc Clin Oncol Educ Book* (2016) 35:e493. doi: 10.1200/EDBK_160766
16. Weber JS. Biomarkers for checkpoint inhibition. *Am Soc Clin Oncol Educ Book* (2017) 37:205–09. doi: 10.14694/EDBK_175463
17. Ancevski Hunter K, Socinski MA, Villaruz LC. PD-L1 testing in guiding patient selection for PD-1/PD-L1 inhibitor therapy in lung cancer. *Mol Diagn Ther* (2018) 22(1):1–10. doi: 10.1007/s40291-017-0308-6
18. Reck M, Rodríguez-Abreu D, Robinson AG, Hui R, Csőszi T, Fülöp A, et al. Updated analysis of Keynote-024: pembrolizumab versus platinum-based chemotherapy for advanced non-small-cell lung cancer with PD-L1 tumor proportion score of 50% or greater. *J Clin Oncol* (2019) 37(7):537–46. doi: 10.1200/JCO.18.00149
19. Mok TSK, Wu YL, Kudaba I, Kowalski DM, Cho BC, Turna HZ, et al. Pembrolizumab versus chemotherapy for previously untreated, PD-L1-expressing, locally advanced or metastatic non-small-cell lung cancer (KEYNOTE-042): a randomised, open-label, controlled, phase 3 trial. *Lancet* (2019) 4;393(10183):1819–30. doi: 10.1016/S0140-6736(18)32409-7
20. Gandhi L, Rodríguez-Abreu D, Gadgeel S, Esteban E, Felip E, De Angelis F, et al. Pembrolizumab plus chemotherapy in metastatic non-small-cell lung cancer. *N Engl J Med* (2018) 31;378(22):2078–92. doi: 10.1056/NEJMoa1801005
21. Piper AJ, Sehgal K, Costa DB, Rangachari D. Can PD-L1 tumor proportion score be used as the key to unlocking the KEYNOTE studies of pembrolizumab in advanced lung cancer? *Transl Lung Cancer Res* (2019) 8 (5):715–22. doi: 10.21037/tlcr.2019.05.12
22. Borghaei H, Paz-Ares L, Horn L, Spigel DR, Steins M, Ready NE, et al. Nivolumab versus docetaxel in advanced nonsquamous non-small-cell lung cancer. *N Engl J Med* (2015) 373(17):1627–39. doi: 10.1056/NEJMoa1507643
23. Brahmer J, Reckamp KL, Baas P, Crinò L, Eberhardt WE, Poddubskaya E, et al. Nivolumab versus docetaxel in advanced squamous-cell non-small-cell lung cancer. *N Engl J Med* (2015) 373(2):123–35. doi: 10.1056/NEJMoa1504627
24. Rittmeyer A, Barlesi F, Waterkamp D, Park K, Ciardiello F, von Pawel J, et al. Atezolizumab versus docetaxel in patients with previously treated non-small-cell lung cancer (OAK): a phase 3, open-label, multicentre randomised controlled trial. *Lancet* (2017) 389(10066):255–65. doi: 10.1016/S0140-6736(16)32517-X
25. Herbst RS, Baas P, Kim DW, Felip E, Pérez-Gracia JL, Han JY, et al. Pembrolizumab versus docetaxel for previously treated, PD-L1-positive, advanced non-small-cell lung cancer (KEYNOTE-010): a randomised controlled trial. *Lancet* (2016) 9;387(10027):1540–50. doi: 10.1016/S0140-6736(15)01281-7
26. Paz-Ares L, Luft A, Vicente D, Tafreshi A, Gümüş M, Mazières J, et al. Pembrolizumab plus chemotherapy for squamous non-small-cell lung cancer. *N Engl J Med* (2018) 22;379(21):2040–51. doi: 10.1056/NEJMoa1810865
27. Antonia SJ, Villegas A, Daniel D, Vicente D, Murakami S, Hui R, et al. Overall survival with durvalumab after chemoradiotherapy in stage III NSCLC. *N Engl J Med* (2018) 379(24):2342–50. doi: 10.1056/NEJMoa1809697
28. Uemura T, Hida T. Durvalumab showed long and durable effects after chemoradiotherapy in stage III non-small cell lung cancer: results of the PACIFIC study. *J Thorac Dis* (2018) 10(Suppl 9):S1108–12. doi: 10.21037/jtd.2018.03.180
29. Clinical Trials. *Nivolumab and ipilimumab* (20219). Available at: https://clinicaltrials.gov/ct2/show/record/NCT03215706 (Accessed May 28, 2020).
30. Hellmann MD, Paz-Ares L, Bernabe Caro R, Zurawski B, Kim SW, Carcereny Costa E, et al. Nivolumab plus ipilimumab in advanced non-small-cell lung cancer. *N Engl J Med* (2019) 21;381(21):2020–31. doi: 10.1056/NEJMoa1910231
31. Fehrenbacher L, Spira A, Ballinger M, Kowanetz M, Vansteenkiste J, Mazieres J, et al. Atezolizumab versus docetaxel for patients with previously treated non-small-cell lung cancer (POPLAR): a multicentre, open-label, phase 2 randomised controlled trial. *Lancet* (2016) 30;387(10030):1837–46. doi: 10.1016/S0140-6736(16)00587-0
32. Reck M, Schenker M, Lee KH, Provencio M, Nishio M, Lesniewski-Kmak K, et al. Nivolumab plus ipilimumab versus chemotherapy as first-line treatment in advanced non-small-cell lung cancer with high tumour mutational burden: patient-reported outcomes results from the randomised, open-label, phase III CheckMate 227 trial. *Eur J Cancer* (2019) 116:137–47. doi: 10.1016/j.ejca.2019.05.008
33. Socinski MA, Jotte RM, Cappuzzo F, Orlandi F, Stroyakovskiy D, Nogami N, et al. Atezolizumab for first-line treatment of metastatic nonsquamous NSCLC. *N Engl J Med* (2018) 378:2288–301. doi: 10.1056/NEJMoa1716948

34. Remon J, Collazo A, Jimenez B. CheckMate 227 trial has not checked the immune-strategy in first-line setting in advanced non-small cell lung cancer. *Transl Cancer Res* (2020) 9(4):2168–70. doi: 10.21037/tcr.2020.03.09
35. Davis AA, Patel VG. The role of PD-L1 expression as a predictive biomarker: an analysis of all US Food and Drug Administration (FDA) approvals of immune checkpoint inhibitors. *J Immunother Cancer* (2019) 26;7(1):278. doi: 10.1186/s40425-019-0768-9
36. Vennapusa B, Baker B, Kowanetz M, Boone J, Menzl I, Bruey JM, et al. Development of a PD-L1 complementary diagnostic immunohistochemistry assay (SP142) for atezolizumab. *Appl Immunohistochem Mol Morphol* (2019) 27(2):92–100. doi: 10.1097/PAI.0000000000000594
37. Hirsch FR, McElhinny A, Stanforth D, Ranger-Moore J, Jansson M, Kulangara K, et al. PD-L1 immunohistochemistry assays for lung cancer: results from phase I of the Blueprint PD-L1 IHC assay comparison project. *J Thorac Oncol* (2017) 12(2):208–22. doi: 10.1016/j.jtho.2016.11.2228
38. Tsao MS, Kerr KM, Kockx M, Beasley MB, Borczuk AC, Botling J, et al. PD-L1 immunohistochemistry comparability study in real-life clinical samples: results of Blueprint phase 2 Project. *J Thorac Oncol* (2018) 13(9):1302–11. doi: 10.1016/j.jtho.2018.05.013
39. Krieger T, Pearson I, Bell J, Doherty J, Robbins P. Targeted literature review on use of tumor mutational burden status and programmed cell death ligand 1 expression to predict outcomes of checkpoint inhibitor treatment. *Diagn Pathol* (2020) 30;15(1):6. doi: 10.1186/s13000-020-0927-9
40. Mansfield AS, Aubry MC, Moser JC, Harrington SM, Dronca RS, Park SS, et al. Temporal and spatial discordance of programmed cell death-ligand 1 expression and lymphocyte tumor infiltration between paired primary lesions and brain metastases in lung cancer. *Ann Oncol* (2016) 27(10):1953–58. doi: 10.1093/annonc/mdw289
41. Fancello L, Gandini S, Pelicci PG, Mazzarella L. Tumor mutational burden quantification from targeted gene panels: major advancements and challenges. *J Immunother Cancer* (2019) 15;7(1):183. doi: 10.1186/s40425-019-0647-4
42. Greillier L, Tomasini P, Barlesi F. The clinical utility of tumor mutational burden in non-small cell lung cancer. *Transl Lung Cancer Res* (2018) 7 (6):639–46. doi: 10.21037/tlcr.2018.10.08
43. Ready N, Hellmann MD, Awad MM, Otterson GA, Gutierrez M, Gainor JF, et al. First-line nivolumab plus ipilimumab in advanced non small cell lung cancer (CheckMate 568): outcomes by programmed death ligand 1 and tumor mutational burden as biomarkers. *J Clin Oncol* (2019) 20;37(12):992–1000. doi: 10.1200/JCO.18.01042
44. Hellmann MD, Ciuleanu TE, Pluzanski A, Lee JS, Otterson GA, Audigier-Valette C, et al. Nivolumab plus ipilimumab in lung cancer with a high tumor mutational burden. *N Engl J Med* (2018) 378(22):2093–104. doi: 10.1056/NEJMoa1801946
45. Allgäuer M, Budczies J, Christopoulos P, Endris V, Lier A, Rempel E, et al. Implementing tumor mutational burden (TMB) analysis in routine diagnostics-a primer for molecular pathologists and clinicians. *Transl Lung Cancer Res* (2018) 7(6):703–15. doi: 10.21037/tlcr.2018.08.14
46. Stenzinger A, Allen JD, Maas J, Stewart MD, Merino DM, Wempe MM, et al. Tumor mutational burden standardization initiatives: Recommendations for consistent tumor mutational burden assessment in clinical samples to guide immunotherapy treatment decisions. *Genes Chromosomes Cancer* (2019) 58 (8):578–88. doi: 10.1002/gcc.22733
47. Gandara DR, Paul SM, Kowanetz M, Schleifman E, Zou W, Li Y, et al. Blood-based tumor mutational burden as a predictor of clinical benefit in non-small-cell lung cancer patients treated with atezolizumab. *Nat Med* (2018) 24 (9):1441–48. doi: 10.1038/s41591-018-0134-3
48. Garrido-Martin EM, Ramos-Paradas J, Hernandez Prieto S, Sanchez E, Rosado A, Caniego-Casas T, et al. Harmonization study of tumour mutational burden determination in non-small-cell lung cancer (NSCLC). *Ann Oncol* (2019) 30(suppl_5):v851–934. doi: 10.1093/annonc/mdz394.002
49. Bremnes RM, Busund LT, Kilvær TL, Andersen S, Richardsen E, Paulsen EE, et al. The role of tumor-infiltrating lymphocytes in development, progression, and prognosis of non-small cell lung cancer. *J Thorac Oncol* (2016) 11(6):789–800. doi: 10.1016/j.jtho.2016.01.015
50. Daud AI, Loo K, Pauli ML, Sanchez-Rodriguez R, Sandoval PM, Taravati K, et al. Tumor immune profiling predicts response to anti-PD-1 therapy in human melanoma. *J Clin Invest* (2016) 1;126(9):3447–52. doi: 10.1172/JCI87324
51. Lizotte PH, Ivanova EV, Awad MM, Jones RE, Keogh L, Liu H, et al. Multiparametric profiling of non-small-cell lung cancers reveals distinct immunophenotypes. *JCI Insight* (2016) 8;1(14):e89014. doi: 10.1172/jci.insight.89014
52. Tumeh PC, Harview CL, Yearley JH, Shintaku IP, Taylor EJ, Robert L, et al. PD-1 blockade induces responses by inhibiting adaptive immune resistance. *Nature* (2014) 27;515(7528):568–71. doi: 10.1038/nature13954
53. Wang H, Guo J, Shang X, Wang Z. Less immune cell infiltration and worse prognosis after immunotherapy for patients with lung adenocarcinoma who harbored STK11 mutation. *Int Immunopharmacol* (2020) 84:106574. doi: 10.1016/j.intimp.2020.106574
54. Barrera-Rodriguez R. Importance of the Keap1-Nrf2 pathway in NSCLC: Is it a possible biomarker? *Biomed Rep* (2018) 9:375–82. doi: 10.3892/br.2018.1143
55. Tong YH, Zhang B, Fan Y, Lin NM. Keap1-Nrf2 pathway: A promising target towards lung cancer prevention and therapeutics. *Chronic Dis Transl Med* (2015) 22;1(3):175–86. doi: 10.1016/j.cdtm.2015.09.002
56. Hung YP, Redig A, Hornick JL, Sholl LM. ARID1A mutations and expression loss in non-small cell lung carcinomas: clinicopathologic and molecular analysis. *Mod Pathol* (2020) 33:2256–68. doi: 10.1038/s41379-020-0592-2
57. Choo JR, Tan CS, Soo RA. Treatment of EGFR T790M-positive non-small cell lung cancer. *Target Oncol* (2018) 13(2):141–56. doi: 10.1007/s11523-018-0554-5
58. Ward MC, Prabhu RS, Burri SH. Osimertinib in EGFR mutation–positive advanced NSCLC. *N Engl J Med* (2018) 29;378(13):1262–63. doi: 10.1056/NEJMc1801669
59. Lam VK, Zhang J. Blood-based tumor mutation burden: continued progress toward personalizing immunotherapy in non-small cell lung cancer. *J Thorac Dis* (2019) 11(6):2208–11. doi: 10.21037/jtd.2019.05.68
60. Van Campenhout C, Meléndez B, Remmelink M, Salmon I, D'Haene N. Blood tumor mutational burden: are we ready for clinical implementation? *J Thorac Dis* (2019) 11(Suppl 15):S1906–8. doi: 10.21037/jtd.2019.07.60
61. Peters S, Cho BC, Reinmuth N, Lee KH, Luft A, Ahn MJ, et al. (2019). Tumor mutational burden (TMB) as a biomarker of survival in metastatic non-small cell lung cancer (mNSCLC): Blood and tissue TMB analysis from MYSTIC, a Phase III study of first-line durvalumab plus tremelimumab vs chemotherapy, in: *AACR Annual Meeting* (2019). 79(13 suppl). p. CT074. doi: 10.1158/1538-7445.AM2019-CT074
62. Rizvi NA, Cho BC, Reinmuth N, Lee KH, Luft A, Ahn MJ, et al. Blood tumor mutational burden (bTMB) and tumor PD-L1 as predictive biomarkers of survival in MYSTIC: First-line durvalumab (D) ± tremelimumab (T) versus chemotherapy (CT) in metastatic (m) NSCLC. *J Clin Oncol* (2019) suppl:9016. doi: 10.1200/JCO.2019.37.15_suppl.9016
63. Meyo MT, Jouinot A, Giroux-Leprieur E, Fabre E, Wislez M, Alifano M, et al. Predictive value of soluble PD-1, PD-L1, VEGFA, CD40 ligand and CD44 for nivolumab therapy in advanced non-small cell lung cancer: a case-control study. *Cancers (Basel)* (2020) 18;12(2):473. doi: 10.3390/cancers12020473
64. Zhang J, Gao J, Li Y, Nie J, Dai L, Hu W, et al. Circulating PD-L1 in NSCLC patients and the correlation between the level of PD-L1 expression and the clinical characteristics. *Thorac Cancer* (2015) 6(4):534–38. doi: 10.1111/1759-7714.12247
65. Ricciuti B, Champagne C, Jones G, Lazarus TS, Adeni AE, Cheng ML, et al. Early plasma circulating tumor DNA (ctDNA) changes to predict response to first-line pembrolizumab +/- chemotherapy in non-small cell lung cancer (NSCLC). *J Clin Oncol* (2020) 38(15 suppl):3518. doi: 10.1200/JCO.2020.38.15
66. Jia N, Sun Z, Gao X, Cheng Y, Zhou Y, Shen C, et al. Serial monitoring of circulating tumor dna in patients with metastatic colorectal cancer to predict the therapeutic response. *Front Genet* (2019) 10:470. doi: 10.3389/fgene.2019.00470
67. Daassi D, Mahoney KM, Freeman GJ. The importance of exosomal PD-L1 in tumour immune evasion. *Nat Rev Immunol* (2020) 20:209–15. doi: 10.1038/s41577-019-0264-y
68. Kugeratski FG, Kalluri R. Exosomes as mediators of immune regulation and immunotherapy in cancer. *FEBS J* (2020) 10:1–26. doi: 10.1111/febs.15558
69. Chen G, Huang AC, Zhang W, Zhang G, Wu M, Xu W, et al. Exosomal PD-L1 contributes to immunosuppression and is associated with anti-PD-1 response. *Nature* (2018) 560(7718):382–86. doi: 10.1038/s41586-018-0392-8
70. Tanizaki J, Haratani K, Hayashi H, Chiba Y, Nakamura Y, Yonesaka K, et al. Peripheral blood biomarkers associated with clinical outcome in non-small

cell lung cancer patients treated with nivolumab. *J Thorac Oncol* (2018) 13 (1):97–105. doi: 10.1016/j.jtho.2017.10.030

71. Diem S, Schmid S, Krapf M, Flatz L, Born D, Jochum W, et al. Neutrophil-to-Lymphocyte ratio (NLR) and Platelet-to-Lymphocyte ratio (PLR) as prognostic markers in patients with non-small cell lung cancer (NSCLC) treated with nivolumab. *Lung Cancer* (2017) 111:176–81. doi: 10.1016/j.lungcan.2017.07.024
72. Templeton AJ, McNamara MG, Šeruga B, Vera-Badillo FE, Aneja P, Ocaña A, et al. Prognostic role of neutrophil-to-lymphocyte ratio in solid tumors: a systematic review and meta-analysis. *J Natl Cancer Inst* (2014) 29;106(6): dju124. doi: 10.1093/jnci/dju124
73. Takeda T, Takeuchi M, Saitoh M, Takeda S. Neutrophil-to-lymphocyte ratio after four weeks of nivolumab administration as a predictive marker in patients with pretreated non-small-cell lung cancer. *Thorac Cancer* (2018) 9 (10):1291–99. doi: 10.1111/1759-7714.12838
74. Liu J, Li S, Zhang S, Liu Y, Ma L, Zhu J, et al. Systemic immune-inflammation index, neutrophil-to-lymphocyte ratio, platelet-to-lymphocyte ratio can predict clinical outcomes in patients with metastatic non-small-cell lung cancer treated with nivolumab. *J Clin Lab Anal* (2019) 33(8):e22964. doi: 10.1002/jcla.22964
75. Meyer C, Cagnon L, Costa-Nunes CM, Baumgaertner P, Montandon N, Leyvraz L, et al. Frequencies of circulating MDSC correlate with clinical outcome of melanoma patients treated with ipilimumab. *Cancer Immunol Immunother* (2014) 63(3):247–57. doi: 10.1007/s00262-013-1508-5

8

Long Progression-Free Survival of Immunotherapy for Lung Adenocarcinoma with Epidermal Growth Factor Receptor Mutation

Jianfeng Peng[1], *Xianguang Zhao*[2], *Kaikai Zhao*[3,4] *and Xiangjiao Meng*[2*]

[1] *Department of Radiation Oncology, Shandong Cancer Hospital Affiliated to Shandong First Medical University, Jinan, China,* [2] *Department of Radiation Oncology, Shandong Cancer Hospital, Jinan, China,* [3] *Department of Radiation Oncology, The First Affiliated Hospital of China Medical University, Shenyang, China,* [4] *Department of Radiation Oncology, Yantai Affiliated Hospital of Binzhou Medical University, Yantai, China*

Correspondence:
Xiangjiao Meng
mengxiangjiao@126.com

Background: Immune checkpoint inhibitors (ICIs) have been clinically proven to be efficient in non-small cell lung cancer (NSCLC). However, it has also been found that immunotherapy is not effective for all patients. For instance, some patients with epidermal growth factor receptor (EGFR) mutation tumors have a low overall response rate to ICIs. As a result, we retrospectively analyzed the efficacy of anti-programmed death-ligand 1 (anti-PD-L1) blockade (atezolizumab) treatment for a patient with EGFR mutation, and we explored the interaction between immunotherapy and EGFR mutations in NSCLC.

Case Presentation: A patient, 62-year-old non-smoking female, with lung adenocarcinoma was initially misdiagnosed as EGFR wild type and received a third-line treatment with atezolizumab, experiencing partial response (PR) and progression-free survival (PFS) for 23 months. She had later been confirmed with EGFR L858R mutation prior to taking atezolizumab. On top of that, the patient developed T790M mutation after being administered with atezolizumab instead of EGFR tyrosine kinase inhibitors (TKIs). She started with osimertinib, although the lesion continued to progress. Tumor mutational burden (TMB), PD-L1 expression, and tumor-infiltrating lymphocytes (TILs) had been tested for further analysis.

Conclusion: The case report and literature review indicate that ICIs might be more effective for L858R mutation than for other EGFR mutant subtypes, which correlates with certain potential predictors such as TMB and concurrent PD-L1 plus $CD8^+$ TIL expression. However, there is no report on progression from non-primary EGFR T790M mutation to T790M mutation of patients who neither previously suffered from EGFR-TKIs nor responded to osimertinib. This case report will offer some information to guide the investigation on how to identify those who can benefit from immunotherapy and those who do not respond to EGFR-TKIs among the patients with EGFR mutations.

Keywords: non-small cell lung cancer (NSCLC), immunotherapy, EGFR mutation, EGFR-TKIs, biomarkers

INTRODUCTION

Immunotherapy using monoclonal antibodies directed at checkpoint proteins has become the newest treatment modality in lung cancer, including PD-1, programmed death-ligand 1 (PD-L1), and CTLA4 (1). Previous studies have shown better overall survival (OS) with immune checkpoint inhibitors (ICIs) compared with second- or third-line docetaxel (2). Compared with traditional cytotoxic chemotherapy, ICI monotherapy or combination therapy has shown to be a reliable and safe first- and second-line therapy for non-small cell lung cancer (NSCLC) without driver gene mutations (3–6). Thus, National Comprehensive Cancer Network (NCCN) guidelines recommends them as first-line and second-line treatments for NSCLC patients.

However, single-agent ICIs do not appear to have a striking advantage over cytotoxic agents in NSCLC harboring epidermal growth factor receptor (EGFR) mutations (2). As a major molecular subtype in Asian lung cancer patients, EGFR mutation accounts for 40% of lung adenocarcinoma, of which the two most common mutations are exon 19 deletion (60%) and L858R missense replacement (35%) (7). The specific criteria of the choice of EGFR tyrosine kinase inhibitors (TKIs) and ICIs for NSCLC patients with EGFR mutation appear to be the focus and challenge of the current research.

This case report describes a lung adenocarcinoma patient who achieved long progression-free survival (PFS) with an EGFR mutation treated with atezolizumab.

CASE PRESENTATION

A 62-year-old non-smoking woman with cough and chest tightness was initially found to have space-occupying lesions in her lungs in a physical examination at another hospital. Then she came to our hospital for further treatment. At this time, she had an Eastern Cooperative Oncology Group (ECOG) performance status of 1. And she had no relevant medical or surgical history. Enhanced CT showed a 3.0 × 3.0 cm mass in the left lower lung with diffuse miliary metastases in both lungs and no distant lymph node metastasis. The clinical stage was T1cN0M1a, and the pathological puncture diagnosis was lung adenocarcinoma in December 2016. She refused the gene test and received first-line treatment: pemetrexed 0.5 mg/m^2 d1 + cisplatin 75 mg/m^2 d1, q3w, for six cycles from January 2017 to June 2017. From July 2017 to April 2018, pemetrexed was given 0.8 d1, q3w, for nine cycles, and the best response was stable disease (SD) (**Figure 1**). In May 2018, CT reexamination revealed multiple vertebral metastases in the spine, and the efficacy was evaluated as progressive disease (PD). Therefore, second-line treatment regimen was used: docetaxel 120 mg d1, q21d, five cycles, from May 2018 to September 2018. Then CT reexamination after the end of treatment showed that the response was PD.

This time, the patient expressed a strong desire for treatment, and we had full discussions with the patient and her family to determine the next step of treatment. On October 22, 2018, we performed genetic testing on the patient using PCR, and the results showed that EGFR, ALK, and ROS1 were all wild types (**Figure 2A**). Atezolizumab treatment was initiated on November 2, 2018, based on the results of the OAK clinical trial (6) and the guidelines. After two cycles, CT showed partial response (PR) (**Figure 3**).

At cycle 18 of atezolizumab, free triiodothyronine (FT3) decreased to 3.62 pmol/L, and the patient was treated with the addition of levothyroxine sodium tablet 50 μg qd po. Liver metastasis occurred, and lung disease progressed on October 13, 2020 (**Figure 2C**). PFS was as long as 23 months. The clinical stage at this time was T2aN0M1c. After discussion of the multidisciplinary team (MDT), pathological puncture and genetic testing were conducted again for the patient, and the results showed EGFR L858R and T790M mutations (**Figure 2B**). Research by Hsu et al. suggested that mutations in EGFR are associated with a higher

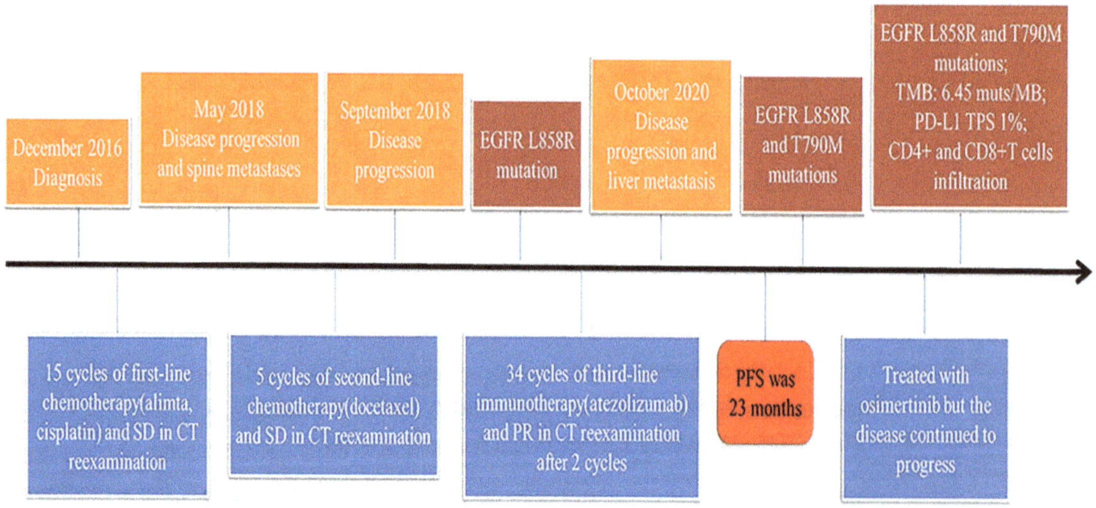

FIGURE 1 | Timeline of disease status and corresponding treatment regimens.

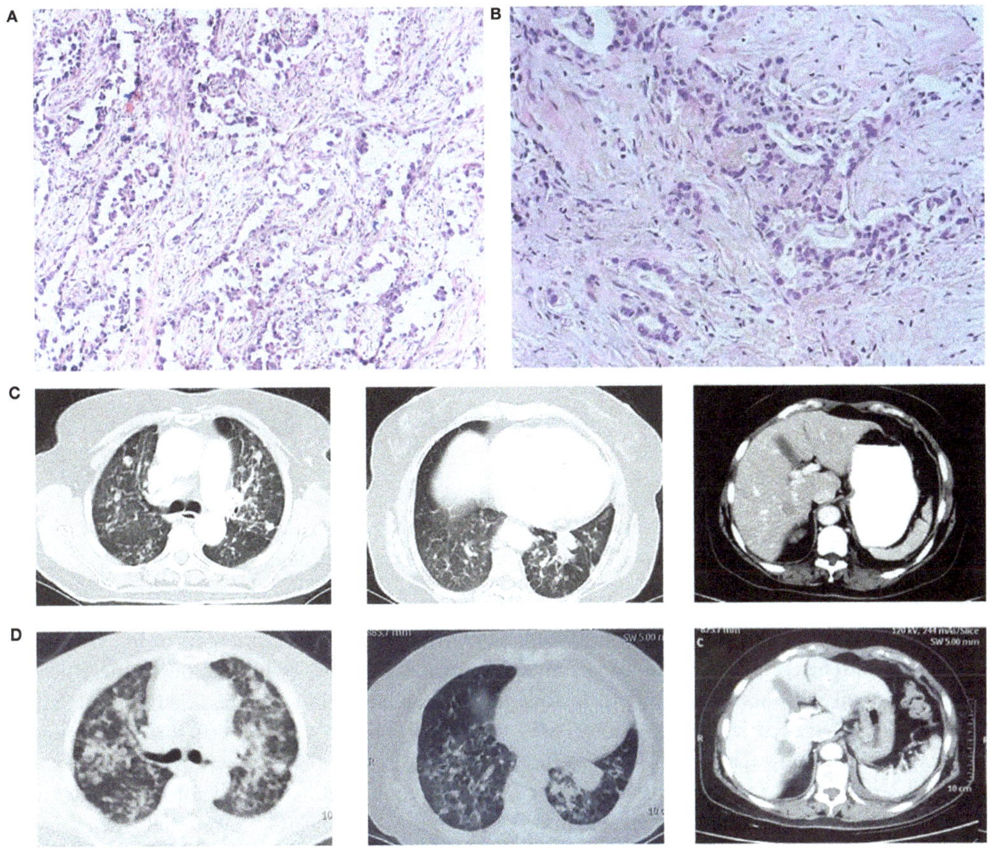

FIGURE 2 | **(A)** Pathological biopsy on October 22, 2018. **(B)** Pathological biopsy on November 11, 2020. **(C)** Lung lesion progression and liver metastasis on October 13, 2020. **(D)** Lesion progression in March 2021 after osimertinib treatment.

rate of miliary lung metastases (8); for the sake of precision, we redid genetic testing on the patient's 2018 pathological specimen using a more accurate next-generation sequencing (NGS) (9), and we found that the patient had the EGFR L858R mutation prior to the use of atezolizumab. Then the patient was treated with osimertinib in view of $EGFR^{T790M}$, but the follow-up CT until March 2021 showed that the lesion continued to progress (**Figure 2D**).

In order to explore why the patient responded well to atezolizumab but not to osimertinib, we performed the whole gene test (825 gene) by NGS and immunohistochemistry (IHC). At this time, the patient carried EGFR L858R, T790M, and TP53 R282W mutations; and her plasma sample had a low tumor mutational burden (TMB) of 6.45 muts/Mb. IHC showed PD-L1 tumor proportion score (TPS) <1% (antibody was 22C3), but the expression of PD-L1 in immune cells was 5%. In addition, $CD4^+$ and $CD8^+$ T cells were highly infiltrated (**Figure 4**).

DISCUSSION

Atezolizumab, a kind of ICIs, is a humanized monoclonal antibody that can specifically bind to PD-L1 to alter the immune escape mechanism of tumors and plays a role in anti-tumor activity (10). Several clinical trials have shown that ICIs can significantly prolong PFS and OS in tumors, whereas the benefit is limited to patients with EGFR wild type and ALK wild type. The OAK study subgroup showed that the patients with EGFR mutation received similar OS benefit with atezolizumab and docetaxel (6), which is consistent with the results of the CheckMate 057 and Keynote 010 trials (5, 11).

In this case, the patient with EGFR L858R mutation who was not pretreated with EGFR-TKIs was treated with atezolizumab. She obtained an extremely long PFS, although previous studies show different results. Some clinical trials have shown that certain EGFR mutant subtypes of tumors do respond to ICIs; for example, Hastings et al. observed that patients with EGFR L858R mutation receiving immunotherapy showed similar response rates and OS as patients with EGFR wild-type lung cancer, but they had much worse PFS (12). Her longer PFS may be related to some biomarkers. The predictive biomarkers such as PD-L1 TPS in cancer cells and microsatellite instability (13) have been approved by the U.S. Food and Drug Administration (FDA) for determining suitable advanced NSCLC patients that can benefit from ICIs (13). Moreover, other markers, including TMB, tumor-infiltrating lymphocytes (TILs), and other components of tumor microenvironment (TME), are being

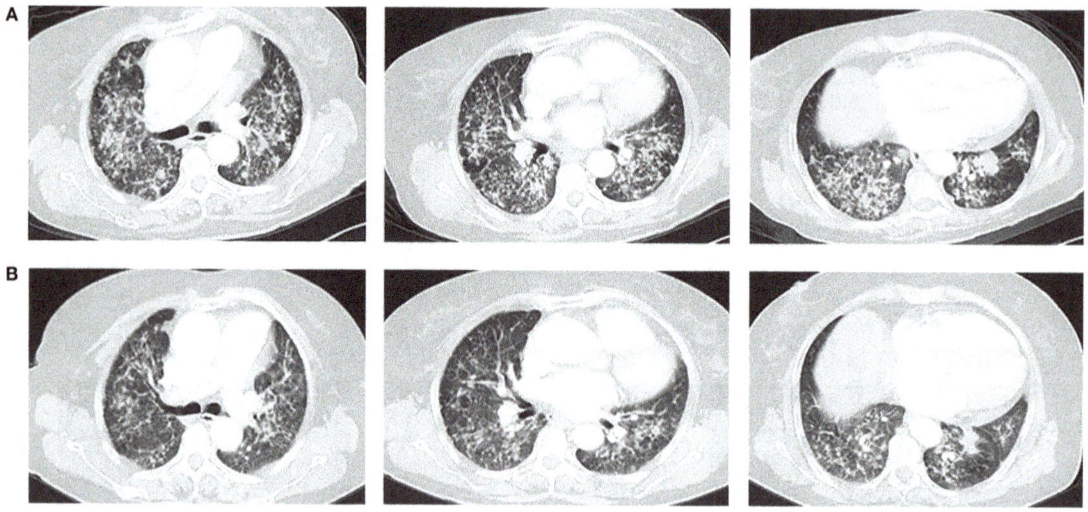

FIGURE 3 | **(A)** Chest CT on October 25, 2018. **(B)** Chest CT on December 21, 2018. The response was partial response (PR).

actively investigated (13). High level of PD-L1 expression, TMB, and CD8^{+} TIL is associated with benefits of blocking PD-L1 and may lead to better PFS, OS, and response rates (13, 14). In this case, genetic testing and IHC of this patient showed low TMB level and low PD-L1 expression but a high level of CD8^{+} TILs, which is a beneficial advantage for patient receiving immunotherapy. CD8^{+} T cell can specifically recognize tumor antigens to kill tumors directly or target cells indirectly by secreting cytokines (15). In addition, previous studies have concluded that the expression of PD-L1 on both dendritic cells and macrophages is in relation to the efficacy of ICIs (16, 17). This patient's PD-L1 expression in immune cells takes 5%, which might be one of the reasons for the response to atezolizumab. Furthermore, this patient was pretreated with multiline chemotherapeutic agents before receiving atezolizumab. Results from the ATLANTIC showed that when durvalumab is used as a third-line treatment or above, NSCLC patients who are with EGFR mutations and have at least 25% of tumor cells with PD-L1

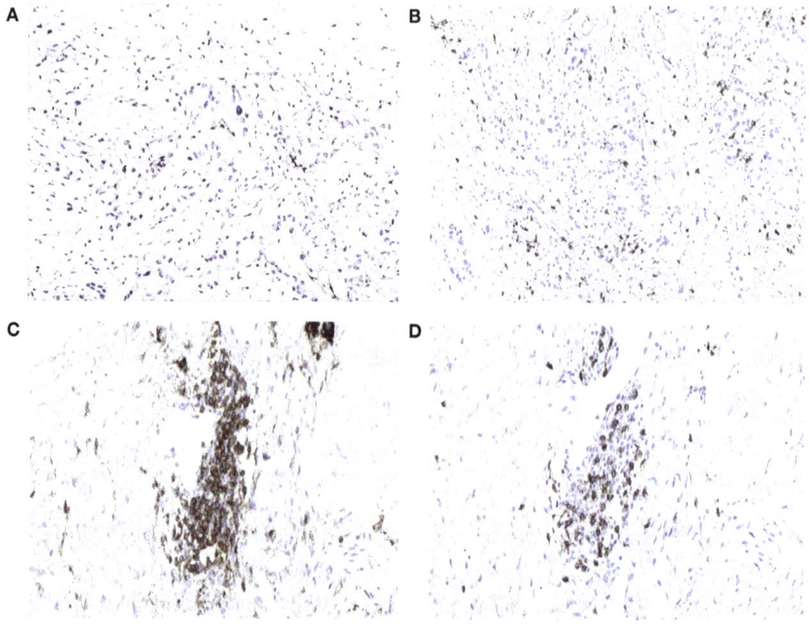

FIGURE 4 | **(A)** Programmed death-ligand 1 (PD-L1) tumor proportion score (TPS) <1%. **(B)** High infiltration of CD8^{+} tumor-infiltrating lymphocytes (TILs). **(C)** Presence of large numbers of CD4^{+} T cells in the stroma of the tumor. **(D)** Presence of large numbers of CD8^{+} T cells in the stroma of the tumor.

expression could benefit from durvalumab with an objective response rate of 12.2% (9/74 patients, 95% CI 5.7–21.8). The objective response rate in patients accounting for less than 25% of tumor cells with PD-L1 expression is only 3.6% (1/28 patients, 95% CI 0.1–18.3) (18). Therefore, for this patient, further studies are needed to confirm whether NSCLC harboring EGFR L858R mutations with a high degree of $CD8^+$ TILs might benefit from atezolizumab or even obtain longer PFS after having multiline chemotherapy. In addition, the whole gene testing of the patient revealed that she also carried the TP53 R282W mutation, which is considered to be a positive gene (19). Previous studies have found that TP53 mutation increases the expression of PD-L1, thus making patients more likely to benefit from immunotherapy (20). Wu and his team found that TP53 mutations not only triggered these changes but also increased the proportion of $CD8^+$ T cells (21), which is consistent with this case. However, a clinical retrospective study has shown a contrasting result, suggesting that TP53 mutation is negatively correlated with immunotherapy efficacy (22). Therefore, subsequent studies are needed to confirm the correlation between TP53 mutation and immunotherapy and to clarify the relevant mechanisms.

Moreover, T790M mutations are a common resistance mutation, causing about 60% resistance to EGFR-TKIs (23). T790M mutations can be divided into two types—primary or acquired. Acquired T790M mutation is usually the resistant gene after the first or second generation of EGFR-TKIs, and both primary and secondary mutations have shown good responses to osimertinib (a type of third-generation EGFR-TKIs) therapy (24, 25). The patient presented in this report with non-primary EGFR T790M mutation who developed T790M mutation after ICIs rather than EGFR-TKIs, and she had a complete failure to respond to osimertinib. It has not been previously reported whether immunotherapy will induce new EGFR mutations or affect the efficacy of osimertinib. In addition, it is also worth exploring if high $CD8^+$ TILs cause the above effect. A retrospective study conducted by Su et al. reports a high proportion of $PD\text{-}L1^+/CD8^+$ cases in advanced NSCLC patients who were *de novo* resistant to first-line EGFR-TKIs. These patients, despite their poor response to EGFR-TKIs, exhibited higher immunogenicity, which, as a result, may benefit from immunotherapy (26). Another retrospective study performed by Yoshiya et al. also found that EGFR-TKIs as first-line treatment may have less benefit in EGFR-mutated tumors with both high expression of PD-L1 and $CD8^+$ TILs (27). However, in their study, high $CD8^+$ TIL (cohort 4) had longer PFS than low $CD8^+$ TILs (cohort 2) under the same low expression level of PD-L1 can be observed (27). Due to the small sample sizes of these two groups, further studies are needed to be conducted to confirm the relationship between $CD8^+$ TILs and the efficacy of EGFR-TKIs. In addition, it has been reported that the relative EGFR mutation abundance also could affect the therapeutic effect of using EGFR-TKI (28, 29). NGS of plasma performed prior to the application of osimertinib showed a mutation frequency of only 0.9% for EGFR T790M. The results of the study of Wang et al. showed that patients with low T790M mutation frequency are more likely to develop resistance and thus fail to benefit from osimertinib treatment (30).

However, there is one limitation to this case. Due to the insufficient pathological samples of patients saved before immunotherapy, we only performed genetic tests and could not perform IHC, so we did not know the levels of TMB, PD-L1 expression, and TILs before immunotherapy. For our subsequent studies, it is necessary to pay attention to the dynamic changes of biomarkers.

CONCLUSION

At present, how to select immunotherapy regimens for NSCLC patients with EGFR mutations is still controversial, but it is undeniable that some mutant subtypes do respond to ICIs, which may be due to the different effects of EGFR mutation subtypes on PD-L1 expression, TMB, and TME, thus affecting the efficacy of ICIs. However, we do not know much about whether ICIs or $CD8^+$ TILs affect the EGFR pathway and the efficacy of EGFR-TKIs. We need to further study this, so as to provide reference value for the selection of drug regimens for NSCLC with EGFR mutations in the future.

AUTHOR CONTRIBUTIONS

XM designed the study, edited, and approved the final manuscript. KZ and XZ collected clinical data and performed histological analysis. JP collected and analyzed the data and drafted the manuscript. All authors contributed to the article and approved the submitted version.

REFERENCES

1. Bunn PAJr. Karnofsky Award 2016: A Lung Cancer Journey, 1973 to 2016. *J Clin Oncol* (2017) 35(2):243–52. doi: 10.1200/JCO.2016.70.4064
2. Soo RA, Lim SM, Syn NL, Teng R, Soong R, Mok TSK, et al. Immune Checkpoint Inhibitors in Epidermal Growth Factor Receptor Mutant non-Small Cell Lung Cancer: Current Controversies and Future Directions. *Lung Cancer* (2018) 115:12–20. doi: 10.1016/j.lungcan.2017.11.009
3. Bylicki O, Barazzutti H, Paleiron N, Margery J, Assie JB, Chouaid C. First-Line Treatment of Non-Small-Cell Lung Cancer (NSCLC) With Immune Checkpoint Inhibitors. *BioDrugs* (2019) 33(2):159–71. doi: 10.1007/s40259-019-00339-4
4. Lee CK, Man J, Lord S, Cooper W, Links M, Gebski V, et al. Clinical and Molecular Characteristics Associated With Survival Among Patients Treated With Checkpoint Inhibitors for Advanced Non-Small Cell Lung Carcinoma: A Systematic Review and Meta-Analysis. *JAMA Oncol* (2018) 4(2):210–6. doi: 10.1001/jamaoncol.2017.4427
5. Borghaei H, Paz-Ares L, Horn L, Spigel DR, Steins M, Ready NE, et al. Nivolumab Versus Docetaxel in Advanced Nonsquamous Non-Small-Cell Lung Cancer. *N Engl J Med* (2015) 373(17):1627–39. doi: 10.1056/NEJMoa1507643
6. Rittmeyer A, Barlesi F, Waterkamp D, Park K, Ciardiello F, von Pawel J, et al. Atezolizumab Versus Docetaxel in Patients With Previously Treated non-Small-Cell Lung Cancer (OAK): A Phase 3, Open-Label, Multicentre Randomised Controlled Trial. *Lancet* (2017) 389(10066):255–65. doi: 10.1016/s0140-6736(16)32517-x
7. Chan BA, Hughes BG. Targeted Therapy for non-Small Cell Lung Cancer: Current Standards and the Promise of the Future. *Transl Lung Cancer Res* (2015) 4(1):36–54. doi: 10.3978/j.issn.2218-6751.2014.05.01

8. Hsu F, Nichol A, Toriumi T, De Caluwe A. Miliary Metastases are Associated With Epidermal Growth Factor Receptor Mutations in Non-Small Cell Lung Cancer: A Population-Based Study. *Acta Oncol* (2017) 56(9):1175–80. doi: 10.1080/0284186X.2017.1328128
9. Xuan J, Yu Y, Qing T, Guo L, Shi L. Next-Generation Sequencing in the Clinic: Promises and Challenges. *Cancer Lett* (2013) 340(2):284–95. doi: 10.1016/j.canlet.2012.11.025
10. Dhillon S, Syed YY. Atezolizumab First-Line Combination Therapy: A Review in Metastatic Nonsquamous NSCLC. *Target Oncol* (2019) 14(6):759–68. doi: 10.1007/s11523-019-00686-w
11. Herbst RS, Baas P, Kim DW, Felip E, JL P-G, Han JY, et al, Pembrolizumab Versus Docetaxel for Previously Treated, PD-L1-Positive, Advanced non-Small-Cell Lung Cancer (KEYNOTE-010): A Randomised Controlled Trial. *Ann Oncol* (2015) 387: (10027):1540–50. doi: 10.1016/S0140-6736(15)01281-7
12. Hastings K, Yu HA, Wei W, Sanchez-Vega F, DeVeaux M, Choi J, et al. EGFR Mutation Subtypes and Response to Immune Checkpoint Blockade Treatment in non-Small-Cell Lung Cancer. *Ann Oncol* (2019) 30(8):1311–20. doi: 10.1093/annonc/mdz141
13. Bustamante-Alvarez JG, Owen DH. Biomarkers for Immunotherapy. *Thorac Surg Clin* (2020) 30(2):207–14. doi: 10.1016/j.thorsurg.2020.01.010
14. Yu Y, Zeng D, Ou Q, Liu S, Li A, Chen Y, et al. Association of Survival and Immune-Related Biomarkers With Immunotherapy in Patients With non-Small Cell Lung Cancer: A Meta-Analysis and Individual Patient-Level Analysis. *JAMA Netw Open* (2019) 2(7):e196879. doi: 10.1001/jamanetworkopen.2019.6879
15. Simoni Y, Becht E, Fehlings M, Loh CY, Koo SL, Teng KWW, et al. Bystander CD8(+) T Cells are Abundant and Phenotypically Distinct in Human Tumour Infiltrates. *Nature* (2018) 557(7706):575–9. doi: 10.1038/s41586-018-0130-2
16. Lin H, Wei S, Hurt EM, Green MD, Zhao L, Vatan L, et al. Host Expression of PD-L1 Determines Efficacy of PD-L1 Pathway Blockade-Mediated Tumor Regression. *J Clin Invest* (2018) 128(2):805–15. doi: 10.1172/JCI96113
17. Tang H, Liang Y, Anders RA, Taube JM, Qiu X, Mulgaonkar A, et al. PD-L1 on Host Cells is Essential for PD-L1 Blockade-Mediated Tumor Regression. *J Clin Invest* (2018) 128(2):580–8. doi: 10.1172/JCI96061
18. Garassino MC, Cho B-C, Kim J-H, Mazières J, Vansteenkiste J, Lena H, et al. Durvalumab as Third-Line or Later Treatment for Advanced Non-Small-Cell Lung Cancer (ATLANTIC): An Open-Label, Single-Arm, Phase 2 Study. *Lancet Oncol* (2018) 19(4):521–36. doi: 10.1016/s1470-2045(18)30144-x
19. Assoun S, Theou-Anton N, Nguenang M, Cazes A, Danel C, Abbar B, et al. Association of TP53 Mutations With Response and Longer Survival Under Immune Checkpoint Inhibitors in Advanced Non-Small-Cell Lung Cancer. *Lung Cancer* (2019) 132:65–71. doi: 10.1016/j.lungcan.2019.04.005
20. Serra P, Petat A, Maury JM, Thivolet-Bejui F, Chalabreysse L, Barritault M, et al. Programmed Cell Death-Ligand 1 (PD-L1) Expression Is Associated With RAS/TP53 Mutations in Lung Adenocarcinoma. *Lung Cancer* (2018) 118:62–8. doi: 10.1016/j.lungcan.2018.02.005
21. Dong ZY, Zhong WZ, Zhang XC, Su J, Xie Z, Liu SY, et al. Potential Predictive Value of TP53 and KRAS Mutation Status for Response to PD-1 Blockade Immunotherapy in Lung Adenocarcinoma. *Clin Cancer Res* (2017) 23 (12):3012–24. doi: 10.1158/1078-0432.CCR-16-2554
22. Carlisle JW, Nho NT, Kim C, Chen Z, Li S, Hill C, et al. Impact of TP53 Mutations on Efficacy of PD-1 Targeted Immunotherapy in Non-Small Cell Lung Cancer (NSCLC). *J Clin Oncol* (2018) 36(15_suppl):e21090-0. doi: 10.1200/JCO.2018.36.15_suppl.e21090
23. Li X, Lian Z, Wang S, Xing L, Yu J. Interactions Between EGFR and PD-1/PD-L1 Pathway: Implications for Treatment of NSCLC. *Cancer Lett* (2018) 418:1–9. doi: 10.1016/j.canlet.2018.01.005
24. Wang S, Yan B, Zhang Y, Xu J, Qiao R, Dong Y, et al. Different Characteristics and Survival in non-Small Cell Lung Cancer Patients With Primary and Acquired EGFR T790M Mutation. *Int J Cancer* (2019) 144(11):2880–6. doi: 10.1002/ijc.32015
25. Li H, Zhang S, Cheng Y. Advanced Research on T790M Mutation in non-Small Cell Lung Cancer. *Zhongguo Fei Ai Za Zhi* (2013) 16(6):314–20. doi: 10.3779/j.issn.1009-3419.2013.06.08
26. Su S, Dong ZY, Xie Z, Yan LX, Li YF, Su J, et al. Strong Programmed Death Ligand 1 Expression Predicts Poor Response and De Novo Resistance to EGFR Tyrosine Kinase Inhibitors Among NSCLC Patients With EGFR Mutation. *J Thorac Oncol* (2018) 13(11):1668–75. doi: 10.1016/j.jtho.2018.07.016
27. Matsumoto Y, Sawa K, Fukui M, Oyanagi J, Izumi M, Ogawa K, et al. Impact of Tumor Microenvironment on the Efficacy of Epidermal Growth Factor Receptor-Tyrosine Kinase Inhibitors in Patients With EGFR-Mutant non-Small Cell Lung Cancer. *Cancer Sci* (2019) 110(10):3244–54. doi: 10.1111/cas.14156
28. Zhou Q, Zhang XC, Chen ZH, Yin XL, Yang JJ, Xu CR, et al. Relative Abundance of EGFR Mutations Predicts Benefit From Gefitinib Treatment for Advanced Non-Small-Cell Lung Cancer. *J Clin Oncol* (2011) 29(24):3316–21. doi: 10.1200/JCO.2010.33.3757
29. Li X, Cai W, Yang G, Su C, Ren S, Zhao C, et al. Comprehensive Analysis of EGFR-Mutant Abundance and its Effect on Efficacy of EGFR Tkis in Advanced NSCLC With EGFR Mutations. *J Thorac Oncol* (2017) 12 (9):1388–97. doi: 10.1016/j.jtho.2017.06.006
30. Wang Y, He Y, Tian P, Wang W, Wang K, Chuai S, et al. Low T790M Relative Allele Frequency Indicates Concurrent Resistance Mechanisms and Poor Responsiveness to Osimertinib. *Transl Lung Cancer Res* (2020) 9(5):1952–62. doi: 10.21037/tlcr-20-915

9

ERAP2 is Associated with Immune Infiltration and Predicts Favorable Prognosis in SqCLC

Zhenlin Yang[1†], He Tian[1†], Fenglong Bie[1†], Jiachen Xu[2], Zheng Zhou[1], Junhui Yang[3], Renda Li[1], Yue Peng[1], Guangyu Bai[1], Yanhua Tian[4], Ying Chen[5], Lei Liu[1], Tao Fan[1], Chu Xiao[1], Yujia Zheng[1], Bo Zheng[6], Jie Wang[2], Chunxiang Li[1], Shugeng Gao[1*] and Jie He[1*]*

[1] Department of Thoracic Surgery, National Cancer Center/National Clinical Research Center for Cancer/Cancer Hospital, Chinese Academy of Medical Sciences, Peking Union Medical College, Beijing, China, [2] Department of Medical Oncology, National Cancer Center/National Clinical Research Center for Cancer/Cancer Hospital, Chinese Academy of Medical Sciences, Peking Union Medical College, Beijing, China, [3] Genetron Health (Beijing) Co. Ltd., Beijing, China, [4] Department of Thoracic Surgery/Head & Neck Medical Oncology, The University of Texas (UT) MD Anderson Cancer Center, Houston, TX, United States, [5] Department of Thoracic Surgery I, The Third Affiliated Hospital of Kunming Medical University (Yunnan Cancer Hospital, Yunnan Cancer Center), Kunming, China, [6] Department of Pathology, National Cancer Center/National Clinical Research Center for Cancer/Cancer Hospital, Chinese Academy of Medical Sciences, Peking Union Medical College, Beijing, China

***Correspondence:**
Jie He
prof.jiehe@gmail.com
Shugeng Gao
gaoshugeng@cicams.ac.cn
Chunxiang Li
lichunxiang@cicams.ac.cn

[†]These authors have contributed equally to this work and share the first authorship*

Background: Immunotherapy has been proven effective among several human cancer types, including Squamous cell lung carcinoma (SqCLC). ERAP2 plays a pivotal role in peptide trimming of many immunological processes. However, the prognostic role of ERAP2 and its relationship with immune cell infiltration in SqCLC remains unclear.

Methods: The differential expression of ERAP2 was identified *via* GEO and TCGA databases. We calculated the impact of ERAP2 on clinical prognosis using the Kaplan-Meier plotter. TIMER was applied to evaluate the abundance of immune cells infiltration and immune markers. SqCLC tissue microarrays containing 190 patients were constructed, and we performed immunohistochemical staining for ERAP2, CD8, CD47, CD68, and PD-L1 to validate our findings in public data.

Results: In the GEO SqCLC database, ERAP2 was upregulated in patients with better survival (p=0.001). ERAP2 expression in SqCLC was significantly lower than that of matched normal samples (p<0.05) based on TCGA SqCLC data. Higher expression of ERAP2 was significantly associated with better survival in SqCLC patients from TCGA (p=0.007), KM-plotter (p=0.017), and our tissue microarrays (TMAs) (p=0.026). In univariate and multivariate Cox analysis of SqCLC TMAs, high ERAP2 expression was identified as an independent protective factor for SqCLC patients (Univariate Cox, HR=0.659, range 0.454-0.956, p<0.05. Multivariate Cox, HR=0.578, range 0.385-0.866, p<0.05). In TIMER, ERAP2 was positively correlated with several immune markers (CD274, p=1.27E-04; CD68, p=5.88E-08) and immune infiltrating cells ($CD8^+$ T cell, p=4.09E-03; NK cell, p=1.00E-04). In our cohort, ERAP2 was significantly correlated with $CD8^+$ tumor-infiltrating lymphocytes (TILs) (p=0.0029), and patients with higher ERAP2 expression had a higher percentage of PD-L1 positive patients (p=0.049) and a higher $CD8^+$ TILs level (p=0.036).

Conclusions: For the first time, our study demonstrates that higher expression of ERAP2 is tightly associated with the immuno-supportive microenvironment and can predict a favorable prognosis in SqCLC. Meanwhile, ERAP2 may be a promising immunotherapeutic target for patients with SqCLC.

Keywords: ERAP2, squamous cell lung cancer (SqCLC), prognosis, immune microenvironment, biomarker

INTRODUCTION

According to the newest data published in 2021, lung cancer has the highest mortality rate among all cancer types and is a significant health care concern throughout the world (1). Approximately 85% of lung cancer can be classified into a histological subtype generally known as non-small cell lung cancer (NSCLC), 25% to 30% of which is squamous cell lung cancer (SqCLC) (2). SqCLC had specific clinicopathologic characteristics, including male gender, older age, smoker preference, comorbidities, and centrally located tumors (3). Patients with SqCLC are usually diagnosed at an advanced stage, and the 5-year overall survival rate of advanced SqCLC was less than 20%.

Even though standard platinum-based chemotherapy is the mainstay of first-line treatment for most SqCLC patients (4), there are still many patients who cannot receive satisfying outcomes (5). Additionally, different from lung adenocarcinoma (LUAD), which has greatly benefited from targeted therapies against driver mutations such as epidermal growth factor receptor (EGFR) mutations, etc., inroads in targeted therapy are rare in SqCLC (6, 7). Over the past few decades, the limited therapeutic options rendered SqCLC a challenging-to-treat disease. The introduction of immunotherapy, particularly blockers of the PD-1 axis, into the treatment of NSCLC has revolutionized the therapeutic stand-care of this recalcitrant disease, yielding significant survival benefits (8). However, only a minority of SqCLC patients have achieved sustained benefits. Primary and acquired resistances are common phenomena in SqCLC immunotherapy (9). The immunotherapy of SqCLC is still in its infancy, and more immune-related treatments are warranted.

ERAP2 (Endoplasmic Reticulum Aminopeptidase 2), located on chromosome 5q15, belongs to the oxytocinase subfamily of M1 aminopeptidases and is closely related to ERAP1 (endoplasmic Reticulum Aminopeptidase 1), a homologous enzyme of it (10). Both ERAP2 and ERAP1 mainly participate in the final trimming of peptides that will be loaded on MHC-I (Major Histocompatibility Complex class I) molecules at the cell surface for $CD8^+$ T cells/Natural Killer (NK) cells recognition (11, 12). The length of some peptides entering ER is not suitable for being loaded onto MHC I molecule and thus will be trimmed by ERAP1/2 (13). In the immune-evading tumor, malfunction ERAP2 can undermine tumor-associated antigenic episodes while the immune checkpoints are over-expressed, thus anti-tumor T cell response is suspended (14). Previous studies have highlighted that ERAPs are potential targets for enhancing T/NK cell-mediated immunogenicity of malignant cells for developing anti-tumor immunotherapy (15, 16). In addition, Lim et al. has proved that in bladder cancer patients receiving anti-PD-L1 therapy, ERAP2 expression can stratify overall survival (17). The deficiencies in the expression and function of ERAPs have been demonstrated in multiple tumor types, including lung cancer (18–20). So far, the biological roles of ERAP2 in SqCLC have remained unclear.

This study explored the predictive value and immune-related roles of ERAP2 in SqCLC using public databases. We validated our conclusions in a large-scale SqCLC tissue-microarray with long-term follow-up data. We aimed to illustrate the biological functions of ERAP2 in SqCLC and provide novel clues for administering immunotherapy in SqCLC.

MATERIALS AND METHODS

Bioinformatic Mining of ERAP2

Using R software, we obtained differentially expressed genes (DEGs) from patients with distinct survival in the GEO dataset (GSE30219). GSE30219 dataset contained 61 SqCLC patients, whose median survival time (59 months) was used to stratify groups with better and worse survival. Totally 11 DEGs ($p<0.05$) of the two groups were extracted using the R package limma. The list of DEGs and corresponding logFC values were shown in **Figure 1A**. Using GEPIA (http://gepia2.cancer-pku.cn/#index), an online analysis website containing pan-cancer transcriptome data from TCGA (https://portal.gdc.cancer.gov/), we explored the ERAP2 expression level among multiple cancer types and paired normal samples (**Figure 1B**), in which the SqCLC dataset included 486 tumor samples and 338 normal samples (Red Arrow in **Figure 1B**).Using patients with follow-up data from the GEO dataset (GSE30219), we performed survival analysis in SqCLC stratified by ERAP2 expression. KM-plotter (http://www.kmplot.com/lung/) was used to validate the prognostic effect of ERAP2 in SqCLC that we found in the GEO dataset.

Tissue Microarray Construction and IHC Staining

Following the IRB (Institutional Review Board) approval, formalin-fixed, paraffin-embedded tissue microarrays (TMAs) were created using SqCLC samples collected from patients who underwent surgery from April 2010 to August 2011 in the

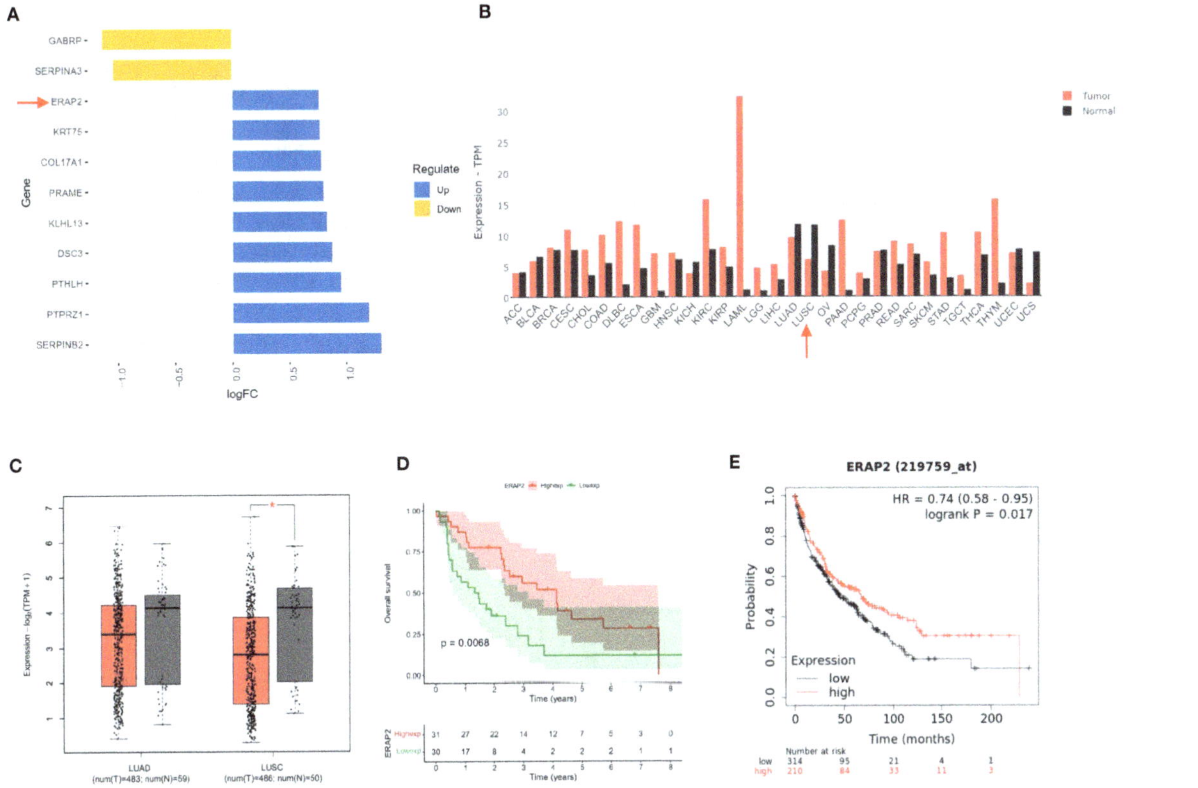

FIGURE 1 | Bioinformatic mining of ERAP2. **(A)** High and low expression genes of SqCLC patients with better survival based on GEO dataset GSE30219. The length of the bar represents the log (fold change) of gene expression between patients with different survival. Orange, low expression genes in patients with better survival. Blue, high expression genes in patients with longer survival. **(B)** ERAP2 expression profiles across all 31 tumor types and paired normal tissues based on TCGA data. The height of the bar represents the median expression of certain tumor types or normal samples. Red, tumor; Black, normal tissue. Arrow, ERAP2 expression in SqCLC. ACC, Adrenocortical carcinoma; BLCA, Bladder Urothelial Carcinoma; BRCA, Breast invasive carcinoma; CESC, Cervical squamous cell carcinoma and endocervical adenocarcinoma; CHOL, Cholangiocarcinoma; COAD, Colon adenocarcinoma; DLBC, Lymphoid Neoplasm Diffuse Large B-cell Lymphoma; ESCA, Esophageal carcinoma; GBM, Glioblastoma multiforme; HNSC, Head and Neck squamous cell carcinoma; KICH, Kidney Chromophobe; KIRC, Kidney renal clear cell carcinoma; KIRP, Kidney renal papillary cell carcinoma; LAML, Acute Myeloid Leukemia; LGG, Brain Lower Grade Glioma; LIHC, Liver hepatocellular carcinoma; LUAD, Lung adenocarcinoma; LUSC, Lung squamous cell carcinoma; OV, Ovarian serous cystadenocarcinoma; PAAD, Pancreatic adenocarcinoma; PCPG, Pheochromocytoma and Paraganglioma; PRAD, Prostate adenocarcinoma; READ, Rectum adenocarcinoma; SARC, Sarcoma; SKCM, Skin Cutaneous Melanoma; STAD, Stomach adenocarcinoma; TGCT, Testicular Germ Cell Tumors; THCA, Thyroid carcinoma; THYM, Thymoma; UCEC, Uterine Corpus Endometrial Carcinoma; USC, Uterine Carcinosarcoma. **(C)** ERAP2 expression in LUAD and LUSC based on data in GEPIA. Left, LUAD. Right, LUSC. Red, tumor sample. Grey, normal sample. Asterisk, p value<0.05; Centerline, median; box limits, upper and lower quartiles; points, outliers. **(D)** K-M curve showing the overall survival of SqCLC patients stratified by ERAP2 expression in the GEO dataset. Red, ERAP2 high expression group. Green, ERAP2 low expression group. **(E)** K-M curve showing the overall survival of SqCLC patients stratified by ERAP2 expression in the KM-Plotter dataset. Red, ERAP2 high expression group. Black, ERAP2 low expression group.

Department of Thoracic Surgery, Cancer Hospital, Chinese Academy of Medical Sciences and Peking Union Medical College. The TMAs contained 190 SqCLC tumor samples. The tumor tissues were fixed by formalin and embedded in paraffin. We took two 2-mm cores from each sample to constitute the TMAs, and then 4-μm thick TMA sections were manufactured. All manual process was conducted by professional pathological technicians from the Department of Pathology of our hospital. All specimens in the 3 TMAS were diagnosed, selected, and confirmed by two certified pathological clinicians.

We performed immunohistochemistry (IHC) of several markers on the TMA, including ERAP2, PD-L1, CD47, CD8, and CD68. We incubated the TMAs with the primary antibodies against ERAP2 (Sigma, HPA034498), PD-L1 (Abcam, 28-8), CD47 (Abcam, EPR21794), CD8 (CST, D8A8Y), and CD68 (Abcam, KP1), and then with the secondary antibodies and 3, 3'-diaminobenzidine (DAB).

Two independent pathologists without prior knowledge of our research evaluated the IHC staining results. ERAP2 expression was scored using a combined method (21). Negative, weak, moderate, and strong intensities were scored as 0, 1, 2, and 3, respectively. The percentage of cells that stained at each intensity score was estimated visually. The ultimate score for each specimen was calculated as the sum of the percentage of stained cells multiplied by the intensity scores. For instance, a sample with 10% negative staining, 40% moderate staining, and

50% strong staining would be assessed a score of 2.3 (0.1×0 + 0.4×2 + 0.5×3 = 2.3). All samples were scored twice independently by two pathologists who were blinded to our study. For PD-L1 and CD47, membranous tumor proportion score (TPS) was applied, during which TPS ≥ 1% and TPS ≥ 5% were set as the positive standard for the two markers, respectively. Co-expression of PD-L1 and CD47 was defined as samples positive in both PD-L1 and CD47. For CD8 and CD68, we calculated the number of CD8-positive TILs and CD68-positive macrophages under six high-power fields and took the average for each specimen.

Survival Analysis

Overall survival (OS) was used to evaluate the prognosis in both public data and our SqCLC cohort. OS was determined as the time from the diagnosis of SqCLC to the patient's death, independent from the cause of death. For OS of our cohort, patients who were alive on September 20, 2018, were defined as censored data. The K-M curve was applied to analyze the survival data of patients. We used the R software package "RMS" to portray the Nomogram for patients based on several clinicopathological factors and immune biomarkers, including ERAP2 expression level. In our model, the total point of a patient was generated based on facts from each element and had corresponding 1-year, 2-year, and 3-year survival rates.

Gene Function Analysis

Based on TCGA (502 samples) and GEO dataset GSE30219 (61 samples) SqCLC transcription data, we used gene enrichment analysis to explore the function of ERAP2-related differentially expressed genes. The enrichment analysis method was described in the previous research (22). The gene enrichment analysis was performed using the following database and gene set: Gene Ontology (GO, c5.all.v7.4.symbols.gmt [Gene ontology]), Kyoto Encyclopedia of Genes and Genomes (KEGG, c2.cp.kegg.v7.4.symbols.gmt [Curated]), Immunologic signatures (c7.all.v7.4.symbols.gmt [Immunologic signatures]). R software was used to visualize the results of gene function enrichment analysis. Based on the above-mentioned TCGA and GEO transcriptome dataset, we classified patients into ERAP2 high and low expression groups using the median ERAP2 expression value and performed differentially expressed genes (DEGs)analysis between them ($p<0.05$, R package "edgeR" and "limma" were for TCGA data and GEO data, respectively). Then we conducted GO and KEGG enrichment analysis based on the DEGs and drew the bubble charts.

Immune-Associated Exploration of ERAP2

To identify the potential connection between each two factors of the TMAs, we performed pairwise association analysis. For ERAP2, we classified all SqCLC TMAs patients into high and low expression groups according to the median staining score. The expression of other immune markers was evaluated based on their cut-off values (CD8, CD68: median. PD-L1: 1% and 10%. CD47: 5% and 20%).

We also explored the immune-associated function of ERAP2 in public data using TIMER (http://timer.comp-genomics.org). With this tool, we study the associations between the expression of ERAP2 and several immune markers in SqCLC, including CD68, CD8A, CTLA4, FOXP3, CD274, and CD4. We also explored the relationship between ERAP2 expression and immune cell infiltration levels in SqCLC, including $CD8^{+}$T cell, M0 macrophage, regulatory T cell, M1 macrophage, activated NK cell, and M2 macrophage. CIBERSORT (23) algorithm was applied by TIMER for analysis.

Statistical Analysis

All data were managed using R software (R x64 4.0.2 Version) and GraphPad Prism 8. An independent-sample was used to make comparisons of continuous and categorical variables between groups. The univariate/multivariate Cox proportional hazard models were used to assess the prognosis. The Kaplan–Meier method was applied to evaluate survival, and the log-rank test was used to determine significance. We used Spearman correlation to explore the associations between variables. We regarded a two-tailed p-value <0.05 as statistically significant.

RESULTS

Bioinformatic Mining of ERAP2

We used the GEO dataset GSE30219 (containing SqCLC patients) and classified the patients into better and worse survival groups. DEGs were acquired based on the two groups. According to the p-value and fold-change (FC), we showed 11 DEGs in **Figure 1A**. ERAP2 upregulated in patients with better survival (p-value=0.001, logFC=0.767). According to previous studies, ERAP2 was closely related with CD8 T cell, NK cell, and several immune process (13), indicating it may play important roles in cancer immunology. We then profiled the expression of ERAP2 in multiple cancer types and matched normal tissues by GEPIA2, as shown in **Figure 1B**. We then drew boxplots to show more details on the expression of ERAP2 for NSCLC. We found that ERAP2 expression in SqCLC was statistically lower than that in paired normal tissues (**Figure 1C**), suggesting that the deficiency of ERAP2 might participate in the carcinogenesis of SqCLC. Further, using the GEO dataset GSE30219 (**Figure 1D**) and KM-plotter (http://kmplot.com/analysis/index.php?p=service&cancer=lung) (**Figure 1E**), we drew K-M curves stratified by ERAP2 expression, exhibiting that patients with high ERAP2 expression had longer overall survival in SqCLC ($p<0.05$).

Prognostic Roles of ERAP2 in Our Cohort

To validate the prognostic impact of ERAP2 on SqCLC, we established an independent SqCLC cohort, including a total of 190 SqCLC patients, and the tumor samples were retrospectively collected to constitute TMAs. The clinicopathological information of our cohort is shown in **Table 1**. Most patients were males (183, 96.32%) and smokers (176, 92, 63%). According to the 8th AJCC (American Joint Committee on Cancer) Staging Manual (24), there were 34 (17.89%) stage I patients, 70 (36.84%) stage II patients, and 86 (45.26%) stage III patients at diagnosis. At the last follow-up, 112 (58.95%) patients were dead, while the

TABLE 1 | Clinicopathological characteristics of SqCLC patients in tissue microarrays.

Characteristics	Groups	Number of patients (%)
Gender	Male	183 (96.32%)
	Female	7 (3.68%)
Age	≤60 years old	88 (46.32%)
	>60 years old	102 (53.68%)
Smoking	Yes	176 (92.63%)
	No	14 (7.37%)
T stage	T1	25 (13.16%)
	T2	99 (52.11%)
	T3	45 (23.68%)
	T4	21 (11.05%)
N stage	N0	64 (33.68%)
	N1	67 (35.26%)
	N2	59 (31.05%)
TNM stage	I	34 (17.89%)
	II	70 (36.84%)
	III	86 (45.26%)
Tumor diameter*	≤4.5mm	98 (51.58%)
	>4.5mm	92 (48.42%)

The median of tumor diameter is 4.5mm.

left 78 (41.05%) patients were alive or censored. The median follow-up time was 66.5 months.

IHC of ERAP2 on our TMAs was conducted, and we calculated an IHC score for each specimen as the sum of the percentage of stained cells multiplied by the staining intensity. The standard of staining intensity was displayed in **Figure 2A**. The median IHC score of ERAP2 is 1.375, and we classified the samples into high and low ERAP2 expression subgroups using the median score as the cut-off value. Representative images of high expression and low expression of ERAP2 were shown in **Figure 2B**. We profiled the demographic information for each patient annotated for the expression level of ERAP2, and the distributions of characteristic features did not show a noticeable difference between ERAP2 high and low expression subgroups (**Figure 2C**). K-M curve exhibited that in our cohort, patients with ERAP2 high expression had significantly longer overall survival than the ERAP2 low expression subgroup (**Figure 2D**).

To further explore the prognostic marker of SqCLC, firstly we performed a univariate analysis in our cohort (**Figure 2E** and **Table 2**). Then we conducted the multivariate analysis using the variables that were proved to be statistically significant in univariate analysis (**Figure 2F** and **Table 3**). ERAP2 was identified as an independent protective factor for SqCLC (Univariate, HR =0.659, 95% CI, 0.454-0.956, p-value=0.028; Multivariate, HR =0.523, 95% CI, 0.353-0.775, p value=0.001). The ERAP2 score and clinical information of each sample in our cohort was recorded in **Supplementary Data 1**.

Construction of Nomogram

The 190 SqCLC patients with complete clinical information and follow-up survival time from our cohort were used to establish a prognostic nomograph using R software with the RMS package (**Figure 3**). All clinicopathological factors and immune markers expression status were included in the nomogram model. In the nomogram, the ERAP2 expression was a decisive parameter among all immune markers, for which score 0 represented 100 points and scored three indicated 0 points. The T stage behaved like a very effective indicator among clinicopathological factors, and T3 represented 100 points. The weight of gender, tumor diameter, PD-L1, and CD68+ macrophages were relatively low compared to other indicators. Total points over 700 could predict a survival rate <50% in 1-year survival, a survival rate <20% in 2-year survival, and a survival rate <10% in 3-year survival.

Exploration of ERAP2-Related Function by Pathway Enrichment

Based on SqCLC data from TCGA (**Figures 4A–C**) and GEO (**Figures 4D–F**), we analyzed signaling pathway enrichment for patients with ERAP2 expression levels. We revealed that high ERAP2 expression was synergistic with several immune-promoting biological processes. In both TCGA and GEO databases, high ERAP2 expression was enriched in the natural killer cell-mediated cytotoxicity pathway and T cell receptor signaling pathway, consistent with previous studies. In the TCGA database, high ERAP2 expression was also enriched in the positive regulation of lymphocyte differentiation, T cell activation terms, and positive regulation of innate immune response, suggesting that high ERAP2 expression was correlated with the immune active environment. In the GEO database, high ERAP2 expression was enriched in the PI3K-Akt signaling pathway, JAK-STAT pathway, and the Toll-like receptor pathway, arousing our interest in the molecular network about ERAP2.

Immune-Related Exploration of ERAP2 in Public Data

Inspired by the pathway enrichment analysis results, we further explored the correlations between the expression of ERAP2 and several immune markers in public data using TIMER (an online tool). In **Figure 5A**, we showed the association between the expression level of ERAP2 and CD68, CD8A, CTLA4, FOXP3, CD274 (PD-L1), and CD4, in which ERAP2 was positively correlated with these markers and all the correlations were statistically significant (p=5.88e-08 for CD68, p=4.35e-14 for CD8A, p=1.28e-15 for CTLA4, p=1.65e-14 for FOXP3, p=1.27e-04 for CD274, p=9.98e-14 for CD4), indicating that ERAP2 may enhance the antitumor immune response.

We then characterized the interactions between ERAP2 expression and immune cell infiltration levels in SqCLC samples (**Figure 5B**). Several immune cells were selected, including $CD8^+$ T cells, M0 macrophages, regulatory T cells, M1 macrophages, activated NK cells, and M2 macrophages. ERAP2 expression was significantly positively correlated to the infiltration levels ($CD8^+$ T cells, p=4.09e-03; M0 macrophages, p=1.93e-02; regulatory T cells, p=2.29e-02; M1 macrophages, p=2.16e-08; activated NK cells, p=1.00e-04; M2 macrophages, p=1.24e-06), consistent with previous findings in our study, further suggesting that ERAP2 may act as a tumor suppressor in SqCLC in an immune-promoting manner.

Immune-Related Exploration of ERAP2 in Our Cohort

We evaluated the IHC expression level of PD-L1, CD47, CD8, and CD68 in our cohort, and as shown in **Figure 6A**, pairwise

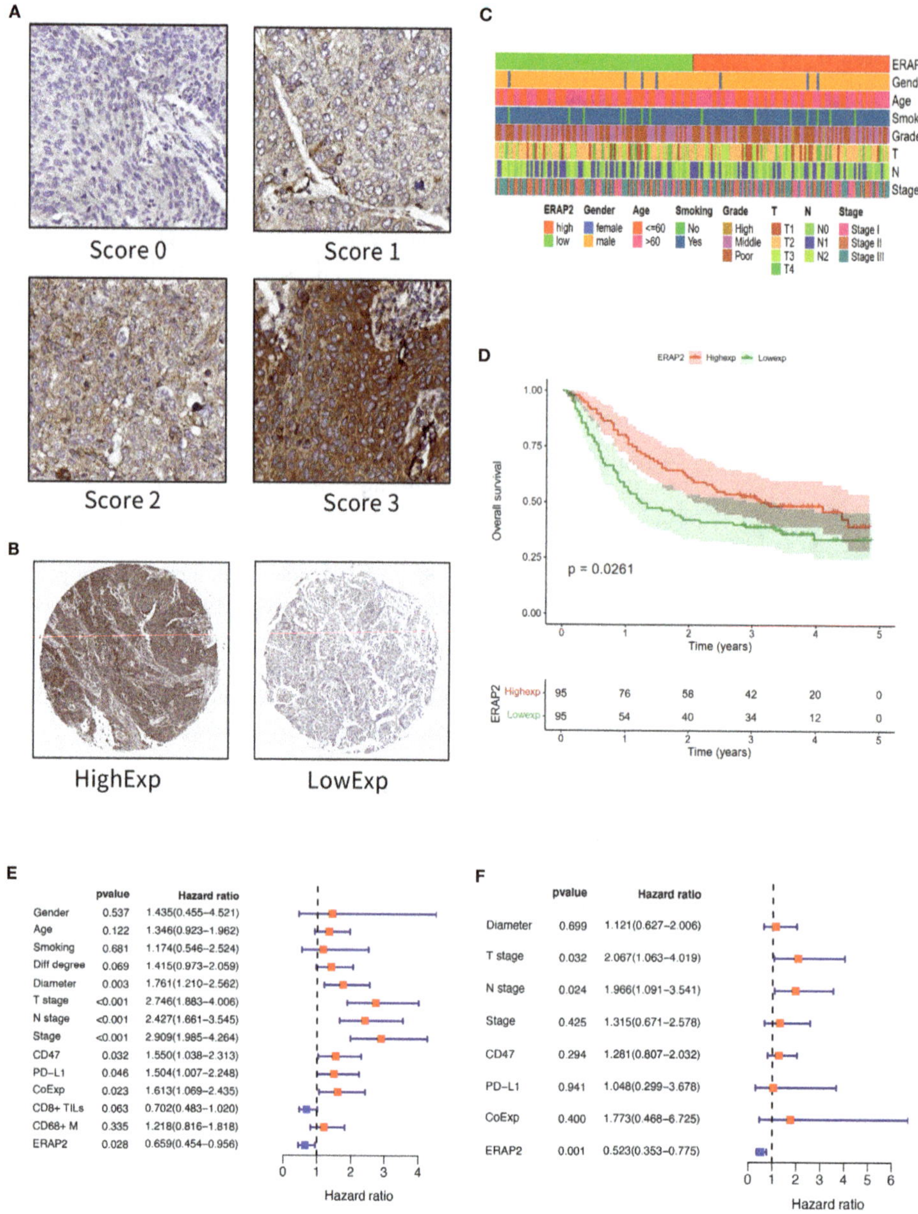

FIGURE 2 | ERAP2 expression in SqCLC tumor microarray (TMA). **(A)** ERAP2 staining intensity scoring standard. ERAP2 expression was graded into 4 categories: 0, 1, 2, and 3 according to the staining intensity. The larger number represented higher ERAP2 staining intensity (100×). The final score of samples is evaluated by multiplying the grade and corresponding area percentages. **(B)** Example of high and low ERAP2 expression in TMA. Left, high expression sample. Right, low expression sample (20×). **(C)** Clinicopathological information related heatmap of SqCLC TMA. **(D)** K-M curve showing the overall survival in SqCLC TMA stratified by ERAP2 expression. Red, ERAP2 high expression group. Green, low expression group. **(E)** Univariate analysis forest plot of clinicopathological factors, ERAP2 expression, and other immune markers' expression in SqCLC TMA. CoExp, PD-L1, and CD47 co-expression. CD8+ TILs, CD8+ tumor infiltration lymphocytes. CD68+ M, CD68+ infiltration macrophages infiltration level. The red square represents risk factors for prognosis, while the blue square represents protective factors for patients. **(F)** Multivariate analysis forest plot of factors, which could predict the overall survival in the univariate analysis. CoExp, PD-L1, and CD47 co-expression. CD8+ TILs, CD8+ tumor infiltration lymphocytes. The red square represents risk factors for prognosis, while the blue square represents protective factors for patients.

correlation analysis was performed for all clinicopathological factors and molecular markers. We found that ERAP2 expression was significantly correlated with CD8$^+$ TILs (Spearman r=0.22, p=0.0029, **Figure 6B**). Applying the median staining score of ERAP2 expression as the cut-off value (median=1.375), we classified all 190 SqCLC patients of our cohort into two groups and compared the expression levels CD47 and PD-L1 and the infiltrating density of CD8$^+$ TILs

TABLE 2 | Univariate Cox Regression of Prognostic Factors in SqCLC.

	OS	
	HR (95% CI)	**p**
Age		0.122
≤60y	1.000	
>60y	1.346 (0.923-1.962)	
Gender		0.537
Female	1.000	
Male	1.435 (0.455-4.521)	
Smoking		0.681
No	1.000	
Yes	1.174 (0.546-2.524)	
Tumor Diameter		0.003
≤median	1.000	
>median	1.761 (1.210-2.562)	
T stage		1.56E-07
T1+T2	1.000	
T3+T4	2.746 (1.883-4.006)	
N stage		0.000
N0+N1	1.000	
N2	2.427 (1.661-3.545)	
TNM Stage		0.000
I+II	1.000	
III	2.090 (1.985-4.264)	
CD47 expression		0.032
Low	1.000	
High	1.55 (1.038-2.313)	
PD-L1 expression		0.046
Negative	1.000	
Positive	1.504 (1.007-2.248)	
PD-L1 and CD47 co-expression		0.023
No	1.000	
Yes	1.163 (1.069-2.435)	
CD8+ TILs level		0.063
Low	1.000	
High	0.702 (0.483-1.02)	
CD68+Macrophage infiltration level		0.335
Low	1.000	
High	1.218 (0.816-1.818)	
ERAP2 expression		0.028
Low	1.000	
High	0.659 (0.454-0.956)	

All p values were two sides and less than 0.05 were considered significant.
SqCLC, Squamous cell lung cancer; OS, overall survival; HR, hazard ratio; CI, confidence interval.
Low and high expression was classified as the median except for CD47 (1% as cut-off value).

TABLE 3 | Multivariate Cox Regression of Prognostic Factors in SqCLC.

	OS	
	HR (95% CI)	**p**
Diameter		0.699
≤60y	1.000	
>60y	1.121 (0.627-2.006)	
T stage		0.032
T1+T2	1.000	
T3+T4	2.067 (1.063-4.019)	
N stage		0.024
N0+N1	1.000	
N2	1.966 (1.091-3.541)	
TNM stage		0.425
I+II	1.000	
III	1.315 (0.671-2.578)	
CD47 expression		0.294
Negative	1.000	
Positive	1.281 (0.807-2.032)	
PD-L1 expression		0.941
Negative	1.000	
Positive	1.048 (0.299-3.678)	
PD-L1 and CD47 co-expression		0.400
No	1.000	
Yes	1.773 (0.468-6.725)	
ERAP2 expression		0.001
Low	1.000	
High	0.523 (0.353-0.775)	

All p values were two sides and less than 0.05 were considered significant.
SqCLC, Squamous cell lung cancer; OS, overall survival; HR, hazard ratio; CI, confidence interval.
Low and high expression was classified as the median except for CD47 (1% as cut-off value).

and $CD68^+$ Macrophages of them (**Figure 6C**). In the ERAP2 high expression group, the expression level of PD-L1 was significantly higher ($p<0.05$), meanwhile, the infiltrating density of $CD8^+$ TILs were also considerably higher in the ERAP2 high expression group ($p<0.05$). ERAP2 expression in positive groups was significantly higher than in negative groups for all three immune markers, implying ERAP2 may exert significant functions in anti-tumor immunity. The representative images of each one patient from the ERAP2 high and low expression group (**Figure 6D**). In addition, we distributed all the patients of our cohort into positive and negative groups according to the status of PD-L1 (10% TPS as cutoff value), the status of PD-L1/CD47 co-expression (co-expression criteria: 1% for PD-L1 and 5% for CD47) and infiltrating density of $CD8^+$ TILs (median as cutoff value). We compared the ERAP2 expression levels between the groups (**Figure 6E**).

DISCUSSION

SqCLC has been a refractory disease for decades, with few inroads in targeted therapy, and only a minority of SqCLC patients have achieved sustained benefits from immunotherapy (5, 25). Based on public databases and our SqCLC cohort (190 patients), our study identified ERAP2 as a favorable prognostic indicator and potential enhancer for ICIs in SqCLC.

It is reasonable for us to believe that ERAP2 may exert a significant role in SqCLC. Using GEO and TCGA data, we found ERAP2 was lowly expressed in SqCLC and was significantly associated with longer survival. As an endoplasmic reticulum-settled enzyme, ERAP2 is responsible for the final trimming of peptides represented by the major histocompatibility complex (MHC) class I molecules (13). Previous researcher has demonstrated that ERAP2 enzyme function could affect T cell and NK cell responses towards normal and cancer cells as well as the synthesis of inflammatory cytokines (26). Since ERAP2 is deeply involved in the generation and destruction of immunopeptidome, its deficiency can lead to disorders in anti-

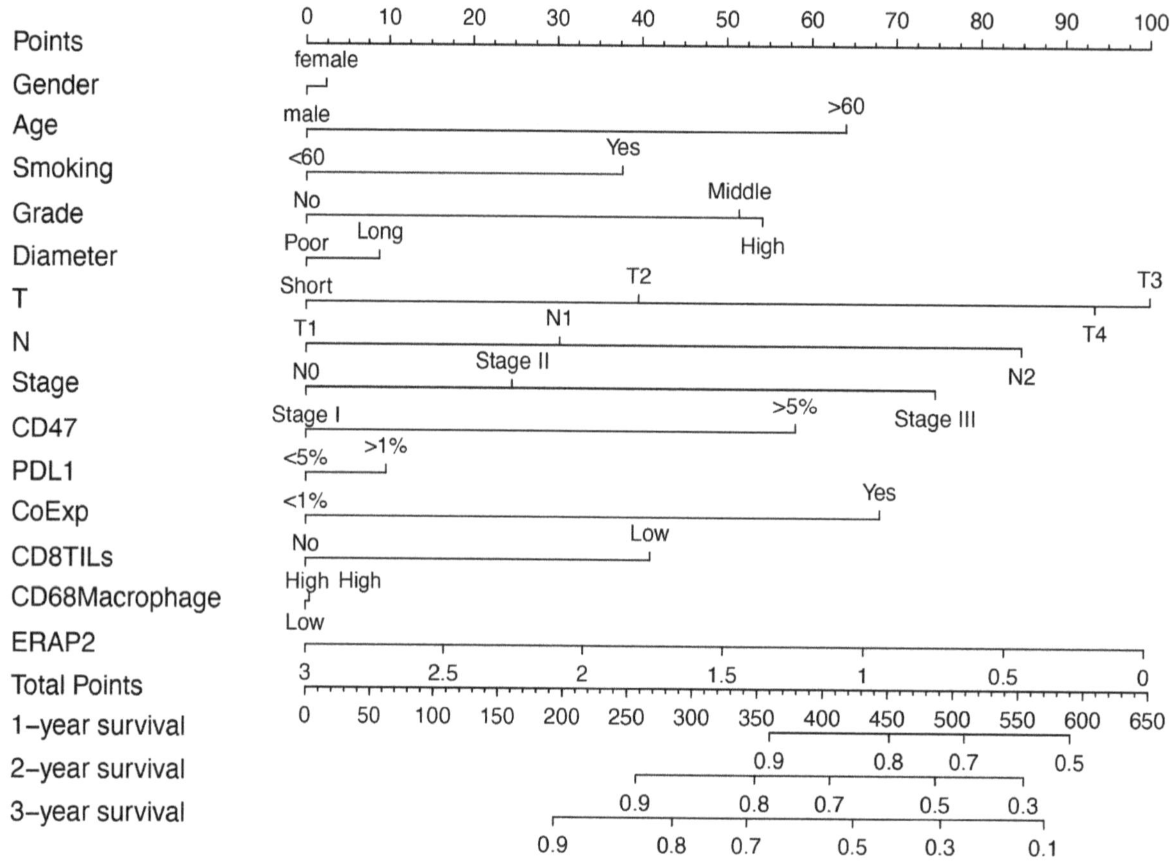

FIGURE 3 | Prognostic nomogram based on the clinicopathological factors, ERAP2 expression, and other immune markers predicting the 1-year, 2-year, and 3-year overall survival rate in our SqCLC cohort. T, T stage. N, N stage. CoExp, PD-L1and CD47 co-expression. CD8TILs, CD8+ tumor infiltration lymphocytes. CD68 Macrophage, CD68+ infiltration macrophages.

tumor immunity activation. Considering our findings in the public database, we speculated that ERAP2 is of great worth in SqCLC.

We are the first to illustrate the predictive value of ERAP2 in SqCLC. The predictive value of ERAP2 was validated in SqCLC TMAs with high quality. All patients in our cohort accepted no pre-surgery treatments, and the most recent patient was diagnosed in 2011, offering a long enough follow-up period. In our cohort, ERAP2 expression was positively related to overall survival, consistent with what we found in the public database, providing further evidence for the definition of ERAP2 as a prognostic indicator in SqCLC. Moreover, using multivariate analysis, we confirmed that ERAP2 expression was an independent prognostic factor for SqCLC individuals based on our cohort.

Based on previous research, we hypothesized that the positive predictive function of ERAP2 in SqCLC derived from its ability to prevent immune evasion by modulating immune recognition (27) because improper trimming of peptides in ER is one of the strategies that cancer cells avoid the attack from the immune system (28). In 2021, Mpakali et al. (14) reported that ERAP2 can trim the peptides that enter the ER and are too long to fit into MHC I molecule. However, while trimming peptides, ERAP2 can also destroy tumor-associated antigenic peptides destined for loading on MHC I, thus affecting avoiding T cell response.

Little was known about how ERAP2 behaves in lung cancer. In 2014, Zhou et al. (29) reported that ERAP2 rs2248374/rs2549782-AG haplotype was significantly associated with increased NSCLC risk, while ERAP2 rs2248374/rs2549782-GT haplotype individuals tended to indicate a reduced risk. In 2021, Wis´niewski et al. (30) asserted that the extent of ERAP2 presence could affect the anti-cancer response of ERAP1 in NSCLC. To our knowledge, there has been no study focusing on the ERAP2 expression in lung cancer so far, and the area of ERAP2 in SqCLC has never been set foot in.

One of the highlight conclusions of our study is that in both public data and our cohort, high expression of ERAP2 is correlated with the immunoreactive tumor microenvironment, which is favorable for administering immunotherapy in SqCLC. Due to its malignant nature and intricate genomic architecture, many SqCLC patients are marginalized in the prosperity of immunotherapy, failing to obtain sustained benefits from ICIs

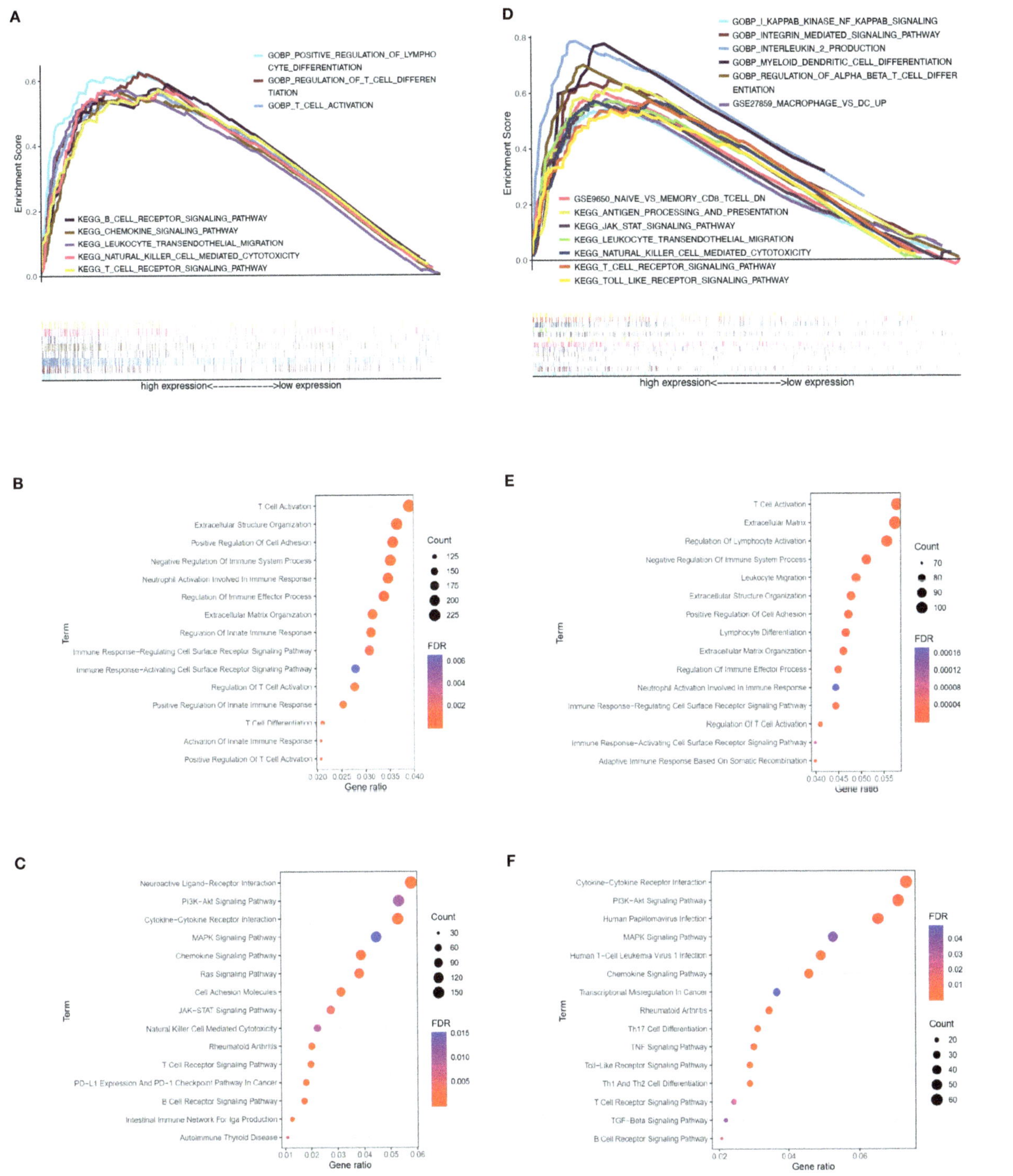

FIGURE 4 | Pathway enrichment analysis of patients with different ERAP2 expression level in SqCLC public data. **(A)** Enrichment analysis based on TCGA SqCLC data. Upper: pathways, terms, or gene sets enriched in ERAP2 high expression group. **(B)** Representative GO terms and pathways enriched in DEGs between high and low ERAP2 expression groups based on TCGA SqCLC data. **(C)** Representative KEGG terms and pathways enriched in DEGs between high and low ERAP2 expression groups based on TCGA SqCLC data. **(D)** Enrichment analysis based on GEO SqCLC data. Upper: pathways, terms, or gene sets enriched in ERAP2 high expression group. **(E)** Representative GO terms and pathways enriched in DEGs between high and low ERAP2 expression groups based on GEO SqCLC data. **(F)** Representative KEGG terms and pathways enriched in DEGs between high and low ERAP2 expression groups based on GEO SqCLC data.

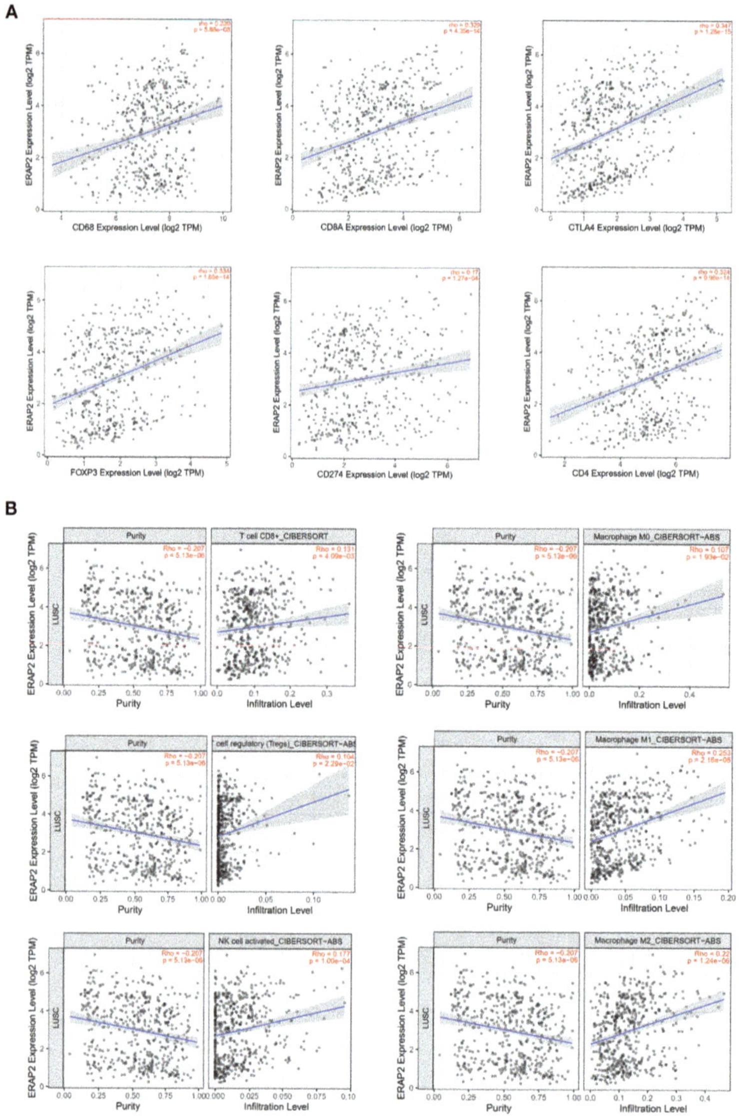

FIGURE 5 | Immune associations about ERAP2 expression using public data (TIMER). **(A)** Correlations between the expression of ERAP2 and immune markers in SqCLC. Top: CD68, CD8A, CTLA4. Bottom: FOXP3, CD274, CD4. The correlation coefficient and p-value are in the top right corner of each picture. **(B)** Correlations between ERAP2 expression and immune cell infiltration level in SqCLC. Top CD8+ T cell, M0 macrophage. Middle: regulatory T cell regulatory, M1 macrophage. Bottom: Activated NK cell, M2 macrophage.

(31). In the realm of SqCLC, methods that can boost immunotherapy efficacy are demanding. The tumor microenvironment (TME) is an integral component of cancer, composed of various cell types crucial to tumor immunology (32). The TME infrastructure and the interactions between cancer cells and TME during cancer initiation and progression could dictate the response to immunotherapy (33). In our study, high ERAP2 expression was associated with high levels of multiple immune markers and cells, including PD-L1, CD47, $CD8^+$ TILs, $CD68^+$ Macrophages, and NK cells which were positive indicators for immunotherapy. Our findings of ERAP2 and NK cells were consistent with previous studies (13, 15), while we are the first to illustrate the associations between ERAP2 and other immune cells and markers. The positive association between ERAP2 and FOXP3 aroused our interest. Although FOXP3 was previously reported to promote tumor growth and metastasis in NSCLC (34), there were also researches asserting that tumoral FOXP3 had the potential to suppress tumor function in SqCLC (35). The involvements between FOXP3 and tumor immunity have not been clearly illustrated, and current results of tumor FOXP3 are inconsistent and inconclusive (36). The ERAP2 high expression group harbored an immune-active TME, suggesting the feasibility of immune-related treatments among SqCLC with ERAP2 high expression

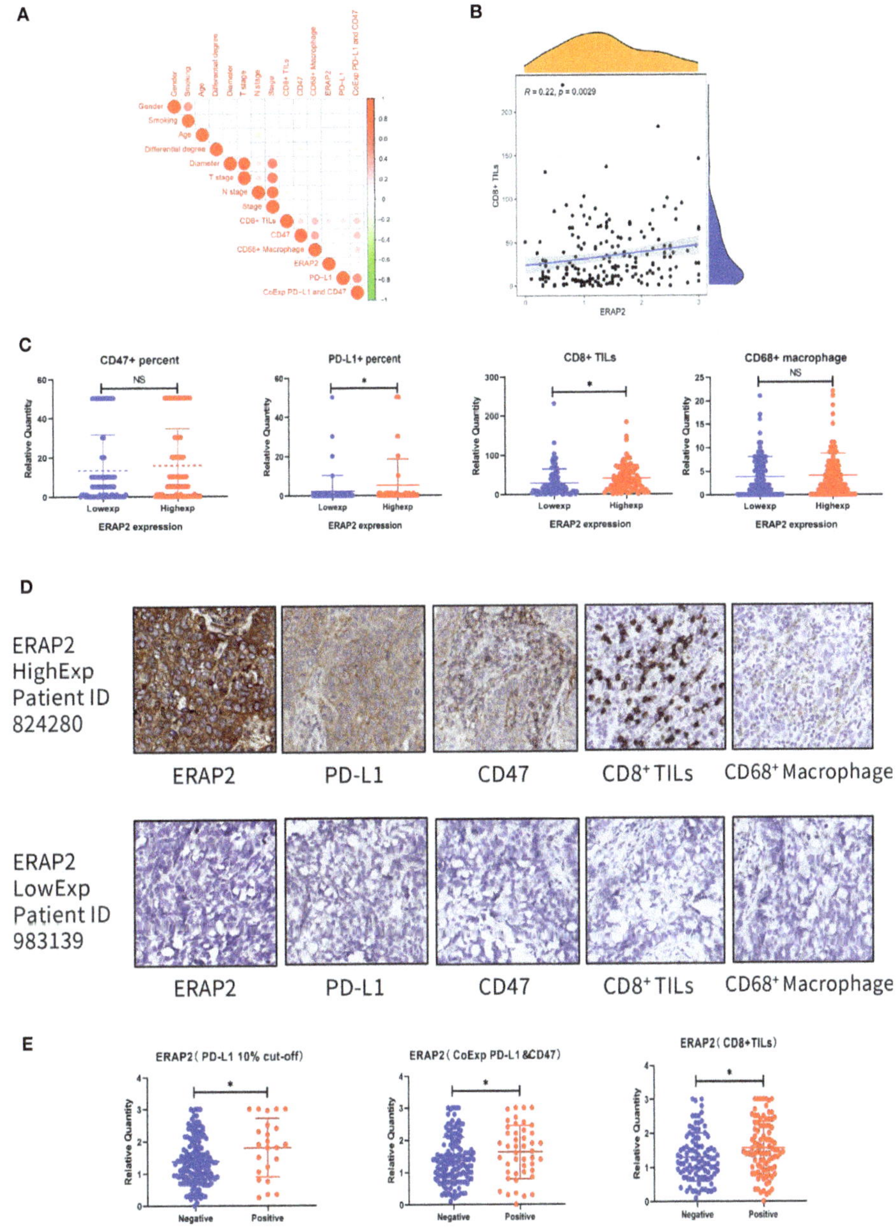

FIGURE 6 | Association between ERAP2 expression and multiple immune markers in our SqCLC TMA. **(A)** Associations among all clinicopathological and immune markers in SqCLC TMAs. The circle color represents the correlational tendency. The circle size represents the statistical significance. Red, positive correlation. Green, negative correlation. Larger circle represents the lower p-value. **(B)** Correlation between ERAP2 expression and CD8+ TILs. Spearman relevant coefficient = 0.22, p-value=0.0029. **(C)** The relative quantity of immune markers in ERAP2 high and low expression patients of SqCLC TMAs. From left to right: CD47, PD-L1, CD8, and CD68. Blue, ERAP2 low expression group. Red, ERAP2 high expression group. Asterisk, p-value<0.05. **(D)** IHC images of representative patients in the ERAP2 high and low expression group (100×). Upper: representative patient with high ERAP2 expression. Lower: representative patient with low ERAP2 expression. From left to right: ERAP2, PD-L1, CD47, $CD8^+$ TILs and $CD68^+$ Macrophages. **(E)** The relative quantity of ERAP2 among patients with different immune marker statuses. From left to right: PD-L1, PD-L1 and CD47 co-expression, CD8+ TILs. Asterisk, p-value < 0.05.

and the potentiality of ERAP2 as a biomarker for SqCLC immunotherapy. ERAP2 was also involved in autoimmune diseases, such as ankylosing spondylitis (34), whose etiology is unclear. The immune activation process during pre-eclampsia was also reported to be engaged with the differential expression of ERAP1/2 (37), suggesting the importance of ERAP2 in the immune system (38).

Under the pandemic of SARS-CoV-2, ERAP2 abnormity is related to the unfavorable clinical outcomes of COVID-19 infected patients, while ERAP2 may also inspire the development of the vaccine. Recently, ERAP2 was reported to participate in the virus antigen presentation process of COVID-19 (39, 40). ERAP2 and its homolog ERAP1 constituted an efficient filter to epitope presentation by greatly limiting the diversity of virus antigenic peptides sequences produced, suggesting the promising value of ERAP2 in SARS-CoV-2 immunogenicity studies and vaccine design (41). The rs150892504 mutations in the ERAP2 gene were believed to be a genetic factor related to severe life-threatening complications in individuals infected with coronavirus (42). Since ERAP2 was involved in the renin-angiotensin system (RAS), ERAP2 dysfunction was hypothesized to exacerbate the symptomatology and prognosis of the SARS-CoV-2.

Several limitations existed in our study. First, our TMAs only contained tumor tissue of each patient, lacking the data of matched normal samples. Secondly, we only performed IHC to a limited number of immune markers, which were far from enough to represent the whole ecosystem of TME. Third, we did not validate our findings at the transcriptional level because there were no fresh or fresh frozen samples.

In conclusion, our study is the first to intensively illustrate the role of ERAP2 in lung cancer. We identified ERAP2 as a positive prognostic biomarker for SqCLC and revealed its potentiality in predicting immunotherapy response, offering novel ideas for the administration of ICIs in SqCLC.

FOOTNOTE

The authors are accountable for all aspects of the work in ensuring that questions related to the accuracy or integrity of any part of the word are approximately investigated and resolved.

Written informed consents for the publication of details relating to any participant were obtained from that person.

AUTHOR CONTRIBUTIONS

JH, SG, and CL were responsible for conception and design. JH, SG, JW, CL, and BZ offered administrative support. HT and ZY provided study materials and clinical resources. HT, FB, and ZZ were responsible for the collection and assembly of data. HT, ZY, FB, and JY were responsible for data analysis. JX, RL, YP, GB, YT, YC, LL, TF, CX, and YZ were responsible for data interpretation. All authors were contributed to the writing and final approval of the manuscript.

ACKNOWLEDGMENTS

We appreciate the technical support of Cunming Hu from Outdo Biotech Co., LTD., Shanghai, and we appreciated the TCGA and GEO organization for providing us with solid public data.

REFERENCES

1. Siegel RL, Miller KD, Fuchs HE, Jemal A. Cancer Statistics, 2021. *CA Cancer J Clin* (2021) 71(1):7–33. doi: 10.3322/caac.21654
2. Herbst RS, Morgensztern D, Boshoff C. The Biology and Management of non-Small Cell Lung Cancer. *Nature* (2018) 553(7689):446–54. doi: 10.1038/nature25183
3. Friedlaender A, Banna G, Malapelle U, Pisapia P, Addeo A. Next Generation Sequencing and Genetic Alterations in Squamous Cell Lung Carcinoma: Where Are We Today? *Front Oncol* (2019) 9:166. doi: 10.3389/fonc.2019.00166
4. Hanna N, Johnson D, Temin S, Baker S Jr, Brahmer J, Ellis PM, et al. Systemic Therapy for Stage IV Non-Small-Cell Lung Cancer: American Society of Clinical Oncology Clinical Practice Guideline Update. *J Clin Oncol* (2017) 35 (30):3484–515. doi: 10.1200/JCO.2017.74.6065
5. Yang CY, Yang JC, Yang PC. Precision Management of Advanced Non-Small Cell Lung Cancer. *Annu Rev Med* (2020) 71:117–36. doi: 10.1146/annurev-med-051718-013524
6. Reck M, Rabe KF. Precision Diagnosis and Treatment for Advanced Non-Small-Cell Lung Cancer. *N Engl J Med* (2017) 377(9):849–61. doi: 10.1056/NEJMra1703413
7. Stewart PA, Welsh EA, Slebos RJC, Fang B, Izumi V, Chambers M, et al. Proteogenomic Landscape of Squamous Cell Lung Cancer. *Nat Commun* (2019) 10(1):3578. doi: 10.1038/s41467-019-11452-x
8. Doroshow DB, Sanmamed MF, Hastings K, Politi K, Rimm DL, Chen L, et al. Immunotherapy in Non-Small Cell Lung Cancer: Facts and Hopes. *Clin Cancer Res* (2019) 25(15):4592–602. doi: 10.1158/1078-0432.CCR-18-1538
9. Somasundaram A, Burns TF. The Next Generation of Immunotherapy: Keeping Lung Cancer in Check. *J Hematol Oncol* (2017) 10(1):87. doi: 10.1186/s13045-017-0456-5
10. Fierabracci A, Milillo A, Locatelli F, Fruci D. The Putative Role of Endoplasmic Reticulum Aminopeptidases in Autoimmunity: Insights From Genomic-Wide Association Studies. *Autoimmun Rev* (2012) 12(2):281–8. doi: 10.1016/j.autrev.2012.04.007
11. Saveanu L, Carroll O, Lindo V, Del Val M, Lopez D, Lepelletier Y, et al. Concerted Peptide Trimming by Human ERAP1 and ERAP2 Aminopeptidase Complexes in the Endoplasmic Reticulum. *Nat Immunol* (2005) 6(7):689–97. doi: 10.1038/ni1208
12. López de Castro JA. How ERAP1 and ERAP2 Shape the Peptidomes of Disease-Associated MHC-I Proteins. *Front Immunol* (2018) 9:2463. doi: 10.3389/fimmu.2018.02463
13. Haroon N, Inman RD. Endoplasmic Reticulum Aminopeptidases: Biology and Pathogenic Potential. *Nat Rev Rheumatol* (2010) 6(8):461–7. doi: 10.1038/nrrheum.2010.85
14. Mpakali A, Stratikos E. The Role of Antigen Processing and Presentation in Cancer and the Efficacy of Immune Checkpoint Inhibitor Immunotherapy. *Cancers (Basel)* (2021) 13(1):6–7. doi: 10.3390/cancers13010134
15. Cifaldi L, Lo Monaco E, Forloni M, Giorda E, Lorenzi S, Petrini S, et al. Natural Killer Cells Efficiently Reject Lymphoma Silenced for the Endoplasmic Reticulum Aminopeptidase Associated With Antigen Processing. *Cancer Res* (2011) 71(5):1597–606. doi: 10.1158/0008-5472.CAN-10-3326
16. Cifaldi L, Romania P, Falco M, Lorenzi S, Meazza R, Petrini S, et al. ERAP1 Regulates Natural Killer Cell Function by Controlling the Engagement of Inhibitory Receptors. *Cancer Res* (2015) 75(5):824–34. doi: 10.1158/0008-5472.CAN-14-1643
17. Lim YW, Chen-Harris H, Mayba O, Lianoglou S, Wuster A, Bhangale T, et al. Germline Genetic Polymorphisms Influence Tumor Gene Expression and Immune Cell Infiltration. *Proc Natl Acad Sci USA* (2018) 115(50):E11701–e11710. doi: 10.1073/pnas.1804506115
18. Babaie F, Hosseinzadeh R, Ebrazeh M, Seyfizadeh N, Aslani S, Salimi S, et al. The Roles of ERAP1 and ERAP2 in Autoimmunity and Cancer Immunity: New Insights and Perspective. *Mol Immunol* (2020) 121:7–19. doi: 10.1016/j.molimm.2020.02.020
19. Compagnone M, Cifaldi L, Fruci D. Regulation of ERAP1 and ERAP2 Genes and Their Disfunction in Human Cancer. *Hum Immunol* (2019) 80(5):318–24. doi: 10.1016/j.humimm.2019.02.014
20. Fruci D, Giacomini P, Nicotra MR, Forloni M, Fraioli R, Saveanu L, et al. Altered Expression of Endoplasmic Reticulum Aminopeptidases ERAP1 and ERAP2 in Transformed non-Lymphoid Human Tissues. *J Cell Physiol* (2008) 216(3):742–9. doi: 10.1002/jcp.21454

21. Chang KP, Hao S-P, Chang J-H, Wu C-C, Tsang N-M, Lee Y-S, et al. Macrophage Inflammatory Protein-3alpha is a Novel Serum Marker for Nasopharyngeal Carcinoma Detection and Prediction of Treatment Outcomes. *Clin Cancer Res* (2008) 14(21):6979–87. doi: 10.1158/1078-0432.CCR-08-0090
22. Ma S, Sun S, Geng L, Song M, Wang W, Ye Y, et al. Caloric Restriction Reprograms the Single-Cell Transcriptional Landscape of Rattus Norvegicus Aging. *Cell* (2020) 180(5):984–1001.e22. doi: 10.1016/j.cell.2020.02.008
23. Newman AM, Steen CB, Liu CL, Gentles AJ, Chaudhuri AA, Scherer F, et al. Determining Cell Type Abundance and Expression From Bulk Tissues With Digital Cytometry. *Nat Biotechnol* (2019) 37(7):773–82. doi: 10.1038/s41587-019-0114-2
24. Chansky K, Detterbeck FC, Nicholson AG, Rusch VW, Vallières E, Groome P, et al. The IASLC Lung Cancer Staging Project: External Validation of the Revision of the TNM Stage Groupings in the Eighth Edition of the TNM Classification of Lung Cancer. *J Thorac Oncol* (2017) 12(7):1109–21. doi: 10.1016/j.jtho.2017.04.011
25. Socinski MA, Obasaju C, Gandara D, Hirsch FR, Bonomi P, Bunn PA Jr, et al. Current and Emergent Therapy Options for Advanced Squamous Cell Lung Cancer. *J Thorac Oncol* (2018) 13(2):165–83. doi: 10.1016/j.jtho.2017.11.111
26. Stratikos E, Stamogiannos A, Zervoudi E, Fruci D. A Role for Naturally Occurring Alleles of Endoplasmic Reticulum Aminopeptidases in Tumor Immunity and Cancer Pre-Disposition. *Front Oncol* (2014) 4:363. doi: 10.3389/fonc.2014.00363
27. Lee ED. Endoplasmic Reticulum Aminopeptidase 2, a Common Immunological Link to Adverse Pregnancy Outcomes and Cancer Clearance? *Placenta* (2017) 56:40–3. doi: 10.1016/j.placenta.2017.03.012
28. Jhunjhunwala S, Hammer C, Delamarre L. Antigen Presentation in Cancer: Insights Into Tumour Immunogenicity and Immune Evasion. *Nat Rev Cancer* (2021) 21(5):298–312. doi: 10.1038/s41568-021-00339-z
29. Zhou J, Ma Q, Guo C, Shi L, Yao Y, Yu J, et al. A Study on the Relationship Between Endoplasmic Reticulum Aminopeptidase2 Genetic Polymorphisms and non-Small Cell Lung Cancer in Yunnan Han Population. *Zhonghua Jie He He Hu Xi Za Zhi* (2014) 37(12):909–14. doi: 10.1016/s0169-5002(96)90254-8
30. Wiśniewski A, Sobczyński M, Pawełczyk K, Porębska I, Jasek M, Wagner M, et al. Polymorphisms of Antigen-Presenting Machinery Genes in Non-Small Cell Lung Cancer: Different Impact on Disease Risk and Clinical Parameters in Smokers and Never-Smokers. *Front Immunol* (2021) 12:664474. doi: 10.3389/fimmu.2021.664474
31. Hai J, Zhang H, Zhou J, Wu Z, Chen T, Papadopoulos E, et al. Generation of Genetically Engineered Mouse Lung Organoid Models for Squamous Cell Lung Cancers Allows for the Study of Combinatorial Immunotherapy. *Clin Cancer Res* (2020) 26(13):3431–42. doi: 10.1158/1078-0432.CCR-19-1627
32. Pitt JM, Marabelle A, Eggermont A, Soria J-C, Kroemer G, Zitvogel L. Targeting the Tumor Microenvironment: Removing Obstruction to Anticancer Immune Responses and Immunotherapy. *Ann Oncol* (2016) 27 (8):1482–92. doi: 10.1093/annonc/mdw168
33. Murciano-Goroff YR, Warner AB, Wolchok JD. The Future of Cancer Immunotherapy: Microenvironment-Targeting Combinations. *Cell Res* (2020) 30(6):507–19. doi: 10.1038/s41422-020-0337-2
34. Yang S, Liu Y, Li M-Y, Ng CSH, Yang S-L, Wang S, et al. FOXP3 Promotes Tumor Growth and Metastasis by Activating Wnt/β+-Catenin Signaling Pathway and EMT in non-Small Cell Lung Cancer. *Mol Cancer* (2017) 16 (1):124. doi: 10.1186/s12943-017-0700-1
35. Won KY, Kim HK, Kim GY, Min Song J, Lim S-J. Hippo Pathway and Tumoral FOXP3 Expression Correlate With Tumor Growth in Squamous Cell Carcinoma of the Lung. *Pathol Res Pract* (2020) 216(7):153003. doi: 10.1016/j.prp.2020.153003
36. Jia H, Qi H, Gong Z, Yang S, Ren J, Liu Y, et al. The Expression of FOXP3 and its Role in Human Cancers. *Biochim Biophys Acta Rev Cancer* (2019) 1871 (1):170–8. doi: 10.1016/j.bbcan.2018.12.004
37. Seamon K, Kurlak LO, Warthan M, Stratikos E, Strauss JF 3rd, Mistry HD, et al. The Differential Expression of ERAP1/ERAP2 and Immune Cell Activation in Pre-Eclampsia. *Front Immunol* (2020) 11:396. doi: 10.3389/fimmu.2020.00396
38. Paladini F, Fiorillo MT, Tedeschi V, Mattorre B, Sorrentino R. The Multifaceted Nature of Aminopeptidases ERAP1, ERAP2, and LNPEP: From Evolution to Disease. *Front Immunol* (2020) 11:1576. doi: 10.3389/fimmu.2020.01576
39. Saulle I, Vanetti C, Goglia S, Vicentini C, Tombetti E, Garziano M, et al. A New ERAP2/Iso3 Isoform Expression Is Triggered by Different Microbial Stimuli in Human Cells. Could It Play a Role in the Modulation of SARS-CoV-2 Infection? *Cells* (2020) 9(9):5–9. doi: 10.3390/cells9091951
40. Saulle I, Vicentini C, Clerici M, Biasin M. Antigen Presentation in SARS-CoV-2 Infection: The Role of Class I HLA and ERAP Polymorphisms. *Hum Immunol* (2021) 82(8):551–60. doi: 10.1016/j.humimm.2021.05.003
41. Stamatakis G, Samiotaki M, Mpakali A, Panayotou G, Stratikos E. Generation of SARS-CoV-2 S1 Spike Glycoprotein Putative Antigenic Epitopes *in Vitro* by Intracellular Aminopeptidases. *J Proteome Res* (2020) 19(11):4398–406. doi: 10.1021/acs.jproteome.0c00457
42. Malkova A, Kudlay D, Kudryavtsev I, Starshinova A, Yablonskiy P, Shoenfeld Y. Immunogenetic Predictors of Severe COVID-19. *Vaccines (Basel)* (2021) 9 (3):5. doi: 10.3390/vaccines9030211

10

Concordance of PD-L1 Status Between Image-Guided Percutaneous Biopsies and Matched Surgical Specimen in Non-Small Cell Lung Cancer

Liang Zhao[1†], Peiqiong Chen[2†], Kaili Fu[1†], Jinluan Li[1], Yaqing Dai[1], Yuhuan Wang[2], Yanzhen Zhuang[2], Long Sun[3], Haojun Chen[3] and Qin Lin[1*]*

[1] *Department of Radiation Oncology, The First Affiliated Hospital of Xiamen University, Teaching Hospital of Fujian Medical University, Xiamen, China,* [2] *Department of Pathology, The First Affiliated Hospital of Xiamen University, Teaching Hospital of Fujian Medical University, Xiamen, China,* [3] *Department of Nuclear Medicine & Minnan PET Center, The First Affiliated Hospital of Xiamen University, Teaching Hospital of Fujian Medical University, Xiamen, China*

Correspondence:
Haojun Chen
leochen0821@foxmail.com
Qin Lin
linqin05@163.com

[†]These authors have contributed equally to this work

Objective: Programmed death-ligand 1 (PD-L1) expression status is a crucial index for identifying patients who will benefit from anti-programmed cell death protein 1 (PD-1)/PD-L1 therapy for non-small cell lung cancer (NSCLC). However, the concordance of Tumor Proportion Score (TPS) between biopsies and matched surgical specimens remains controversial. This study aims to evaluate the concordance of PD-L1 expression between image-guided percutaneous biopsies and matched surgical specimens.

Method: We evaluated 157 patients diagnosed with operable NSCLC on both surgical tissue sections and matched lung biopsies retrospectively. The patients underwent either regular computed tomography (CT)-guided biopsy (n = 82) or positron emission tomography (PET)/CT-guided biopsy (n = 75). The concordance between surgical specimens and lung biopsies for PD-L1 TPS was evaluated using Cohen's kappa (κ) coefficient.

Results: Immunohistochemical expression of PD-L1 was evaluated in both surgical resected specimens and matched biopsies in the eligible 138 patients. The concordance rate of PD-L1 expression between surgical tissue sections and matched biopsies was fairly high at 84.1% (116/138), and the κ value was 0.73 (95% CI: 0.63–0.83, $P < 0.001$). The concordance rate was higher for tissue sections from PET/CT-guided biopsy than for tissue sections from CT-guided biopsy [88.6% (62/70, κ value: 0.81) vs 79.4% (54/68, κ value: 0.66)].

Conclusion: PD-L1 TPS was strongly concordant between surgical specimens and matched lung biopsies. Thus, the routine evaluation of PD-L1 expression in diagnostic percutaneous biopsies could be reliable for identifying patients who will benefit from anti-PD-1/PD-L1 immunotherapy.

Keywords: programmed death-ligand 1 (PD-L1), biopsy, surgical resected specimen, PET/CT, non-small cell lung cancer

INTRODUCTION

Lung cancer is the leading cause of cancer-related death worldwide, and it is projected to account for over 22% of deaths in 2020 in the United States (1). Non-small cell lung cancer (NSCLC) accounts for about 80% of lung cancers. NSCLC has poor prognosis, but immunotherapy has markedly improved survival in patients with advanced NSCLC without driver alterations. In the KEYNOTE-024 and KEYNOTE-042 phase III clinical trials, programmed cell death protein 1 (PD-1)-targeted immunotherapy significantly improved the overall survival (OS) rate compared with standard therapy in advanced NSCLC (2, 3). Based on these studies, the FDA approved pembrolizumab as the first-line treatment for advanced NSCLC patients with a Tumor Proportion Score (TPS) of ≥50% (based on KEYNOTE-024) and 1% (based on KEYNOTE-042), respectively.

Other immunotherapies targeted against PD-1 or programmed death-ligand 1 (PD-L1), such as nivolumab, atezolizumab, and durvalumab (**Supplemental Table 1**), also showed OS benefit with similar PD-L1 cut-off values (4, 5). Thus, determining PD-L1 expression status may help select patients who will optimally benefit from immunotherapy. Immunohistochemistry (IHC) has been widely used to evaluate PD-L1 status in both clinical trials and routine clinical practice. Currently, PD-L1 testing is mainly performed on biopsy samples, which may not be representative of the whole tumor. Thus, the concordance of TPS between lung biopsies and matched surgical specimens remains controversial (6), which may result in decreased confidence on the reliability of biopsies for PD-L1 testing.

Image-guided percutaneous biopsy is currently widely used as it is minimally invasive and is associated with fewer complications. CT-guided biopsy is the most common approach for sampling of lung lesions, but it has varying diagnostic performance depending upon the target organ and type of needle used (7, 8). Meanwhile, ^{18}F-FDG PET/CT provides both anatomic structures and metabolic features and has therefore been suggested to improve the diagnostic accuracy of image-guided biopsy (9–12). We have previously reported the importance of PET/CT-guided biopsy for patient evaluation at various stages of cancers (9, 13, 14). Applying PET/CT information to image-guided biopsy may facilitate accurate histopathological diagnosis and help with staging. However, only few studies to date have compared the reliability and reproducibility of PET/CT-guided biopsy with corresponding resected surgical specimens. Moreover, the use of PD-L1 as a biomarker for determining sensitivity to PD-1/PD-L1 checkpoint blockades has raised concerns on the reliability of biopsy samples compared with surgical specimens. Thus, the present study aimed to evaluate the concordance of immunohistochemical expression of PD-L1 between image-guided biopsies and matched surgical specimens.

MATERIALS AND METHODS

Patient Population

The study protocol was discussed and approved by the institutional review board of the First Affiliated Hospital of Xiamen University (ID, KY2017-001), and written informed consent was obtained from all patients.

We retrospectively evaluated 157 patients with operable NSCLC who underwent both diagnostic percutaneous lung biopsy and surgical resection at the First Affiliated Hospital of Xiamen University, between December 2016 and October 2019. The exclusion criteria were as follows: (i) history of chemotherapy or radiotherapy before biopsy and surgery and (ii) incomplete preoperative clinical record, including data on body mass index, smoking history, blood routine examination, and blood biochemistry examination. Of the 157 patients, 82 underwent CT-guided biopsy, while the other 75 patients underwent ^{18}F-FDG PET/CT-guided biopsy. Eventually, 138 matched biopsy and surgical resection specimens were obtained for further IHC analysis of PD-L1 expression. There were 72 men and 66 women in the derivation cohort, and the median patient age was 63 years (range: 25–81 years). In total, 53 (38.4%) patients were current or former smokers. All patients were staged or restaged according to the 8th International Association for the Study of Lung Cancer staging system based on postoperative pathological result. Overall, 61 (44.2%) patients had stages II–III disease, and majority (n = 116, 84.1%) had non-squamous histology. The clinicodemographic characteristics of the 138 patients are summarized in **Table 1**.

Image-Guided Percutaneous Biopsy

Diagnostic percutaneous lung biopsy was performed under either CT guidance or ^{18}F-FDG PET/CT guidance. ^{18}F-FDG PET/CT protocol and imaging analysis were performed as previously described (15). The imaging modality was determined based on discussions with the referring oncologists. The biopsy target was decided by the referring oncologists and interventional radiologists based on the results of ^{18}F-FDG PET/CT or CT scan.

Image-guided biopsy was performed with an 18G or 20G semiautomatic core needle (Coaxial Achieve, Bard, IL, USA) with coaxial guide needle. The percutaneous biopsy was performed by a board-certified interventional radiologist following a step-by-step technique as previously described (8, 13). Briefly, the patients were positioned in a supine or prone position in accordance with factors such as the location of FDG-avid lesion, shortest skin-to-target distance, and optimal needle path. Interventions were conducted under aseptic conditions after administration of local anesthesia using 2.0% lidocaine. The needle was introduced in a stepwise manner under fused PET/CT and CT imaging guidance. Three or four specimens were obtained from each patient, after which histopathological examination and immunohistochemical staining were performed on each specimen. After the biopsy, the patients were observed by referring oncologists for at least 24 h, and the patients were asked to report any abnormality.

Immunohistochemistry

The samples were prepared and stained as previously described (15). In brief, formalin-fixed, paraffin-embedded tumor tissues were sliced into 4 μm-thick sections. For IHC detection of PD-L1, we used the BenchMark GX automated slide stainer (SP263,

TABLE 1 | Clinicodemographic characteristics of the study patients.

Characteristic	Number	%
Age (years)		
<65	79	57.2%
≥65	59	42.8%
Median (range)	63 (25–81)	
Sex		
Male	72	52.2%
Female	66	47.8%
Smoking history		
Nonsmoker	85	61.6%
Smoker	53	38.4%
Histology		
Squamous cell carcinoma	22	15.9%
Adenocarcinoma	116	84.1%
Clinical stage (International Association for the Study of Lung Cancer 8th)		
I	77	55.8%
II/III	61	44.2%
Tumor size (cm)		
≤3	94	68.1%
>3	44	31.9%
Derived neutrophil–lymphocyte ratio		
<3	133	96.4%
≥3	5	3.6%
Lactate dehydrogenase (U/L)		
<240	129	93.5%
≥240	9	6.5%
Body mass index		
<25	102	73.9%
≥25	36	26.1%

Ventana, Oro Valley, AZ, USA) to stain the sections with the PD-L1 antibody according to the manufacturer's recommended protocol. Positive control (placenta) and negative control samples were run simultaneously.

The immunostained tissue sections were scored according to the PD-L1 scoring algorithm (16, 17) by three independent experienced pathologists who were blinded to the clinical data. Discrepancies in the PD-L1 score were resolved by reviewing the slides again. The cut-off values for PD-L1 expression were set to 1 and 50%.

Statistical Analysis

All statistical analyses were conducted using the SPSS 22.0 statistical analysis software (IBM, Armonk, NY, USA). For continuous data, we used the t-test or the Wilcoxon test for analyses, as appropriate. The concordance of PD-L1 TPS between surgical specimens and lung biopsies was evaluated using Cohen's kappa (κ) coefficient (18, 19). The relative strength of agreement was interpreted as follows: κ <0, poor; 0.01–0.20, slight; 0.21–0.40, fair; 0.41–0.60, moderate; 0.61–0.80, substantial; and 0.81–1.00, almost perfect (18, 19). Between group comparisons were performed using the chi-squared test, Yates' correction of chi-squared test, or Fisher's exact test. The correlation between different variables was analyzed using the non-parametric Spearman's rank test. All tests were two-sided, and a P value lower than 0.05 was considered statistically significant.

RESULTS

The diagnostic success rates of CT- and PET/CT-guided biopsy were 82.9% (68/82) and 93.3% (70/75), respectively. There were 11 central and 146 peripheral NSCLCs. Fourteen (8.9%) patients underwent pneumothorax, while 10 (6.4%) patients happened hemoptysis. PD-L1 TPS was <1, 1–49, and ≥50% in 72, 51, and 15 percutaneous biopsy specimens, respectively, and in 58, 63, and 17 surgical resection specimens, respectively (**Figure 1A**). Compared with the whole tumor section, 19 biopsy specimens underestimated the PD-L1 TPS, while only three biopsy section overestimated the TPS. Regarding the concern that biopsy specimens may underestimate the PD-L1 expression, four cases (one with PET/CT-guided biopsy, and three with CT-guided biopsy) in our study showed lower PD-L1 TPS in diagnostic biopsies (1–49%) as compared to the surgical samples (> 50%).

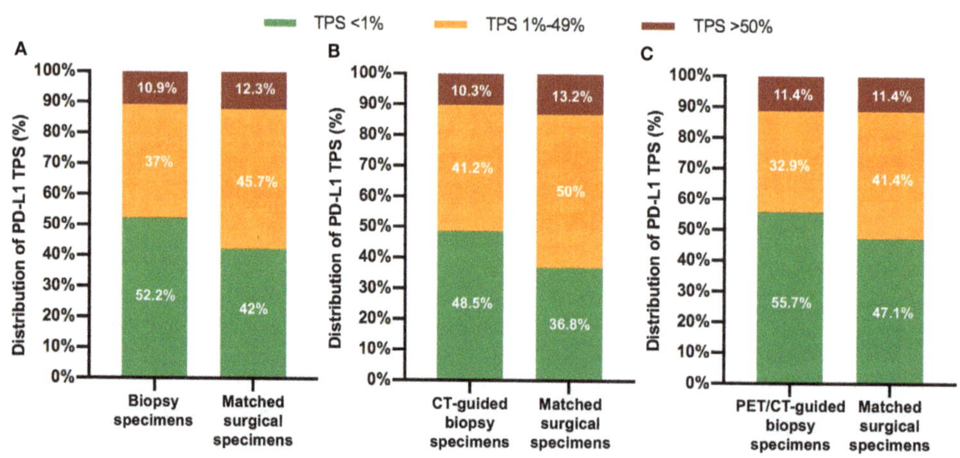

FIGURE 1 | Distribution of PD-L1 Tumor Proportion Score (TPS) for both biopsy specimens and matched surgical specimens in the overall patient population **(A)**, in the CT-guided biopsy group **(B)**, and in the PET/CT-guided biopsy group **(C)**.

The tissue sections from the biopsy and surgical resection in the four cases were further cautiously analyzed by our experienced pathologists, and a highly heterogenous expression of PD-L1 in the surgical specimen was observed in two out of four cases. There was no significant difference in PD-L1 TPS between biopsy and surgical tissue sections (P = 0.24).

The overall concordance rate for PD-L1 TPS between percutaneous biopsy specimens and matched surgical specimens was 84.1% (116/138). The Cohen's κ value was equal to 0.73 (95% CI: 0.63–0.83, P < 0.001), indicating substantial agreement. The concordance rate at a cut-off value of 1% PD-L1 TPS was 88.4%, and the κ value was equal to 0.77. The concordance rate at a cut-off value of PD-L1 TPS 50% also indicated substantial agreement (κ = 0.79). Representative images of concordant and discordant PD-L1 between biopsy and matched surgical specimens are shown in **Figures 2** and **3**, respectively. The Cohen's κ value according to histological subtypes was 0.79 (95% CI: 0.57–1, P < 0.001) for squamous cell carcinoma and 0.71 (95% CI: 0.59–0.83, P < 0.001) for lung adenocarcinoma.

There was no statistical difference in the distribution of PD-L1 TPS between biopsy and surgical specimens (**Figures 1B, C**). The concordance rate for PD-L1 TPS between CT-guided biopsy and matched surgical tissue was 79.4% (54/68), and the Cohen's κ value was 0.66 (95% CI: 0.50–0.82, P < 0.001), which indicated substantial agreement. Meanwhile, the concordance rate between PET/CT-guided biopsy specimen and matched surgical resection specimen was higher at 88.6% (62/70), and the Cohen's κ value was 0.81 (95% CI: 0.68–0.94, P < 0.001), which indicated almost perfect agreement (**Table 2**). PD-L1 TPS was significantly associated with SUVmax on Spearman correction analysis (P = 0.048, **Supplemental Table 2**). Representative ^{18}F-FDG PET/CT images for lung biopsy are shown in **Figure 4**.

As the CT and PET/CT groups had different concordance between percutaneous biopsy and matched surgical specimens, between-group comparisons were performed. The results showed no signifcant difference in the measured PD-L1 TPS between CT-guided biopsies and PET/CT-guided biopsies (P = 0.47). There was no significant difference in the primary clinicodemographic characteristics between the two cohorts (**Supplemental Table 3**).

DISCUSSION

Anti-PD-1/PD-L1 immunotherapy has improved the prognosis of NSCLC. In particular, nivolumab and pembrolizumab have

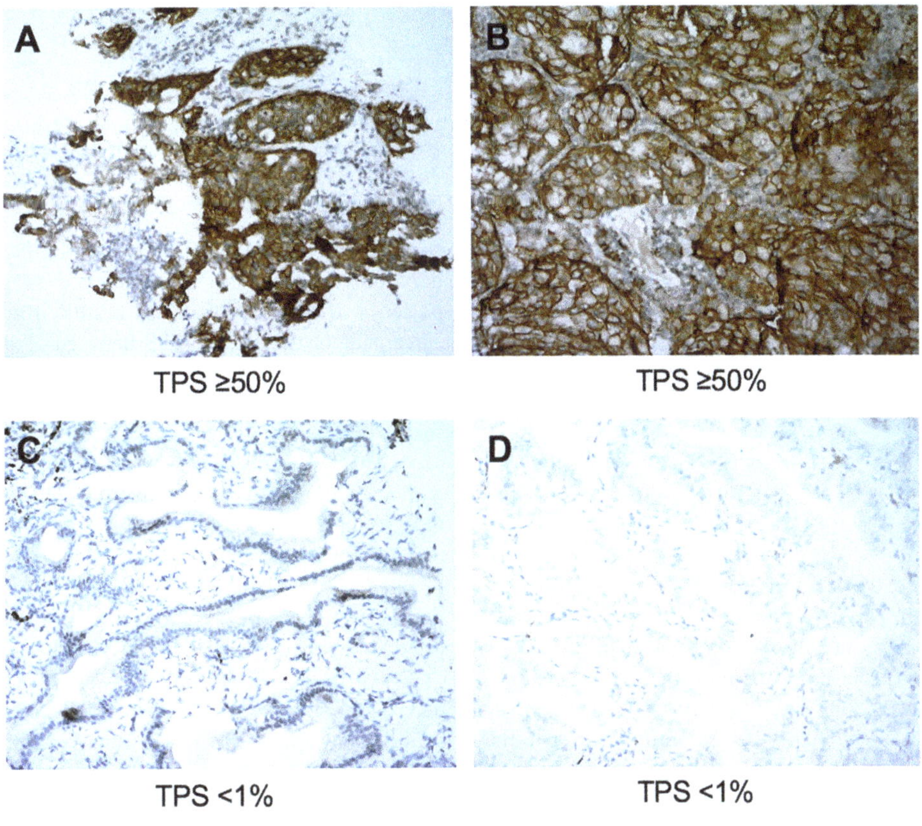

FIGURE 2 | Representative images of concordant cases between biopsy specimens (left panel) and matched surgical resection specimens (right panel). The PD-L1 Tumor Proportion Score (TPS) in the biopsy tumor specimen **(A)** and the corresponding resected tumor **(B)** were both ≥50%. PD-L1 TPS in the biopsy tumor **(C)** and the matched resected specimen **(D)** were both <1%. All images are at ×40 magnification.

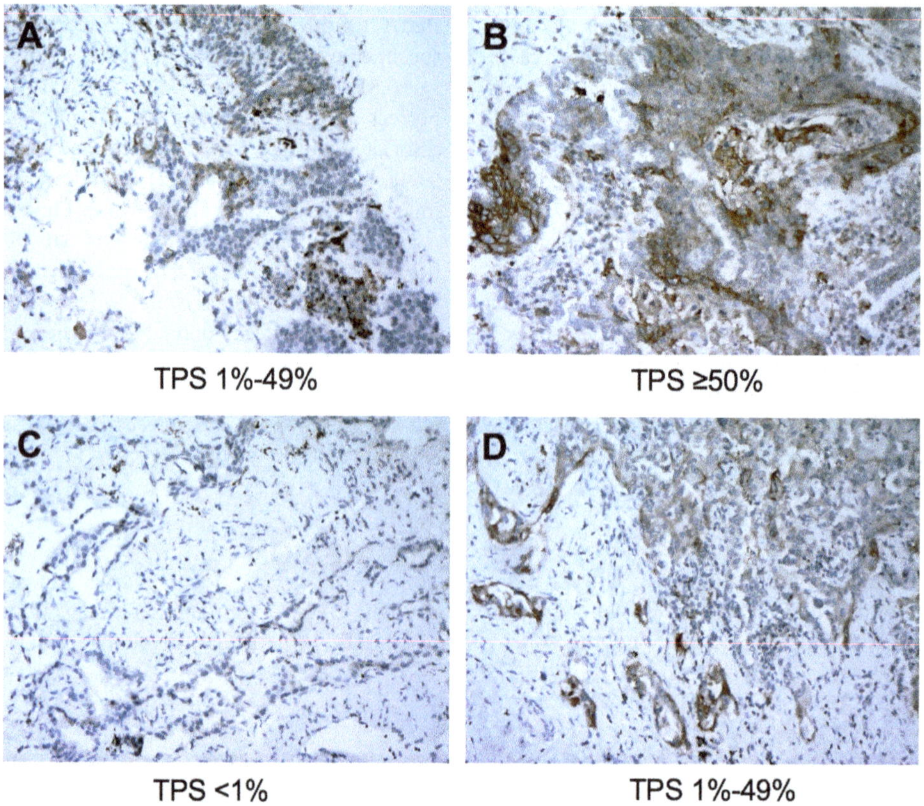

FIGURE 3 | Representative images of discordant cases between biopsy specimens (left panel) and matched resected specimens (right panel). The PD-L1 Tumor Proportion Score (TPS) was 10% in the biopsy tumor specimen **(A)** and was ≥50% in the corresponding resected tumor **(B)**. PD-L1 TPS in the biopsy specimen was <1% **(C)** and was 20% in the matched surgical specimen **(D)**. All images are at ×40 magnification.

TABLE 2 | Cohen's κ for concordance between percutaneous biopsy and matched surgical specimens based on TPS.

PD-L1 cutoff	Cohen's kappa (κ)		
	Overall population (N = 138)	CT group (N = 68)	PET/CT group (N = 70)
Tumor Proportion Score (TPS) ≥1%	0.77	0.7	0.83
TPS ≥50%	0.79	0.72	0.86
Overall	0.73	0.66	0.81

significantly improved the long-term survival of patients with NSCLC (20, 21). Compared to the usual OS rate of 5% with standard chemotherapy, the 5-year OS rate of pembrolizumab treatment was 29.6% in NSCLC patients with a PD-L1 TPS of over 50% in the KEYNOTE-001 study (21). Therefore, determining the PD-L1 TPS may help identify patients who will benefit from PD-1/PD-L1 blockade therapy, allowing for a more individualized treatment approach and avoiding unnecessary treatment. In this study, the percentage of NSCLCs with PD-L1 TPS <1, 1–49, and ≥50% were 42.0, 45.7, and 12.3%, respectively, which was in agreement with the previous publication (22). Accordingly, our study evaluated the concordance of tumor PD-L1 expression between image-guided percutaneous biopsies and matched surgical specimens in patients with NSCLC. Our results indicated substantial agreement of the PD-L1 TPS between surgical specimens and matched lung biopsies. Notably, samples from PET/CT-guided biopsy demonstrated higher success rate and concordance with surgical tissue sections than those from CT-guided biopsy.

PD-L1 testing using surgical specimens is rarely feasible in patients with NSCLC because of diagnosis at the advanced stage. Our results support the reliability of PD-L1 TPS determined using image-guided percutaneous biopsy specimens. These results can help establish PD-L1 expression assessed using image-guided biopsy specimen as a reliable biomarker for predicting benefit from anti-PD-1/PD-L1 immunotherapy.

Previous investigations have shown that intratumoral heterogeneity of PD-L1 expression exists within the entire surgical specimen (23), which may result in low concordance with the results obtained on diagnostic biopsies. As such, the concordance of PD-L1 status between biopsy samples and matched resected specimens varied across previous studies. For example, Tsunoda et al. and Kitazono et al. showed good concordance (24, 25), whereas Ilie et al. and Erik et al. demonstrated poor concordance (6, 26). It is worth noting that

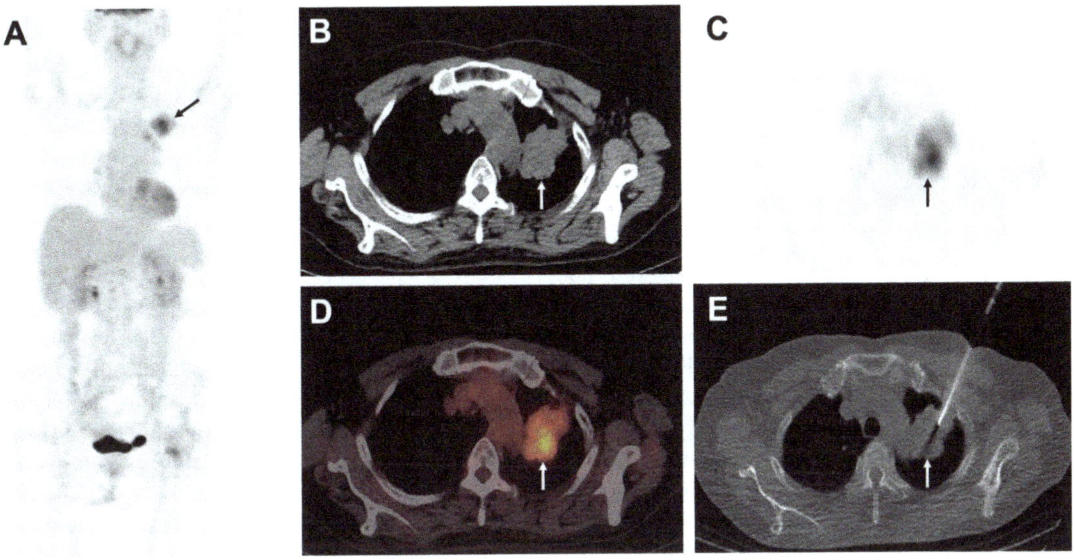

FIGURE 4 | A 58-year-old man with suspected lung carcinoma underwent ^{18}F-FDG PET/CT for tumor staging before treatment. The maximum intensity projection image **(A)** shows intense activity in the left upper lobe of the lung (arrow). Axial view of PET/CT **(B)** CT scan, **(C)** PET image, **(D)**, combined PET/CT image, shows the metabolic active mass (arrow) with atelectasis in its caudal part. Axial view of CT image **(E)** shows biopsy needle positioned into the metabolic active area (arrow). Histological examination confirmed the lung lesion as primary adenocarcinoma.

the biopsy samples in all of these studies were mainly obtained from bronchoscopic biopsy (includes EBUS-TBNA, transbronchial or endobronchial biopsy), and part of the specimen were metastatic lymph nodes instead of primary lung tumors (6, 24–26). Despite being minimally invasive, a tissue core usually is not obtained with bronchoscopic biopsy, limiting a detailed morphologic examination and therefore (27), may affect the observation on PD-L1 expression of tumor cell membrane. In our study, all biopsy specimens were obtained percutaneously using image guidance, which allowed sufficient tissues (generally 3–4 biopsy fragments were obtained for each patient, 8–12 mm * 0.5 mm for each fragment) than bronchoscopic biopsy and tissue microarrays. Although previous study reported a significant difference regarding the number of biopsy tissues between concordant and discordant case (6), we still cannot conclude that more sufficient tissues obtained *via* percutaneous biopsy is the reason for the high PD-L1 concordance observed in our study relative to studies wherein most tissue was obtained with bronchoscopy. Further investigation that comparing percutaneous to bronchoscopic biopsy with respect to PD-L1 testing, is in of itself an important subject matter, but not one addressed in this study.

A successful biopsy procedure must provide a diagnostic sample of tissue, which means the sample of tissue must adequately show the presence of malignancy and specific histopathologic features. Although, PET/CT-guided percutaneously obtained biopsy is not the universal standard of care for image guided biopsies, PET/CT guidance has been widely used to improve the biopsy success rate (9–12). In our study, PET/CT-guided biopsy samples demonstrated a higher success rate (93.3%) than did CT-guided biopsy samples (82.9%), and no significant difference regarding patients' characteristics was observed between those who underwent PET/CT-guided biopsy and CT-guided biopsy. According to our experience, PET/CT-guided biopsy demonstrates the following advantages: First, reducing the frequency of sampling failure can improve biopsy results and patient experiences. Second, resulting in a higher percentage of malignant lesions than did CT-guided biopsy, which could be explained by better identification of the lesion site based on the integration of anatomic structure with metabolic features. For example, we found that ^{18}F-FDG PET/CT-guided biopsy has better accuracy in NSCLC with pulmonary atelectasis in this study (**Figure 4**). Moreover, PET/CT allows identification of FDG-avid lesions that are most accessible to biopsy from among multiple lesions with similar uptake (9–11). Biopsy of the most accessible lesion could simultaneously reduce the risk of complications and minimize the sampling error.

Another important finding of this study is that samples from PET/CT-guided biopsy showed stronger concordance with surgical tissue sections than those from CT-guided biopsy, despite that, there was no significant between-group difference in patient characteristics. Considering the possibility of intra-tumor heterogeneity of PD-L1 expression in NSCLC, sampling the specimen that accurately reflects the PD-L1 status is important (28). Increasing evidence show ^{18}F-FDG uptake in NSCLC samples was positively correlated with PD-L1 expression (29–32), which has been further confirmed in our study. This might be one of the reasons that the FDG uptake of the primary lesion was able to predict the immunotherapy response (33, 34). In some cases, ^{18}F-FDG PET/CT can show the heterogeneity of metabolism in lesions, which are of equal density in CT. Puncture sampling of areas with ^{18}F-FDG-avid focus may help obtain representative specimens for measuring PD-L1 expression.

Compared with previous investigations, our study has the following advantages. First, we compared PD-L1 expression between surgical tissue sections and image-guided percutaneous biopsies in the same group of patients. In the ATLANTIC study that included over 1500 NSCLC patients, PD-L1 expression status was not significantly different between biopsy and surgical samples (35). However, the samples (1,365 samples were obtained by biopsy and 180 by surgical resection) were not matched from the same patients. Second, we used relatively new samples for PD-L1 staining; the specimen in our cohort was less than 3 years old. A previous study showed that samples older than 3 years may show lower PD-L1 TPS on IHC (35). Third, we used SP263 as the antibody for PD-L1 measurement, and the cut-off value was clinically relevant (2–5). SP263 antibody in PD-L1 assay has been reported to have high reliability and reproducibility for NSCLC tumor samples (16, 36, 37). Blueprint PD-L1 IHC Assay Comparability Project Phase 2 consolidates the analytical evidence for interchangeability of the 22C3, SP263, and 28-8 assays because of the similar analytical performance (38).

Despite its advantages, our study also has some notable limitations that need to be addressed. First, our cohort did not include patients with stage IV NSCLC, and all patients had resectable disease. Consequently, the concordant between biopsy samples and matched surgical specimens was mostly applied to early stage NSCLCs, rather than advanced disease. Second, anti-PD-1/PD-L1 immunotherapy to date was mainly used in unresectable NSCLC patients, but the patients in our cohort were treated with surgery rather than immunotherapy. However, the apparent survival benefit of immunotherapy has transformed it from being an alternative modality to being the recommended first-line treatment in the real world. Anti-PD-1/PD-L1 immunotherapy in the neoadjuvant setting also showed encouraging results in patients with resectable lung cancer (39, 40). Third, we did not examine multiple areas of the surgical specimens to evaluate the PD-L1 expression. Since the PD-L1 protein levels in NSCLC reveals heterogeneity within tumors, the PD-L1 expression of the whole tumor in this study may not be fully evaluated. Additionally, this was a retrospective, single-center study with a moderate number of patients. Prospective, multicenter studies with a larger patient population are needed.

In conclusion, PD-L1 expression is concordant between diagnostic percutaneous biopsy samples and matched surgical specimens. Thus, PD-L1 expression in image-guided percutaneous biopsies could be a reliable biomarker for screening patients who will benefit from anti-PD-1/PD-L1 immunotherapy.

AUTHOR CONTRIBUTIONS

LZ, HC, and QL: study conception and design. KF and YD: literature research. KF, PC, YW, and YZ: data acquisition. PC, JL, YD, and LS: data analysis and interpretation. LZ and HC: manuscript drafting. HC and LZ: manuscript editing. All authors contributed to the article and approved the submitted version.

REFERENCES

1. Siegel RL, Miller KD, Jemal A. Cancer statistics, 2020. *CA Cancer J Clin* (2020) 70(1):7–30. doi: 10.3322/caac.21590
2. Reck M, Rodriguez-Abreu D, Robinson AG, Hui R, Csoszi T, Fulop A, et al. Pembrolizumab versus Chemotherapy for PD-L1-Positive Non-Small-Cell Lung Cancer. *N Engl J Med* (2016) 375(19):1823–33. doi: 10.1056/NEJMoa1606774
3. Mok TSK, Wu YL, Kudaba I, Kowalski DM, Cho BC, Turna HZ, et al. Pembrolizumab versus chemotherapy for previously untreated, PD-L1-expressing, locally advanced or metastatic non-small-cell lung cancer (KEYNOTE-042): a randomised, open-label, controlled, phase 3 trial. *Lancet* (2019) 393(10183):1819–30. doi: 10.1016/S0140-6736(18)32409-7
4. Rittmeyer A, Barlesi F, Waterkamp D, Park K, Ciardiello F, von Pawel J, et al. Atezolizumab versus docetaxel in patients with previously treated non-small-cell lung cancer (OAK): a phase 3, open-label, multicentre randomised controlled trial. *Lancet* (2017) 389(10066):255–65. doi: 10.1016/S0140-6736(16)32517-X
5. Shen X, Zhao B. Efficacy of PD-1 or PD-L1 inhibitors and PD-L1 expression status in cancer: meta-analysis. *BMJ* (2018) 362:k3529. doi: 10.1136/bmj.k3529
6. Ilie M, Long-Mira E, Bence C, Butori C, Lassalle S, Bouhlel L, et al. Comparative study of the PD-L1 status between surgically resected specimens and matched biopsies of NSCLC patients reveal major discordances: a potential issue for anti-PD-L1 therapeutic strategies. *Ann Oncol* (2016) 27(1):147–53. doi: 10.1093/annonc/mdv489
7. Nath A, Neyaz Z, Hashim Z, Agrawal V, Richa M. Role of Percutaneous Computed Tomography-guided Lung Biopsy in Non-resolving Consolidation and Identification of Clinical and High-resolution Computed Tomography Characteristics Predicting Outcome. *J Clin Imaging Sci* (2019) 9:48. doi: 10.25259/JCIS_126_2019
8. Chang YY, Chen CK, Yeh YC, Wu MH. Diagnostic feasibility and safety of CT-guided core biopsy for lung nodules less than or equal to 8 mm: A single-institution experience. *Eur Radiol* (2018) 28(2):796–806. doi: 10.1007/s00330-017-5027-1
9. Guo W, Hao B, Chen HJ, Zhao L, Luo ZM, Wu H, et al. PET/CT-guided percutaneous biopsy of FDG-avid metastatic bone lesions in patients with advanced lung cancer: a safe and effective technique. *Eur J Nucl Med Mol Imaging* (2017) 44(1):25–32. doi: 10.1007/s00259-016-3455-9
10. Fei B, Schuster DM. PET Molecular Imaging-Directed Biopsy: A Review. *AJR Am J Roentgenol* (2017) 209(2):255–69. doi: 10.2214/AJR.17.18047
11. Intepe YS, Metin B, Sahin S, Kaya B, Okur A. Our transthoracic biopsy practices accompanied by the imaging process: The contribution of positron emission tomography usage to accurate diagnosis. *Acta Clin Belg* (2016) 71(4):214–20. doi: 10.1080/17843286.2016.1155810
12. Klaeser B, Mueller MD, Schmid RA, Guevara C, Krause T, Wiskirchen J. PET-CT-guided interventions in the management of FDG-positive lesions in patients suffering from solid malignancies: initial experiences. *Eur Radiol* (2009) 19(7):1780–5. doi: 10.1007/s00330-009-1338-1
13. Hao B, Zhao L, Luo NN, Ruan D, Pang YZ, Guo W, et al. Is it sufficient to evaluate bone marrow involvement in newly diagnosed lymphomas using (18)F-FDG PET/CT and/or routine iliac crest biopsy? A new approach of PET/CT-guided targeted bone marrow biopsy. *BMC Cancer* (2018) 18(1):1192. doi: 10.1186/s12885-018-5104-0

14. Guo W, Hao B, Luo N, Ruan D, Guo X, Chen HJ, et al. Early re-staging and molecular subtype shift surveillance of locally recurrent or metastatic breast cancer: A new PET/CT integrated precise algorithm. *Cancer Lett* (2018) 418:221–9. doi: 10.1016/j.canlet.2018.01.019
15. Zhao L, Zhuang Y, Fu K, Chen P, Wang Y, Zhuo J, et al. Usefulness of [(18)F] fluorodeoxyglucose PET/CT for evaluating the PD-L1 status in nasopharyngeal carcinoma. *Eur J Nucl Med Mol Imaging* (2020) 47 (5):1065–74. doi: 10.1007/s00259-019-04654-4
16. Williams GH, Nicholson AG, Snead DRJ, Thunnissen E, Lantuejoul S, Cane P, et al. Inter-observer Reliability of Programmed Cell Death Ligand-1 Scoring Using the VENTANA PD-L1 (SP263) Assay in Non-Small Cell Lung Cancer. *J Thorac Oncol* (2019) 15(4):550–5. doi: 10.1016/j.jtho.2019.11.010
17. Rebelatto MC, Midha A, Mistry A, Sabalos C, Schechter N, Li X, et al. Development of a programmed cell death ligand-1 immunohistochemical assay validated for analysis of non-small cell lung cancer and head and neck squamous cell carcinoma. *Diagn Pathol* (2016) 11(1):95. doi: 10.1186/s13000-016-0545-8
18. Landis JR, Koch GG. The measurement of observer agreement for categorical data. *Biometrics* (1977) 33(1):159–74.
19. Li C, Huang C, Mok TS, Zhuang W, Xu H, Miao Q, et al. Comparison of 22C3 PD-L1 Expression between Surgically Resected Specimens and Paired Tissue Microarrays in Non-Small Cell Lung Cancer. *J Thorac Oncol* (2017) 12 (10):1536–43. doi: 10.1016/j.jtho.2017.07.015
20. Topalian SL, Hodi FS, Brahmer JR, Gettinger SN, Smith DC, McDermott DF, et al. Five-Year Survival and Correlates Among Patients With Advanced Melanoma, Renal Cell Carcinoma, or Non-Small Cell Lung Cancer Treated With Nivolumab. *JAMA Oncol* (2019) 5(10):1411–20. doi: 10.1001/jamaoncol.2019.2187
21. Garon EB, Hellmann MD, Rizvi NA, Carcereny E, Leighl NB, Ahn MJ, et al. Five-Year Overall Survival for Patients With Advanced NonSmall-Cell Lung Cancer Treated With Pembrolizumab: Results From the Phase I KEYNOTE-001 Study. *J Clin Oncol* (2019) 37(28):2518–27. doi: 10.1200/JCO.19.00934
22. Munari E, Zamboni G, Lunardi G, Marchionni L, Marconi M, Sommaggio M, et al. PD-L1 Expression Heterogeneity in Non-Small Cell Lung Cancer: Defining Criteria for Harmonization between Biopsy Specimens and Whole Sections. *J Thorac Oncol* (2018) 13(8):1113–20. doi: 10.1016/j.jtho.2018.04.017
23. Lantuejoul S, Sound-Tsao M, Cooper WA, Girard N, Hirsch FR, Roden AC, et al. PD-L1 Testing for Lung Cancer in 2019: Perspective From the IASLC Pathology Committee. *J Thorac Oncol* (2019) 15(4):499–519. doi: 10.1016/j.jtho.2019.12.107
24. Kitazono S, Fujiwara Y, Tsuta K, Utsumi H, Kanda S, Horinouchi H, et al. Reliability of Small Biopsy Samples Compared With Resected Specimens for the Determination of Programmed Death-Ligand 1 Expression in Non–Small-Cell Lung Cancer. *Clin Lung Cancer* (2015) 16(5):385–90. doi: 10.1016/j.cllc.2015.03.008
25. Tsunoda A, Morikawa K, Inoue T, Miyazawa T, Hoshikawa M, Takagi M, et al. A prospective observational study to assess PD-L1 expression in small biopsy samples for non-small-cell lung cancer. *BMC Cancer* (2019) 19(1):546. doi: 10.1186/s12885-019-5773-3
26. Thunnissen E, Kerr KM, Dafni U, Bubendorf L, Finn SP, Soltermann A, et al. Programmed death-ligand 1 expression influenced by tissue sample size. Scoring based on tissue microarrays' and cross-validation with resections, in patients with, stage I-III, non-small cell lung carcinoma of the European Thoracic Oncology Platform Lungscape cohort. *Mod Pathol* (2019) 33 (5):792–801. doi: 10.1038/s41379-019-0383-9
27. Levy EB, Fiel MI, Hamilton SR, Kleiner DE, McCall SJ, Schirmacher P, et al. State of the Art: Toward Improving Outcomes of Lung and Liver Tumor Biopsies in Clinical Trials-A Multidisciplinary Approach. *J Clin Oncol* (2020) 38(14):1633–40. doi: 10.1200/JCO.19.02322. JCO1902322.
28. McLaughlin J, Han G, Schalper KA, Carvajal-Hausdorf D, Pelekanou V, Rehman J, et al. Quantitative Assessment of the Heterogeneity of PD-L1 Expression in Non-Small-Cell Lung Cancer. *JAMA Oncol* (2016) 2(1):46–54. doi: 10.1001/jamaoncol.2015.3638
29. Wang Y, Zhao N, Wu Z, Pan N, Shen X, Liu T, et al. New insight on the correlation of metabolic status on (18)F-FDG PET/CT with immune marker expression in patients with non-small cell lung cancer. *Eur J Nucl Med Mol Imaging* (2019) 47(5):1127–36. doi: 10.1007/s00259-019-04500-7
30. Kasahara N, Kaira K, Bao P, Higuchi T, Arisaka Y, Erkhem-Ochir B, et al. Correlation of tumor-related immunity with 18F-FDG-PET in pulmonary squamous-cell carcinoma. *Lung Cancer* (2018) 119:71–7. doi: 10.1016/j.lungcan.2018.03.001
31. Kaira K, Shimizu K, Kitahara S, Yajima T, Atsumi J, Kosaka T, et al. 2-Deoxy-2-[fluorine-18] fluoro-d-glucose uptake on positron emission tomography is associated with programmed death ligand-1 expression in patients with pulmonary adenocarcinoma. *Eur J Cancer* (2018) 101:181–90. doi: 10.1016/j.ejca.2018.06.022
32. Lopci E, Toschi L, Grizzi F, Rahal D, Olivari L, Castino GF, et al. Correlation of metabolic information on FDG-PET with tissue expression of immune markers in patients with non-small cell lung cancer (NSCLC) who are candidates for upfront surgery. *Eur J Nucl Med Mol Imaging* (2016) 43 (11):1954–61. doi: 10.1007/s00259-016-3425-2
33. Evangelista L. The prediction of response to immunotherapy in non-small cell lung cancer patients by 18F-FDG PET/CT. *J Thorac Dis* (2019) 11(11):E221–E3. doi: 10.21037/jtd.2019.10.19
34. Grizzi F, Castello A, Lopci E. Is it time to change our vision of tumor metabolism prior to immunotherapy? *Eur J Nucl Med Mol Imaging* (2018) 45 (6):1072–5. doi: 10.1007/s00259-018-3988-1
35. Boothman AM, Scott M, Ratcliffe M, Whiteley J, Dennis PA, Wadsworth C, et al. Impact of Patient Characteristics, Prior Therapy, and Sample Type on Tumor Cell Programmed Cell Death Ligand 1 Expression in Patients with Advanced NSCLC Screened for the ATLANTIC Study. *J Thorac Oncol* (2019) 14(8):1390–9. doi: 10.1016/j.jtho.2019.04.025
36. Ratcliffe MJ, Sharpe A, Midha A, Barker C, Scott M, Scorer P, et al. Agreement between Programmed Cell Death Ligand-1 Diagnostic Assays across Multiple Protein Expression Cutoffs in Non-Small Cell Lung Cancer. *Clin Cancer Res* (2017) 23(14):3585–91. doi: 10.1158/1078-0432.CCR-16-2375
37. Brunnstrom H, Johansson A, Westbom-Fremer S, Backman M, Djureinovic D, Patthey A, et al. PD-L1 immunohistochemistry in clinical diagnostics of lung cancer: inter-pathologist variability is higher than assay variability. *Mod Pathol* (2017) 30(10):1411–21. doi: 10.1038/modpathol.2017.59
38. Tsao MS, Kerr KM, Kockx M, Beasley MB, Borczuk AC, Botling J, et al. PD-L1 Immunohistochemistry Comparability Study in Real-Life Clinical Samples: Results of Blueprint Phase 2 Project. *J Thorac Oncol* (2018) 13(9):1302–11. doi: 10.1016/j.jtho.2018.05.013
39. Yeh J, Marrone KA, Forde PM. Neoadjuvant and consolidation immuno-oncology therapy in stage III non-small cell lung cancer. *J Thorac Dis* (2018) 10(Suppl 3):S451–S9. doi: 10.21037/jtd.2018.01.109
40. Forde PM, Chaft JE, Smith KN, Anagnostou V, Cottrell TR, Hellmann MD, et al. Neoadjuvant PD-1 Blockade in Resectable Lung Cancer. *N Engl J Med* (2018) 378(21):1976–86. doi: 10.1056/NEJMoa1716078

11

GEO Data Mining Identifies OLR1 as a Potential Biomarker in NSCLC Immunotherapy

Bin Liu[1], Ziyu Wang[1], Meng Gu[1], Cong Zhao[1], Teng Ma[1] and Jinghui Wang[1,2*]*

[1] Department of Cellular and Molecular Biology, Beijing Chest Hospital, Capital Medical University, Beijing Tuberculosis and Thoracic Tumor Research Institute, Beijing, China, [2] Department of Medical Oncology, Beijing Chest Hospital, Capital Medical University, Beijing Tuberculosis and Thoracic Tumor Research Institute, Beijing, China

***Correspondence:**
Teng Ma
mateng82913@163.com
Jinghui Wang
jinghuiwang2006@163.com

Non-small cell lung cancer (NSCLC) is the most common type of lung cancer. The tumor immune microenvironment (TME) in NSCLC is closely correlated to tumor initiation, progression, and prognosis. TME failure impedes the generation of an effective antitumor immune response. In this study, we attempted to explore TME and identify a potential biomarker for NSCLC immunotherapy. 48 potential immune-related genes were identified from 11 eligible Gene Expression Omnibus (GEO) data sets. We applied the CIBERSORT computational approach to quantify bulk gene expression profiles and thereby infer the proportions of 22 subsets of tumor-infiltrating immune cells (TICs); 16 kinds of TICs showed differential distributions between the tumor and control tissue samples. Multiple linear regression analysis was used to determine the correlation between TICs and 48 potential immune-related genes. Nine differential immune-related genes showed statistical significance. We analyzed the influence of nine differential immune-related genes on NSCLC immunotherapy, and OLR1 exhibited the strongest correlation with four well-recognized biomarkers (PD-L1, CD8A, GZMB, and NOS2) of immunotherapy. Differential expression of OLR1 showed its considerable potential to divide TICs distribution, as determined by non-linear dimensionality reduction analysis. In immunotherapy prediction analysis with the comparatively reliable tool TIDE, patients with higher OLR1 expression were predicted to have better immunotherapy outcomes, and OLR1 expression was potentially highly correlated with PD-L1 expression, the average of CD8A and CD8B, IFNG, and Merck18 expression, T cell dysfunction and exclusion potential, and other significant immunotherapy predictors. These findings contribute to the current understanding of TME with immunotherapy. OLR1 also shows potential as a predictor or a regulator in NSCLC immunotherapy.

Keywords: non-small cell lung cancer, immunotherapy, tumor microenvironment, PD-L1, immune checkpoint

INTRODUCTION

Lung cancer is one of the most commonly occurring malignancies and is identified as leading cause of cancer-related deaths worldwide. Statistics on cancer reveal that in 2018, more than 2 million patients suffered from lung cancer worldwide, and lung cancer ranked first among all cancer types (1). In China, lung cancer has shown the highest incidence and mortality over the last decade and posed a significant threat to human health (2). Lung cancer comprises nearly 20% of all cancer deaths and its mortality may increase by approximately 40% by 2030 (3). Lung cancer has been subdivided based on pathological classification into two groups: small-cell lung cancer (SCLC) and Non-small cell lung cancer (NSCLC). NSCLC is further stratified into three subsets: adenocarcinoma (the most common type, which comprises 40% of all lung cancer types), squamous cell carcinoma (25%) and large cell carcinoma (about 10%) (4). 75% of NSCLC is diagnosed at the advanced stage, resulting in a five-year survival rate of less than 15% (5). In addition to surgery and chemoradiotherapy, immunotherapy shows promising potential in treatment of NSCLC.

Programmed death-1 (PD-1) and its ligand (PD-L1) antibody based Immunotherapies have recently shown significant advances in the treatment of NSCLC through enhancing the attack of the host immune system on malignant cells (6). However, a number of patients still fail to benefit from these immunotherapies possibly because of tumor immune microenvironment (TME) alterations (7). The tumor microenvironment includes cross-talks among cancer cells, endothelial cells, fibroblasts and immune cells. Previous studies have shown the potential associations between the microenvironment and the effects of immunotherapy (8). The tumor microenvironment presents physical, immunologic, and metabolic barriers to enduring immunotherapy responses, and the suppressive microenvironment of tumors remains one of the limiting factors for immunotherapies. In this study, we screened those genes that enriched in tumor tissue and closely related to the immune microenvironment in NSCLC. Targeting PD-L1, one of the most representative immunotherapy strategies, was studied in relation to the screened microenvironment genes. The response prediction markers of PD-L1 were used as standard and to study the predictive value of each gene as biomarker for host tumor immunity in NSCLC. We aimed to find a highly predictive PD-L1 blockade therapy biomarker for clinical use, or the potential targeting genes, to change the tumor microenvironment for enhanced immunotherapy effects.

MATERIALS AND METHODS

Raw Data

Eligible data sets in GEO were selected according to the following criteria and 11 data sets were obtained as of May 2020 (including 268 cases of control samples, 601 cases of lung tumor samples) (9–18). Data sets details are listed in **Table 1**. The selection criteria are as follows: definite diagnosis with NSCLC; inclusion of control samples in the same data set; samples without any treatment before sequencing; gene expression data based on the Affymetrix platform. After normalization of mRNA data with the limma algorithm in R language, all data sets were merged into a new data set for downstream analysis.

Identification and Analysis of DEGs

Data were analyzed using the limma package in the R language. Details on cutoffs were as follows: Fold change>1 or <−1, and adj. P <0.05. Heatmaps and volcano plots were generated using the limma package and pheatmap respectively. Gene ontology (Go) and Kyoto Encyclopedia of Genes and Genomes (KEGG) analyses with "clusterProfiler" and "org.Hs.eg.db" (the same as below) were performed in R.

Identification of Potential Immune-Related Genes and Analysis

In this study, the algorithm ESTIMATE outputs stromal, immune, and ESTIMATE scores by performing "limma" and "estimate" with merged data sets after normalization (19). The cutoffs for high or low scores were 50% higher or lower. The Venn diagram was drawn with the package "VennDiagram" and an online tool from the Bioinformatics & Systems Biology website. The intersection set of the results of the ESTIMATE

TABLE 1 | The detail of datasets using in this study.

Data Set	Country	Platforms	Diagnosis	Paired	Control	Tumor	Control after filter	Tumor after filter
GSE18842	Spain	GPL570	NSCLC	Part	45	46	45	45
GSE101929	USA	GPL570	NSCLC	Part	34	32	32	30
GSE103888	UK	GPL570	NSCLC	No	6	13	6	13
GSE104636	Switzerland	GPL6244	lung tumor	Yes	9	9	5	0
GSE118370	China	GPL570	LUAD	Yes	6	6	0	1
GSE134381	UK	GPL11532	LUSC/LUAD	Yes	37	37	22	22
GSE19804	China	GPL570	lung tumor	Yes	60	60	60	58
GSE23361	USA	GPL5188	NSCLC	part	7	5	0	1
GSE30219	France	GPL570	lung tumor	No	14	293	14	254
GSE33532	Germany	GPL570	NSCLC	Yes	20	20	20	19
GSE43458	USA	GPL6244	LUAD	part	30	80	18	49

NSCLC, there was clear statement that cancer tissues from NSCLC patients, but pathological classification not included in original article; Lung tumor, there was no clear statement about lung cancer subtype, but small cell lung cancer was excluded; LUAD, articles had a clear statement of lung adenocarcinoma. LUSC, articles had a clear statement of lung squamous cell carcinoma.

scores were considered as control intersection genes and tumor intersect genes off the up-regulated and down-regulated genes respectively. In the subsequent step, the consistently intersecting set was excluded from those tumor intersect genes, and the remaining genes were considered as tumor specific intersect genes. The intersection set of the tumor specific intersect genes and DEGs were identified as potential immune-related genes and used for further analysis.

Identification of Statistically TICs

The normalized data set was employed to estimate the TICs abundance profile by using the CIBERSORT computational method on all control and tumor samples (20). The resulting data set was filtered with a self-compiled script in Perl to exclude invalid data (detail of filtered data set is listed in **Table 1**). The landscape of TICs is shown in a barplot. A heatmap was generated with "pheatmap," and a correlation heatmap was generated using "corrplot." As the filtered data were subjected to a normality test based on skewness and kurtosis rather than its fit in a normal distribution, non-parametric tests were used. For the number of TICs in the control and tumor samples, the differential distributions were analyzed using the Wilcoxon rank-sum test.

Multiple Linear Regression Analysis for Identifying Differential Immune-Related Genes From Potential Immune-Related Genes

The filtered data were used to analyze the effect of gene expression on the TICs distribution. A total of 16 TICs with different distributions were entered as dependent variable and potential immune-related genes entered as independent variables. Predictive factor analysis for TICs distribution was conducted *via* least-squares regression. With both accuracy and computational efficiency considered, adjusted $P< 0.1$ was considered significant in this part. We selected the significantly ones from 48 potential immune-related genes and identified those exhibiting the opposite regression trend in different tissue samples. Those selected genes would be labeled as differential immune-related genes.

Gene Set Enrichment Analysis With Differential Immune-Related Genes

Gene set enrichment analysis (GSEA) was conducted on all differential immune-related genes on the GSEA portal (http://www.broad.mit.edu/GSEA/) with the following parameter settings: probe set collapse = false; phenotype = high vs. low; permutation: sample, permutations = 1000. The gene set size was $15 < n < 500$. We manually discriminated pathways of interest in immune related pathways, microenvironment and metabolic pathways, and classic cancer pathways. The GSEA results were separately shown based on the pathway function.

Non-Linear Dimensionality Reduction

In this study, we selected one differential immune-related gene that is most stable and highly correlated with other well-recognized immunotherapy signatures to perform downstream analysis, which was OLR1 (oxidized low density lipoprotein receptor 1). We determined whether OLR1 was a key gene for the microenvironment and could be a biomarker for immunotherapy. We first analyzed the influence of OLR1 expression to divide the differential immune microenvironment with non-linear dimensionality reduction. We used t-distributed stochastic neighbor embedding (t-SNE) to complete the dimensionality reduction. T-SNE, a non-linear dimensionality reduction technique, is particularly suitable for visualizing high-dimensional data sets. We reduced the dimensionality to two dimensions to reveal the significant difference between the 50% higher OLR1 expression tissue samples and the 50% lower OLR expression tissue samples. The T-SNE plot was completed using the R package "t-SNE."

Prediction of Benefits to Immune Checkpoint Blockade Therapy

We used TIDE, an online prediction tool to predict the responder rate in the samples with higher or lower OLR1 expression under immune checkpoint blockade therapy. TIDE is a novel computational framework that evaluates the potential of tumor immune escape, particularly for melanoma and NSCLC, on the basis of gene expression data (21). Owing to tool limitations, only the top or bottom 50 cases of OLR expression data were selected from the 284 samples. The result was reorganized into a figure with improved readability. We collected predictive indicators and calculated them to explore the details of the predicated therapeutic effect.

Cell Culture

We used BEAS-2B (human normal lung epithelial cell, Cat. 3131C0001000200027), NCI-H460 (human large cell lung cancer cell, Cat. 3111C0001CCC000355), PLA-801D (lung giant cell carcinoma cell, Cat. 3142C0001000000356), A549 (human non-small cell lung cancer cell, Cat. 3111C0001CCC000002), HCC827 (human non-small cell lung cancer cell, Cat. 3111C0001CCC000478), NCI-H1299 (human non-small cell lung cancer cell, Cat. 3111C0001CCC000469), and NCI-H661 (human large cell lung cancer cell, Cat. 3111C0001CCC000357) to detect the basic expression of OLR1 in lung normal and tumor cell lines for verification of data mining results. They were purchased from Chinese National Infrastructure of Cell Line Resource and cultured in PRMI-1640 medium with 10% FBS.

qPCR

RNA was isolated with TRIzol® reagent (Cat.15596018, Thermo Fisher). Reverse-transcription of the RNA was performed with EasyScript First-Strand cDNA Synthesis SuperMix Kit (Cat. AE301-03, TransGen Biotech). The qPCR assay was performed in triplicate with PowerUp SYBE Green Master Mix Kit (Cat.A25741, Applied Biosystems) on an ABI StepOnePlus Real-time PCR system (ABI-7500, Applied Biosystems). The qPCR primer was following: OLR1-F:5′-ACTCTCCATGG TGGTGCCTGG-3′; OLR1-R:5′-GCTTGTTGCCGGGCTGA GATCT-3′; GAPDH-F:5′-GGACTCATGACCACAGTCCA

TGCC-3′; GAPDH-R:5′-TCAGGGATGACCTTGCCC ACAG-3′.

Statistical Methods

Microarray data analysis was performed using the R programming language. The normality of data distributions was assessed using the Shapiro-Wilk test. Data that were nor normally distributed were compared using the Wilcoxon rank-sum test run with GraphPad Prism. Multivariate analysis was performed using multiple linear regression in Eviews. P value < 0.05 was considered significant.

RESULTS

613 Differentially Expressed Genes Were Identified in 11 Data Sets

For this study, 11 data sets were selected based on our screening criteria (**Table 1**). After the data sets were merged and normalized, 601 NSCLC samples and 268 control samples were included. We defined statistical differential significance as P < 0.05 and fold change >10 between the tumor and control samples. A total of 613 differentially expressed genes (DEGs) were identified from 869 samples with 12596 gene expression data. Their gene symbols are listed based on their respective logFC (base 2 logarithm of fold change) values (**Supplementary Table 1**). The results revealed that 200 of the DEGs were highly expressed, whereas the remaining 413 DEGs were down-regulated in tumor tissues (**Figures 1A, B**). GO and KEGG pathway enrichment analyses of up-regulated or down-regulated DEGs were implemented separately. The up-regulated DEGs were enriched in the extracellular matrix structural constituent, glycosaminoglycan binding and growth factor binding (**Supplementary Table 2** and **Figure 1C**). The corresponding signaling pathways were the most enriched (**Supplementary Table 3** and **Figure 1D**). The down-regulated DEGs mainly involved the cytokine-cytokine receptor interaction, transcriptional miss-regulation in cancer, and cell cycle, as well as corresponding gene functions (**Figures 1E, F**).

166 Tumor-Specific Intersect Genes Were Identified Using ESTIMATE Scores, With 48 of Them Identified as Potential Immune-Related Genes by the Intersection With DEGs

ESTIMATE scores were calculated based on immune and stromal scores. We calculated the immune and stromal scores in the tumor and control samples, respectively. The samples were divided into the high-score and low-score groups by the median value of the immune score (or stromal score). For the immune score, 1,457 (1,276) and 359 (31) up-regulated (down-regulated) immune scores genes were identified in the control and tumor samples, respectively. For the stromal score, 461 (203) and 351

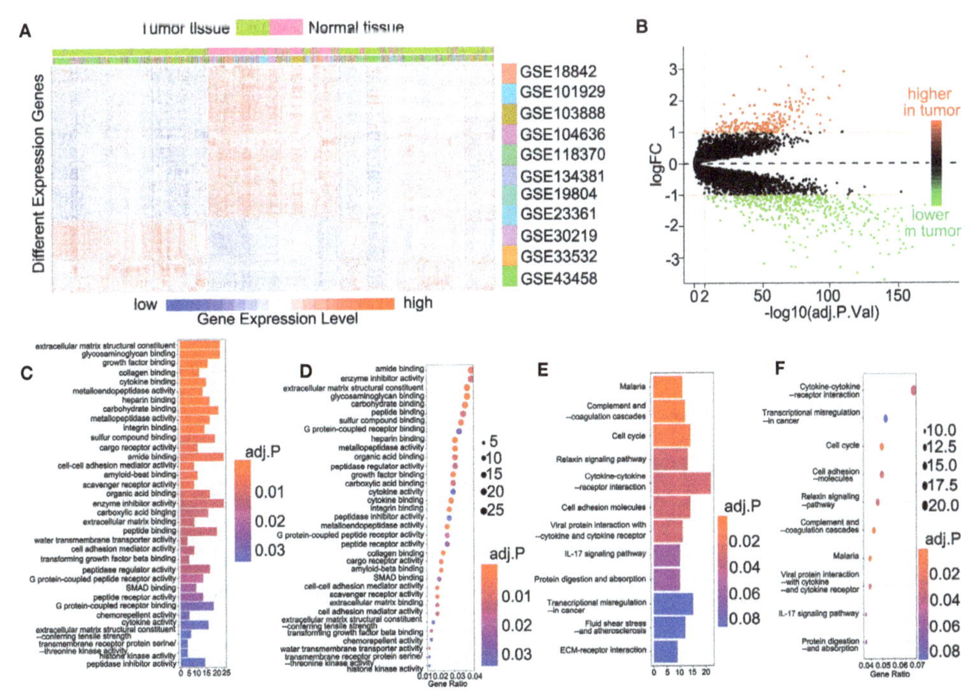

FIGURE 1 | 613 DEGs were identified in 11 datasets. **(A)** Heatmap showed the expression of genes between the tumor and control tissue samples; **(B)** Scatterplot showed the higher or lower DEGs between the tumor and control tissue samples; **(C)** The Go analyses of higher DEGs; **(D)** The KEGG analyses of higher DEGs; **(E)** The Go analyses of lower DEGs; **(F)** The KEGG analyses of lower DEGs.

(30) up-regulated (down-regulated) genes were identified in the control and tumor samples, respectively (**Figure 2A**). The intersection represented the genes with the same trends of up-regulation or down-regulation of immune or stromal score genes in the tumor and control samples. In the control samples, we identified 342 up-regulated immune score genes and 197 down-regulated stromal score genes. Meanwhile, 211 up-regulation immune score genes and 17 down-regulated stromal score genes were found in the tumor samples (**Figure 2A**). A total of 553 up-regulated genes and 214 down-regulated genes were identified in the tumor and control samples (**Figure 2B**). They were regarded as important factors for ESTIMATE scores. Subsequently, 60 up-regulated and two down-regulated genes were duplicates, exhibiting a similar trend of immune or stromal score genes were similar in the tumor and control samples (**Figure 2B**). A concerning finding of this study is that 151 up-regulated and 15 down-regulated ESTIMATE score genes were specifically expressed in the tumor samples (**Supplementary Table 4** and **Figure 2B** with *). Thus, the 166 tumor specific intersect genes were selected for GO enrichment and KEGG pathway analysis. They were enriched in pathways including, immune receptor activity, chemokine activity and receptor binding, receptor ligand activity, glycosaminoglycan binding, phagosome, and lgA immune network (**Supplementary Tables 5** and **6**, **Figures 2C–F**). We then found the intersection of 166 tumor specific intersect genes and 613 DEGs and identified 48 intersected genes (**Supplementary Table 7** and **Figure 2G**).The 48 genes were identified as potential immune-related genes. Potential immune-related genes have significant differences in expression and specific immune effects in the tumor samples.

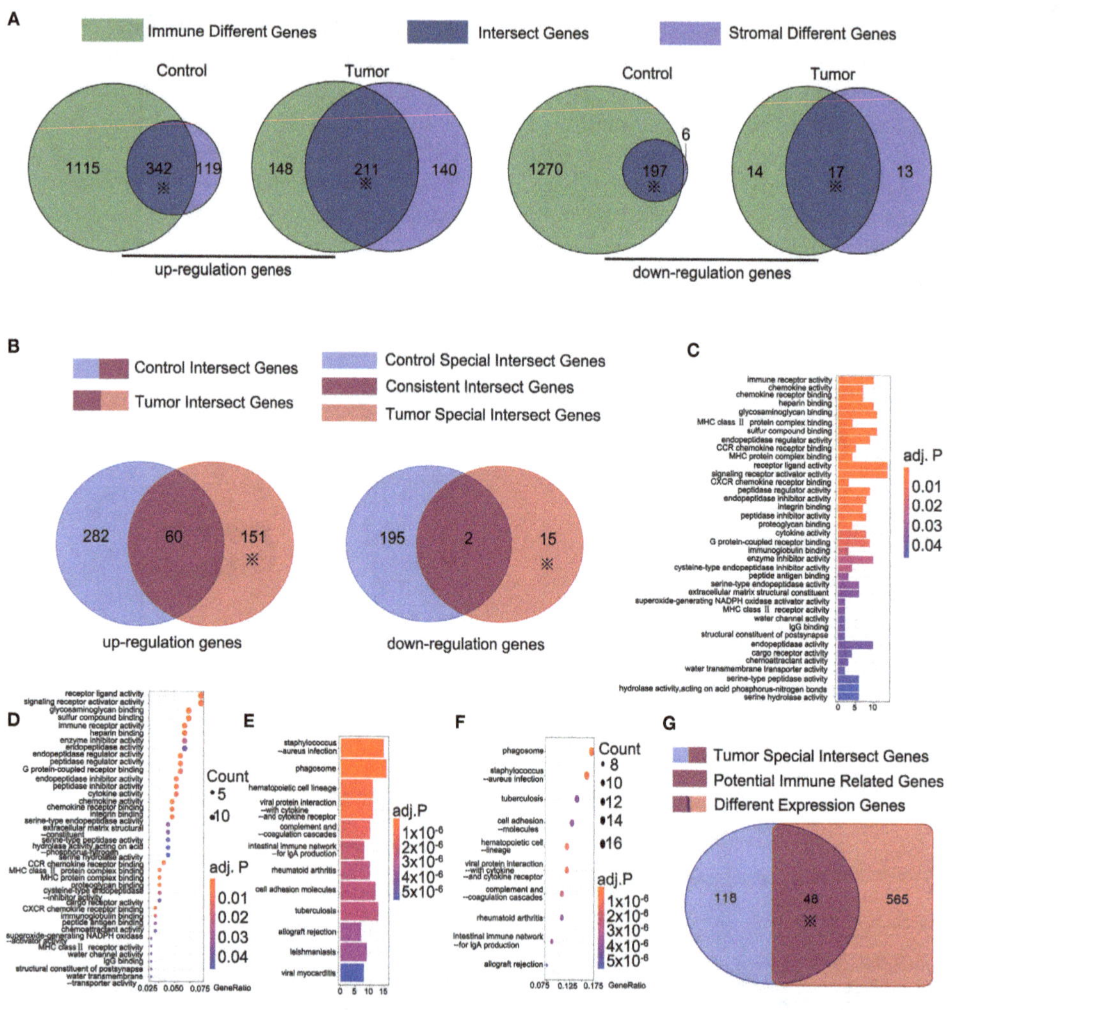

FIGURE 2 | 166 tumor-special intersect genes were identified and 48 of them identified as potential immune-related genes. **(A)** 461 (203) and 351 (30) up-regulated (down-regulated) genes were identified using ESTIMATE in the control and tumor samples. ※ mean this part would be used in following step; **(B)** 151 up-regulated and 15 down-regulated ESTIMATE score genes (total 166 tumor-special intersect genes) were specifically expressed in the tumor samples; **(C)** The Go analyses of 151 up-regulated tumor-special intersect genes; **(D)** The KEGG analyses of 151 up-regulated tumor-special intersect genes; **(E)**. The Go analyses of 15 down-regulated tumor-special intersect genes; **(F)** The KEGG analyses of 15 down-regulated tumor-special intersect genes; **(G)** 48 intersected genes, referred to potential immune-related genes, were identified between 613 DEGs and 166 tumor-special intersect genes.

16 Kinds of TICs Showed Differences in Distribution Between the Tumor and Control Samples

The proportion of tumor-infiltrating immune subsets was analyzed using CIBERSORT in R. A total of 22 TICs profile types in the tumor and control samples were to be constructed. A landscape is presented for preliminary subjective judgment of TICs distributions (**Supplementary Figure 1**). We found that TICs distribution varied based on the kind of TICs. Some of TICs had more immune cells in tumor tissues, whereas others showed the opposite (**Figure 3A**). No significant correlation was found between them with regard to numerical values in both the tumor samples and the control samples (**Figure 3B**). The Mann-Whitney rank-sum test was used to calculate differences in TICs distribution. A significant difference in the distribution of 16 kinds of TICs was found between the tumor and control samples (**Supplementary Table 8** and **Figures 3C–R**).

9 Differentially Expressed Immune-Related Genes Showed Opposite Statistically Significant Regression Trends of TICs Distribution Between the Tumor and Control Samples

We used multiple linear regression with the least square method to calculate the most important genes from 48 potential immune-related genes for differential the distribution of TICs. The control and tumor samples were separated as independent data sets. For an enhanced screen effect, P<0.1 was the level of significance selected. A total of 24 intersected genes were statistically significant both in the tumor and control samples; 16 of these genes showed similar regression trends for some kinds of TICs in both samples (**Supplementary Table 9**), and 9 other genes exhibited the opposite regression trend in different tissue samples (**Supplementary Table 10**). OLR1 showed the same regression trend for resting natural killer (NK) cells and eosinophils; however, it exhibited the opposite regression trend for resting mast cell. Thus, OLR1 was counted separately. The genes showing opposite regression trends between the tumor and control samples were referred to as differential immune-related genes in accordance with the purpose of the study. Subsequently, 9 differential immune-related genes were identified: ADH1B, CHRDL1, DMBT1, MMP, OLR1, PBK, PLA2G1B, SCGB3A1, and TREM1. The potential functions of these genes were analyzed by GSEA. We classified some important pathways into three categories, based on their function for clarity. Some pathways could be activated/repressed by each of the 9 differential immune-related genes (**Figure 4**).

OLR1, One of the Differential Immune-Related Genes, Showed Significant Correlations With Four Known Immunotherapy Biomarkers

Since the data were from 11 data sets merged with different platforms, and some data were lost during merging, we selected only 4 well-recognized biomarkers in the data set with gene expression data: PD-L1, CD8A, GZMB, and NOS2. To reduce potential bias and achieve improved effectiveness, we used only part of the data for downstream analysis. The 284 tumor samples in GSE101929 and GSE30219 with clinical data were used to calculate separately the correlation between 9 differential immune-related genes and 4 known biomarkers. Consequently, OLR1 exhibited the highest correlation with PD-L1, CD8A, GZMB, and NOS2 (**Supplementary Table 11** and **Figures 5A–D**), and each correlation was significant (r>0.4, P<0.0001, moderate intensity). Chi-square test was used to detect whether different expression level of known biomarker was followed by changing of OLR1 expression level. We can found more positive expression for immunotherapy in higher OLR1 group patients (**Supplementary Table 12**). This result suggests the important role of OLR1 in the TME with a changing TICs distribution for immunotherapy prediction.

OLR1 Expression Marked the TICs Distribution

We ran t-SNE to determine the overall distribution of TICs with different levels of OLR1 expression. The OLR1 expression could effectively distinguish the distribution of immune cells (**Figure 5E**). A violin plot of 22 immune cell types shows 14 kinds of immune cells with significantly different distributions between the higher and lower OLR1 expression samples (**Figure 5F**).

OLR1 Affected the Prediction of Clinical Benefits to Immunotherapy in NSCLC Patients

We selected the 50 samples with the highest or lowest OLR1 expression levels from the 284 tumor samples and predicted the responder rate of the immune checkpoint blockade therapy in each group. Among the 50 samples with the lowest OLR1 expression levels, 16 cases were predicted to respond to immune checkpoint blockade therapy. They were also predicted to benefit from immunotherapy. The responder number was 27 in the top 50 OLR1 expression samples. The responder rate was significantly higher in the high OLR1 expression group (**Figure 6A**). We also calculated all indicators of TIDE prediction. OLR1 expression and MSI score exhibited a significant positive correlation. The T cell exclusion potential of the tumor was predicted to be negatively correlated with OLR1 expression. Specifically, a strong positive correlation (r>0.7) was observed between OLR1 expression and the T cell-inflamed signature (Merck18), the average of CD8A and CD8B, both of which were important indicators of immunotherapy (**Supplementary Table 13** and **Figures 6B–E**).

Verification of OLR1 Expression in Lung Normal and Tumor Cell Lines

BEAS-2B was human normal lung epithelial cell. It was used as control cell line comparison with other NSCLC cell lines. The result of qPCR analysis showed a significant reduction in the expression of OLR1 in the most NSCLC cell lines (**Figure 7**). The validation result of cell lines had the same trend as data mining in OLR1 expression.

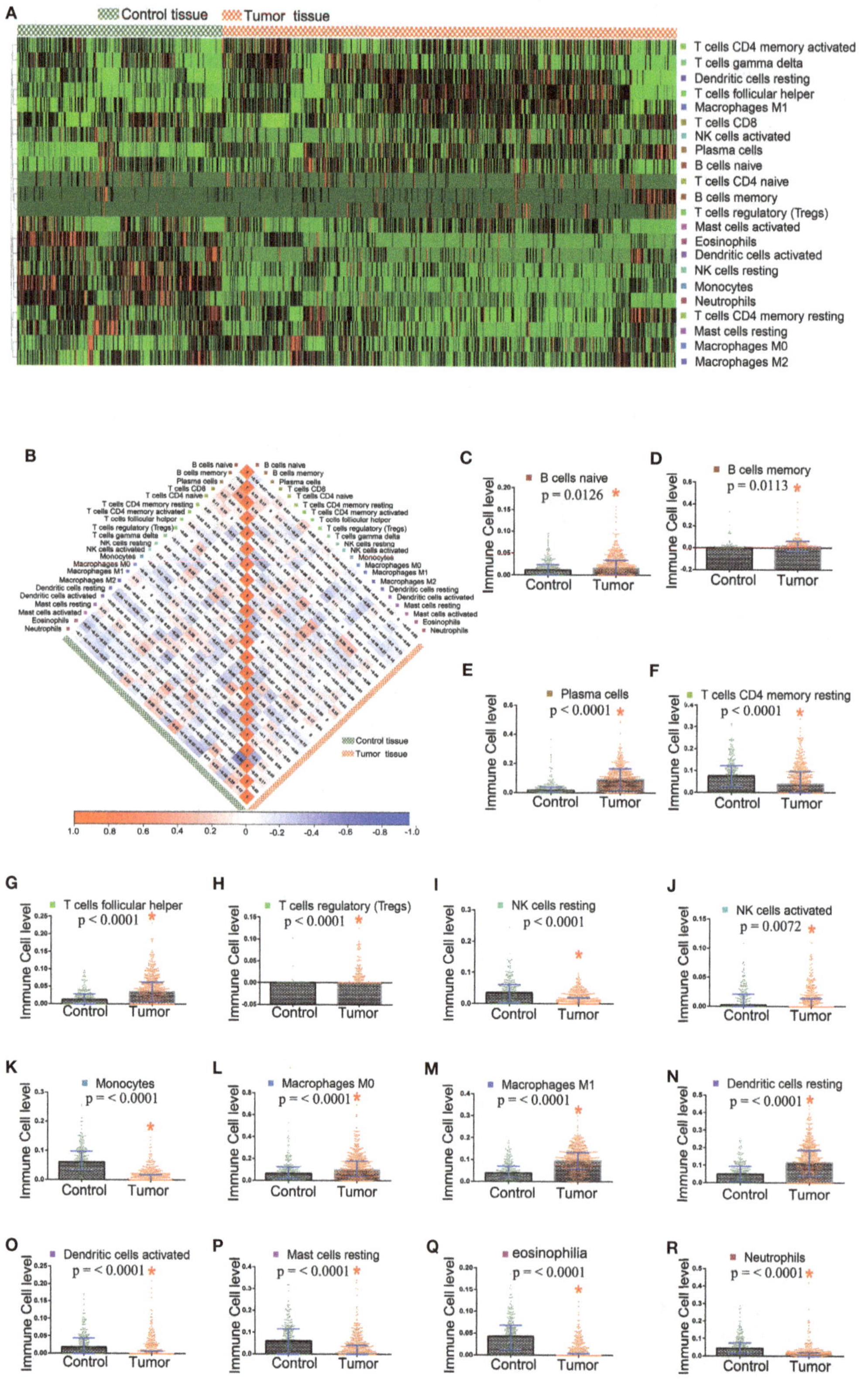

FIGURE 3 | Different distribution of TICs between the tumor and control tissue samples. **(A)** Heatmap showed the distribution state in tumor and control tissue samples; **(B)** The correlation among TICs in the tumor and control tissue samples; **(C–R)** 16 TICs which showed significant difference in the distribution between the tumor and control tissue samples.

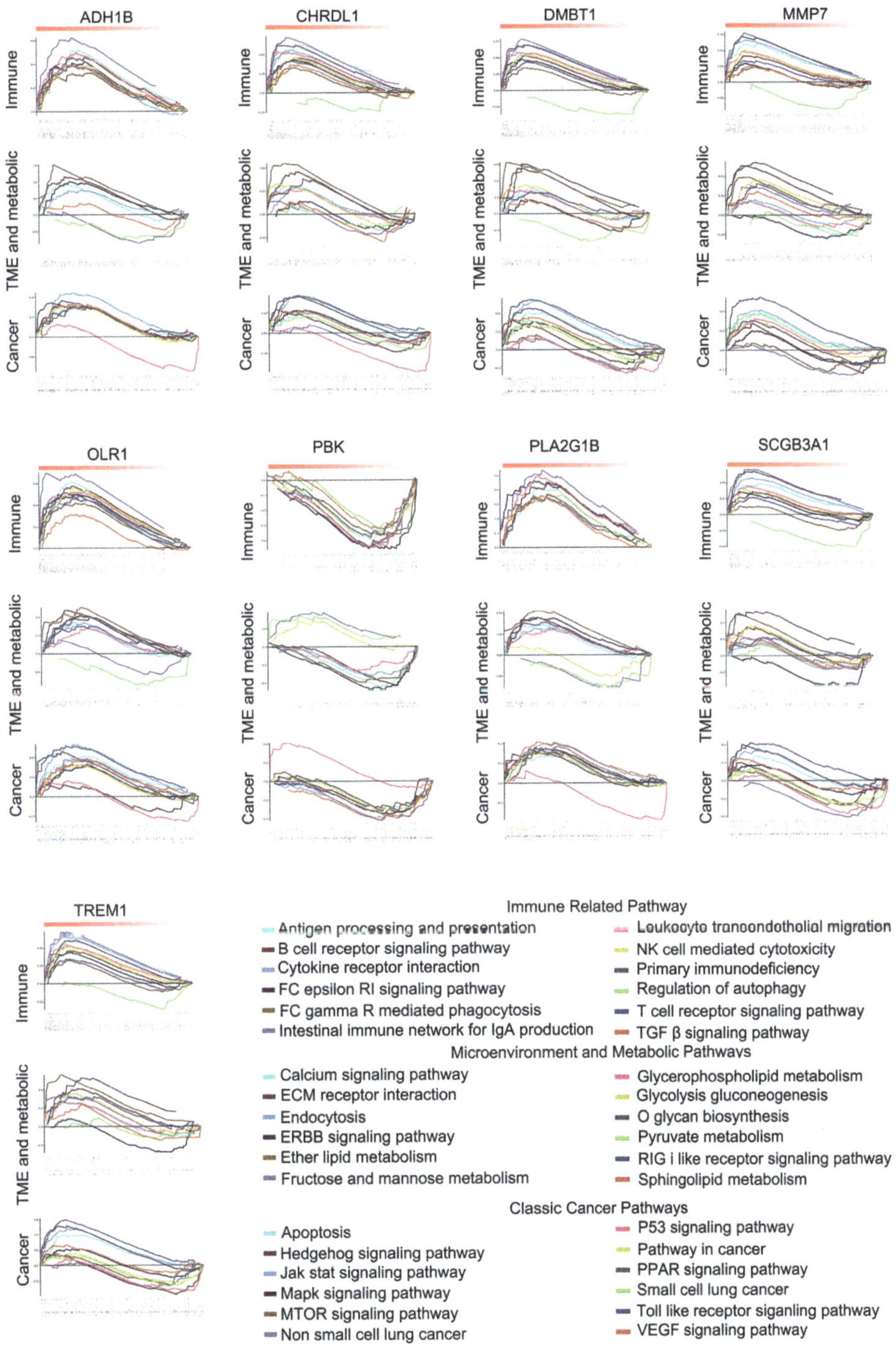

FIGURE 4 | Some pathways could be activated or repressed by each of the 9 differential immune-related genes.

DISCUSSION

In the current study based on GEO data mining, we identified NSCLC microenvironment-related key genes, which show potential as biomarkers for immunotherapy. During the analysis, significant expressions of DEGs were identified between the control and tumor tissue samples; meanwhile, tumor-specific intersect genes also showed significant difference between the immune and stromal components of the tumor samples; further intersection of DEGs and tumor-

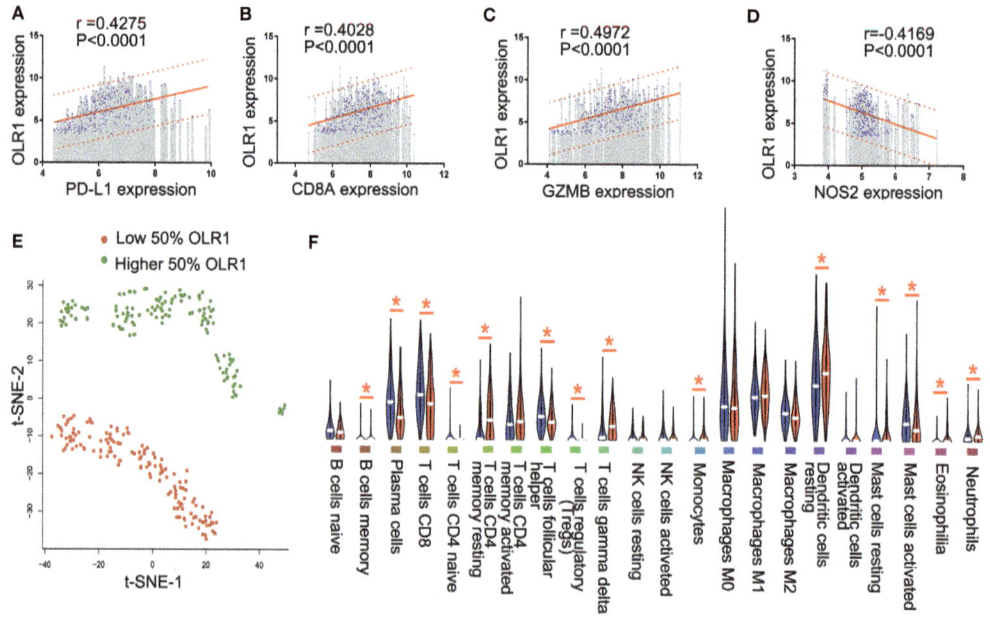

FIGURE 5 | OLR1 showed moderately strong correlations with 4 known immunotherapy biomarkers and its expression marked the TICs distribution. **(A–D)** OLR1 exhibited the highest correlation with PD-L1, CD8A, GZMB, and NOS2; **(E)** OLR1 expression could divide overall status of TICs distribution; **(F)** Violin plot showed the ratio differentiation of 22 kinds of TICs between higher 50% OLR1 expression tumor samples and lower 50% OLR1 expression tumor samples.

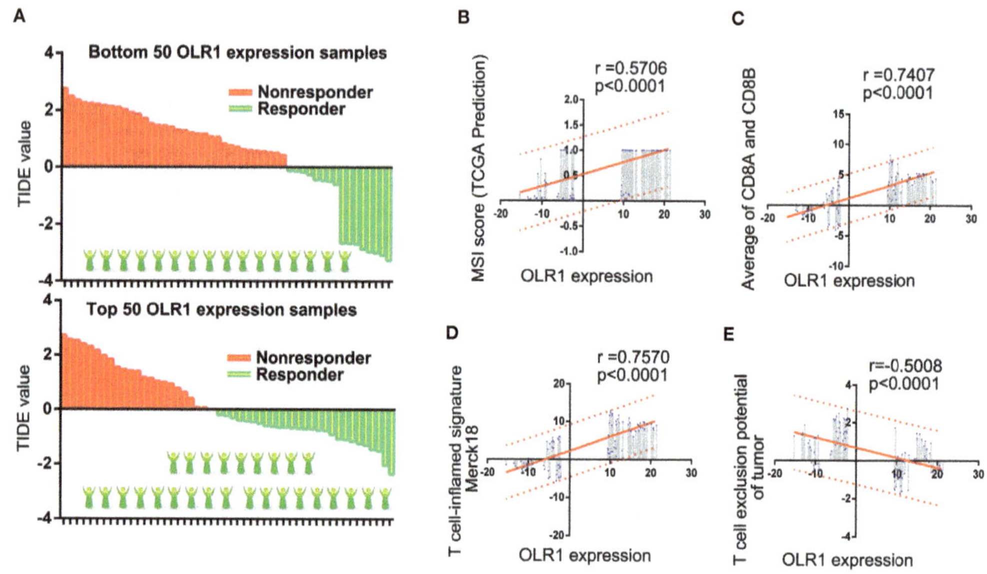

FIGURE 6 | OLR1 may affect the clinical benefits to immunotherapy in NSCLC patients. **(A)** The comparison of responder number in top or bottom OLR1 expression samples. **(B–E)** OLR1 has strong positive correlation with some indicators of TIDE prediction.

specific intersect genes identified potential immune-related genes, both of which were considered different gene expression and significantly affected the ESTIMATE TME scores; finally differential immune-related genes exhibited a significant and opposite correlation with the differential distribution of TICs between the tumor and control samples. OLR1 was considered as a novel potential predictor to immunotherapy of NSCLC.

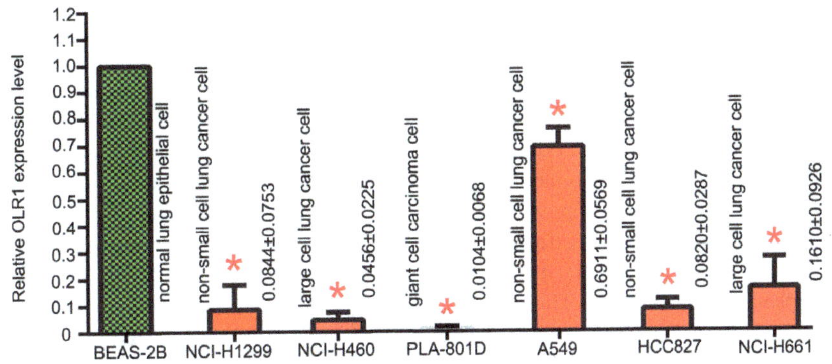

FIGURE 7 | The basic expression level of OLR1 in normal and part NSCLC cell lines.

DEG analysis has been demonstrated as a canonical way to identify novel biomarker genes or novel therapeutic target genes between the normal and tumor samples. In this study, DEG acted as a signature of potential immune-related factors. The screening accuracy of DEGs may be improved using two methods (22). A large sample is expected to improve the screening yield, and analysis with perspective-taking may help improve accuracy based on multiple bioinformatics methods. Other studies randomly chose data sets; in this study, we filtered all GEO data sets by using the selection criteria (see Methods), ultimately including 11 data sets in our analysis cohort. There were 601 tumor samples and 268 control samples across 7 countries and 11 research groups. As our selection criteria, all the 11 data sets should include tumor and normal tissue data for better comparability and higher quality of homogenization data. All data sets were also based on the Affymetrix platform for less data loss in the normalization process. A total of 613 DEGs were identified based on the mRNA array data. These results may be representative and provide an insight in the differences in gene expression in NSCLC. The 613 DEGs were the limited scope for screening in downstream analysis.

The TME is rather complex and largely varies from the microenvironment of normal tissue (7). The TME has been implicated in cancer initiation, development, and treatment resistance. Except for cancer cells, the stromal tumor microenvironment consists of stromal cells and immune cells. The immune cells include T cells, B cells, NK cells, and so on. Stromal cells are the main non-tumor components of the tumor microenvironment (23). Thus, the ESTIMATE algorithm consists of a non-immune "stromal score" parameter and an "immune score" parameter. In this study, the immune and stromal scores, which were determined using ESTIMATE, were used to analyze the infiltration levels of the immune and stromal cells in the tumor and control samples. We focused on genes that specifically regulated the stromal and immune cells in the tumor samples, referred to as the tumor specific intersect gene. We found 166 tumor specific intersect genes in our cohort. They may exhibit cancer-specific effects and show potential to highly regulate the development of the TME in the tumor tissue samples. To determine the type of tumor specific intersect genes with the potential to regulate and control expression; thus the intersecting of the tumor specific intersect genes and DEGs was identified as potential immune-related genes.

Immune cells in TME are the most important defense to eliminate damaged or cancerous cells (23). An established view is that the spatial distribution and the location of immune cells are critical in the immune-oncology field (24). In this study, we tried to identify the differential distributions of immune cells, particularly for TICs. CIBERSORT estimate the abundances of cell types in a mixed cell population based on gene expression data. The CIBERSORT method identified 16 kinds of TICs in our cohort, which were significantly different between the tumor and control samples and not correlated among them. They may each play an independent role in the tumor environment. We explored the correlation between the TICs and 48 potential immune-related genes; the results of multiple non-linear regression analysis indicated that 9 potential immune-related genes with opposite significant correlation between the control and tumor tissue samples. Referred to as differential immune-related genes, those 9 potential immune-related genes, may have tumor tissue-specific functions in the regulation of the immune environment. We evaluated their potential influence on the biological function by using GSEA, and the results showed their potential to activate or inactivate multiple types of signaling pathways, including the immune pathway, microenvironment, and metabolic pathway, and some canonical cancer pathways. The pathways are widely recognized as cancer regulatory mechanisms.

Though much effort has been on identifying genes as biomarkers for immunotherapy, little progress has been made. We thus determined the predicted values for differential immune-related genes in NSCLC. We selected well-recognized biomarkers with gene expression data in our data set (25). PD-L1, also named as B7-H1 or CD274, is the first ligand of PD-1 discovered and widely expressed. It is the main factor responsible for promoting tumor immune evasion (26), and has been a major clinical target for immunotherapy in NSCLC. CD8A is one of the hallmarks of CD8+ T-cell activation signature genes, as well as GZMB (27). NOS2 is the classically activated macrophage transcript (28). They are widely used in multiple studies to predict the efficacy of immunotherapy. In this study, we calculate the relationship between differential immune-related genes and 4 well-recognized immunotherapy biomarkers. OLR1 showed the best correlation with those existing biomarkers and thus was selected to explore its specific relationship with TME. PD-L1 is the most important clinical predictors of immunotherapy and its expression level in tumor tissue determines whether to apply immunotherapy. The NSCLC patient with higher PD-L1 would be believed get better clinical benefit from PD-1/PD-L1 antibody therapy. In this study, there were numerically positive correlations between PD-L1 and OLR1. It may imply that OLR1 could be used as an auxiliary diagnostic marker for immunotherapy. CD8+ activation is the signature event of anti-cancer effect for immune-checkpoint inhibitors. The positive numerically correlation between OLR1 and CD8+ could provide further support for OLR1 plays as a biomarker of immunotherapy. Notably, all analyses were based on gene expression data and all positive or negative correlations just showed statistically significant. However, they have not been assessed in either clinical or experimental models.

Moreover, t-SNE analysis showed a significant difference in the distribution of immune cells with 50% high or low OLR1 expression tumor samples. This finding suggests that OLR1 can distinguish the state of TME by influencing the distribution of immune cells. Fourteen kinds of immune cells changed in OLR1 expression level, and the ratios (low or high) of four well-recognized immunotherapy biomarkers were significantly different between the low and high OLR1 expression groups. Furthermore, we found an interesting result when we compared TILs distribution between "normal vs. tumor" and "lower OLR1 expression vs. higher OLR1 expression" (**Figures 3C–R**, and **Figure 5F**). There were 16 kinds of TILs with different distribution between normal tissue and tumor tissue and 14 kinds of different distribution TILs between lower OLR1 expression tissue and higher OLR1 expression tissue. Ten kinds of TILs were identical in both comparisons. A term TILs (B cells memory, plasma cells, T cells follicular helper and T cells regulatory) have more distribution in tumor tissue (compared with normal tissue) and lower OLR1 expression tissue (compared with higher OLR1 expression tissue), and another term (T cells CD4 memory resting, monocytes, eosinophilia and neutrophils) showed the opposite distribution. It indicates that lower OLR1 expression has close relationship with tumor microenvironment. OLR1 also named LOX1. It was first identified as a scavenger receptor for oxLDL in bovine aortic endothelias cells (29). It is also expressed in macrophages, vascular smooth muscle cells, platelets and tumor cells (30). Its overexpression enhances the migration in breast *via* NF-κB (31). The transcription of OLR1 could be regulated by multiple transcriptional factors, and its activation depended on a wide range of stimuli indicative of dyslipidemia, inflammation and damage initiates several signaling cascades including MAPKs, other protein kinases as well as transcription factors NF-κB and AP-1 (32).

The predictive values of biomarkers should support clinical values. We used TIDE to detect the predictive effect of OLR1 on NSCLC immunotherapy. TIDE is a gene expression biomarker for predicting clinical response to immune checkpoint blockade. Melanoma and NSCLC data are included in the data sets. Given the limitation of the website, we chose 100 tumor samples (top 50 and bottom 50 samples of OLR1 expression in the last cohort) to run the TIDE prediction process. Results showed that the prediction response rate in the top 50 OLR1 expression group was 54% (27/50), which was significantly higher than that in the bottom 50 OLR1 expression group (16/50). In the comparison of other predictive indicators of TIDE, OLR1 expression showed statistical relevance. The results suggested that OLR1 could be used as a biomarker for immunotherapy in NSCLC. As the main disadvantage of data mining study, there are number of limitations of the work. In this study, all analyses used the same data set and all data was from gene expression micro-assay. The single source of data might affect the reliability of the results. Meanwhile, data are derived from multiple countries in this study. Though we set explicit criteria before normalization of data sets, it is inevitable that data missing happens, or some data from different sources may interfere and cancel each other. Therefore, the results might have been biased to a certain degree. In addition, the algorithms are also immature, though we used the well-accepted ones, such as limma, ESTIMATE or CIBERSORT. At last, TIDE, a novel online tool to predict immunotherapy outcome with gene expression data, is used as the last analyses of OLR1 in this research. It is likely that there is no enough evidence for authenticity and reliability of the TIDE prediction results. Those data mining results may change with different data processing or novel algorithm. However, it also provided some clues now for our study and we are trying to validated it experimentally for more evidence. In verification the basic gene expression of OLR1 in multiple NSCLC cell lines, the result showed the significant reduction of OLR1 level in most NSCLC cells than normal lung cell line.

This study explores TME with bioinformatics analysis of public gene expression data sets in NSCLC. Multi-omics data mining shows its reliability in screening meaningful genes in NSCLC with public data sets. The principal findings of this research are that OLR1 played a key role in TME and could predict or potentially be regulated for NSCLC immunotherapy. OLR1 expression was correlated with some well-recognized biomarkers of immunotherapy, including PD-L1, CD8A, GZMB, NOS2, and other predictors. OLR1 expression could divide the differential TICs distribution, and those patients with higher OLR1 expression were predicted to obtain more benefits from immunotherapy in NSCLC. Given the limitations in time and technology, the regulatory role and molecular mechanism of OLR1 were not investigated in depth; regardless, the properties of OLR1 indicate its potential value in NSCLC immunotherapy. We intend to continue this study in future research and explore more clinical data.

AUTHOR CONTRIBUTIONS

Concept and design: TM and JW. Administrative support: MG and ZW. Collection and assembly of data: BL and CZ. Data analysis and interpretation: BL, TM, and JW. Manuscript writing: all authors. Final approval of manuscript: all authors. All authors contributed to the article and approved the submitted version.

REFERENCES

1. Siegel RL, Miller KD, Jemal A. Cancer statistics, 2020. *CA: Cancer J Clin* (2020) 70(1):7–30. doi: 10.3322/caac.21590
2. Chen W, Zheng R, Baade PD, Zhang S, Zeng H, Bray F, et al. Cancer statistics in China, 2015. *CA: Cancer J Clin* (2016) 66(2):115–32. doi: 10.3322/caac.21338
3. Alberg AJ, Brock MV, Samet JM. Epidemiology of lung cancer: looking to the future. *J Clin Oncol Off J Am Soc Clin Oncol* (2005) 23(14):3175–85. doi: 10.1200/JCO.2005.10.462
4. Duruisseaux M, Esteller M. Lung cancer epigenetics: From knowledge to applications. *Semin Cancer Biol* (2018) 51:116–28. doi: 10.1016/j.semcancer.2017.09.005
5. Duma N, Santana-Davila R, Molina JR. Non-Small Cell Lung Cancer: Epidemiology, Screening, Diagnosis, and Treatment. *Mayo Clin Proc* (2019) 94(8):1623–40. doi: 10.1016/j.mayocp.2019.01.013
6. Osmani L, Askin F, Gabrielson E, Li QK. Current WHO guidelines and the critical role of immunohistochemical markers in the subclassification of non-small cell lung carcinoma (NSCLC): Moving from targeted therapy to immunotherapy. *Semin Cancer Biol* (2018) 52(Pt 1):103–9. doi: 10.1016/j.semcancer.2017.11.019
7. Osipov A, Saung MT, Zheng L, Murphy AG. Small molecule immunomodulation: the tumor microenvironment and overcoming immune escape. *J Immunother Cancer* (2019) 7(1):224. doi: 10.1186/s40425-019-0667-0
8. Musetti S, Huang L. Nanoparticle-Mediated Remodeling of the Tumor Microenvironment to Enhance Immunotherapy. *ACS Nano* (2018) 12 (12):11740–55. doi: 10.1021/acsnano.8b05893
9. Calverley DC, Phang TL, Choudhury QG, Gao B, Oton AB, Weyant MJ, et al. Significant downregulation of platelet gene expression in metastatic lung cancer. *Clin Trans Sci* (2010) 3(5):227–32. doi: 10.1111/j.1752-8062.2010.00226.x
10. Fregni G, Quinodoz M, Moller E, Vuille J, Galland S, Fusco C, et al. Reciprocal modulation of mesenchymal stem cells and tumor cells promotes lung cancer metastasis. *EBioMedicine* (2018) 29:128–45. doi: 10.1016/j.ebiom.2018.02.017
11. Hoang LT, Domingo-Sabugo C, Starren ES, Willis-Owen SAG, Morris-Rosendahl DJ, Nicholson AG, et al. Metabolomic, transcriptomic and genetic integrative analysis reveals important roles of adenosine diphosphate in haemostasis and platelet activation in non-small-cell lung cancer. *Mol Oncol* (2019) 13(11):2406–21. doi: 10.1002/1878-0261.12568
12. Kabbout M, Garcia MM, Fujimoto J, Liu DD, Woods D, Chow CW, et al. ETS2 mediated tumor suppressive function and MET oncogene inhibition in human non-small cell lung cancer. *Clin Cancer Res Off J Am Assoc Cancer Res* (2013) 19(13):3383–95. doi: 10.1158/1078-0432.CCR-13-0341
13. Kuo CS, Liu CY, Pavlidis S, Lo YL, Wang YW, Chen CH, et al. Unique Immune Gene Expression Patterns in Bronchoalveolar Lavage and Tumor Adjacent Non-Neoplastic Lung Tissue in Non-Small Cell Lung Cancer. *Front Immunol* (2018) 9:232. doi: 10.3389/fimmu.2018.00232
14. Lu TP, Hsiao CK, Lai LC, Tsai MH, Hsu CP, Lee JM, et al. Identification of regulatory SNPs associated with genetic modifications in lung adenocarcinoma. *BMC Res Notes* (2015) 8:92. doi: 10.1186/s13104-015-1053-8
15. Mitchell KA, Zingone A, Toulabi L, Boeckelman J, Ryan BM. Comparative Transcriptome Profiling Reveals Coding and Noncoding RNA Differences in NSCLC from African Americans and European Americans. *Clin Cancer Res Off J Am Assoc Cancer Res* (2017) 23(23):7412–25. doi: 10.1158/1078-0432.CCR-17-0527
16. Rousseaux S, Debernardi A, Jacquiau B, Vitte AL, Vesin A, Nagy-Mignotte H, et al. Ectopic activation of germline and placental genes identifies aggressive metastasis-prone lung cancers. *Sci Trans Med* (2013) 5(186):186ra66. doi: 10.1126/scitranslmed.3005723
17. Sanchez-Palencia A, Gomez-Morales M, Gomez-Capilla JA, Pedraza V, Boyero L, Rosell R, et al. Gene expression profiling reveals novel biomarkers in nonsmall cell lung cancer. *Int J Cancer* (2011) 129(2):355–64. doi: 10.1002/ijc.25704
18. Xu L, Lu C, Huang Y, Zhou J, Wang X, Liu C, et al. SPINK1 promotes cell growth and metastasis of lung adenocarcinoma and acts as a novel prognostic biomarker. *BMB Rep* (2018) 51(12):648–53. doi: 10.5483/BMBRep.2018.51.12.205
19. Yoshihara K, Shahmoradgoli M, Martinez E, Vegesna R, Kim H, Torres-Garcia W, et al. Inferring tumour purity and stromal and immune cell admixture from expression data. *Nat Commun* (2013) 4:2612. doi: 10.1038/ncomms3612
20. Newman AM, Steen CB, Liu CL, Gentles AJ, Chaudhuri AA, Scherer F, et al. Determining cell type abundance and expression from bulk tissues with digital cytometry. *Nat Biotechnol* (2019) 37(7):773–82. doi: 10.1038/s41587-019-0114-2
21. Jiang P, Gu S, Pan D, Fu J, Sahu A, Hu X, et al. Signatures of T cell dysfunction and exclusion predict cancer immunotherapy response. *Nat Med* (2018) 24 (10):1550–8. doi: 10.1038/s41591-018-0136-1
22. Vougas K, Sakellaropoulos T, Kotsinas A, Foukas GP, Ntargaras A, Koinis F, et al. Machine learning and data mining frameworks for predicting drug response in cancer: An overview and a novel in silico screening process based on association rule mining. *Pharmacol Ther* (2019) 203:107395. doi: 10.1016/j.pharmthera.2019.107395
23. Quail DF, Joyce JA. Microenvironmental regulation of tumor progression and metastasis. *Nat Med* (2013) 19(11):1423–37. doi: 10.1038/nm.3394
24. Holmgaard RB, Schaer DA, Li Y, Castaneda SP, Murphy MY, Xu X, et al. Targeting the TGFbeta pathway with galunisertib, a TGFbetaRI small molecule inhibitor, promotes anti-tumor immunity leading to durable, complete responses, as monotherapy and in combination with checkpoint blockade. *J Immunother Cancer* (2018) 6(1):47. doi: 10.1186/s40425-018-0356-4
25. Camidge DR, Doebele RC, Kerr KM. Comparing and contrasting predictive biomarkers for immunotherapy and targeted therapy of NSCLC. *Nat Rev Clin Oncol* (2019) 16(6):341–55. doi: 10.1038/s41571-019-0173-9
26. Jiang Y, Zhan H. Communication between EMT and PD-L1 signaling: New insights into tumor immune evasion. *Cancer Lett* (2020) 468:72–81. doi: 10.1016/j.canlet.2019.10.013
27. Oja AE, Piet B, van der Zwan D, Blaauwgeers H, Mensink M, de Kivit S, et al. Functional Heterogeneity of CD4(+) Tumor-Infiltrating Lymphocytes With a Resident Memory Phenotype in NSCLC. *Front Immunol* (2018) 9:2654. doi: 10.3389/fimmu.2018.02654
28. Kahn DA, Archer DC, Gold DP, Kelly CJ. Adjuvant immunotherapy is dependent on inducible nitric oxide synthase. *J Exp Med* (2001) 193(11):1261–8. doi: 10.1084/jem.193.11.1261
29. Sawamura T, Kume N, Aoyama T, Moriwaki H, Hoshikawa H, Aiba Y, et al. An endothelial receptor for oxidized low-density lipoprotein. *Nature* (1997) 386(6620):73–7. doi: 10.1038/386073a0
30. Hirsch HA, Iliopoulos D, Joshi A, Zhang Y, Jaeger SA, Bulyk M, et al. A transcriptional signature and common gene networks link cancer with lipid metabolism and diverse human diseases. *Cancer Cell* (2010) 17(4):348–61. doi: 10.1016/j.ccr.2010.01.022
31. Khaidakov M, Mitra S, Kang BY, Wang X, Kadlubar S, Novelli G, et al. Oxidized LDL receptor 1 (OLR1) as a possible link between obesity, dyslipidemia and cancer. *PloS One* (2011) 6(5):e20277. doi: 10.1371/journal.pone.0020277
32. Li D, Saldeen T, Romeo F, Mehta JL. Oxidized LDL upregulates angiotensin II type 1 receptor expression in cultured human coronary artery endothelial cells: the potential role of transcription factor NF-kappaB. *Circulation* (2000) 102(16):1970–6. doi: 10.1161/01.CIR.102.16.1970

12

Exploration of the Tumor-Suppressive Immune Microenvironment by Integrated Analysis in *EGFR*-Mutant Lung Adenocarcinoma

Teng Li[1], *Xiaocong Pang*[2], *Junyun Wang*[3,4], *Shouzheng Wang*[1], *Yiying Guo*[1], *Ning He*[4], *Puyuan Xing*[1*] *and Junling Li*[1*]

[1] *Department of Medical Oncology, National Cancer Center/National Clinical Research Center for Cancer/Cancer Hospital, Chinese Academy of Medical Sciences and Peking Union Medical College, Beijing, China,* [2] *Department of Pharmacy, Peking University First Hospital, Beijing, China,* [3] *CAS Key Laboratory of Genome Sciences and Information, Beijing Institute of Genomics, Chinese Academy of Sciences/China National Center for Bioinformation, Beijing, China,* [4] *Research Institute, GloriousMed Clinical Laboratory (Shanghai) Co., Ltd., Shanghai, China*

***Correspondence:**
Junling Li
lijunling@cicams.ac.cn
Puyuan Xing
xingpuyuan@cicams.ac.cn

Background: Clinical evidence has shown that few non-small cell lung cancer (NSCLC) patients with epidermal growth factor receptor (*EGFR*) mutations can benefit from immunotherapy. The tumor immune microenvironment (TIME) is a significant factor affecting the efficacy of immunotherapy. However, the TIME transformational process in *EGFR*-mutation patients is unknown.

Methods: The mRNA expression and mutation data and lung adenocarcinoma (LUAD) clinical data were obtained from The Cancer Genome Atlas (TCGA) database. Profiles describing the immune landscape of patients with *EGFR* mutations were characterized by differences in tumor mutation burden (TMB), ESTIMATE, CIBERSORT, and microenvironment cell populations-counter (MCP-counter).

Results: In total, the TCGA data for 585 patients were analyzed. Among these patients, 98 had *EGFR* mutations. The TMB was lower in the *EGFR* group (3.94 mut/Mb) than in the *KRAS* mutation group (6.09 mut/Mb, $P < 0.001$) and the entire LUAD (6.58 mut/Mb, $P < 0.001$). The *EGFR* group had a lower population of activated immune cells and an even higher score of immunosuppressive cells. A further inter-group comparison showed that differences in the TMB and tumor-infiltrating lymphocytes were only found between patients with oncogenic mutations and unknown mutation. Meanwhile, there were more myeloid dendritic cells (DCs) in *EGFR* 19del than in L858R-mutation patients and in common mutation patents than in uncommon mutation patients ($P < 0.05$). Additionally, we established a D score, where D = MCP-counter score for cytotoxic T lymphocytes (CTLs)/MCP-counter score for myeloid DCs. Further analysis revealed that lower D scores indicated immune suppression and were negatively related to several immunotherapy biomarkers.

Conclusions: The TIME of *EGFR* mutant NSCLC was immunosuppressive. Myeloid DCs gradually increased in *EGFR* 19del, L858R, and uncommon mutations. The potential role of CTLs and DCs in the TIME of patients requires further investigation.

Keywords: immune microenvironment, lung adenocarcinoma, epidermal growth factor receptor (EGFR) mutation, Bioinformatics & Computational Biology, myeloid dendritic cells (mDCs), cytotoxic T lymphocyte (CTL)

INTRODUCTION

Lung cancer is one of the leading causes of cancer mortality worldwide (1). Nearly 85% of patients with lung cancer are diagnosed with non-small-cell lung cancer (NSCLC). The two main histological subtypes of NSCLC are adenocarcinoma (ADC) and squamous cell carcinoma (SCC). However, ADC and SCC show different characteristic according to the mutation landscape at the molecular level. As reported, the epidermal growth factor receptor (*EGFR*) mutation is one of the most common mutated genes detected in adenocarcinoma. Previous studies have shown that *EGFR* mutations occurred more frequently in females, non-smokers, and Asian patients, and the majority of *EGFR* mutations were deletions in exon 19 or the L858R substitution in exon 21. Other mutations located in exons 18 and 20 are rare but can also cause *EGFR* gene activation (2).

For NSCLC patients harboring a sensitizing *EGFR*-mutation, treatment with *EGFR* tyrosine kinase inhibitors (TKIs) leads to longer progression-free survival (PFS) and has already become the first-line treatment. At present, three generations of *EGFR* TKIs are globally available for the treatment of NSCLC and have significantly improved the prognosis of patients (3–5). However, a significant portion of patients with co-mutations or rare mutations of *EGFR* gain little benefit from TKIs treatment (6). Additionally, almost all patients treated with TKIs eventually experience tumor relapse and acquire resistance. For such patients, the use of TKIs combined with chemotherapy or a monoclonal anti-vascular endothelial growth factor antibody has become the treatment of choice (7). However, the efficacy remains unsatisfactory, and there is still a great need for new treatment strategies.

In recent years, clinical trials have provided unequivocal evidence of the efficacy of immune checkpoint inhibitors (ICIs), so they have become a standard therapy in advanced NSCLC. Still, a major limitation was that patients with sensitizing *EGFR* mutations were excluded from most clinical trials. A meta-analysis demonstrated that ICIs prolonged overall survival in the EGFR wild-type subgroup [hazard ratio, (HR), 0.67], but not in the *EGFR* mutant subgroup (HR, 1.11), and prolonged overall survival in the *KRAS*-mutant subgroup (HR, 0.65), but not in the *KRAS* wild-type subgroup (HR, 0.86) (8). Currently available clinical trial data have shown that single-agent immunotherapy and in combination with TKIs are inappropriate for *EGFR* mutant patients (9). Thus, it is challenging to identify potential patients who could benefit from ICIs and to help patients with specific mutations benefit from immunotherapy.

Recent studies on the tumor immune microenvironment (TIME) suggest that the abundance and location of tumor-infiltrating lymphocytes (TILs) can be a potential predictor of response to ICIs (10). Clinical studies also have confirmed that reversing the TIME might reduce tumor-induced immunosuppression in patients with a mutated *EGFR* (11). All of these studies suggest that we should pay attention to the TIME of mutant lung cancer and seek a breakthrough in treatment. Till now, the immune landscape remains unclear in *EGFR* mutant patients, especially for different mutant subtypes. Therefore, this study aims to explore the TIME in $EGFR^{-mt}$ adenocarcinoma and investigate the specific TIME features within different subgroups. The flow chart of this study is shown in **Figure 1**.

METHODS

Patient Cohort and Genomic Data Processing

The Cancer Genome Atlas (TCGA) lung adenocarcinoma (LUAD) mRNA expression data, mutation data, and clinical information were downloaded from TCGA (http://cancergenome.nih.gov/) and the University of California at Santa Cruz Xena (UCSC Xena; http://xena.ucsc.edu/). For transcriptome data, raw counts and Fragments Per Kilobase of transcripts per Million mapped reads [FPKM] were acquired. The FPKM was then transformed to TPM for further calculation. Genomic alteration was downloaded from the cBioPortal for Cancer Genomics (cBioPortal; http://cbioportal.org).

Common *EGFR* mutations were defined as exon 19 deletion and exon 21 L858R without exon 20 T790M. Uncommon *EGFR* mutations were defined as other oncogenic mutations, such as G719X, S768I, and L861Q in exons 18, 20, and 21, respectively. Except as noted above, others that cannot lead to *EGFR* activation were defined as unknown mutations. Patients with co-mutations of different *EGFR*-mutation status were excluded from all groups.

Analysis of Immune Landscape

Tumor mutational burden (TMB): The TMB was defined as the total number of somatic mutations per megabase (Mb) of the genome examined. The normalized TMB = (whole exome non-synonymous mutations)/(38 Mb).

Estimation of STromal and Immune cells in MAlignant Tumor tissues using Expression data (ESTIMATE): ESTIMATE (12) was used to assess the immune infiltration (ImmuneScore), stromal content (StromalScore), and combined (ESTIMATEScore) of the samples. This kind of scoring can be used to estimate tumor purity. ESTIMATE was downloaded from the MD Anderson Cancer Center database (https://bioinformatics.mdanderson.org).

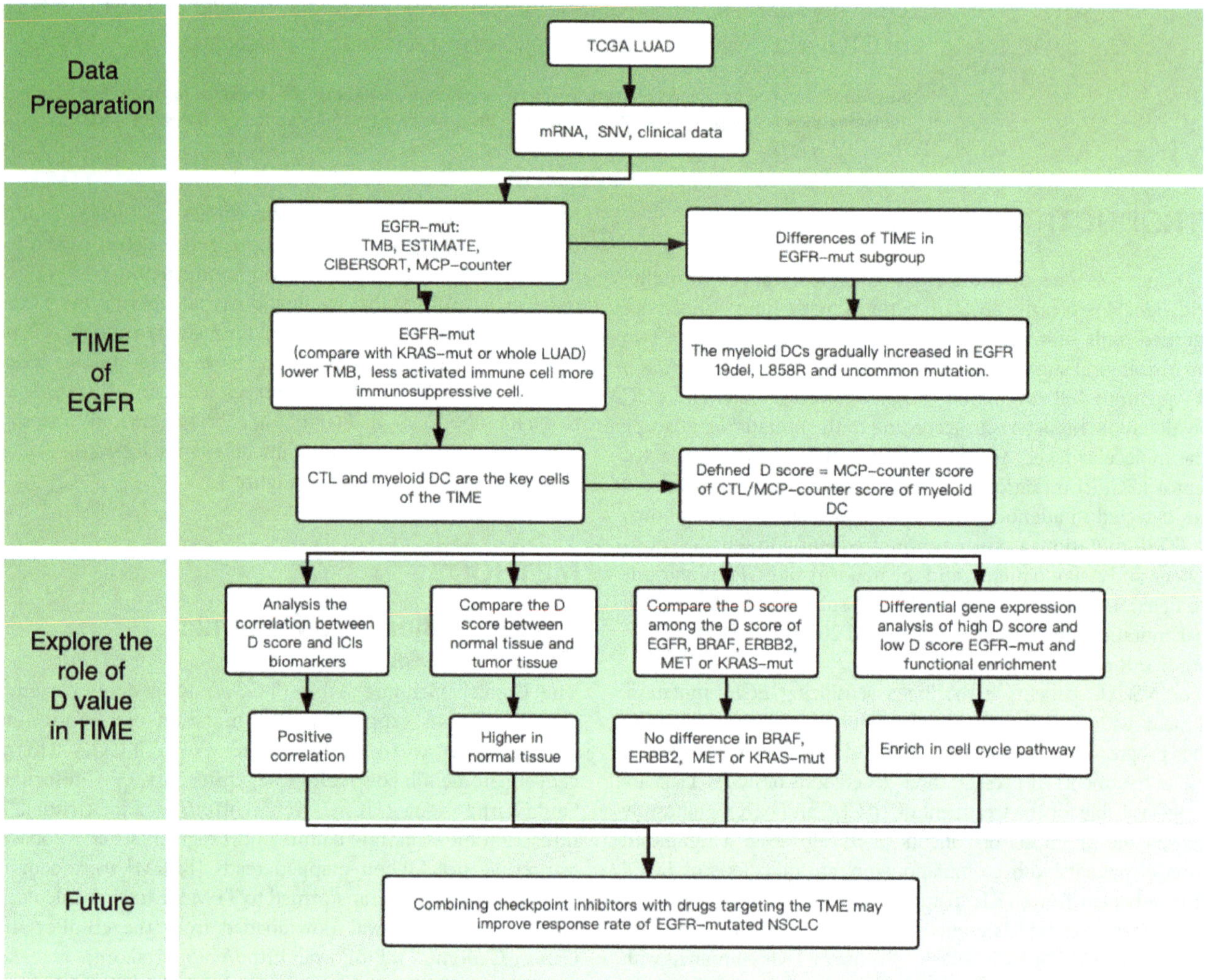

FIGURE 1 | Flowchart of the study design.

CIBERSORT: CIBERSORT (13) is an analytical tool that applies a deconvolution algorithm to estimate the proportions of 22 leucocyte subtypes based on RNA-seq data. Results with a CIBERSORT P-value of <0.05 were used for subsequent calculation. The package 'CIBERSORT' was used to calculate the percentage.

Microenvironment cell populations-counter (MCP-counter): MCP-counter (14) is a computational Method based on the mean marker gene expression that is specifically expressed in the cell type. The eight immune-cell lineage scores were estimated by using the R package MCP-counter algorithm.

Differentially Expressed Genes and Functional Pathways Analysis

Differential gene expression was determined by using the EdgeR software package. Gene Ontology (GO) and Kyoto Encyclopedia of Genes and Genomes (KEGG) enrichment (false discovery rate < 0.05, Foldchange > 1) analysis of differentially expressed genes (DEGs) were performed to search for biological functions and pathways.

Statistical Analysis

The statistical analysis of tumor purity and of the presence of infiltrating stromal/immune cells in tumor tissues was performed by using R packages: MCP-counter and CIBERSORT. Statistical comparisons were evaluated by using the Wilcoxon rank-sum test and Kruskal-Wallis tests. The clinicopathological characteristics were compared by using chi-square test. Correlations were assessed by using Pearson correlational distances. A two-sided P-value of <0.05 was considered to be indicative of statistical significance.

RESULTS

Clinical Characteristics of the Patients

In total, 585 patients data were downloaded from the TCGA data set. Among these, 98 cases involved *EGFR*-mutation. Then, the patients were divided into four groups according to their *EGFR*-mutation type (19del, L858R, uncommon mutation, unknown mutation group). Clinical data were available for 68 of the 98 patients. Baseline characteristics are presented in **Table 1**.

TIME of the Patients With *EGFR* Mutations

Supplementary Figure 1 shows the immune landscape of the *EGFR* mutant group. For further evaluation, we compared the TIME in the *EGFR* group with that in the *KRAS* group, and the whole LUAD. The results showed that the TMB was lower in the *EGFR* group (3.94 mut/Mb) than in the *KRAS* group (6.09 mut/Mb, $P < 0.001$) and in the whole LUAD (6.58 mut/Mb, $P < 0.001$) (**Figure 2A**). For tumor purity, which was inferred from the ESTIMATE purity score, there were no significant differences between the three groups ($P > 0.05$) (**Figure 2B**). For TILs, the *EGFR* group had a lower score of activated immune cells (CD8 T cells, cytotoxic lymphocytes (CTLs), NK cells) and an even higher score of immunosuppressive cells [myeloid dendritic cells (DCs)] according to the MCP-counter results than *KRAS* group and the whole LUAD (**Figure 2D**, $P < 0.05$). The same trend was observed through analysis of the immune-cell proportion by using the CIBERSORT deconvolution Method (**Figure 2C**. $P < 0.05$).

Further Analysis of the TIME in the *EGFR* Mutations Subgroup

Previous studies have suggested that the efficacy of immunotherapy was different among different mutant subtypes. We hypothesized that this may be related to TIME. We then conducted a subgroup analysis to further explore the differences in TIME among different *EGFR* subgroups. Analysis showed that there were significant differences among the four subgroups (19del, L858R, uncommon mutations, unknown mutations) in the TMB, CD8 T cells, and DCs (**Figure 3**). However, there were no differences in the purity scores among the four groups (by ESTIMATE).

To determine the source of the differences, we first classified the *EGFR*-mutation patients into oncogenic and unknown mutation groups according to whether EGFR was activated. The oncogenic group showed a lower TMB, a lower fractions of activated immune subpopulations (by CIBERSORT), and a high abundance of myeloid DCs (by MCP-counter) (**Supplementary Figure 2**, $P < 0.05$). Second, oncogenic *EGFR* mutations can be divided into common and uncommon mutations. There were more myeloid DCs in the common mutations group than in the uncommon mutations group (by MCP-counter). No statistical differences in TMB, tumor purity or fractions of the most immune subgroup were observed between this two groups (**Supplementary Figure 3**, $P < 0.05$). Thirdly, as mentioned above, common *EGFR* mutations include exon 19 deletion and exon 21 L858R. The analysis results showed that there were also no differences in the TMB and ESTIMATE scores between this two subgroups. But a trend toward an immunosuppressive environment was observed in the 19del group. The proportion of resting DCs in the 19del group showed a significant decrease than that in the L858R group (by CIBERSORT, $P < 0.05$) (**Supplementary Figure 4**).

Define a Score (D) Based on the MCP-Counter

Subgroup analysis of clinical trials showed that the efficacy of tumor immunotherapy was better in the KRAS group than in the EGFR group. To further characterize which types of infiltrating cells have important roles in immunotherapy, the compositions of TILs were compared between the *KRAS* and *EGFR* groups. Analysis by MCP-counter (as well as the CIBERSORT results) showed that more abundant CTLs and a lower population of myeloid DCs were observed in the *KRAS*$^{-mt}$ group than in the *EGFR*$^{-mt}$ group (**Supplementary Figure 5**). The results above suggest that CTLs and myeloid DC have an essential role in TIME. According to this result, we built a simplified model (D score) to quantify the generalized TIME state and defined a D score as D = MCP-counter score of CTLs/

TABLE 1 | Demographic characteristics of the patients at baseline.

Characteristics	Type	Total	19del	L858R	Uncommon mutation	Unknown mutation
Age	<=65	33 (48.53%)	11 (42.31%)	9 (50%)	7 (58.33%)	6 (50%)
	>65	32 (47.06%)	12 (46.15%)	9 (50%)	5 (41.67%)	6 (50%)
	Unknown	3 (4.41%)	3 (11.54%)	0 (0%)	0 (0%)	0 (0%)
Gender	FEMALE	49 (72.06%)	22 (84.62%)	15 (83.33%)	9 (75%)	3 (25%)
	MALE	19 (27.94%)	4 (15.38%)	3 (16.67%)	3 (25%)	9 (75%)
Stage	Stage I–II	52 (76.47%)	19 (73.08%)	15 (83.33%)	9 (75%)	9 (75%)
	Stage III–IV	15 (22.06%)	7 (26.92%)	3 (16.67%)	3 (25%)	2 (16.67%)
	Unknown	1 (1.47%)	0 (0%)	0 (0%)	0 (0%)	1 (8.33%)
T	T1–2	58 (85.29%)	26 (100%)	15 (83.33%)	9 (75%)	8 (66.67%)
	T3–4	9 (13.24%)	0 (0%)	3 (16.67%)	2 (16.67%)	4 (33.33%)
	TX	1 (1.47%)	0 (0%)	0 (0%)	1 (8.33%)	0 (0%)
M	M0	47 (69.12%)	17 (65.38%)	15 (83.33%)	7 (58.33%)	8 (66.67%)
	M1	3 (4.41%)	1 (3.85%)	0 (0%)	1 (8.33%)	1 (8.33%)
	Unknown	18 (26.47%)	8 (30.77%)	3 (16.67%)	4 (33.33%)	3 (25%)
N	N0	42 (61.76%)	12 (46.15%)	12 (66.67%)	7 (58.33%)	11 (91.67%)
	N1-3	23 (33.82%)	13 (50%)	6 (33.33%)	3 (25%)	1 (8.33%)
	Unknown	3 (4.41%)	1 (3.85%)	0 (0%)	2 (16.67%)	0 (0%)

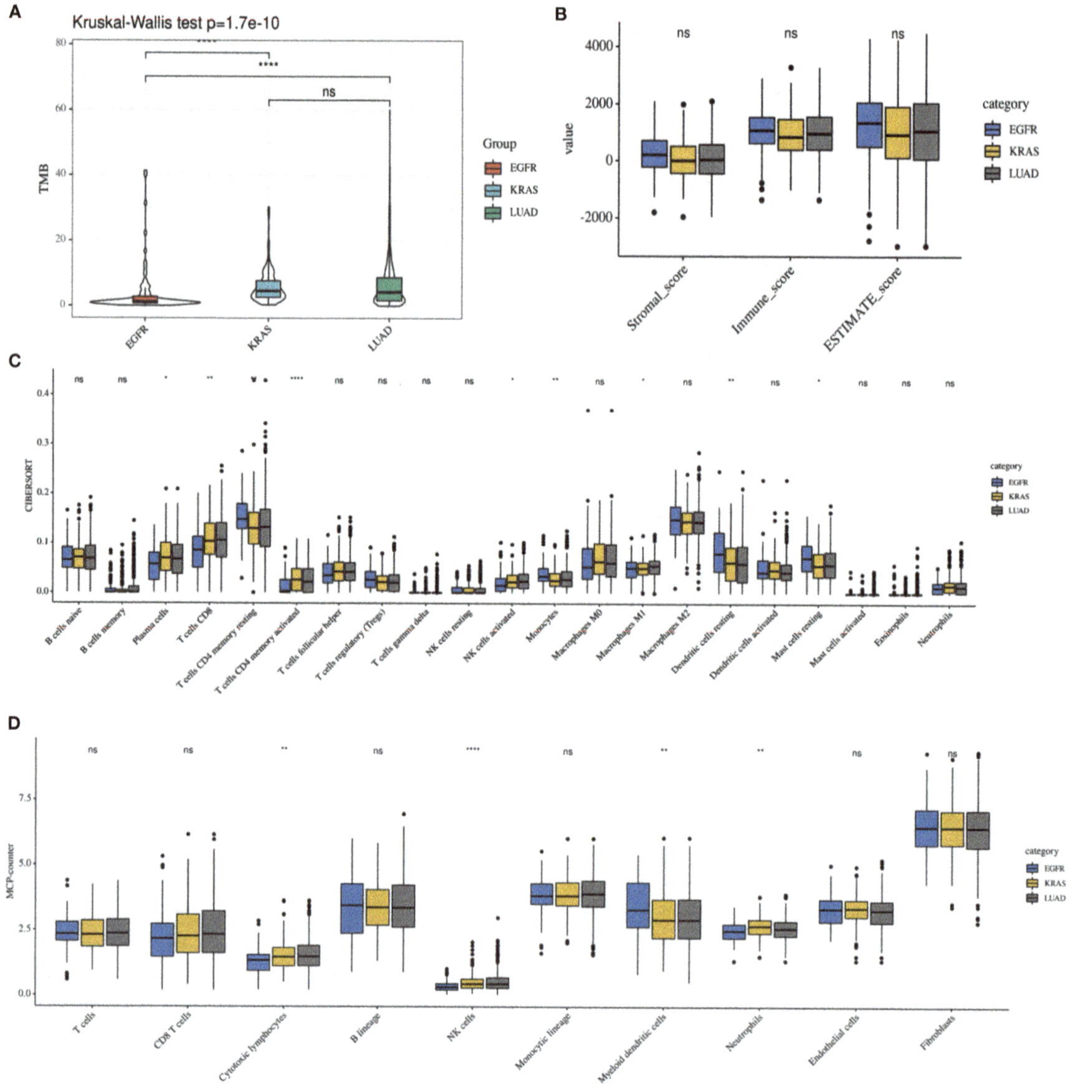

FIGURE 2 | Comparison of the immune landscape of EGFR-mutated group, KRAS-mutated group and the whole lung adenocarcinoma. The TIME of EGFR-mutated NSCLC show an immunosuppressive status with lower **(A)** TMB, a lower score of activated immune cell and an even higher score of immunosuppressive cell, estimated by **(C)** CIBERSORT and **(D)** MCP-counter. No difference was found in tumor purity among three group **(B)**. *P < 0.05, **P < 0.01, and ***P < 0.0001, respectively. ns, not significant.

MCP-counter score of myeloid DCs. The lower the D score, the greater degree of immunosuppression in the TIME. To test the performance of D score, we performed the following analysis.

Functional Enrichment Analysis in Different *EGFR* Mutant Groups Defined by the D Score

To further study the differences in gene expression between different D values, *EGFR*-mutation patients were grouped by D value quartiles, with quartile 1 having the lowest and quartile 3 the highest D level (n = 16 in each group). Differentially expressed genes between the two groups were identified by performing an EdgeR analysis. Among the DEGs identified, 890 were upregulated, and 1373 were downregulated. The DEGs are shown as a volcano plot in **Figure 4A**. The candidate DEG functions and signaling pathway enrichment were analyzed by using GO terms and the KEGG pathway. Overall, 18 KEGG pathways were significantly enriched. The top five KEGG pathways were the cell cycle, viral protein interaction with cytokine and cytokine receptors, cytokine–cytokine receptor interaction, neuroactive ligand–receptor interaction, and hematopoietic cell lineage (**Figure 4B**). The organelle fission GO term was the top GO term, followed by nuclear division, receptor ligand activity chromosome segregation, and chromosomal region (**Figure 4C**).

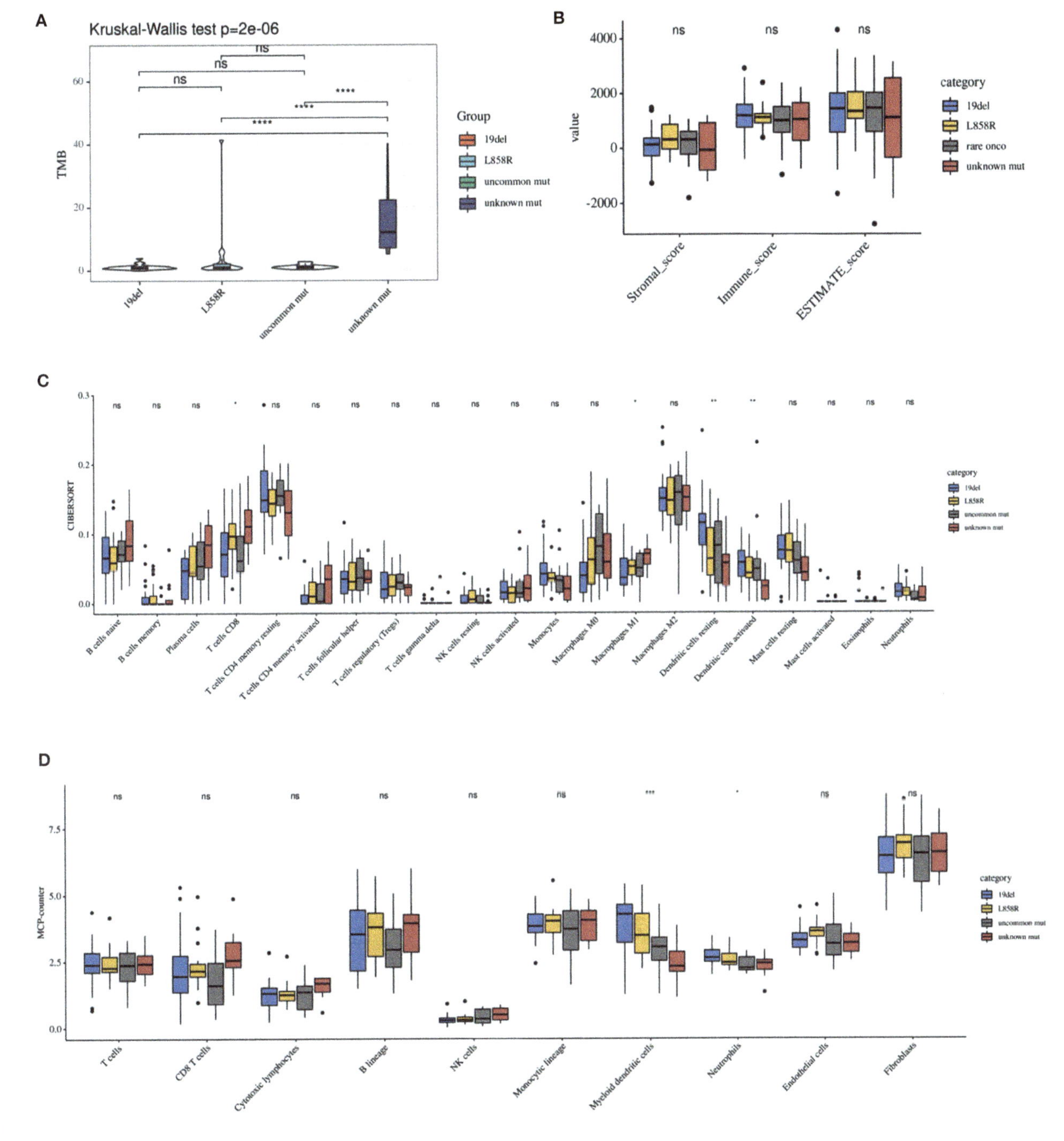

FIGURE 3 | Comparison of the immune landscape among 19del, L858R, uncommon mutation and unknown mutation group. **(A)** TMB, **(B)** ESTIMATE, **(C)** CIBERSORT, **(D)** MCP-counter. Only significant difference in myeloid DC cells was presented among different groups estimated by **(C)** CIBERSORT and **(D)** MCP-counter. *P < 0.05, **P < 0.01, ***P < 0.001 and ****P < 0.0001, respectively. ns, not significant.

Exploration of D Score Among Patients With Different Driver Mutation

Since it remained uncertain whether NSCLC with targetable drivers will benefit from immunotherapy, we further calculated the D value of different mutation subgroups, including *EGFR*, *BRAF*, *ERBB2*, *KRAS*, and *MET* mutations. The results showed that the average D values were 0.37, 0.47, 0.56, 0.57, and 0.51 in patients with EGFR, *BRAF*, *ERB*B2, *KRAS*, and *MET* mutations. Inter-group analysis showed that the D value was lower in the *EGFR* group than in the other rare mutation groups ($P < 0.05$) except for the *MET* mutation. However, there were no significant differences in the D values among the *BRAF*, *ERBB2*, *KRAS*, and *MET* mutations (**Figure 5**).

Clinical Characteristics and Immune-Cell Infiltration of Different D score Groups in LUAD

To examine the significance of the D score, we further studied its role among all TCGA-LUAD patients. We first compared the D score between tumors and normal tissues from TCGA. The results showed that the D value was higher in normal tissue than in tumor tissue, which was consistent with expectations (**Figure 6A**, $P <$ 0.001). We then compared the clinicopathological features and immune landscape characteristics of different LUAD patients by their D scores. For further analysis, the median D score was selected as the cutoff value. The patients were divided into two groups: the high (D > 0.51, n = 252) group and low (D ≤ 0.51, n = 251) D group. We found there were no significant differences in the D scores of the samples among the clinicopathological features groups, including T, N, M, Stage, Grade, and Age ($P > 0.05$) (**Supplementary Table 1**). We also observed that the tumor purity difference between the patients in the high- and low-D groups was not significant (median ESTIMATE score, $P > 0.05$). However, the immunescore was higher for the high-D group, as expected ($P < 0.05$) (**Figure 6B**).

Because the D score reflected the immunosuppressive environment based on T cells and DCs, we decided to explore whether the levels of other immune cells in different D groups were consistent with expectations. The different immune cell distribution between the high- and low-D groups is shown in **Figures 6C, D**. In addition to CD8+T cells and DCs, we observed that the high-D group had higher infiltration of activated T cells CD4 memory activated, T- cells follicular helper, NK cells activated, and macrophages M1 according to CIBERSORT ($P <$ 0.05). In contrast, the low-D group had higher infiltration of Ts cells CD4 memory resting, T cells regulatory (Tregs), and monocytes and mast cells resting ($P < 0.05$) (**Figure 6C**). Similar to this result, we found that a variety of T-cell MCP-counter scores decreased in the low-D group ($P < 0.05$) (**Figure 6D**).

Relationship Between the D Score and Predictive Biomarkers for Immunotherapy

Immunotherapy is currently a first-line treatment for lung adenocarcinoma. However, it remains challenging to identify immune resistance and the beneficiary groups. To explore the predictive role of the D value in immunotherapy, we further explored the relationship between the D score and predictive biomarkers for ICIs. First, we found a positive correlation between D scores and TMB (r = 0.30, $P < 0.001$), which suggests that the lower the D value, the lower the TMB, and the less likely it is to benefit from immunotherapy. In addition, we further explored the association between different patient groups defined by the D score and immune checkpoints. We found that lower mRNA expression levels of PDCD1, CD274, PDCD1LG2, LAG3, TIGIT, and IDO1 were observed in the low-D score patients (**Figures 7A–F**, $P < 0.05$). The results also suggest that a lower D value is a good indicator of immunosuppression and a potentially negative biomarker for immunotherapy.

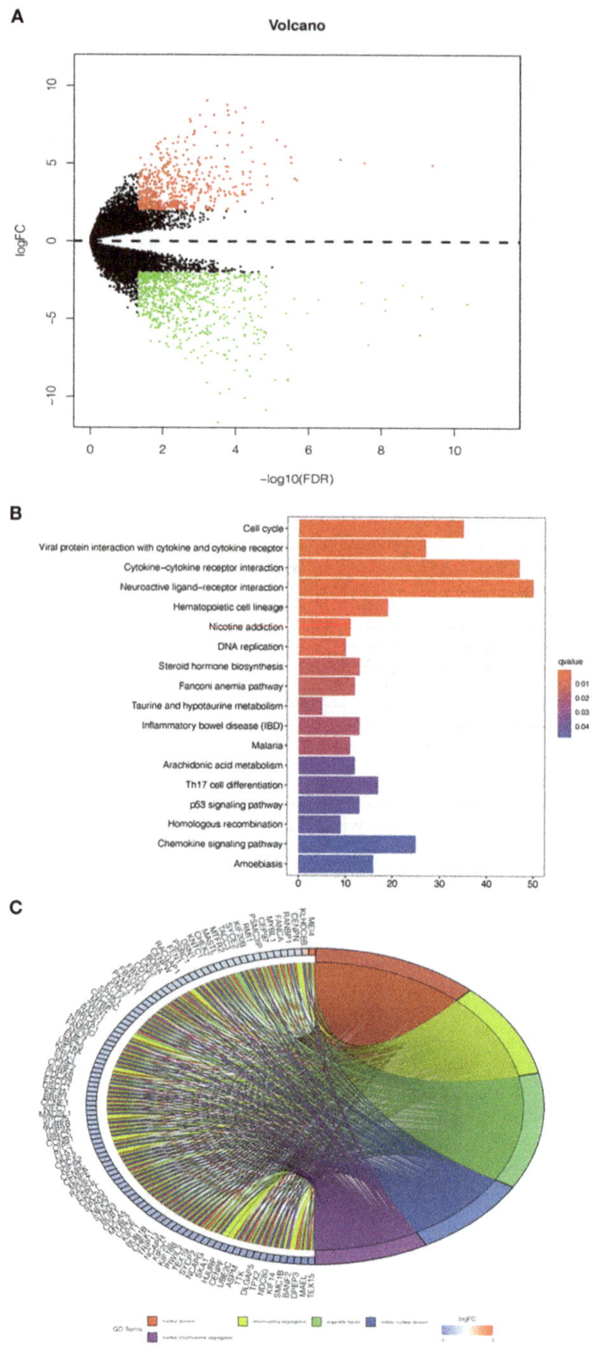

FIGURE 4 | Analysis of differentially expressed genes (DEGs) from the D value of EGFR-mut group quartile 1 compared with quartile 3. **(A)** Volcano plot showing DEGs between higher D score group and lower D score group. **(B)** Top 10 enrichments of up-regulated DEGs by KEGG analyses. **(C)** Gene Ontology analyses of DEGs according to their biological process.

DISCUSSION

Although ICIs have demonstrated clinical activity in a variety of tumors, resistance of cancer to ICI therapy remains a major

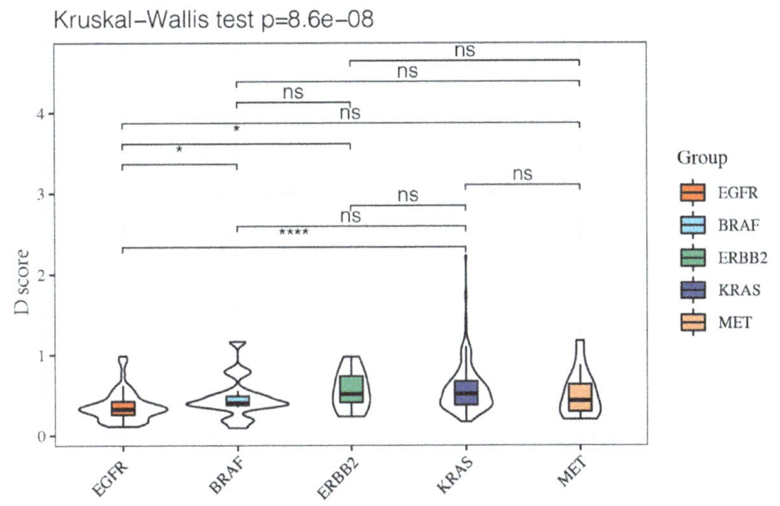

FIGURE 5 | The D value of EGFR group was lower than rare mutation group except MET mutation and there was no significant difference among BRAF, ERBB2, KRAS and MET mutation. *P < 0.05 and ****P < 0.0001, respectively. ns, not significant.

clinical problem (15). From a clinical perspective, resistance to PD-(L)1 inhibitors can be classified into three distinct scenarios: primary resistance, secondary resistance, and progression after treatment discontinuation (16). The mechanisms of primary resistance to immunotherapy include tumor-cell intrinsic (for example, absence of antigenic proteins) and tumor-cell extrinsic (for example, absence of T cells and infiltration of immunosuppressive cells) (17), which can interact with each other. Increasing evidence has suggested that identifying immunophenotyping will help predict outcomes of immunotherapy and provide a novel direction for overcoming resistance (18, 19). On the basis of the above, we conducted the present study. **Figure 8** is a schematic representation of the findings presented in this article.

In this study, we characterized four aspects to describe the immune landscape of patients with *EGFR* mutations. The first aspect is the TMB. Previous studies have shown that the TMB is an important criterion for successful immunotherapy. Our findings suggest that the TMB was lower for the *EGFR* group than for the *KRAS* group and the whole LUAD. In an open-label, randomized, phase 3 trial (CheckMate 227), the researchers demonstrated longer PFS time in NSCLC patients with a high TMB (defined as ≥10 mut/Mb), regardless of PD-L1 expression or tumor type (HR, 0.58; 95% CI, 0.41–0.81) (20). However, in our study, only 12.5% of the *EGFR* patients had TMB of >10mut/Mb. Seventy-eight percent of patients in the *EGFR* group had TMB of <5mut/Mb. This finding partly explains the reason for the poor curative effect in the $EGFR^{-mt}$ group. The second aspect is the ESTIMATE score. The higher the ESTIMATE score, the lower the tumor purity. Our study showed that there were no significant differences in tumor purity among the three groups, which was inferred by using the ESTIMATE purity score. The third and fourth aspects were CIBERSORT and MCP-counter. Both of these tools are mathematical Methods to estimate TILs. A previous study suggested that immune-cell infiltration was associated with antitumor activity. It has been reported that high stromal infiltration of CD8+ ICs and CD4+ ICs was associated with better overall survival by analyzing 139 nivolumab-treated NSCLC simple tumor tissue specimens (21). In our study, compared with KRAS and the whole LUAD group, the TIME in the *EGFR* mutant patients showed a trend of diminishing activated TILs and increasing numbers of immunosuppressive cells. Some previous experimental studies have reported similar results. Although there are artificial intelligence approaches to calculate the absolute count of immune cells, these Methods and tools are still evolving. At present, the most commonly used Method to quantify the number and type of immune cells is by immunohistochemistry (IHC). A study based on 245 Chinese NSCLC patients showed that lower immune infiltration was associated with *EGFR* mutations in adenocarcinoma samples through IHC staining of CD8 (22). Similarly, a French study also confirmed this conclusion; the researchers found that the expression of PD-L1 was decreased, and the density of CD8+T lymphocytes was lower in patients with *EGFR* mutations in lung cancer through IHC. In addition, with the development of technology in recent years, some new technologies, such as Digital Spatial Profiling, have also gradually shown the advantages of quantifying the tumor microenvironment, but it has not been widely used (23). Clinically, our results are also consistent with clinical evidence showing that compared with *KRAS*-mutant patients, patients with *EGFR* mutations-mutant are difficult to rarely benefit from immunotherapy (8).

In the era of molecular targeted therapy, different subtypes of *EGFR* mutations may cause different TKIs sensitivity. However, it remains undetermined if there are differences in the TIMEs and ICI efficacies among different *EGFR*-mutation subtypes. In a registration study, a total of 125 *EGFR*-mutation patients treated

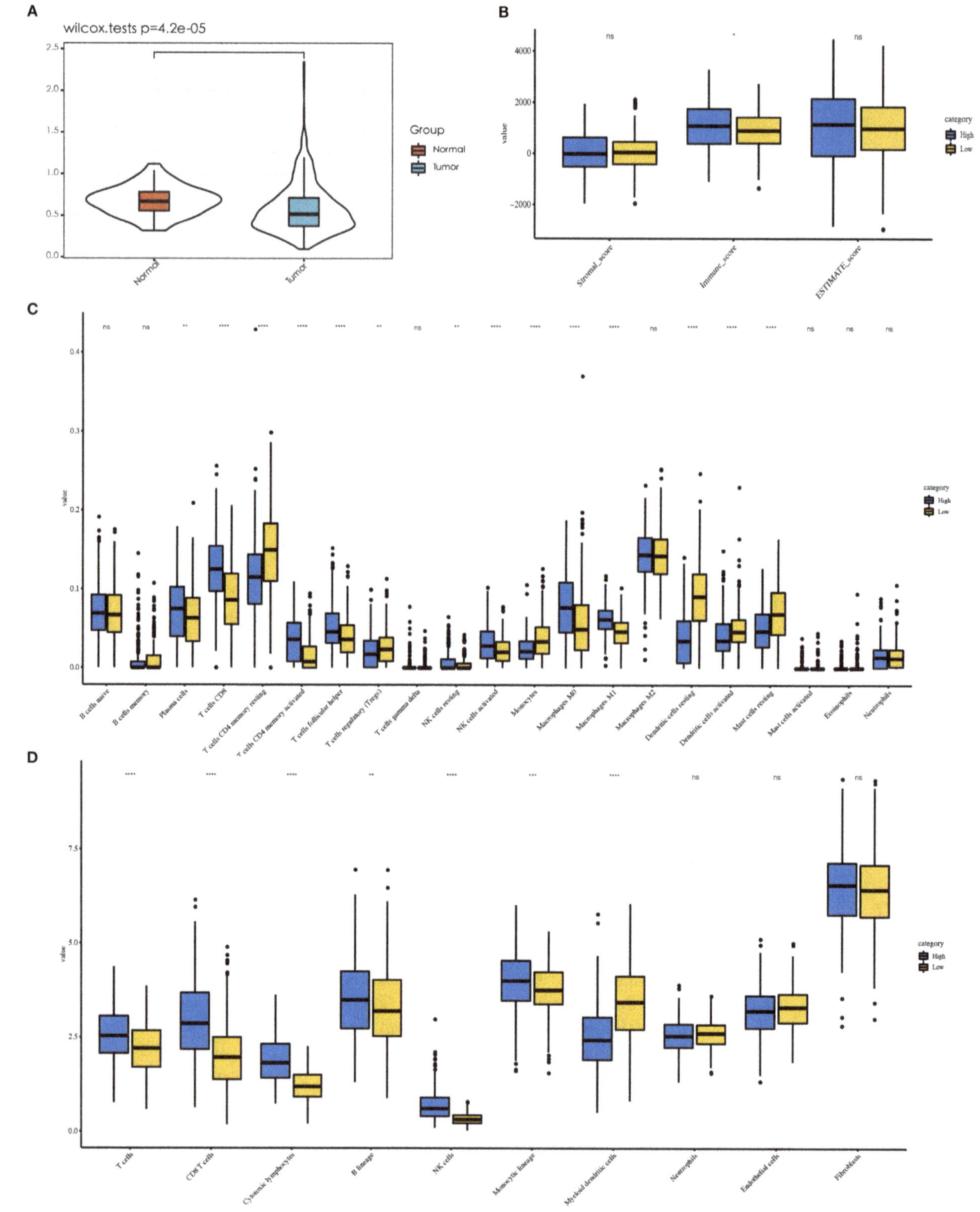

FIGURE 6 | Explore the role of D value in LUAD. Tumor tissue showed a lower D value than normal tissue **(A)**. No difference in tumor purity was observed between high-D and low-D group **(B)**. Less abundant of activated immune cell were observed in low-D group by CIBERSORT **(C)** as well as the result MCP-counter **(D)**. *P < 0.05, **P < 0.01, ***P < 0.001 and ****P < 0.0001, respectively. ns, not significant.

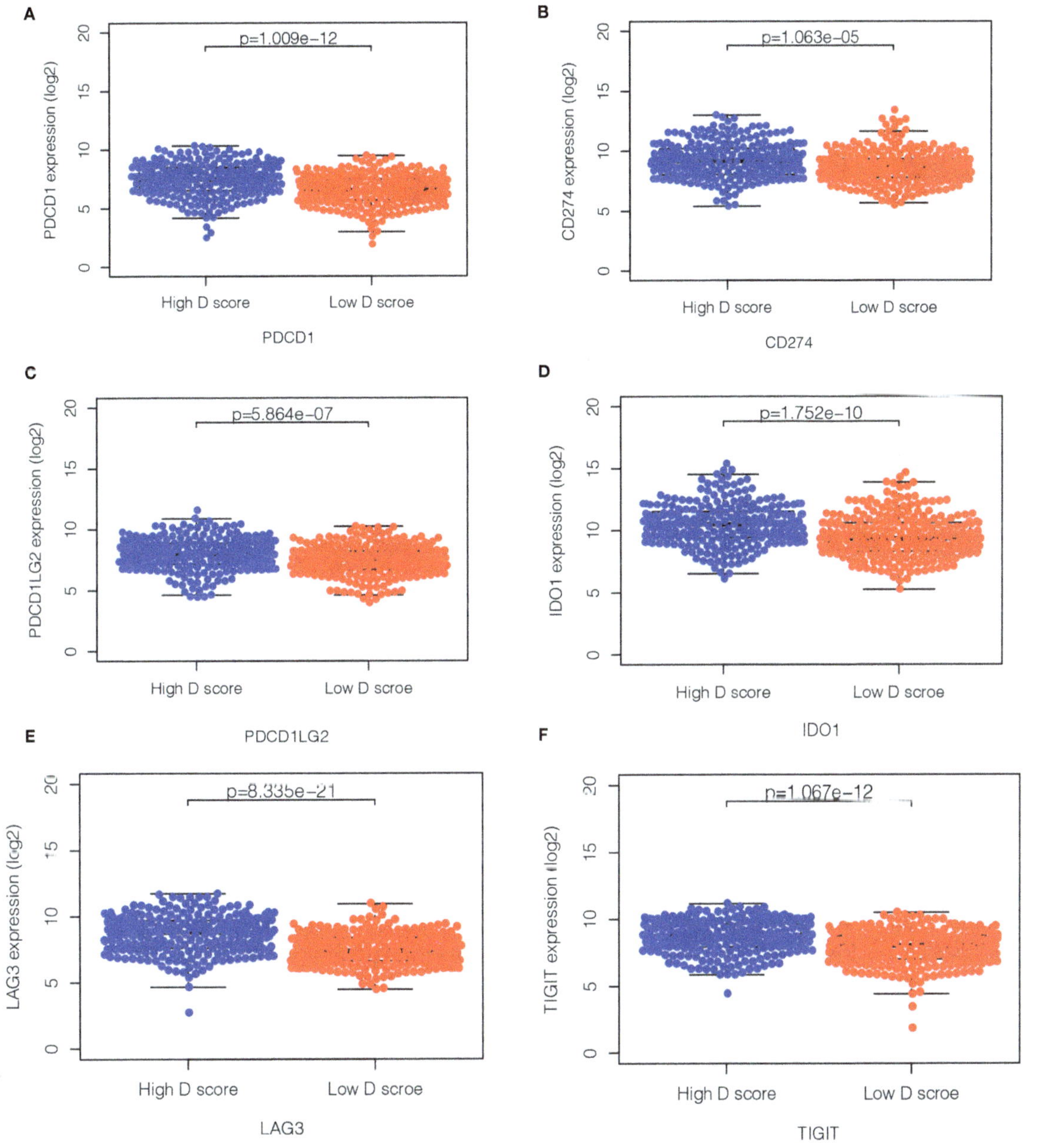

FIGURE 7 | Relationship between the D score and the expression of immune checkpoint. **(A–F)** the distribution of mRNA level of PDCD1, CD274, PDCD1LG2, LAG3, TIGIT and IDO1 in high- and low-D score groups.

with ICIs were included. That study showed that different *EGFR*-patient subgroups had different PFS and OS durations. The median PFS was 1.4 months for patients with T790 single or multiple mutations, 1.8 months for patients with the exon 19del mutation, 2.5 months for patients with the exon21 L858R mutation, and 2.8 months for patients with other mutations ($P < 0.001$) (24). In the present study, we also observed differences in the immune landscapes among the 19del, 21L85R, uncommon-mutant, and unknown-mutant groups. Through a further inter-group comparison, we found that differences in the TMB and TILs were only found between patients with oncogenic mutations and unknown mutations. No significant differences were observed in the activated immune cells between 19del patients and L858R-mutation patients or between common mutation and uncommon mutation patients. However, the myeloid DCs increased in the 19del group relative to those in the L858R group and in the common mutation group relative to those in the uncommon group. These findings indicated that, from an immunological perspective, oncogenic mutation might be an important factor

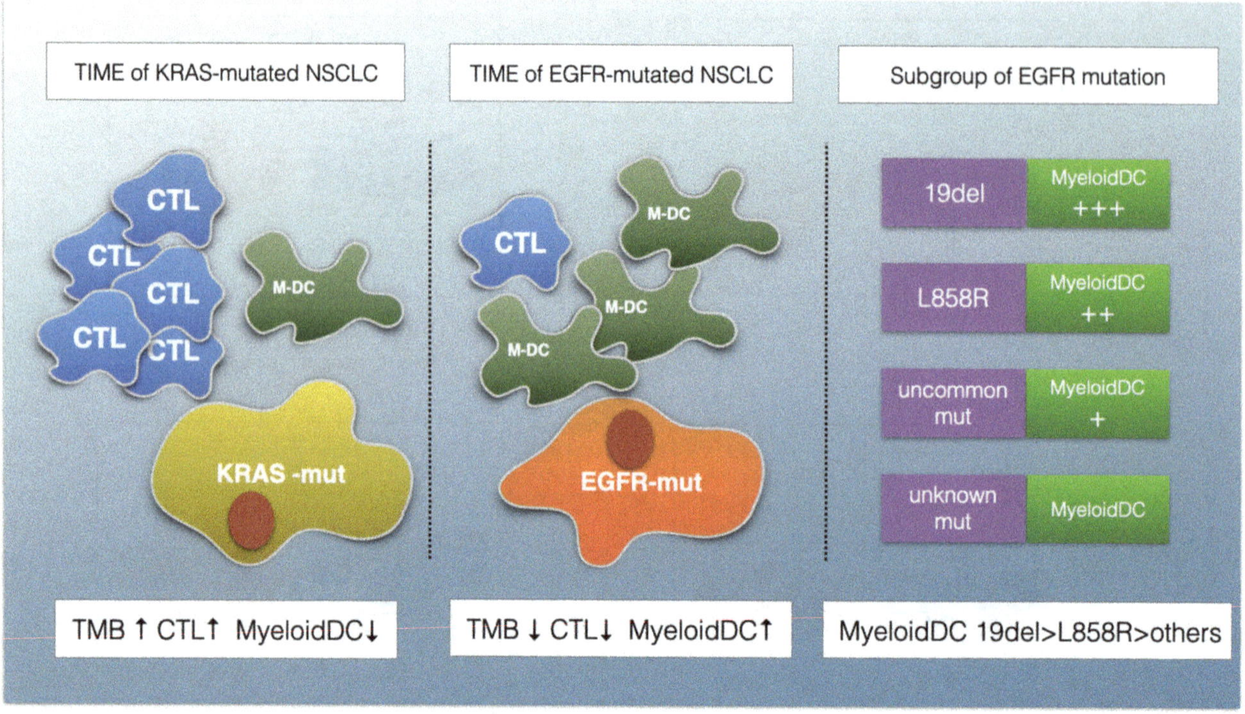

FIGURE 8 | A schematic summarizing the major findings of this study. The TIME of EGFR-mutated NSCLC show an immunosuppressive status with lower TMB, fewer cytotoxic T cells (CTLs) and more myeloid DC (M-DC) cells compared with KRAS-mutated NSCLC. The myeloid DCs increased in EGFR 19del compared with L858R mutation patients, and in common mutation patents compared with uncommon mutations.

for cellular immune suppression. Targeting DC therapy may be an interesting future direction for *EGFR*-mutation patients.

As is known, the tumor microenvironment is a complex and dynamic system formed by stromal, immune, and inflammatory cells and the extracellular matrix (ECM) (18). In our research, to further identify the key immune cells in the TIME, we analyzed the TILs in the KRAS and *EGFR* groups, including CIBERSORT and MCP-counter results, and we finally determined through inter-group comparisons that activated T cells and resting DCs were the key analysis factors. Various studies have proven the significant functions of T cells in the antitumor process. The role of DCs has been gradually recognized in recent years. Previous studies have shown that DCs are central to the initiation of antigen-specific immunity and tolerance. In the TIME, DCs acquire, process, and present tumor-associated antigens on major histocompatibility complex molecules and provide co-stimulation and soluble factors to shape T-cell responses (25). For the above reasons, we defined D = MCP-counter score of CTLs/MCP-counter score of myeloid DCs. Considering that the MCP-counter score presents as the geoMETric mean of marker gene expression (26), the D value, as a further calculation of the MCP-counter score, might have good clinical application and promotional value by validation through multiple IHC analyses with tyramide signal amplification or DSP technology in the future.

An interesting result of D value analysis was that the differential genes were mainly enriched in the cell cycle pathway when the low-D-score group was compared with the high-D-score group for *EGFR*-mutation patients. Although previous clinical trials have shown that necitumumab, an anti-EGFR antibody combined with abemaciclib (a CDK4/6 inhibitor), did not produce an additive effect over single-agent activity in patients with stage IV NSCLC, no clinical studies have been conducted to explore the effectiveness of immunotherapy combined with a CDK4/6 inhibitor (22). Some basic studies have established that CDK4/6 inhibitors could enhance T-cell activation and induce a T-cell inflamed TME (23, 24). Based on our analysis results, the combination of ICIs with a cell cycle-related drug may be a potential therapeutic option for *EGFR*-mutation patients. However, this hypothesis needs to be confirmed.

Mutation features comprise an important signature of LUAD. In addition to classical mutations, some other mutations have gained increasing attention from researchers. Although ICIs have shown promising benefit in NSCLC, the efficacy of ICIs in NSCLC patients with rare mutations remains largely unknown. Previous reports have shown how different mutations affect the microenvironmental phenotype of tumors, which in turn affects the sensitivity of tumors to immunotherapy. For example, the TIME has been shown to have less immune-cell infiltration in *STK11*-mutation patients who have a worse prognosis after immunotherapy (27). A similar phenomenon was also observed in patients with *KEAP1* mutations, despite a high

TMB level (28). Our data shows that the D scores of *BRAF*, *ERBB2*, *MET*, or *KRAS* were very similar, suggesting that they may have similar TIMEs in some ways. On the one hand, this result is consistent with previous real-world study data showing that ICI efficacies against *BRAF*-, *HER2*-, *MET*-, or *RET*-NSCLC patients were close to the efficacy observed in unselected NSCLC patients (29). On the other hand, our results support the application of ICIs from a TIME viewpoint.

Although immunotherapy has greatly improved the prognosis of patients with lung cancer, screening patients who are potentially effective or resistant to treatment remains challenging (30). Through early detection of potential biomarkers, we can choose individualized strategies for patients who may be resistant to immunotherapy, which may help to prolong the survival time (31). In our study, a lower D score was shown to be a new indicator of immunosuppression. This result was further verified by analyzing the TMEs of the high- and low-D groups in the whole LUAD population. Just as we expected, we observed less activated and more resting immune cells in the low-D group through analysis of immune cells. To further clarify the role of the D value in clinical practice, we further investigated the relationship between the D score and the well-studied immunotherapy predictive biomarkers. We found that low-D score patients had significantly lower levels of immune checkpoint gene expression and TMB. These novel findings suggest that the D score may be a predictive biomarker for immunotherapy response. This possibility needs to be confirmed in future prospective clinical studies.

In conclusion, the TIME of $EGFR^{-mt}$ NSCLC was found to be immunosuppressive. Myeloid DCs were higher in *EGFR* 19del patients than in L858R mutation patients and in common mutation patients than in uncommon mutations. CTLs and DCs have key roles in the TIME and may be potential predictors of immunotherapy efficacy. Certain aspects of the findings require further validation and qualification in a large longitudinal population study in the future.

AUTHOR CONTRIBUTIONS

Conception and design: TL and XP. Development of methodology: JW and YG. Analysis and interpretation of data (e.g., statistical analysis, biostatistics, computational analysis): NH and SW. Writing, review, and/or revision of the manuscript: TL and JW. Administrative, technical, or material support (i.e., reporting or organizing data, constructing databases): XP. Study supervision: PX and JL. All authors contributed to the article and approved the submitted version.

REFERENCES

1. Sung H, Ferlay J, Siegel RL, Laversanne M, Soerjomataram I, Jemal A, et al. Global Cancer Statistics 2020: GLOBOCAN Estimates of Incidence and Mortality Worldwide for 36 Cancers in 185 Countries. *CA Cancer J Clin* (2021) 71:209–49. doi: 10.3322/caac.21660
2. Sharma SV, Bell DW, Settleman J, Haber DA. Epidermal Growth Factor Receptor Mutations in Lung Cancer. *Nat Rev Cancer* (2007) 7:169–81. doi: 10.1038/nrc2088
3. Lee CK, Davies L, Wu YL, Mitsudomi T, Inoue A, Rosell R, et al. Gefitinib or Erlotinib vs Chemotherapy for EGFR Mutation-Positive Lung Cancer: Individual Patient Data Meta-Analysis of Overall Survival. *J Natl Cancer Inst* (2017) 109:djw279. doi: 10.1093/jnci/djw279
4. Sequist LV, Yang JC, Yamamoto N, O'Byrne K, Hirsh V, Mok T, et al. Phase III Study of Afatinib or Cisplatin Plus Pemetrexed in Patients With Metastatic Lung Adenocarcinoma With EGFR Mutations. *J Clin Oncol* (2013) 31:3327–34. doi: 10.1200/JCO.2012.44.2806
5. Gregorc V, Lazzari C, Karachaliou N, Rosell R, Santarpia M. Osimertinib in Untreated Epidermal Growth Factor Receptor (EGFR)-Mutated Advanced Non-Small Cell Lung Cancer. *Transl Lung Cancer Res* (2018) 7:S165–70. doi: 10.21037/tlcr.2018.03.19
6. Yang JC, Schuler M, Popat S, Miura S, Heeke S, Park K, et al. Afatinib for the Treatment of NSCLC Harboring Uncommon EGFR Mutations: A Database of 693 Cases. *J Thorac Oncol* (2020) 15:803–15. doi: 10.1016/j.jtho.2019.12.126
7. Saito H, Fukuhara T, Furuya N, Watanabe K, Sugawara S, Iwasawa S, et al. Erlotinib Plus Bevacizumab Versus Erlotinib Alone in Patients With EGFR-Positive Advanced Non-Squamous Non-Small-Cell Lung Cancer (NEJ026): Interim Analysis of an Open-Label, Randomised, Multicentre, Phase 3 Trial. *Lancet Oncol* (2019) 20:625–35. doi: 10.1016/S1470-2045(19)30035-X
8. Lee CK, Man J, Lord S, Cooper W, Links M, Gebski V, et al. Clinical and Molecular Characteristics Associated With Survival Among Patients Treated With Checkpoint Inhibitors for Advanced Non-Small Cell Lung Carcinoma: A Systematic Review and Meta-Analysis. *JAMA Oncol* (2018) 4:210–6. doi: 10.1001/jamaoncol.2017.4427
9. Yang JC, Shepherd FA, Kim DW, Lee GW, Lee JS, Chang GC, et al. Osimertinib Plus Durvalumab Versus Osimertinib Monotherapy in EGFR T790M-Positive NSCLC following Previous EGFR TKI Therapy: CAURAL Brief Report. *J Thorac Oncol* (2019) 14:933–9. doi: 10.1016/j.jtho.2019.02.001
10. Mazzaschi G, Madeddu D, Falco A, Bocchialini G, Goldoni M, Sogni F, et al. Low PD-1 Expression in Cytotoxic CD8(+) Tumor-Infiltrating Lymphocytes Confers an Immune-Privileged Tissue Microenvironment in NSCLC with a Prognostic and Predictive Value. *Clin Cancer Res* (2018) 24:407–19. doi: 10.1158/1078-0432.CCR-17-2156
11. Socinski MA, Jotte RM, Cappuzzo F, Orlandi F, Stroyakovskiy D, Nogami N, et al. Atezolizumab for First-Line Treatment of Metastatic Nonsquamous NSCLC. *N Engl J Med* (2018) 378:2288–301. doi: 10.1056/NEJMoa1716948
12. Yoshihara K, Shahmoradgoli M, Martinez E, Vegesna R, Kim H, Torres-Garcia W, et al. Inferring Tumour Purity and Stromal and Immune Cell Admixture From Expression Data. *Nat Commun* (2013) 4:2612. doi: 10.1038/ncomms3612
13. Chen B, Khodadoust MS, Liu CL, Newman AM, Alizadeh AA. Profiling Tumor Infiltrating Immune Cells with CIBERSORT. *Methods Mol Biol* (2018) 1711:243–59. doi: 10.1007/978-1-4939-7493-1_12
14. Becht E, Giraldo NA, Lacroix L, Buttard B, Elarouci N, Petitprez F, et al. Estimating the Population Abundance of Tissue-Infiltrating Immune and Stromal Cell Populations Using Gene Expression. *Genome Biol* (2016) 17:218. doi: 10.1186/s13059-016-1070-5
15. Kalbasi A, Ribas A. Tumour-Intrinsic Resistance to Immune Checkpoint Blockade. *Nat Rev Immunol* (2020) 20:25–39. doi: 10.1038/s41577-019-0218-4
16. Kluger HM, Tawbi HA, Ascierto ML, Bowden M, Callahan MK, Cha E, et al. Defining Tumor Resistance to PD-1 Pathway Blockade: Recommendations From The First Meeting of The SITC Immunotherapy Resistance Taskforce. *J Immunother Cancer* (2020) 8:e000398. doi: 10.1136/jitc-2019-000398
17. Sharma P, Hu-Lieskovan S, Wargo JA, Ribas A. Primary, Adaptive, and Acquired Resistance to Cancer Immunotherapy. *Cell* (2017) 168:707–23. doi: 10.1016/j.cell.2017.01.017
18. Ladanyi A, Timar J. Immunologic and Immunogenomic Aspects of Tumor Progression. *Semin Cancer Biol* (2020) 60:249–61. doi: 10.1016/j.semcancer.2019.08.011

19. Thorsson V, Gibbs DL, Brown SD, Wolf D, Bortone DS, Ou Yang TH, et al. The Immune Landscape of Cancer. *Immunity* (2018) 48:812–30.e814.
20. Hellmann MD, Ciuleanu TE, Pluzanski A, Lee JS, Otterson GA, Audigier-Valette C, et al. Nivolumab Plus Ipilimumab in Lung Cancer with a High Tumor Mutational Burden. *N Engl J Med* (2018) 378:2093–104. doi: 10.1056/NEJMoa1801946
21. Niemeijer AN, Sahba S, Smit EF, Lissenberg-Witte BI, de Langen AJ, Thunnissen E. Association of Tumour and Stroma PD-1, PD-L1, CD3, CD4 and CD8 Expression With DCB and OS to Nivolumab Treatment in NSCLC Patients Pre-Treated With Chemotherapy. *Br J Cancer* (2020) 123:392–40. doi: 10.1038/s41416-020-0888-5
22. Zhang XC, Wang J, Shao GG, Wang Q, Qu X, Wang B, et al. Comprehensive Genomic and Immunological Characterization of Chinese Non-Small Cell Lung Cancer Patients. *Nat Commun* (2019) 10:1772. doi: 10.1038/s41467-019-09762-1
23. Kulasinghe A, Taheri T, O'Byrne K, Hughes BGM, Kenny L, Punyadeera C. Highly Multiplexed Digital Spatial Profiling of the Tumor Microenvironment of Head and Neck Squamous Cell Carcinoma Patients. *Front Oncol* (2020) 10:607349. doi: 10.3389/fonc.2020.607349
24. Mazieres J, Drilon A, Lusque A, Mhanna L, Cortot AB, Mezquita L, et al. Immune Checkpoint Inhibitors for Patients With Advanced Lung Cancer and Oncogenic Driver Alterations: Results From The IMMUNOTARGET Registry. *Ann Oncol* (2019) 30:1321-8. doi: 10.1093/annonc/mdz167
25. Wculek SK, Cueto FJ, Mujal AM, Melero I, Krummel MF, Sancho D. Dendritic Cells in Cancer Immunology and Immunotherapy. *Nat Rev Immunol* (2020) 20:7–24. doi: 10.1038/s41577-019-0210-z
26. Sturm G, Finotello F, Petitprez F, Zhang JD, Baumbach J, Fridman WH, et al. Comprehensive Evaluation of Transcriptome-Based Cell-Type Quantification Methods for Immuno-Oncology. *Bioinformatics* (2019) 35:i436–45. doi: 10.1093/bioinformatics/btz363
27. Wang H, Guo J, Shang X, Wang Z. Less Immune Cell Infiltration and Worse Prognosis After Immunotherapy for Patients With Lung Adenocarcinoma Who Harbored STK11 Mutation. *Int Immunopharmacol* (2020) 84:106574. doi: 10.1016/j.intimp.2020.106574
28. Marinelli D, Mazzotta M, Scalera S, Terrenato I, Sperati F, D'Ambrosio L, et al. KEAP1-Driven Co-Mutations in Lung Adenocarcinoma Unresponsive to Immunotherapy Despite High Tumor Mutational Burden. *Ann Oncol* (2020) 31:1746–54. doi: 10.1016/j.annonc.2020.08.2105
29. Guisier F, Dubos-Arvis C, Vinas F, Doubre H, Ricordel C, Ropert S, et al. Efficacy and Safety of Anti-PD-1 Immunotherapy in Patients With Advanced Non Small Cell Lung Cancer With BRAF, HER2 or MET Mutation or RET-Translocation. GFPC 01-2018. *J Thorac Oncol* (2020) 15:628–36. doi: 10.1016/j.jtho.2019.12.129
30. Litchfield K, Reading JL, Puttick C, Thakkar K, Abbosh C, Bentham R, et al. Meta-Analysis of Tumor- and T Cell-Intrinsic Mechanisms of Sensitization to Checkpoint Inhibition. *Cell* (2021) 184:596–614.e514. doi: 10.1016/j.cell.2021.01.002
31. Camidge DR, Doebele RC, Kerr KM. Comparing and Contrasting Predictive Biomarkers for Immunotherapy and Targeted Therapy of NSCLC. *Nat Rev Clin Oncol* (2019) 16:341–55. doi: 10.1038/s41571-019-0173-9

13

Nivolumab in Non-Small Cell Lung Cancer: Real World Long-Term Survival Results and Blood-Based Efficacy Biomarkers

Sameh Daher[1‡], Yaacov R. Lawrence[1‡], Elizabeth Dudnik[2‡], Ekaterina Hanovich[3], Damien Urban[1], Nir Peled[2†], Rossie Navon[1], Raya Leibowitz[1†], Ariel Hammerman[4], Erez Battat[4], Teodor Gottfried[1], Amir Onn[1] and Jair Bar[1] on behalf of the Israel Lung Cancer Group*

[1] Thoracic Cancer Unit, Institute of Oncology, Sheba Medical Center, Tel HaShomer, Israel, [2] Thoracic Cancer Unit, Davidoff Cancer Center, Rabin Medical Center, Petah Tikva, Israel, [3] Institute of Oncology, Shamir Medical Center, Zerifin, Israel, [4] Department of Pharmaceutical Technology Assessment, Clalit Health Services Headquarters, Tel Aviv, Israel

***Correspondence:**
Sameh Daher
sameh.daher@sheba.gov.il

†Present address:
Nir Peled,
Oncology Center, Shaare Zedek Medical Center, Jerusalem, Israel
Raya Leibowitz,
Institute of Oncology, Shamir Medical Center, Zerifin, Israel

‡These authors have contributed equally to this work

Objectives: We aimed to examine clinical data and baseline blood test results as potential predictive biomarkers for benefit from nivolumab, in advanced non-small cell lung cancer patients (NSCLC).

Materials and Methods: A chart review was performed of 108 advanced NSCLC patients who commenced treatment with nivolumab between 2015-6 at three Israeli cancer centers, and for whom laboratory tests results were available. Data collected included sex, age, ECOG-PS, histology and number of previous lines of treatment. Baseline blood test results collected: absolute lymphocyte and neutrophil count (ANC), white blood cells (WBC), hemoglobin, platelets, albumin and lactate dehydrogenase (LDH). Neutrophil to Lymphocyte Ratio and 'derived NLR' (dNLR = (ANC/[WBC-ANC])) were calculated. Disease control at six months (DC6) was defined as any tumor shrinkage or stable disease during the first six months of nivolumab treatment. The association between clinical/laboratory variables and survival was tested with a Cox proportional hazard model. Data cut-off occurred in November 2019.

Results: 35 patients (32.4%) achieved DC6. Median overall survival (OS) of entire study population was 5.4 months. Four year survival rate was 16%. Achievement of DC6 strongly correlated with longer OS (HR 0.12, 95% C.I. 0.07-0.21, $p<0.001$). In univariate and multivariate analysis, dNLR, albumin and LDH correlated significantly with OS. No variables correlated significantly with DC6 in multivariate analysis. Based on albumin and LDH, we produced a score called CLAS (combined LDH and albumin score), including four prognostic groups of patients. Patients having low albumin and high LDH had the worst prognosis.

Conclusion: In real-life setting, long-term efficacy of nivolumab in advanced line treatment of NSCLC is consistent with clinical trials. Response or stability of disease during first six months of treatment is associated with prolonged survival. We propose a novel score (CLAS) that may be useful for predicting outcome in nivolumab-treated NSCLC patients, but further validation is required.

Keywords: nivolumab, NSCLC, long term survival, real life data, biomarker

INTRODUCTION

Lung cancer is the leading cause of cancer -related death worldwide (1). Immune checkpoint inhibitors (ICI) for treatment of NSCLCdemonstrated superior survival of patients treated with the anti-PD-1 antibody nivolumab compared with docetaxel after failure of platinum-based chemotherapy (2–4). Pembrolizumab, another PD-1 inhibitor, and atezolizumab, an anti-PD-L1 inhibitor, have both also demonstrated significantly better overall survival (OS) in similarly designed trials, comparing each of them with 2nd-line docetaxel (5, 6).

Based on these trials, in 2015 nivolumab has received US Food and Drug Administration agency (FDA) and European Medicines Agency (EMA) approval for second-line treatment of NSCLC. Atezolizumab is similarly approved by FDA and EMA, while pembrolizumab is approved only for the treatment of patients with PD-L1 positive tumors (as included in the KEYNOTE 010 trial) (5). Response rate (RR) for each of these drugs in the 2nd line setting is roughly 15-20%. Combined updated OS results from checkmate 017 and checkmate 057 show 13.4% OS rate at five years follow-up (3). In a landmark analysis of OS by response category at six months in checkmate 017 and checkmate 057, the OS rate at four years in nivolumab treated patients with CR/PR was 58%, and 19% for patients with SD at six months (3).

Efforts are being undertaken to identify biomarkers predicting response to immunotherapeutic agents (7). PD-L1 expression level and tumor mutational burden (TMB) are predictive for benefit from immunotherapy but are not always available and their predictive accuracy is limited (7–11). Additional molecular biomarkers are being investigated, such as STK11/LKB1 and KRAS (12–15). STK11/LKB1 genomic alterations were associated with shorter PFS and shorter OS in first line ICI treated NSCLC patients (12). On the other hand, several studies showed similar efficacy of ICI in KRAS mutant compared with KRAS wild type NSCLC patients (14, 15).

Numerous studies are onging, aiming to identify immune-related gene signatures correlating with clinical benefit from ICI. One of these assessed the utility of the 18-gene expression tumor inflammation signature in predicting ICI treatment outcome, and found it to predict clinical benefit of ICI in several tumors, including NSCLC (16). Another study reported predictability of selected gene signatures and genes for discriminating patients with durable clinical benefit from ICI from those with non durable benefit. These signatures and genes included the M1 signature, peripheral T cell signature, CD137 and PSMB9 mRNA expression (17). An additional study identified two signatures predicting outcome from ICI in chemotherapy-refractory advanced NSCLC patients, one reflecting the degree of immune infiltration and upregulation of interferon-gamma-induced genes, and a second reflected the epithelial-to-mesenchymal transition status (18).

Potential predictive biomarkers from the tumor microenvironment are being investigated in the PIONeeR study. The analysis for its first 100 patients, presented recently, suggested a predictive value for PDL1 positive cell density and density of cytotoxic T cells and immunosuppressive cells (regulatory T cells and myeloid-derived suppressor cells) in the tumor (19).

Levels of peripheral blood components, blood cells and various circulating molecules are an accessible potential non-invasive source of predictive biomarkers in NSCLC patients, and possibly relevant also for ICI-treated patients. Some of these biomarkers are validated prognostic markers for cancer in various scenarios. For example, high levels of serum lactate dehydrogenase (LDH) has been associated with poorer cancer-specific survival in several malignancies, including lung, colorectal and prostate cancer (20). Another example is albumin serum levels, known to be a robust predictor of survival in cancer patients in general and NSCLC patients in particular (21, 22). Interestingly, retrospective studies have demonstrated a correlation between high serum LDH levels at baseline and lower response rate (RR), and shorter (PFS) and OS in several types of cancer treated with anti-PD-1 and anti-PD-L1 antibodies (23–25). Hemoglobin levels can also serve as prognostic or potentially a predictive biomarker; several studies have demonstrated that anemia is linked to poorer prognosis in NSCLC patients (26, 27).

A number of studies investigated the peripheral blood cellular components as biomarkers of ICI efficacy. For ipilimumab-treated melanoma patients, improved OS and PFS were associated with low absolute neutrophil count, low neutrophil-to-lymphocyte ratio and high lymphocyte levels (28, 29). In a retrospective study including 607 pembrolizumab-treated melanoma patients, baseline elevated eosinophil count and elevated lymphocyte count were both associated with improved OS (30). Retrospective studies demonstrated elevated pre-treatment neutrophil-to-lymphocyte ratio (NLR) to be associated with shorter OS and PFS and with lower response rates in ICI-treated metastatic NSCLC patients (31–33). High NLR has been shown to be associated with decreased OS in a retrospective study analyzing the records of metastatic NSCLC patients enrolled on a number of phase I immunotherapy trials at the MD Anderson Cancer Center (32). However, NLR may not be relevant for all patients; a study demonstrated that in NSCLC, low NLR was correlated with favorable OS and PFS for patients with TMB > 10, while in patients with TMB ≤ 10, the differences between high and low NLR were not significant (33).

Conceivably, combining such biomarkers may derive a more accurate predictive or prognostic score. A group from Gustave Roussy analyzed data from a retrospective study of ICI *versus* chemotherapy for NSCLC patients and compiled a Lung Immune Prognostic Index (LIPI) (34). In this study, LIPI was correlated with worse outcomes for immunotherapy but not for chemotherapy. Other studies examining the applicability of LIPI in NSCLC and in solid tumors other than NSCLC reported results supporting its correlation with outcomes in ICI-treated patients (35, 36). In contrast, an exploratory pooled analysis of clinical studies of immunotherapy and targeted therapies for advanced NSCLC patients has shown LIPI to be associated with OS and PFS irrespective of treatment, emphasizing its prognostic rather than predictive role (37).

We report here real-world long-term survival results of NSCLC patients treated with nivolumab as a second or later treatment line in three Oncology centers, with a median follow-up of four years. We have comprehensively assessed clinical data and baseline blood levels of LDH, albumin and complete blood count results, as potential predictive biomarkers for benefit from nivolumab.

MATERIALS AND METHODS

Study Conduct

This is a retrospective pharmacoepidemiological study, conducted, analyzed and reported according to REporting of studies Conducted using Observational Routinely collected health Data (RECORD) guidelines, the Strengthening the Reporting of OBservational studies in Epidemiology (STROBE), and ROCORD-pharmacoepidemiological research (RECORD-PE) guidelines (38–40). A chart review was performed of patients with advanced NSCLC that fit the study inclusion criteria.

Patients

Inclusion criteria were age of 18 years and above, progression on first-line platinum-based chemotherapy, treatment at one of three participating Israeli cancer centers (Sheba Medical center (MC), Rabin MC and Shamir MC), administration of at least one cycle of nivolumab, with treatment commencing during 2015-2016. Exclusion criteria was lack of blood test results from the relevant time window (**Figure S1, Supplementary Data**).

Data Collection

Data collected included sex, age, Eastern Cooperative Oncology Group performance status (ECOG-PS), histology and number of previous lines of treatment. Baseline blood test results collected included: absolute lymphocyte count (ALC), absolute neutrophil count (ANC), white blood cells (WBC), hemoglobin (HGB), platelets (PLT), albumin (ALB) and LDH. Baseline blood tests were defined as those performed prior to and within two weeks of the first nivolumab treatment. These parameters were categorized as high or low relative to the median of the study cohort, except for LDH, categorized as normal or above the upper limit of normal for the relevant clinical laboratory and albumin, categorized as normal or below the lower limit of normal for the relevant clinical laboratory. LIPI calculation is based on LDH greater than upper limit of normal (ULN) and 'derived NLR' (dNLR, calculated by: (ANC/[WBC-ANC])) > 3. Three risk groups were characterized: good: none of these factors, intermediate: one factor, poor: two factors. NLR, dNLR and LIPI score were calculated. In addition, CLAS ("Combined LDH and Albumin Score") was defined as a suggested novel score and calculated as described in the results section.

Tumor assessments were performed by the treating physicians based on computerized tomography (CT) scans performed as part of the standard of care. CT scans were usually performed at two-three months intervals, at the treating physicians' discretion. Two major outcomes have been assessed in our study: Disease control at six months (DC6) and OS. DC6 was defined as either present (any tumor shrinkage at any time during the first six months after initiating nivolumab treatment, or no change in tumors' size for at least six months after starting nivolumab) or absent (any tumor growth or death at any time within the first six months).

OS was defined as time from initiation of nivolumab treatment until death, or censored at the last date patient was known to be alive.

Statistics

Variables analyzed as categorial included sex and histology. In addition, LDH was redefined as a binary variable based upon whether the values being above or below the upper-limit of normal, and ALB was redefined as a binary variable based upon whether the values were above or below the lower-limit of normal. Variables analyzed as continuous included age, HGB, WBC, ANC, ALC and PLT. Variables analyzed as ordinal were ECOG-PS and number of previous lines.

The impact of covariates on survival was assessed using a Cox proportional hazard model. Multivariate analysis incorporated putative covariates found at univariate analysis to be significant at $p < 0.1$. Statistical comparisons were performed using Chi-squared test for categorical data and t-test for continuous variables. All p-values were two-sided, and $p < 0.05$ was considered statistically significant. The goodness-of-fit of different models were compared by examining pseudo-R^2 values. Calculations were performed using Stata (version I/C 16.0, StataCorp). Data cut-off was at November 2019.

Ethics

The study was approved by the institutional ethics committees of each of the participating centers. (Shamir Medical Center (MC): IRB #8993-11; Rabin Medical Center (MC): IRB #0391-14; Shamir MC: IRB #0062-17).

Investigators had complete access to the database of population included in the study. No patient identifying information was included in the study database.

RESULTS

Patient Characteristics

A total of 108 patients treated with nivolumab were included in this study, mostly men (65%). Out of the study cohort, 35 patients (32.4%) had achieved DC6. More patients in the non-DC6 group had ECOG-PS of two or higher compared with DC group (p=0.030). The two groups were balanced in terms of other parameters (**Table 1**). Median follow-up was 48.7 months (IQR 47.4m - 53.0m).

Survival and DC6 Analysis

The median OS of the entire study population was 5.4 months (95% CI 3.9-7.4, **Figure 1**).

Survival rates after one, two, three and four years were as follows: 34%, 27%, 19% and 16%, respectively.

Of patients that have achieved DC6, 46% were alive at data cut-off, compared to 1% of patients that did not achieve DC6. In addition, Patients with DC6 demonstrated longer OS compared to patients without DC6 (HR 0.12, 95% confidence interval (CI) 0.07-0.21, p<0.001; **Figure 2**).

Biomarkers

We next tested the effects of the variables collected (demographic, hematological and biochemical) on OS. On univariate analysis, ECOG-PS and baseline values of WBC, ANC, NLR, dNLR, LDH and albumin were significantly correlated with OS. Due to overlap with dNLR, the variables WBC, ANC and NLR were not included in the multivariate analyses. On multivariate analysis, dNLR, albumin and LDH significantly correlated with OS (**Table 2** and **Figures 3A, B**), with high dNLR, low albumin and high LDH being adverse factors correlating with shorter survival. The statistical value of albumin and LDH was more significant than that of dNLR.

Regarding the binomial outcome DC6; age, ECOG-PS and baseline values of WBC, ANC, NLR, dNLR and albumin were all correlated with DC6 on univariate analysis. However, none of the investigated factors were found to be significant on multivariate analysis (**Table S1, Supplementary Data**).

We aimed to validate the prognostic role of LIPI in our cohort. Indeed, in our cohort LIPI was independently associated with OS (HR 1.8, 95% CI, 1.35-2.49, p < 0.001), leading to median OS for poor, intermediate and good LIPI of 2.1 months, 6.4 months, and 9.8 months, respectively (**Figure 4**). Therefore, our data provide further validation of the prognostic value of LIPI for nivolumab-treated advanced NSCLC patients.

Of the parameters examined in our study, baseline LDH and albumin levels were found to be most significantly correlated with survival. We attempted to produce a predictive score by combining these two variables, naming it 'CLAS'. CLAS includes four prognostic groups of patients: high LDH + low albumin (CLAS 0), low LDH + low albumin (CLAS 1), high LDH + high albumin (CLAS 2), low LDH + high albumin (CLAS 3). Indeed, patients classified as CLAS 0 had the worst survival (p<0.001), while patients with CLAS 2 had better survival than patients with CLAS 1, suggesting that low albumin is worse than high LDH (**Figure 3C**).

DISCUSSION

Based on long-term (four years) follow up of our cohort, we report now real-world data of survival of a set of NSCLC patients treated with 2nd-line or higher ICI. In our study, the median OS of nivolumab-treated patients compares unfavorably with the

TABLE 1 | Baseline patient and disease characteristics.

Baseline patient/disease characteristics	All study cohort (108)	DC6 (35)	Non-DC6 (73)	P Value
Age – median (range), years	68 (40-96)	66 (40-85)	69 (43-96)	0.090
Sex – men – n (%)	70 (65%)	23 (66%)	47 (64%)	0.890
ECOG-PS – n (%)				0.030
0	4 (4%)	3 (9%)	1 (1%)	
1	46 (42%)	17 (48%)	29 (40%)	
2	40 (37%)	11 (31%)	29 (40%)	
3	17 (16%)	3 (9%)	14 (19%)	
Unknown	1 (1%)	1 (3%)	0 (0%)	
Histology – n (%)				0.220
Adenocarcinoma	64 (59%)	22 (63%)	42 (57%)	
Squamous cell carcinoma	29 (27%)	10 (28%)	19 (26%)	
NSCLC other*	15 (14%)	3 (9%)	12 (17%)	
No. of previous anticancer treatment lines$ - n (%)				0.440
0	12 (11%)	0 (0%)	12 (17%)	
1	79 (73%)	31 (88%)	48 (66%)	
2	10 (9%)	1 (3%)	9 (12%)	
≥3	7 (7%)	3 (9%)	4 (5%)	

*DC6, Disease Control 6; ECOG-PS, Eastern Cooperative Oncology Group performance status; NSCLC, Non Small Cell Lung Carcinoma. *Other histologies included: large cell neuroendocrine (6), large cell undifferentiated (3), adenosquamous (1), NSCLC non-otherwise-specified (NOS; 5). $ Treatment lines for advanced disease prior to nivolumab treatment.*

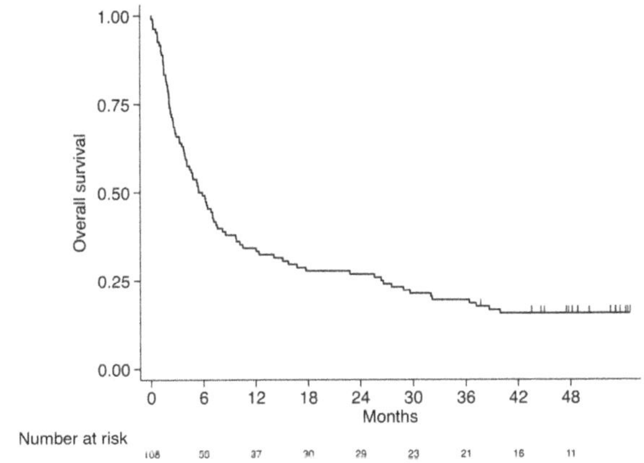

FIGURE 1 | Kaplan–Meier curve for overall survival (entire study cohort, n=108). Median OS 5.4 months (95% CI 3.9-7.4).

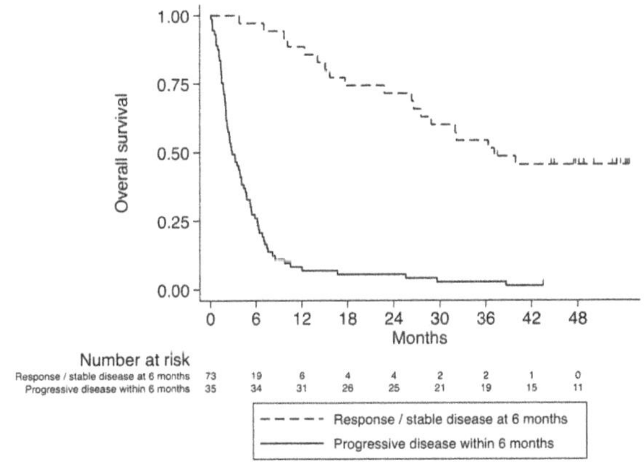

FIGURE 2 | Kaplan–Meier curve for overall survival stratified according to DC6 (n=35) *vs.* non-DC6 (n=73) patients. HR 0.12, 95% confidence interval (CI) 0.07-0.21, p<0.001.

TABLE 2 | Univariate and multivariate analysis for OS of the parameters investigated.

	Univariate Analysis		Multivariate Analysis	
	HR (95% C.I.)	P value	HR (95% C.I.)	P value
Age	1.02 (0.99 - 1.04)	0.148		
Sex	1.18 (0.76 - 1.83)	0.455		
ECOG-PS	**1.46 (1.12 - 1.89)**	**0.005**	1.31 (0.91 - 1.89)	0.141
Histology				
Adenocarcinoma	Comparator			
Squamous	1.02 (0.63 - 1.65)	0.933		
Other	1.47 (0.81 - 2.65)	0.207		
HGB	0.94 (0.83 - 1.05)	0.270		
WBC	**1.12 (1.06 - 1.18)**	**<0.001**		
ANC	**1.15 (1.09 - 1.22)**	**<0.001**		
ALC	0.97 (0.73 - 1.30)	0.860		
PLT	1.00 (1.00 - 1.00)	0.119		
LDH	**1.15 (1.06 - 1.25)**	**0.001**	**1.12 (1.03 - 1.22)**	**0.006**
ALB	**0.33 (0.20 - 0.52)**	**<0.001**	**0.36 (0.20 - 0.63)**	**<0.001**
NLR	**1.05 (1.02 - 1.07)**	**<0.001**		
dNLR	**1.18 (1.10 - 1.27)**	**<0.001**	**1.12 (1.01 - 1.24)**	**0.032**
Number of Previous Lines	0.85 (0.63 - 1.13)	0.260		

Statistically significant values are highlighted as bold. Due to overlap with dNLR, the variables WBC, ANC and NLR were not included in the multivariate analysis. HR, Hazard Ratio; C.I., Confidence Interval; ECOG-PS, Performance Status; HGB, Hemoglobin; WBC, White Blood Cells; ANC, Absolute Neutrophil Count; ALC, Absolute Lymphocyte Count; PLT, Platelets; LDH, Lactate Dehydrogenase; ALB, Albumin; NLR, Neutrophil to Lymphocyte Ratio; dNLR, derived Neutrophil to Lymphocyte Ratio. HR for LDH reflects LDH as calculated for each 100 international units per liter (IU/L). Number of patients with missing data: ECOG-PS: 1, HGB: 2, WBC: 3, ANC: 3, ALC: 4, PLT: 3, LDH: 28 and ALB: 26.

median OS of 9.2 months and 12.2 months for patients with squamous and non-squamous NSCLC in CheckMate 017 and CheckMate 057 trials, respectively (2–4), as may be expected when comparing real-world data to clinical trial data. DC6 was found to be a strong predictor of OS in our cohort, consistent with published data analysis from these two checkmate trials (3). We also report baseline dNLR, ALB and LDH to be significantly and strongly associated with OS for these patients, with none of the examined variables found to be associated with DC6 on multivariate analysis. LIPI score was significantly correlated with survival as well, with poor LIPI group of patients having the worst outcomes, consistent with previous publications. Based on our data, we have produced a score we named CLAS combining ALB and LDH, which demonstrated strong correlation with survival, with low baseline albumin and high baseline LDH correlating with worst outcome. CLAS requires further validation in larger cohorts to clarify its contribution to the management of advanced NSCLC patients.

The relatively shorter median OS in our study may be attributed to the inclusion of patients with ECOG-PS 2/3 that constituted 52% (57 patients) of our cohort, while the randomized studies included only ECOG-PS 0/1 patients. Furthermore, 16% of the patients in our study were heavily pretreated, receiving nivolumab as a later than 2nd treatment line. It should be noted that despite these poor prognostic characteristics, the long-term survival curve looks similar, with 16% long term survivors at data cut-off, consistent with data from the previously mentioned checkmate trials (2–4).

The two parameters outstanding from our data, which were included in the suggested 'CLAS' reflect tumor burden (LDH) and the patients' nutritional status (ALB). The three variables that make up CLAS and LIPI score (LDH, albumin,

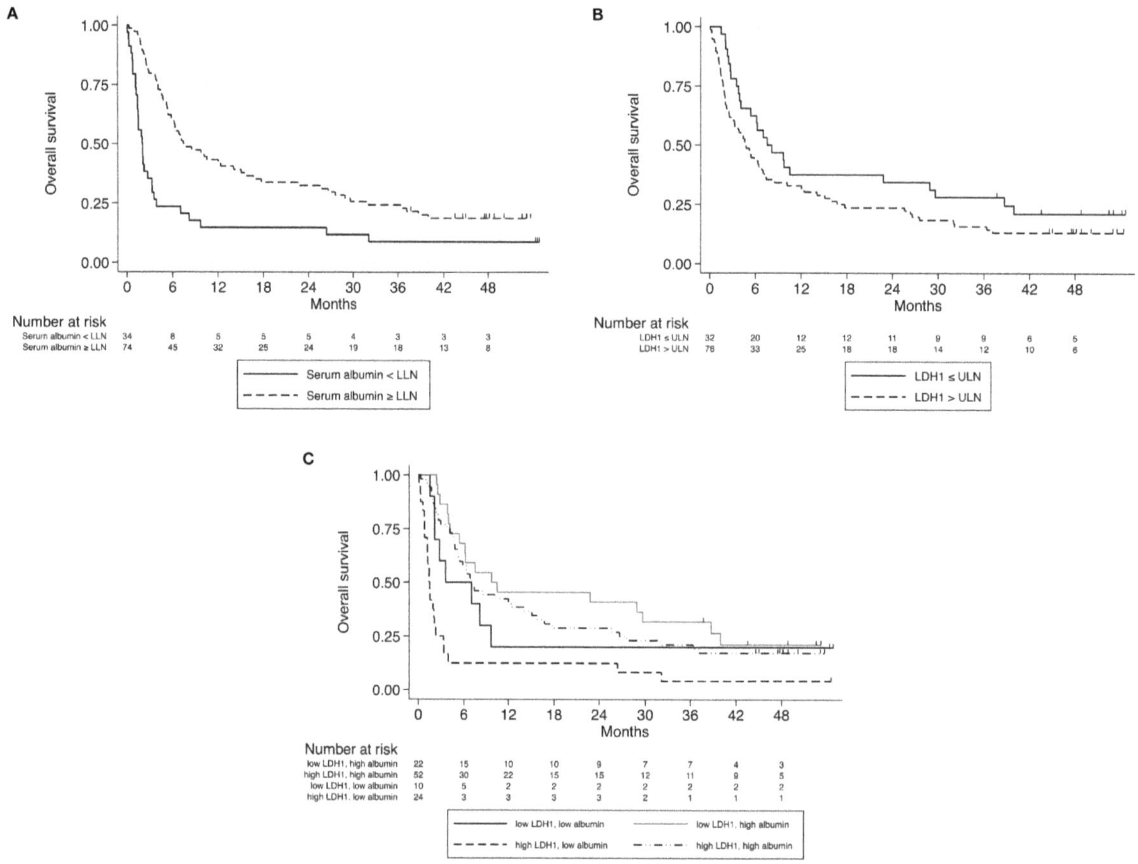

FIGURE 3 | **(A)** Kaplan–Meier curve for overall survival stratified according to Albumin level at baseline (normal or below the lower limit of normal, n=108). **(B)** Kaplan–Meier curve for overall survival stratified according to LDH level at baseline (above upper limit of normal\below upper limit of normal, n=108). **(C)** Kaplan–Meier curves for overall survival stratified according to combined Albumin and LDH levels at baseline. **(A)** HR 0.33, 95% CI (0.20 - 0.52), p<0.001 **(B)** HR 1.15, 95% CI (1.06 - 1.25), p=0.001 **(C)** P<0.001.

dLNR) surprisingly performed better than ECOG-PS as predictors of OS. Despite the recognized validity of ECOG-PS as a strong prognostic factor, the inter-observer variability of this parameter may limit its usefulness in some cases (41). An important question relates to the predictive value of these parameters regarding chemotherapy treatment. Clinical and laboratory factors found to be prognostic in IO-treated NSCLC patients should be examined in parallel in large cohorts of chemotherapy-treated NSCLC patients, all treated with a similar type of chemotherapy. Such analyses would allow the assessment of the role of these factors as potentially predictive for outcome with IO treatments *versus* being general prognostic biomarkers.

A limitation of the study is its retrospective nature, with recognized drawbacks in terms of data accuracy and non-regular follow-up intervals. Furthermore, radiological response to treatment was based on investigators' assessment and not on RECIST. In addition, the relevance of this cohort can be questioned, as most patients are now treated front-line with ICI (either as monotherapy or combined with chemotherapy). We raise here the possibility CLAS score could be applicable in the first-line setting as well, and examining our score in this setting is justified.

Another limitation is the relatively small size of the study, and the lack of a validation cohort to assess the accuracy of the suggested CLAS classifier. Such a validation cohort with equivalent prolonged follow up will be available in the future. However, our data of correlates of long-term survival allows insight into factors correlating with significant ICI efficacy, potentially with the postulated chance of cure. A larger data set is required for comparing the utility of LIPI and CLAS.

In conclusion, unlike median OS, the real life long-term efficacy of nivolumab in the advanced line setting in NSCLC is similar to data from published randomized trials. In addition, we propose a novel score we named 'CLAS' based on baseline albumin and LDH results as a potentially useful score for predicting outcome in nivolumab-treated NSCLC patients. The simple and unbiased measurement of these values adds to their apparent clinical applicability. This score needs further validation before any practical conclusions can be reached. Furthermore, we suggest categorization of patients on immunotherapy according to disease control after six months of treatment to be a simple and

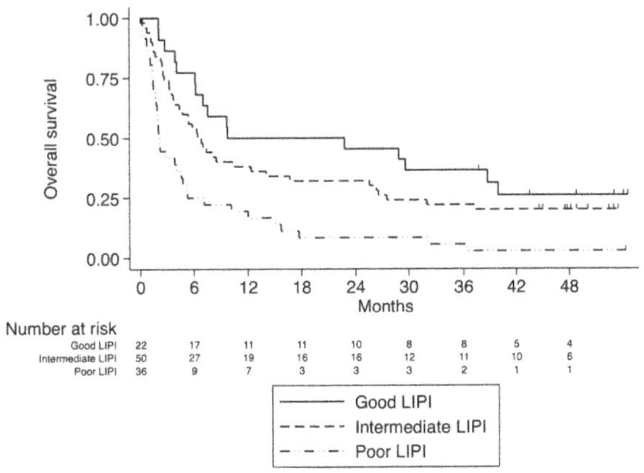

FIGURE 4 | Kaplan–Meier curves for overall survival stratified according to LIPI score. Median OS for poor, intermediate and good LIPI was 2.1 months, 6.4 months, and 9.8 months, respectively, P<0.001.

useful tool for similar studies. DC6 reflects the survival benefit of responding patients as well as of those with prolonged stability, and marks them as having a good chance for durable response and prolonged survival. Thus, this parameter should be further investigated as a surrogate factor for OS in ICI studies.

AUTHOR CONTRIBUTIONS

SD: Conceptualization, Methodology, Investigation, Writing - original draft. YL: Formal analysis, Data curation, Writing - Review & Editing. ED: Conceptualization, Methodology, Investigation, Writing - Review & Editing. EH: Investigation, Writing - Review & Editing. DU: Conceptualization, Methodology, Writing - Review & Editing. NP: Conceptualization, Methodology, Writing - Review & Editing. RN: Resources, Writing - Review & Editing. RL: Conceptualization, Methodology, Writing - Review & Editing. AH: Resources, Data curation, Writing - Review & Editing. EB: Resources, Data curation, Writing - Review & Editing. TG: Resources, Formal analysis, Writing - Review & Editing. AO: Conceptualization, Methodology, Writing - Review & Editing. JB: Conceptualization, Methodology, Validation, Supervision, Project administration, Writing - Review & Editing. All authors contributed to the article and approved the submitted version.

REFERENCES

1. Torre LA, Bray F, Siegel RL, Ferlay J, Lortet-Tieulent J, Jemal A. Global Cancer Statistics, 2012. *CA Cancer J Clin* (2015) 65:87–108. doi: 10.3322/caac.21262
2. Brahmer J, Reckamp KL, Baas P, Crinò L, Eberhardt WEE, Poddubskaya E, et al. Nivolumab *Versus* Docetaxel in Advanced Squamous-Cell Non-Small-Cell Lung Cancer. *N Engl J Med* (2015) 373:123–35. doi: 10.1056/NEJMoa1504627
3. Brahmer J, Horn L, Hossein B, Ramalingam S, Pluzanski A, Burgio MA, et al. O.02 Long-Term Survival Outcomes With Nivolumab (NIVO) in Pts With Previously Treated Advanced Non-Small Cell Lung Cancer (NSCLC): Impact of Early Disease Control and Response. *J Thorac Oncol* (2019) 14:S1152–3. doi: 10.1016/j.jtho.2019.09.089
4. Borghaei H, Paz-Ares L, Horn L, Spigel DR, Steins M, Ready NE, et al. Nivolumab *Versus* Docetaxel in Advanced Nonsquamous Non-Small-Cell Lung Cancer. *N Engl J Med* (2015) 373:1627–39. doi: 10.1056/NEJMoa1507643
5. Herbst RS, Baas P, Kim DW, Felip E, Pérez-Gracia JL, Han JY, et al. Pembrolizumab *Versus* Docetaxel for Previously Treated, PD-L1-Positive, Advanced Non-Small-Cell Lung Cancer (KEYNOTE-010): A Randomised Controlled Trial. *Lancet* (2016) 387:1540–50. doi: 10.1016/S0140-6736(15)01281-7
6. Rittmeyer A, Barlesi F, Waterkamp D, Park K, Ciardiello F, von Pawel J, et al. Atezolizumab *Versus* Docetaxel in Patients With Previously Treated Non-Small-Cell Lung Cancer (OAK): A Phase 3, Open-Label, Multicentre Randomised Controlled Trial. *Lancet* (2017) 389:255–65. doi: 10.1016/S0140-6736(16)32517-X
7. Manson G, Norwood J, Marabelle A, Kohrt H, Houot R. Biomarkers Associated With Checkpoint Inhibitors. *Ann Oncol* (2016) 27:1199–206. doi: 10.1093/annonc/mdw181
8. Reck M, Rodriguez-Abreu D, Robinson AG, Hui R, Csőszi T, Fülöp A, et al. Pembrolizumab *Versus* Chemotherapy for PD-L1-Positive Non-Small-Cell Lung Cancer. *N Engl J Med* (2016) 375:1823–33. doi: 10.1056/NEJMoa1606774
9. Patel SP, Kurzrock R. Pd-L1 Expression as a Predictive Biomarker in Cancer Immunotherapy. *Mol Cancer Ther* (2015) 14:847–56. doi: 10.1158/1535-7163.MCT-14-0983
10. Rizvi NA, Hellmann MD, Snyder A, Kvistborg P, Makarov V, Havel JJ, et al. Mutational Landscape Determines Sensitivity to PD-1 Blockade in Non-Small Cell Lung Cancer. *Sci (80-)* (2015) 348:124–8. doi: 10.1126/science.aaa1348
11. Johnson DB, Frampton GM, Rioth MJ, Yusko E, Xu Y, Guo X, et al. Targeted Next Generation Sequencing Identifies Markers of Response to PD-1 Blockade. *Cancer Immunol Res* (2016) 4:959–67. doi: 10.1158/2326-6066.CIR-16-0143
12. Skoulidis F, Arbour KC, Hellmann MD, Patil PD, Marmarelis ME, Awad MM, et al. Association of STK11/LKB1 Genomic Alterations With Lack of Benefit From the Addition of Pembrolizumab to Platinum Doublet Chemotherapy in Non-Squamous Non-Small Cell Lung Cancer. *J Clin Oncol* (2019) 37:102. doi: 10.1200/JCO.2019.37.15_suppl.102
13. Lee CK, Man J, Lord S, Cooper W, Links M, Gebski V, et al. Clinical and Molecular Characteristics Associated With Survival Among Patients Treated With Checkpoint Inhibitors for Advanced Non-Small Cell Lung Carcinoma: A Systematic Review and Meta-Analysis. *JAMA Oncol* (2018) 4:210–6. doi: 10.1001/jamaoncol.2017.4427
14. Passiglia F, Cappuzzo F, Alabiso O, Bettini AC, Bidoli P, Chiari R, et al. Efficacy of Nivolumab in Pre-Treated Non-Small-Cell Lung Cancer Patients Harbouring KRAS Mutations. *Br J Cancer* (2019) 120:57–62. doi: 10.1038/s41416-018-0234-3

15. Jeanson A, Tomasini P, Souquet-Bressand M, Brandone N, Boucekine M, Grangeon M, et al. Efficacy of Immune Checkpoint Inhibitors in KRAS-Mutant Non-Small Cell Lung Cancer (Nsclc). *J Thorac Oncol* (2019) 14:1095–101. doi: 10.1016/j.jtho.2019.01.011
16. Damotte D, Warren S, Arrondeau J, Boudou-Rouquette P, Mansuet-Lupo A, Biton J, et al. The Tumor Inflammation Signature (TIS) Is Associated With Anti-PD-1 Treatment Benefit in the CERTIM Pan-Cancer Cohort. *J Transl Med* (2019) 17:1–11. doi: 10.1186/s12967-019-2100-3
17. Hwang S, Kwon AY, Jeong JY, Kim S, Kang H, Park J, et al. Immune Gene Signatures for Predicting Durable Clinical Benefit of Anti-PD-1 Immunotherapy in Patients With Non-Small Cell Lung Cancer. *Sci Rep* (2020) 10:1–10. doi: 10.1038/s41598-019-57218-9
18. Thompson JC, Hwang WT, Davis C, Deshpande C, Jeffries S, Rajpurohit Y, et al. Gene Signatures of Tumor Inflammation and Epithelial-to-Mesenchymal Transition (EMT) Predict Responses to Immune Checkpoint Blockade in Lung Cancer With High Accuracy. *Lung Cancer* (2020) 139:1–8. doi: 10.1016/j.lungcan.2019.10.012
19. Barlesi F, Greillier L, Monville F, Foa C, le Treut J, Audigier-Valette C, et al. Lba53 Precision Immuno-Oncology for Advanced Non-Small Cell Lung Cancer (NSCLC) Patients (Pts) Treated With PD1/L1 Immune Checkpoint Inhibitors (Icis): A First Analysis of the PIONeeR Study. *Ann Oncol* (2020) 31: S1183. doi: 10.1016/j.annonc.2020.08.2286
20. Wulaningsih W, Holmberg L, Garmo H, Malmstrom H, Lambe M, Hammar N, et al. Serum Lactate Dehydrogenase and Survival Following Cancer Diagnosis. *Br J Cancer* (2015) 113:1389–96. doi: 10.1038/bjc.2015.361
21. Gupta D, Lis CG. Pretreatment Serum Albumin as a Predictor of Cancer Survival: A Systematic Review of the Epidemiological Literature. *Nutr J* (2010) 9. doi: 10.1186/1475-2891-9-69
22. Espinosa E, Feliu J, Zamora P, González Barón M, Sánchez JJ, Ordón ez A, et al. Serum Albumin and Other Prognostic Factors Related to Response and Survival in Patients With Advanced Non-Small Cell Lung Cancer. *Lung Cancer* (1995) 12:67–76. doi: 10.1016/0169-5002(95)00407-r
23. Diem S, Kasenda B, Spain L, Martin-Liberal J, Marconcini R, Gore M, et al. Serum Lactate Dehydrogenase as an Early Marker for Outcome in Patients Treated With Anti-PD-1 Therapy in Metastatic Melanoma. *Br J Cancer* (2016) 114:256–61. doi: 10.1038/bjc.2015.467
24. Cona MS, Lecchi M, Cresta S, Damian S, Del Vecchio M, Necchi A, et al. Combination of Baseline LDH, Performance Status and Age as Integrated Algorithm to Identify Solid Tumor Patients With Higher Probability of Response to Anti PD-1 and PD-l1 Monoclonal Antibodies. *Cancers (Basel)* (2019) 11. doi: 10.3390/cancers11020223
25. Kataoka Y, Hirano K, Narabayashi T, Hara S, Fujimoto D, Tanaka T, et al. P1.07-004 Predictive Biomarkers of Response to Nivolumab in Non–Small Cell Lung Cancer: A Multicenter Retrospective Cohort Study. *J Thorac Oncol* (2017) 12:S1996. doi: 10.1016/j.jtho.2017.09.922
26. Manegold C. The Causes and Prognostic Significance of Low Hemoglobin Levels in Tumor Patients, Strahlenther. *Onkol* (1998) 174 Suppl 4:17—19.
27. Aoe K, Hiraki A, Maeda T, Katayama H, Fujiwara K, Tabata M, et al. Serum Hemoglobin Level Determined at the First Presentation Is a Poor Prognostic Indicator in Patients With Lung Cancer. *Intern Med* (2005) 44:800–4. doi: 10.2169/internalmedicine.44.800
28. Ferrucci PF, Ascierto PA, Pigozzo J, Del Vecchio M, Maio M, Antonini Cappellini GC, et al. Baseline Neutrophils and Derived Neutrophilto-Lymphocyte Ratio: Prognostic Relevance in Metastatic Melanoma Patients Receiving Ipilimumab. *Ann Oncol* (2016) 27:732–8. doi: 10.1093/annonc/mdw016
29. Martens A, Wistuba-Hamprecht K, Foppen MG, Yuan J, Postow MA, Wong P, et al. Baseline Peripheral Blood Biomarkers Associated With Clinical Outcome of Advanced Melanoma Patients Treated With Ipilimumab. *Clin Cancer Res* (2016) 22:2908–18. doi: 10.1158/1078-0432.CCR-15-2412
30. Weide B, Martens A, Hassel JC, Berking C, Postow MA, Bisschop K, et al. Baseline Biomarkers for Outcome of Melanoma Patients Treated With Pembrolizumab. *Clin Cancer Res* (2016) 22:5487–96. doi: 10.1158/1078-0432.CCR-16-0127
31. Preeshagul IR, Sullivan KM, Paul D, Seetharamu N. The Utilization of Pre-Treatment Neutrophil to Lymphocyte Ratio as a Predictive Marker for Response to Nivolumab Therapy in Non Small Cell Lung Cancer. *J Clin Oncol* (2017) 35:e20634–4. doi: 10.1200/JCO.2017.35.15_suppl.e20634
32. Maymani H, Hess K, Groisberg R, Hong DS, Naing A, Piha-Paul S, et al. Predicting Outcomes in Patients With Advanced Non-Small Cell Lung Cancer Enrolled in Early Phase Immunotherapy Trials. *Lung Cancer* (2018) 120:137–41. doi: 10.1016/j.lungcan.2018.03.020
33. Ren F, Zhao T, Liu B, Pan L. Neutrophil–Lymphocyte Ratio (NLR) Predicted Prognosis for Advanced Non-Small-Cell Lung Cancer (NSCLC) Patients Who Received Immune Checkpoint Blockade (ICB). *Onco Targets Ther* (2019) 12:4235–44. doi: 10.2147/OTT.S199176
34. Mezquita L, Auclin E, Ferrara R, Charrier M, Remon J, Planchard D, et al. Association of the Lung Immune Prognostic Index With Immune Checkpoint Inhibitor Outcomes in Patients With Advanced Non-Small Cell Lung Cancer. *JAMA Oncol* (2018) 4:351–7. doi: 10.1001/jamaoncol.2017.4771
35. Ruiz-Banobre J, Areses-Manrique MC, Mosquera-Martinez J, Cortegoso A, Afonso-Afonso FJ, de Dios-Alvarez N, et al. Evaluation of the Lung Immune Prognostic Index in Advanced Non-Small Cell Lung Cancer Patients Under Nivolumab Monotherapy. *Transl Lung Cancer Res* (2019) 8:1078–85. doi: 10.21037/tlcr.2019.11.07
36. Meyers DE, Stukalin I, Vallerand IA, Lewinson RT, Suo A, Dean M, et al. The Lung Immune Prognostic Index Discriminates Survival Outcomes in Patients With Solid Tumors Treated With Immune Checkpoint Inhibitors. *Cancers (Basel)* (2019) 11. doi: 10.3390/cancers11111713
37. Kazandjian D, Gong Y, Keegan P, Pazdur R, Blumenthal GM. Prognostic Value of the Lung Immune Prognostic Index for Patients Treated for Metastatic Non-Small Cell Lung Cancer. *JAMA Oncol* (2019) 5:1481–5. doi: 10.1001/jamaoncol.2019.1747
38. Benchimol EI, Smeeth L, Guttmann A, Harron K, Moher D, Petersen I, et al. The REporting of Studies Conducted Using Observational Routinely-Collected Health Data (RECORD) Statement. *PloS Med* (2015) 12:e1001885. doi: 10.1371/journal.pmed.1001885
39. von Elm E, Altman DG, Egger M, Pocock SJ, Gøtzsche PC, Vandenbroucke JP. The Strengthening the Reporting of Observational Studies in Epidemiology (STROBE) Statement: Guidelines for Reporting Observational Studies. *Epidemiology* (2007) 18(6):800–4. doi: 10.1097/EDE.0b013e3181577654
40. Langan SM, Schmidt SA, Wing K, Ehrenstein V, Nicholls SG, Filion KB, et al. The Reporting of Studies Conducted Using Observational Routinely Collected Health Data Statement for Pharmacoepidemiology (RECORD-PE). *BMJ* (2018) 363. doi: 10.1136/bmj.k3532
41. Sørensen JB, Klee M, Palshof T, Hansen HH. Performance Status Assessment in Cancer Patients. An Inter-Observer Variability Study. *Br J Cancer* (1993) 67:773–5. doi: 10.1038/bjc.1993.140

14

Immune Checkpoint Inhibitors Plus Single-Agent Chemotherapy for Advanced Non-Small-Cell Lung Cancer after Resistance to EGFR-TKI

*Haiyi Deng†, Xinqing Lin†, Xiaohong Xie†, Yilin Yang, Liqiang Wang, Jianhui Wu, Ming Liu, Zhanhong Xie, Yinyin Qin and Chengzhi Zhou**

State Key Laboratory of Respiratory Disease, National Clinical Research Centre for Respiratory Disease, Guangzhou Institute of Respiratory Health, First Affiliated Hospital, Guangzhou Medical University, Guangzhou, China

***Correspondence:**
Chengzhi Zhou
doctorzcz@163.com

†These authors have contributed equally to this work

Purpose: Platinum-based chemotherapy remains the classic treatment option for patients with advanced non-small-cell lung cancer (NSCLC) who progress while receiving treatment with epidermal growth factor receptor-tyrosine kinase inhibitors (EGFR-TKIs). In this study, we analyzed real-world outcomes of treatment with immune checkpoint inhibitors (ICIs) combined with platinum-free chemotherapy in patients with NSCLC after developing resistance to EGFR-TKIs.

Methods: This retrospective study included patients with mutation-positive NSCLC after developing resistance to EGFR-TKIs. Patients who received chemotherapy alone plus ICIs with or without anti-angiogenic drugs (cohort A) or platinum-based chemotherapy (cohort B) between February 2019 and August 2020 were enrolled. Clinical characteristics, EGFR mutation status, response to therapy, and adverse events (AEs) were retrospectively analyzed.

Results: Seventeen patients were eligible and included in the analysis, including 8 in cohort A and 9 in cohort B. After a median follow-up of 7.6 months, the median progression-free survival was 6.5 months [95% confidence interval (CI), 6.1 to 7.0] in cohort A and 3.6 months (95% CI, 1.3–5.8) in cohort B (hazard ratios, 0.22; 95% CI, 0.05–0.93; P = 0.039). The overall response and disease control rates were 50% and 100% in cohort A, and 22% and 89% in cohort B, respectively. Adverse events of grade 3 or higher occurred in 25% of the patients in cohort A and in 33.3% of the patients in cohort B.

Conclusion: ICIs plus platinum-free, single-agent chemotherapy provides promising progression-free survival and overall response rate benefit, along with a low rate of severe AEs in patients with EGFR-TKI-resistant advanced NSCLC.

Keywords: epidermal growth factor receptor gene (EGFR), immune checkpoint inhibitor, immunotherapy, non-small-cell lung cancer, single-agent chemotherapy

INTRODUCTION

Lung cancer is the first-leading cause of cancer-related death worldwide (1). The vast majority (85%) of lung cancer cases are non-small-cell lung cancer (NSCLC), and approximately 50% of them harbor epidermal growth factor receptor gene (EGFR) mutations in Asia (2). Multiple clinical studies have confirmed the significant response of patients with EGFR mutation to EGFR-tyrosine kinase inhibitors (EGFR-TKIs) (3). According to the current guidelines, the use of EGFR-TKIs has been recommended for the first-line treatment of advanced NSCLC with EGFR mutation. However, these patients develop resistance to EGFR-TKIs after 9–14 months. Approximately 50% of the patients with resistance to first- and second-generation TKIs have T790M mutations, which can be treated with third-generation TKIs (4). Unfortunately, these patients also develop resistance to third-generation EGFR-TKIs after approximately 1 year. According to the guidelines, chemotherapy is generally selected for follow-up treatment of T790M-negative or T790M-positive patients with resistance to third-generation TKIs; however, the efficacy of this regimen is unsatisfactory.

Immune checkpoint inhibitors (ICIs) offer a survival benefit to NSCLC patients without EGFR mutation, but not to those with EGFR mutations (5). The potential benefits of ICIs to patients with resistance to EGFR-TKIs are currently being explored. A meta-analysis showed that ICI alone does not exert a better effect than chemotherapy for patients who have progressed after treatment with TKIs (6). A phase II study (CT18, NCT03513666) of toripalimab combined with pemetrexed and carboplatin showed favorable efficacy (7). IMpower 150, which enrolled patients with EGFR mutation, demonstrated that ICI combined with chemotherapy and an anti-angiogenic drug prolonged progression-free survival (PFS) *versus* chemotherapy plus an anti-angiogenic drug (8). However, these two clinical studies also showed higher proportion of grades 3–5 adverse events (AEs).

A study showed that the immunomodulatory effects of pemetrexed or paclitaxel appeared to be reduced when combined with platinum (9). In addition, CheckMate 9LA confirmed that dual immunotherapy combined with limited chemotherapy exerts a good effect (10). The addition of chemotherapy to immunotherapy should not be restricted to the regimen of four courses of platinum-based chemotherapy. Our previous study proposed the concept of "chemo-reform": the addition of post-reform chemotherapy to immunotherapy, including single-drug chemotherapy (without platinum), platinum alone, low-dose chemotherapy, chemotherapy with adjusted course, or cycle interval–adjusted chemotherapy (11). This retrospective study was designed to assess the efficacy and safety of ICIs combined with single-drug chemotherapy without platinum in patients with EGFR-TKI-resistant advanced NSCLC in a real-world setting.

PATIENTS AND METHODS

Patients

Eligible patients with incurable NSCLC were treated with ICIs combined with single-drug chemotherapy without platinum, with or without anti-angiogenic treatment (cohort A) or platinum-containing chemotherapy (cohort B) at the First Affiliated Hospital of Guangzhou Medical University (Guangzhou, China) between February 2019 and August 2020. All patients had incurable advanced or metastatic NSCLC [unresectable stage III or IV according to the 8th edition TNM classification (12)]. Patients had to have sensitizing EGFR mutations [exon 19 deletions (Del19); exon 21 L858R mutation (L858R)] detected at the initial biopsy, clinical or radiological progression after at least one treatment with EGFR-TKIs, and no mutations that can be targeted for treatment. There was no upper limit regarding the number of prior treatments with EGFR-TKIs or systemic therapies. This study was approved by the local Ethics Committee of the First Affiliated Hospital of Guangzhou Medical University.

Data Collection and Outcome Assessment

The following information was retrospectively collected from the medical records of the patients: patient demographics, prior treatments with EGFR-TKIs or systemic therapies, lines of immunotherapy, Eastern Cooperative Oncology Group (ECOG) performance status (PS), EGFR mutation type, programmed death-ligand 1 (PD-L1) tumor proportion score (TPS), tumor imaging, tumor response to therapy, and AEs. The ECOG PS was evaluated prior to treatment. PD-L1 expression was tested by anti-human PD-L1 (Dako 22C3) according to the manufacturer's recommendations, using 4–5 μm formalin-fixed and paraffin-embedded (FFPE) sections. The cutoff value was 1% for PD-L1 positivity or negativity (PD-L1+/−). Tumor response was assessed in accordance with the Response Evaluation Criteria in Solid Tumors (RECIST version 1.1) (13). The objective response rate (ORR) was defined as the percentage of patients who exhibited response (complete or partial). The disease control rate (DCR) corresponds to all cases with complete response (CR), partial response (PR), and stable disease (SD). PFS was defined as the time from therapy initiation to disease progression or death. AEs were graded according to the National Cancer Institute Common Terminology Criteria for Adverse Events, version 4.0.

Statistical Analysis

Continuous and categorical data were summarized as medians (ranges) and frequencies (percentages), respectively. An independent-samples t-test or the Mann-Whitney U test was used to analyze continuous variables. Differences in categorical variables were assessed using either Chi-square ($\chi2$) or Fisher's exact test. We used the binomial exact method to evaluate the ORR and DCR with 95% confidence intervals (CIs). The Kaplan–Meier method was used to evaluate PFS with 95% CI. Statistical tests were two-sided, and a P-value <0.05 denoted statistically significant difference. Statistical analyses were performed using the IBM SPSS Statistics version 25.0 (Armonk, NY, USA) software.

RESULTS

Patients

In total, 17 patients were eligible and enrolled in the study. Patients' demographics are summarized in **Tables 1** and **2**. The median age of all patients was 59 (range: 42–73)years; nine patients (52.9%) were males and 82.4% had never smoked. All patients were adenocarcinoma. EGFR mutation status in the initial biopsy was Del19 and L858R in 11 and 6 patients, respectively. Nine patients were positive for the T790M mutation. Third or later lines were reported in 76.5% of patients, and 11 patients were treated with at least two EGFR-TKIs. For the 14 participants with available PD-L1 TPS values, 6 (42.8%), 4 (28.6%), and 4 (28.6%) patients had TPS values less than 1%, 1–49%, and ≥50%.

Cohort A included 8 (47.1%) patients and cohort B had 9 (52.9%) patients. In the cohort A, 2 patients received ICI combined with single agent chemotherapy and 6 patients received ICI

TABLE 1 | Characteristics of patients at baseline.

Characteristics	Cohort A (N = 8)	Cohort B (N = 9)	P value
Age,y; median (Range)	66 (53-73)	58 (42-71)	0.18
Sex (male/ female)	4/4	5/4	1
Smoking status			0.58
Current/former	2 (25)	1 (11.1)	
Never	6 (75)	8 (88.9)	
ECOG PS (at initiation of ICI/chemotherapy)			0.58
0	2 (25)	1 (11.1)	
1	6 (75)	8 (88.9)	
Disease status			0.47
III B	1 (12.5)	0	
IV	7 (87.5)	9 (100)	
Site of metastasis (at initiation of ICI/ chemotherapy)			
Brain	3 (37.5)	4 (44.4)	1
Liver	3 (37.5)	2 (22.2)	0.62
EGFR mutation status (initial biopsy/pre-TKI)			1
Del19	5 (62.5)	6 (66.7)	
L858R	3 (37.5)	3 (33.3)	
T790M status (rebiopsy/ post-TKI)			0.64
Positive	5 (62.5)	4 (44.4)	
Negative	3 (37.5)	5 (55.6)	
Prior treatment lines			0.57
1	2 (25)	2 (22.2)	
2	3 (37.5)	6 (66.7)	
3	3 (37.5)	1 (11.1)	
PD-L1 TPS			0.11
<1%	3 (37.5)	3 (33.3)	
1-49%	4 (50)	0	
≥50%	1 (12.5)	3 (33.3)	
Unknown	0	3 (33.3)	

ECOG PS, Eastern Cooperative Oncology Group performance status; EGFR, epidermal growth factor receptor gene; ICI, immune checkpoint inhibitor; TKI, tyrosine kinase inhibitor; Del19, exon 19 deletions; PD-L1 TPS, programmed death-ligand 1 tumor proportion score.

TABLE 2 | Characteristics of patients with EGFR-TKIs resistance who received immunotherapy or chemotherapy.

Patients	Gender	Age	Smoking status	EGFR mutation	T790M status (post-TKI)	Prior treatment lines	PFS on first TKI (months)	PD-L1 Expression level (%)	Response to ICI or chemotherapy
A-1	Female	54	Never	Del19	Negative	3	6.0	50	SD
A-2	Female	58	Never	L858R	Negative	1	10.3	2	SD
A-3	Female	68	Never	L858R	Positive	2	6.7	2	SD
A-4	Male	53	Former	Del19	Positive	3	9.7	<1	PR
A-5	Male	70	Former	L858R	Negative	1	4.6	<1	PR
A-6	Male	66	Never	Del19	Positive	2	11.9	10	PR
A-7	Male	66	Never	Del19	Positive	3	10.3	<1	SD
A-8	Female	73	Never	Del19	Positive	2	7.4	5	PR
B-1	Female	70	Never	L858R	Negative	2	3.7	<1	SD
B-2	Female	55	Never	Del19	Positive	2	8.1	<1	SD
B-3	Female	42	Never	Del19	Negative	1	4.6	80	PR
B-4	Male	59	Never	L858R	Negative	1	4.9	80	PR
B-5	Female	59	Never	Del19	Negative	2	6.1	<1	PD
B-6	Male	57	Never	Del19	Negative	2	9.5	NA	SD
B-7	Male	58	Never	Del19	Positive	2	10.9	NA	SD
B-8	Male	71	Former	L858R	Positive	2	12.2	NA	SD
B-9	Male	48	Never	Del19	Positive	3	7.6	50	SD

EGFR, epidermal growth factor receptor gene; Del19, exon 19 deletions; TKI, tyrosine kinase inhibitor; PFS, progression-free survival; PD-L1 , programmed death-ligand 1; ICI, immune checkpoint inhibitor, A-, cohort A; B-, cohort B; NA, unknown.

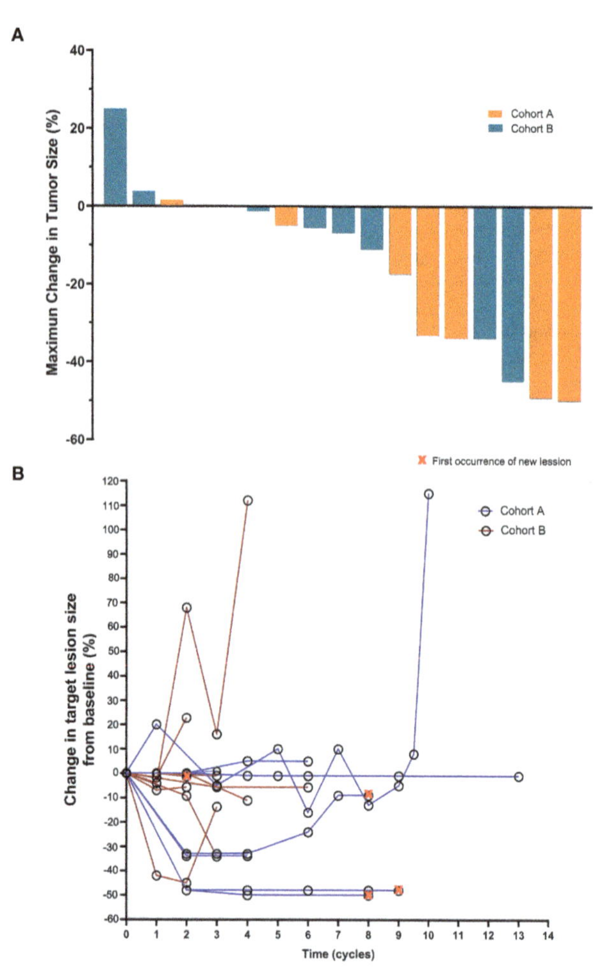

FIGURE 1 | Maximum percent change from baseline in the sum of the diameter of the longest target lesion according to the Response Evaluation Criteria in Solid Tumors (RECIST) version 1.1 in patients with measurable disease at baseline **(A)**. Positive and negative change in tumor size indicates tumor growth and reduction, respectively. Percent change in target lesion tumor burden from baseline and throughout the course of immunotherapy **(B)**.

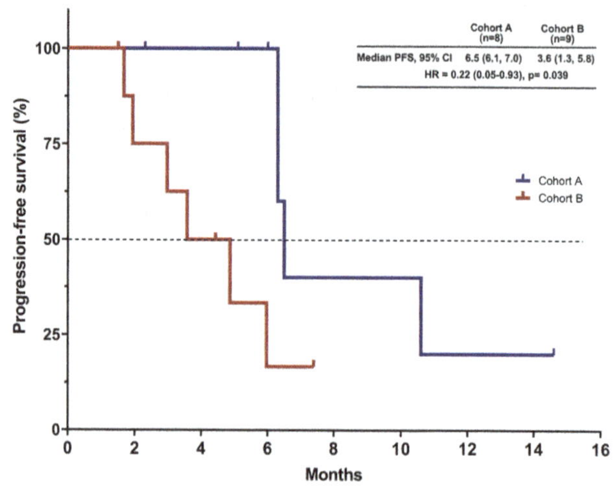

FIGURE 2 | Kaplan–Meier curve for progression-free survival (PFS). CI, confidence interval; HR, hazard ratio.

combined with single-agent chemotherapy and anti-angiogenesis therapy. Baseline demographic and disease characteristics were no significant difference between groups (**Table 1**).

Efficacy

A total of 17 patients were evaluable for response. Partial responses were observed in 4 of 8 patients in cohort A and in 2 of 9 patients in cohort B. None of the patients had CR as their best reponse. The confirmed ORR was 50% (95% CI, 16–84) in cohort A and 22% (95% CI, 3–60) in cohort B (P = 0.34; **Table 2** and **Figure 1**). The DCR was 100% in cohort A and 88.9% in cohort B. The overall median follow-up for this analysis was 7.6 months. With 10 events of progression or death, the median PFS was 6.5 months (95% CI, 6.1 to 7.0) in cohort A and 3.6 months (95% CI, 1.3–5.8) in cohort B [hazard ratios (HR) for PFS, 0.22; 95% CI, 0.05–0.93; P = 0.039; **Figure 2**]. The 6-month PFS rate was 60.0% in cohort A and 16.7% in cohort B. During the follow-up, the median overall survival was not reached.

Safety

A summary of the safety data of all treated patients is shown in **Table 3**. During treatment, AEs of any grade, regardless of attribution to treatment by the investigator, occurred in all patients. AEs of grade 3 or higher occurred in 25% of the patients in cohort A and in 33.3% of the patients in cohort B. There was no occurrence of toxicity-related deaths. None of the AEs led to discontinuation of treatment with ICIs in cohort A. The most common AEs in cohort A were anemia (75%), constipation (75%), and fatigue (50%), and the most common AEs in cohort B were anemia (77.8%) and decreased neutrophil count (33.3%).

DISCUSSION

The results of this study involving patients with advanced NSCLC patients after TKI acquired resistance showed that ICIs plus platinum-free chemotherapy, as compared with platinum-containing chemotherapy, prolonged median progression-free survival by 2.9 months (6.5 *vs.* 3.6 months).The risk of disease progression or death was 22% lower in cohort A than in cohort B. The ORR was higher in the in cohort A than in cohort B (50% *vs.* 22%). To our knowledge, this is the first study to demonstrate the efficacy and safety of immunotherapy combined with platinum-free chemotherapy in such patients.

The subsequent therapy of EGFR positive patients after TKI resistance is a conundrum. *In vitro*, PD-1 inhibitor prolonged the survival of mice with EGFR-mutant lung cancer by enhancing effector T cell function and reducing the level of tumor-promoting cytokines (14). However, previous studies showed ICI monotherapy has no survival benefit than docetaxel in the

TABLE 3 | Adverse Events of Any Cause.

Event	Cohort A (N = 8)		Cohort B (N = 9)	
	Any Grade	Grade 3 or 4	Any Grade	Grade 3 or 4
Any event	8 (100)	2 (25)	9 (100)	3 (33.3)
Anemia	6 (75)	2 (25)	7 (77.8)	1 (11.1)
Constipation	6 (75)	0	0	0
Fatigue	4 (50)	0	1 (11.1)	0
Decreased appetite	3 (37.5)	0	2 (22.2)	0
Skin reactions	3 (37.5)	0	2 (22.2)	0
Peripheral edema	3 (37.5)	0	1 (11.1)	0
Mucosal inflammation	3 (37.5)	0	1 (11.1)	0
Hyperthyroidism	2 (25)	0	1 (11.1)	0
Diabetes	2 (25)	0	0	0
Hepatitis	2 (25)	0	2 (22.2)	1 (11.1)
Dizziness	2 (25)	0	0	0
Neutrophil count decreased	1 (12.5)	0	3 (33.3)	1 (11.1)
Pneumonitis	1 (12.5)	0	0	0
Vomiting	1 (12.5)	0	0	0
Hypothyroidism	1 (12.5)	0	0	0
Nephritis	1 (12.5)	0	0	0

treatment of TKI resistant NSCLC patients (6), which may be associated with low rates of concurrent PD-L1 expression and CD8(+) TILs within the tumor microenvironment (15). Chemotherapy and immunotherapy had synergistic effects by upregulating PD-L1 expression (16).

Platinum-based chemotherapy is regarded as the standard treatment for EGFR-TKI resistant patients and is an appropriate comparator for this study. Although there were confounding effects compared with historical data, the outcomes of cohort B were consistent with the expectations based on previous studies (17, 18). Also, the outcomes of cohort A were consistent with that reported in the CT18 study (ORR: 50%; median PFS: 7 months) in advanced NSCLC patients received toripalimab combined with chemotherapy after resistance to prior EGFR TKIs (7). Nevertheless, 75% of patients enrolled in our study had received third or later lines of therapy, including four patients with T790M positive and resistance to third-generation TKIs. In the cohort A, 6/8 patients received received ICI plus chemotherapy and anti-angiogenesis therapy, of which 4 cases (66.7%) achieved PR. IMpower150 (8) included patients with EGFR mutation treated with ACP (atezolizumab + carboplatin + paclitaxel) or BCP (carboplatin + paclitaxel + bevacizumab) or ABCP (atezolizumab + carboplatin + paclitaxel +bevacizumab). Our ORR appeared to be numerically higher than those reported in these three subgroups (16% *vs.* 18% *vs.* 24%, respectively). The numerically lower PFS in cohort A, compared with that of ABCP group in IMpower150 study, may be explained in part by the inclusion of 2 patients who received ICI-chemotherapy without anti-angiogenic drugs.

The adverse-event profile observed in our study was as expected on the basis of the known events, and no new safety signals were found. The present results reveal that the proportion of grade ≥3 AEs (25%) in cohort A was numerically lower than those reported in the CT18 (55%) (7) and IMpower150 (ACP *vs.* BCP *vs.* ABCP, 57% *vs.* 57% *vs.* 64%, respectively) studies (8). Additionally, there were no grade 3–5 immune-related AEs recorded in our study. The majority of AEs were resolved or improved and were manageable.

This study had some limitations. Firstly, it was a retrospective study performed in a real-world setting, with potential for bias. We did not perform subgroup analysis due to a small sample size. We are currently conducting relevant prospective clinical studies (NCT04316351, NCT04310943). Secondly, the present findings provide only a narrow time window with limited follow-up of some patients. As a result, we did not calculate OS, and were able to analyze ORR and PFS as measures of short-term efficacy. The follow-up results will provide a more comprehensive analysis.

In conclusion, we showed a clinically meaningful survival benefit and a lower rate of severe AEs in patients treated with ICIs plus "chemo-reform". These clinically relevant data support the use of immunotherapy combined with single-drug chemotherapy may be a new treatment option for patients with advanced NSCLC after developing resistance to EGFR-TKIs. Prospective clinical studies are needed for further validation.

AUTHOR CONTRIBUTIONS

HD, XL, XX, and CZ designed the study. HD, YY, LW, and JW collected the patients' data. HD, XL, ZX, ML, and YQ analyzed the data. HD, XL, XX, and CZ drafted and revised the manuscript. All authors contributed to the article and approved the submitted version.

ACKNOWLEDGMENTS

We sincerely thank the participating patients and all medical staff members.

REFERENCES

1. Sung H, Ferlay J, Siegel RL, Laversanne M, Soerjomataram I, Jemal A, et al. Global Cancer Statistics 2020: GLOBOCAN Estimates of Incidence and Mortality Worldwide for 36 Cancers in 185 Countries. *CA: Cancer J Clin* (2021) 71(3):209–249. doi: 10.3322/caac.21660
2. Midha A, Dearden S, McCormack R. EGFR Mutation Incidence in non-Small-Cell Lung Cancer of Adenocarcinoma Histology: A Systematic Review and Global Map by Ethnicity (Mutmapii). *Am J Cancer Res* (2015) 5(9):2892–911.
3. Zhang Y, Sheng J, Yang Y, Fang W, Kang S, He Y, et al. Optimized Selection of Three Major EGFR-TKIs in Advanced EGFR-Positive non-Small Cell Lung Cancer: A Network Meta-Analysis. *Oncotarget* (2016) 7(15):20093–108. doi: 10.18632/oncotarget.7713
4. Wang ZF, Ren SX, Li W, Gao GH. Frequency of the Acquired Resistant Mutation T790 M in non-Small Cell Lung Cancer Patients With Active Exon 19Del and Exon 21 L858R: A Systematic Review and Meta-Analysis. *BMC Cancer* (2018) 18(1):148. doi: 10.1186/s12885-018-4075-5
5. Lee CK, Man J, Lord S, Links M, Gebski V, Mok T, et al. Checkpoint Inhibitors in Metastatic EGFR-Mutated Non-Small Cell Lung Cancer-A Meta-Analysis. *J Thorac Oncol* (2017) 12(2):403–7. doi: 10.1016/j.jtho.2016.10.007
6. Cavanna L, Citterio C, Orlandi E. Immune Checkpoint Inhibitors in EGFR-Mutation Positive TKI-Treated Patients With Advanced non-Small-Cell Lung Cancer Network Meta-Analysis. *Oncotarget* (2019) 10(2):209–15. doi: 10.18632/oncotarget.26541
7. Zhang J, Zhou C, Zhao Y, Mu X, Zhou J, Bao Z, et al. A PII Study of Toripalimab, a PD-1 mAb, in Combination With Chemotherapy in EGFR Plus Advanced NSCLC Patients Failed to Prior EGFR TKI Therapies. *J Thorac Oncol* (2019) 14(10):S292–S. doi: 10.1016/j.jtho.2019.08.587
8. Reck M, Mok TSK, Nishio M, Jotte RM, Cappuzzo F, Orlandi F, et al. Atezolizumab Plus Bevacizumab and Chemotherapy in non-Small-Cell Lung Cancer (IMpower150): Key Subgroup Analyses of Patients With EGFR Mutations or Baseline Liver Metastases in a Randomised, Open-Label Phase 3 Trial. *Lancet Respir Med* (2019) 7(5):387–401. doi: 10.1016/s2213-2600(19)30084-0
9. Schaer DA, Geeganage S, Amaladas N, Lu ZH, Rasmussen ER, Sonyi A, et al. The Folate Pathway Inhibitor Pemetrexed Pleiotropically Enhances Effects of Cancer Immunotherapy. *Clin Cancer Res* (2019) 25(23):7175–88. doi: 10.1158/1078-0432.Ccr-19-0433
10. Paz-Ares L, Ciuleanu TE, Cobo M, Schenker M, Zurawski B, Menezes J, et al. First-Line Nivolumab Plus Ipilimumab Combined With Two Cycles of Chemotherapy in Patients With non-Small-Cell Lung Cancer (CheckMate 9LA): An International, Randomised, Open-Label, Phase 3 Trial. *Lancet Oncol* (2021) 22(2):198–211. doi: 10.1016/s1470-2045(20)30641-0
11. Deng H, Zhou C. From CheckMate 227 to CheckMate 9LA: Rethinking the Status of Chemotherapy in the Immunotherapy Era-Chemo-Free or Chemo-Reform? *Transl Lung Cancer Res* (2021) 10(4):1924–7. doi: 10.21037/tlcr-21-179
12. Goldstraw P, Chansky K, Crowley J, Rami-Porta R, Asamura H, Eberhardt WE, et al. The IASLC Lung Cancer Staging Project: Proposals for Revision of the TNM Stage Groupings in the Forthcoming (Eighth) Edition of the TNM Classification for Lung Cancer. *J Thorac Oncol* (2016) 11(1):39–51. doi: 10.1016/j.jtho.2015.09.009
13. Eisenhauer EA, Therasse P, Bogaerts J, Schwartz LH, Sargent D, Ford R, et al. New Response Evaluation Criteria in Solid Tumours: Revised RECIST Guideline (Version 1.1). *Eur J Cancer (Oxford England: 1990)* (2009) 45 (2):228–47. doi: 10.1016/j.ejca.2008.10.026
14. Akbay EA, Koyama S, Carretero J, Altabef A, Tchaicha JH, Christensen CL, et al. Activation of the PD-1 Pathway Contributes to Immune Escape in EGFR-Driven Lung Tumors. *Cancer Discovery* (2013) 3(12):1355–63. doi: 10.1158/2159-8290.CD-13-0310
15. Gainor JF, Shaw AT, Sequist LV, Fu X, Azzoli CG, Piotrowska Z, et al. EGFR Mutations and ALK Rearrangements Are Associated With Low Response Rates to PD-1 Pathway Blockade in Non-Small Cell Lung Cancer: A Retrospective Analysis. *Clin Cancer Res* (2016) 22(18):4585–93. doi: 10.1158/1078-0432.CCR-15-3101
16. Xue Y, Gao S, Gou J, Yin T, He H, Wang Y, et al. Platinum-Based Chemotherapy in Combination With PD-1/PD-L1 Inhibitors: Preclinical and Clinical Studies and Mechanism of Action. *Expert Opin Drug Delivery* (2021) 18(2):187–203. doi: 10.1080/17425247.2021.1825376
17. Soria JC, Wu YL, Nakagawa K, Kim SW, Yang JJ, Ahn MJ, et al. Gefitinib Plus Chemotherapy *Versus* Placebo Plus Chemotherapy in EGFR-Mutation-Positive non-Small-Cell Lung Cancer After Progression on First-Line Gefitinib (IMPRESS): A Phase 3 Randomised Trial. *Lancet Oncol* (2015) 16 (8):990–8. doi: 10.1016/s1470-2045(15)00121-7
18. Goldberg SB, Oxnard GR, Digumarthy S, Muzikansky A, Jackman DM, Lennes IT, et al. Chemotherapy With Erlotinib or Chemotherapy Alone in Advanced non-Small Cell Lung Cancer With Acquired Resistance to EGFR Tyrosine Kinase Inhibitors. *Oncologist* (2013) 18(11):1214–20. doi: 10.1634/theoncologist.2013-0168

15

The Correlation Between SPP1 and Immune Escape of EGFR Mutant Lung Adenocarcinoma was Explored by Bioinformatics Analysis

Yi Zheng[1], Shiying Hao[2], Cheng Xiang[1], Yaguang Han[1], Yanhong Shang[3], Qiang Zhen[1], Yiyi Zhao[1], Miao Zhang[1] and Yan Zhang[1]*

[1] Department of Oncology, Shijiazhuang People's Hospital, Shijiazhuang, China, [2] Department of Cardiothoracic Surgery, Standford University, Stanford, CA, United States, [3] Department of Oncology, Affiliated Hospital of Hebei University, Baoding, China

***Correspondence:**
Yan Zhang
zhangyan201810@163.com

Background: Immune checkpoint inhibitors have achieved breakthrough efficacy in treating lung adenocarcinoma (LUAD) with wild-type epidermal growth factor receptor (EGFR), leading to the revision of the treatment guidelines. However, most patients with EGFR mutation are resistant to immunotherapy. It is particularly important to study the differences in tumor microenvironment (TME) between patients with and without EGFR mutation. However, relevant research has not been reported. Our previous study showed that secreted phosphoprotein 1 (SPP1) promotes macrophage M2 polarization and PD-L1 expression in LUAD, which may influence response to immunotherapy. Here, we assessed the role of SPP1 in different populations and its effects on the TME.

Methods: We compared the expression of SPP1 in LUAD tumor and normal tissues, and in samples with wild-type and mutant EGFR. We also evaluated the influence of SPP1 on survival. The LUAD data sets were downloaded from TCGA and CPTAC databases. Clinicopathologic characteristics associated with overall survival in TCGA were assessed using Cox regression analysis. GSEA revealed that several fundamental signaling pathways were enriched in the high SPP1 expression group. We applied CIBERSORT and xCell to calculate the proportion and abundance of tumor-infiltrating immune cells (TICs) in LUAD, and compared the differences in patients with high or low SPP1 expression and wild-type or mutant EGFR. In addition, we explored the correlation between SPP1 and CD276 for different groups.

Results: SPP1 expression was higher in LUAD tumor tissues and in people with EGFR mutation. High SPP1 expression was associated with poor prognosis. Univariate and multivariate cox analysis revealed that up-regulated SPP1 expression was independent indicator of poor prognosis. GSEA showed that the SPP1 high expression group was mainly enriched in immunosuppressed pathways. In the SPP1 high expression group, the infiltration of CD8+ T cells was lower and M2-type macrophages was higher. These results were also observed in patients with EGFR mutation. Furthermore, we found that the SPP1 expression was positively correlated with CD276, especially in patients with EGFR mutation.

Conclusion: SPP1 levels might be a useful marker of immunosuppression in patients with EGFR mutation, and could offer insight for therapeutics.

Keywords: immune checkpoint inhibitors, lung adenocarcinoma, epidermal growth factor receptor, tumor microenvironment, secreted phosphoprotein 1, tumor-infiltrating immune cells

INTRODUCTION

Lung cancer has become one of the most serious threats to human health, and its global morbidity and mortality rank first among all cancer types (1). Approximately 85% of lung cancers are non-small cell lung cancer (NSCLC), and lung adenocarcinoma (LUAD) accounts for 40%–50% of NSCLC. In China, 50%–60% of patients with LUAD also have epidermal growth factor receptor (EGFR) mutation. Epidermal growth factor receptor-tyrosine kinase inhibitor (EGFR-TKI) targeted therapy has been recommended for treating patients with EGFR sensitive mutations and such therapy has significantly improved survival in advanced NSCLC (2, 3). However, EGFR-TKI resistance has been observed in patients with NSCLC, which is challenging the prognosis of the disease (4).

Recently, immune checkpoint inhibitors (ICIs), represented by programmed cell death-1 (PD-1) and programmed cell death-ligand 1(PD-L1) monoclonal antibodies, have presented a new approach for NSCLC treatment (5, 6). ICIs achieve long-term disease control in patients who have developed an anti-tumor response, by activating the body's immune system for tumor cell recognition and removal (7). However, ICIs had poor efficacy and adverse effects in patients with EGFR mutation or secondary T790M mutation (8–10).

The IMpower 150 study found that a combination of atezolizumab, bevacizumab, and chemotherapy improved overall survival (OS) in patients with EGFR mutation (11). This study was the first randomized phase III trial of immunotherapy that showed a benefit in patients with EGFR mutation, suggesting that "primary drug resistance" could be reversed. *In-vitro* studies showed that the non-inflammatory tumor microenvironment (TME) changed in EGFR-mutated NSCLC after partial drug intervention, improving the efficacy of immunotherapy (12). Hence, there might be a connection between the EGFR-mutated NSCLC immune microenvironment and the mechanism of primary resistance to ICIs. Exploring the microenvironment characteristics may improve our knowledge of drug resistance mechanism and offer clues to reversing resistance.

Osteopontin (OPN, encoded by SPP1) is a secreted phosphorylated glycoprotein, which is produced by T, NK and other immune cells, myeloid cells, osteoblasts, bone cells, epithelial cells, etc. (13, 14). It is also a kind of multifunctional cytokine. Previously, we found that lung adenocarcinoma cells induced M2 polarization of macrophages through SPP1, and activation of T cells were observed after SPP1 silencing (15). However, the role of SPP1 mediated immunosuppression in patients with EGFR mutations remains unclear. What is more, the B7 family is important in regulating T cell immune response. PD-1 and B7-H3 (CD276) are both members of B7/CD28 family and had similar effects in TME (16). The up-regulated of CD276 expression can promote immune escaping of tumor cells, including inhibit the proliferation of T cells, reduce the secretion of IFN-γ, tumor necrosis factor-alpha (TNF-α), and other cytokines (16). As a co-inhibitory molecule of T cell, CD276 is an attractive target for cancer immunotherapy (17, 18).

In this study, we explored the TME of patients with EGFR mutation, which has been highlighted for its potential impact on the resistance of ICIs. We analyzed SPP1 expression in LUAD with or without EGFR mutation, and explored its association with clinicopathologic characteristics and patient outcomes. We further evaluated the differences in the tumor-infiltrating immune cells (TICs) in the immune microenvironment between groups with different levels of SPP1 expression, and those with or without EGFR mutation. In addition, the correlation between SPP1 and CD276 for different groups was compared. A study workflow is presented in **Figure 1**.

MATERIALS AND METHODS

Data Acquisition

LUAD patient datasets were downloaded from The Cancer Genome Atlas (TCGA, https://portal.gdc.cancer.gov/) (19, 20), including transcriptome RNA-seq gene expression profiles (Level 3), and clinical information. A total of 497 tumor tissues and 54 adjacent tissues were included. We compared SPP1 protein expression in 102 normal and 109 cancer tissues, using The Clinical Proteomic Tumor Analysis Consortium (CPTAC, https://proteomics.cancer.gov/programs/cptac) (21, 22). We collected the mutation information of TCGA cohort from UCSC Xena database (https://xenabrowser.net/datapages/) (23), in which there are 472 cases with mutation information available including 409 EGFR wild-type and 63 EGFR mutant cases. Additionally, survival of patients with LUAD was analyzed in relation to SPP1 expression in TCGA and CPTAC databases.

Cox Regression Analysis and GSEA

Univariate and multivariate cox regression analysis was performed in 435 patients (missing clinical information were excluded) to screen factors significantly associated with OS in TCGA. Gene Set Enrichment Analysis (GSEA) (http://software.broadinstitute.org/gsea/) was performed to determine the biological differences and pathways affected by differential

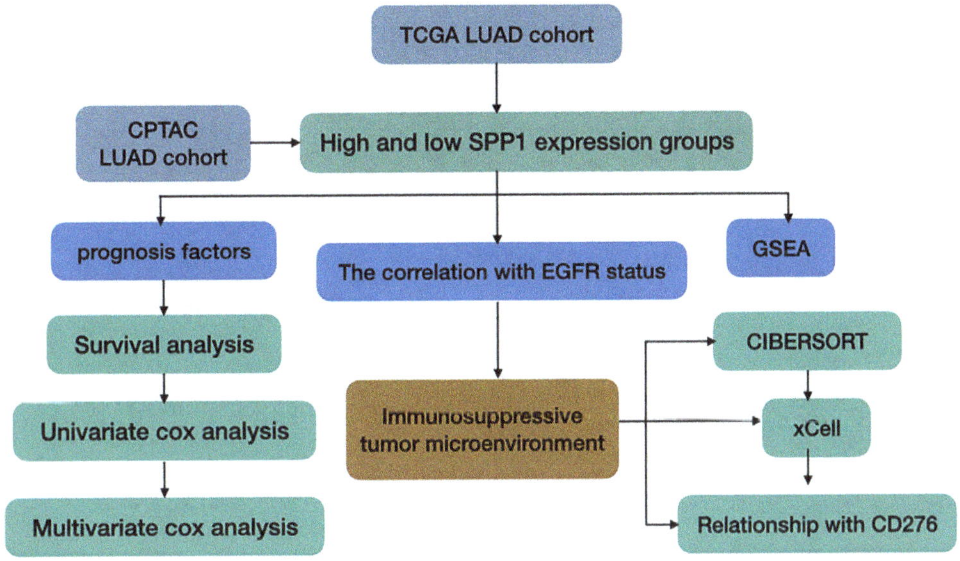

FIGURE 1 | Study workflow.

expression of SPP1 (one-fourth cutoff) in Gene Set c2(c2.cp.Kegg.v7.0.symbols) and c5(c5.all.v7.0.symbols). The number of random sample permutations was set at 1000. The significance threshold was $P < 0.05$ and false discovery rate (FDR) < 0.25.

Correlation With TICs and CD276

CIBERSORT(http://cibersort.stanford.edu/) is an immune cell infiltrating assessment analysis tool (24, 25). We assessed the influence of SPP1 expression and EGFR mutation to 22 types of immune cells by CIBERSORT. The filter criteria of each sample is set as the $P < 0.05$, which indicating that the inferred proportion of each TICs subtype are accurate and suitable for further analysis. We calculated the correlation between different immune cells, and marked those with $P < 0.05$. xCell is a gene signatures-based method, which performs cell type enrichment analysis from gene expression data for 64 immune and stroma cell types (26). To verify the results of CIBERSORT, we downloaded the results of immune cell abundance in TCGA LUAD by xCell algorithm from TIMER database (http://timer.cistrome.org/) (27). Besides, the correlation between SPP1 and CD276 for different groups was calculated using Spearman correlation coefficients.

Statistical Analysis

Statistical analysis of data from TCGA and CPTAC were performed using R-3.6.1. The independent samples t-test or Wilcoxon's rank sum-tests were used to compare continuous variables between two groups. Kruskal-Wallis one-way analysis of variance followed by a posthoc Kruskal-Dunn test with BH's method for adjusting for multiple comparisons. Prism8 software was used to plot the survival curves using the Kaplan-Meier method, and the log-rank test was used to compare the survival curves. Uni- and multi-variate analyses were performed using Cox proportional hazard models, where $P < 0.05$ was considered statistically significant. The correlation between SPP1 and CD276 was calculated using Spearman's correlation coefficient (R), with $P < 0.01$ was considered statistically significant.

RESULTS

SPP1 Expression and OS Differences

LUAD cohorts consisted of a total of 477 patients in TCGA and 109 patients in CPTAC. The clinical characteristics between low and high SPP1 expression groups were listed in **Table 1** and **Supplementary Table 1**. SPP1 expression was significantly higher in tumor tissues than in adjacent tissues, regardless of RNA or protein level (**Figures 2A, B**, $P < 0.001$). SPP1 expression was higher in EGFR-mutated tumor samples than in wild-type samples (**Figure 2C**, $P = 0.017$). The median level of SPP1 expression was used to dichotomize patients into high- or low-expression groups, and Kaplan-Meier survival analysis was performed separately for TCGA and CPTAC. Increased SPP1 expression was significantly correlated with poor OS, and the median OS of the TCGA cohort was 4.73 *vs.* 3.37 (**Figure 2D**; HR:1.48 95%CI 1.10-2.00; $P= 0.009$). Median OS was not achieved in CPTAC cohort, but differences were observed (**Figure 2E**; HR: 3.40 95%CI 1.15-10.08; $P = 0.047$). In addition, subgroup analysis of TCGA LUAD showed that patients with EGFR mutation in SPP1 high-expression group had a poor prognosis (**Supplementary Figure 1A**; HR: 1.62 95% CI 0.90-2.93; $P = 0.055$). There was no difference in survival between wild and mutant EGFR patients in SPP1 low-expression group (**Supplementary Figure 1B**; HR: 1.17 95%CI 0.56-2.44; $P = 0.662$).

TABLE 1 | The clinical characteristics of patients in TCGA.

	Total	SPP1 low expression	SPP1 high expression	P-value
Patients	477	238	239	–
Age				0.853
≤65	224 (49%)	111 (48%)	113 (50%)	
>65	234 (51%)	119 (52%)	115 (50%)	
Gender				0.967
female	260 (55%)	129 (54%)	131 (55%)	
male	217 (45%)	109 (46%)	108 (45%)	
Stage				0.291
stageI	257 (55%)	138 (59%)	119 (51%)	
stageII	109 (23%)	51 (22%)	58 (25%)	
stageIII	78 (17%)	33 (14%)	45 (19%)	
stageIV	25 (5%)	12 (5%)	13 (6%)	
T stage				0.38
T1	159 (34%)	86 (36%)	73 (31%)	
T2	255 (54%)	120 (51%)	135 (57%)	
T3+T4	60 (13%)	30 (13%)	30 (13%)	
N stage				0.005
N0	307 (66%)	169 (73%)	138 (59%)	
N1	87 (19%)	34 (15%)	53 (23%)	
N2+N3	71 (15%)	28 (12%)	43 (18%)	
M stage				0.349
M0	324 (68%)	155 (66%)	169 (71%)	
M1	24 (5%)	11 (5%)	13 (5%)	
Mx	125 (26%)	69 (29%)	56 (24%)	
EGFR				0.176
wild	409 (87%)	210 (89%)	199 (84%)	
mutation	63 (13%)	26 (11%)	37 (16%)	

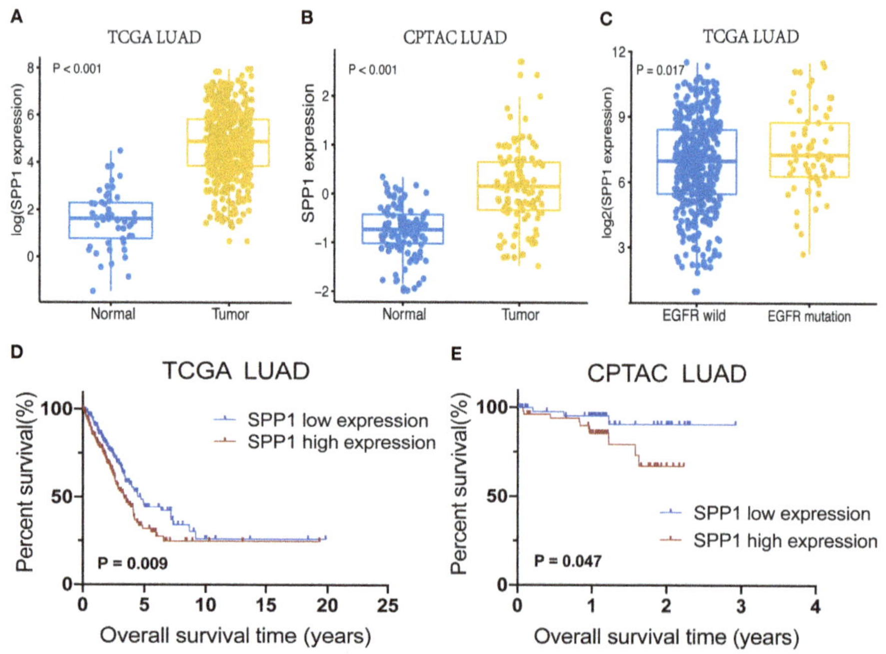

FIGURE 2 | SPP1 expression differences and survival outcomes in LUAD. **(A)** SPP1 RNA expression levels in Normal *vs*. Tumor samples. **(B)** Expression of SPP1 protein in Normal *vs*. Tumor samples. **(C)** SPP1 RNA expression in EGFR wild-type *vs*. EGFR mutant samples. **(D)** Kaplan–Meier survival curves for high and low SPP1 expression groups in TCGA. **(E)** Kaplan–Meier survival curves for high and low SPP1 expression groups in CPTAC.

Identification of Independent Prognostic Factors

A Cox proportional hazards model including differentiation age, gender, stage, T stage, N stage, EGFR status and SPP1 expression was used. The resulted of univariate and multivariate analysis revealed that different SPP1 expression in patients was significantly associated with OS. Moreover, early tumor stage, and T stage are also the independent factors of favorable prognosis (**Figures 3A, B**).

SPP1 Expression Mediates Immune Escape

To interrogate potential signaling pathways related to SPP1 gene in LUAD, we used GSEA analysis (**Figure 4**). We found that the high SPP1 expression group was significantly associated with extracellular matrix (ECM) receptor interaction (NES = 1.737, $P = 0.028$), Fc gamma r mediated phagocytosis (NES = 1.813, $P = 0.010$), glycolysis and gluconeogenesis (NES = 1.770, $P = 0.006$), and the Toll like receptor (TLR) signaling pathway (NES = 2.025, $P < 0.001$). Meanwhile, GO analysis showed that the high SPP1 expression group was positively associated with integrin-mediated cell adhesion (NES = 2.008, $P < 0.001$), interleukin 6 production (NES = 1.960, $P < 0.001$), Nik Nf-Kappa B (NF-κB) signaling (NES – 1.961, P – 0.044), and phagocytosis (NES = 2.043, $P < 0.001$).

Effect of SPP1 on TME

Previous analyses suggested that TICs could be markers of response to ICIs in several cancers (28). In this study, we examined how EGFR mutation and SPP1 expression are related to immune infiltration in LUAD. TCGA LUAD tumor samples (n = 477) were analyzed by CIBERSORT and 368 cases in the wild-type group and 63 cases in the mutant group met the CIBERSORT screening criteria. The results showed that EGFR mutations contribute to reducing the infiltration of CD4+ T cells, CD8+ T cells, M1 macrophages and other immune effector cells in the TME (**Figure 5A**). Taken together, these results indicate that EGFR mutations confer immunosuppressive effects. Additionally, 207 cases in the SPP1 low-expression group and 233 cases in the SPP1 high-expression group met the screening criteria. The results show that high SPP1 expression may play a role in regulating macrophage polarization to the M2 phenotype, reducing TICs such as CD8+ T cells, B cells, follicular helper T cells, NK cells, and activated dendritic cells (**Figure 5B**). These results support the contentions that SPP1 promotes host tumor immune tolerance and immune escape. The correlation heat map (**Figure 5C**) reveals that the different TIC subpopulations are weakly or moderately correlated. Subgroup analysis showed that the proportion of CD8+ T cells infiltration was the highest in patients with wild-type EGFR in SPP1 low-expression group, and the lowest in patients with EGFR mutation in SPP1 high-expression group (**Figure 5D**, P < 0.001). The infiltration of

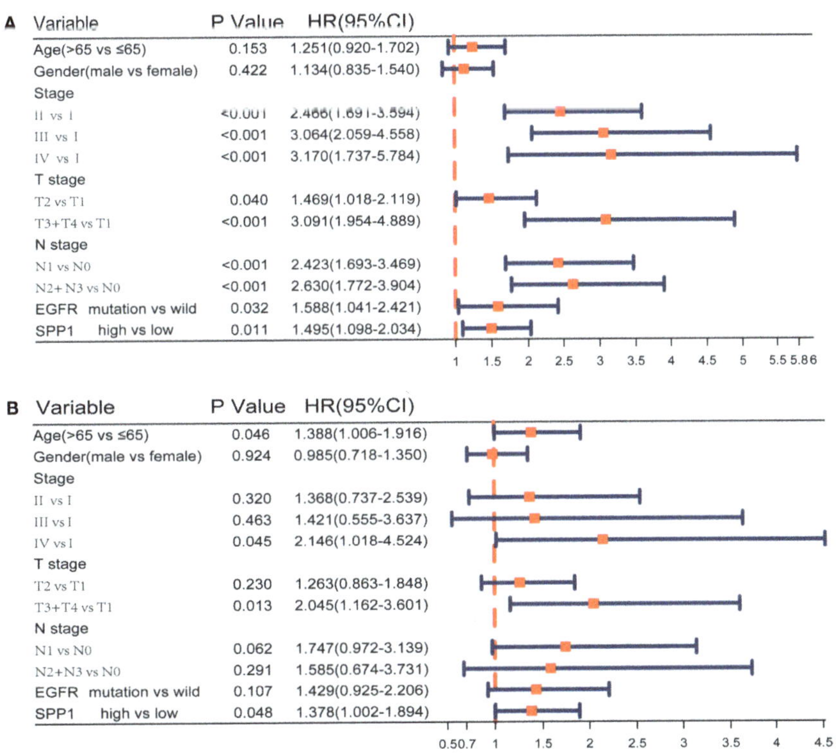

FIGURE 3 | SPP1 was an independent prognostic biomarker in TCGA. **(A, B)** Univariate and Multivariate Cox analysis of SPP1 expression and other clinicopathological factors.

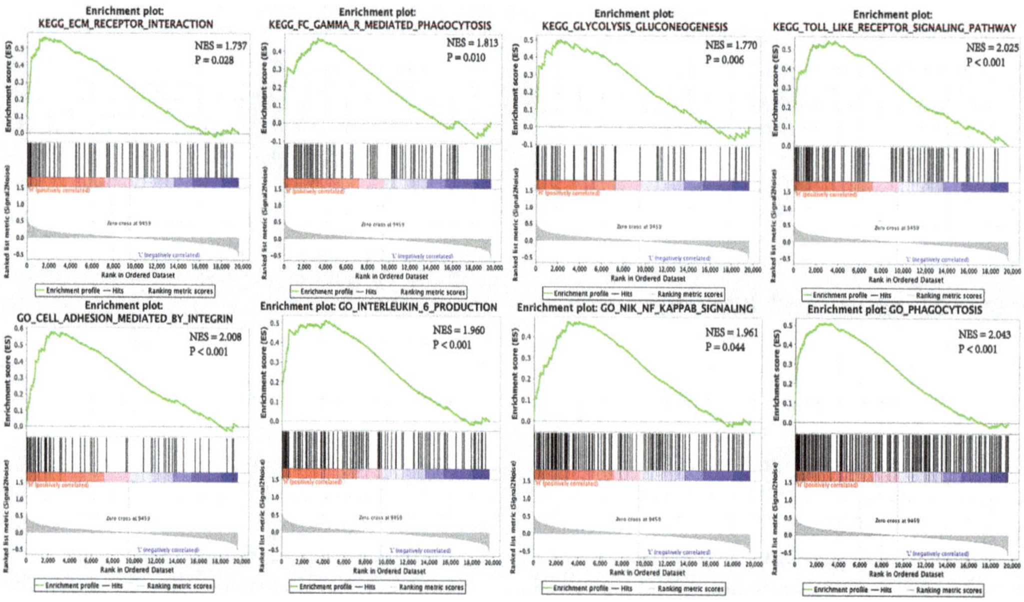

FIGURE 4 | GSEA for high and low SPP1 expression samples.

M2 macrophages was the most in patients with EGFR mutation in SPP1 high-expression group, and the least in patients with wild type EGFR in SPP1 low-expression group (**Figure 5E**, P = 0.071).

xCell results showed that the abundance of CD8+ T cells was less (P = 0.009) and M2 macrophages was more (P = 0.073) in patients with EGFR mutation (**Figure 6A**). There were more CD8+ T cells (P = 0.036) and less M2 macrophages (P = 0.018) in SPP1 low-expression group (**Figure 6B**). The abundance of CD8+ T cells was the highest in EGFR wild-type patients with SPP1 low-expression group (**Figure 6C**). M2-type macrophages in SPP1 high-expression group with EGFR mutation was higher than those of the group with SPP1 low-expression and EGFR wild type (**Figure 6D**, P = 0.073). And we compared CD8 and M2 between the group (SPP1 high and EGFR mutation) and the group (SPP1 low and EGFR wild) in supplement **Figure 2**. Moreover, we found that the SPP1 expression was positively correlated with CD276, especially in patients with EGFR mutation (**Figures 6E–G**).

DISCUSSION

Immunotherapy can eliminate tumor cells through the body's immune system and bring long-term survival benefits to patients with NSCLC, significantly ushering in a new era of antitumor therapy. EGFR mutation is a predictor of the therapeutic effects of EGFR-TKIs in patients with LUAD (2, 3). However, it was once considered as a marker of immune resistance (9, 29–31). Here, we recognized the characteristics of TICs in LUAD using bioinformatics analysis. The immune-tolerant TME is more likely to correlate with patients harboring EGFR mutation. Additionally, the observed outcomes indicate that SPP1 may be a potential indicator for patients nonresponsive to ICIs.

In this study, we showed that the SPP1 expression is significantly higher in LUAD tumor tissues and in patients with EGFR mutation. Several previous studies showed SPP1 expression is directly related to CD8+ T cell activation (32, 33), and M2 macrophage polarization (15). Consistently, we found that SPP1 expression was negatively correlated with CD8+ T cell numbers and positively correlated with M2 macrophage numbers. By applying two methods for immunocyte enrichment or proportion analysis, we can find that M2 macrophages enriched more (CD8+ T cells enriched less) in SPP1 high group or EGFR mutation group, and the phenomenon seems more obvious in the group with both SPP1 high and EGFR mutation, which indicated that tumors with both SPP1 high and EGFR mutation tend to show immune evasion phenotype. Therefore, we speculate that SPP1 might cause immune resistance in NSCLC with EGFR mutation.

OPN involved in many physiological and pathological processes, including inflammatory, angiogenesis, tumor metastasis, immune suppression in TME (34, 35). GSEA analysis results indicate the involvement of extracellular matrix (ECM) receptor interaction, Fc gamma r mediated phagocytosis, TLR signaling pathway, integrin- mediated cell adhesion, interleukin 6 production, NF-κB signaling, and phagocytosis in the high SPP1 expression group. OPN is an important component of ECM, regulating matrix interactions and cell adhesion (13). It plays a key role in tumor cell migration by interacting with integrins and CD44 (36). The interaction between OPN and CD44 transmembrane glycoprotein

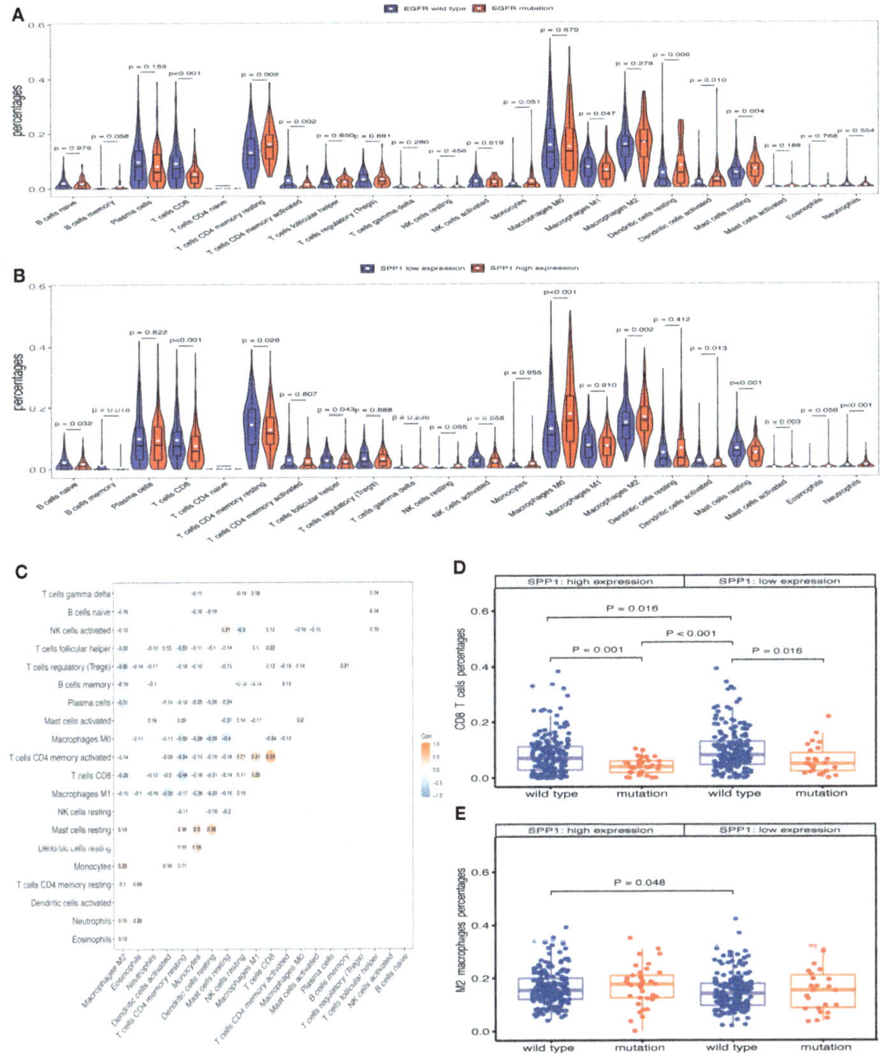

FIGURE 5 | SPP1-related immune infiltration alteration. **(A)** Violin plot showing the ratio differentiation of 22 kinds of TICs in EGFR wild-type and mutant samples. Wilcoxon rank sum was used for the significance test. **(B)** Violin plot showing the ratio differentiation of 22 kinds of TICs in low and high SPP1 expression groups. **(C)** The correlation between different TICs subpopulations. **(D)** Differences in CD8+ T cells infiltration between EGFR mutation and wild-type patients with SPP1 high- or low-expression group. **(E)** Differences in M2 macrophages infiltration between EGFR mutation and wild-type patients with SPP1 high- or low-expression group.

suppressed the CD8+ T cell activation and IFN-γ production. OPN regulation by TLR and NF-κB signaling can reshape the immune inflammatory environment (37, 38). IL-6 binds to IL-6R and activates the Janus kinase (JAK)-STAT3 pathway and the JAK-SHP-2-mitogen-activated protein (MAP) kinase pathway *via* gp130 (39). Previously, it was shown that activation of the JAK/STAT3 pathway can suppress the immune response (40) and that this pathway is activated in patients with EGFR mutation (41). However, it is not clear whether anti-OPN agents, combined with ICIs, can reverse primary resistance in EGFR mutated NSCLC. Therefore, increased SPP1 expression is consistent with a role in immunosuppression, indicating a possible mechanism through which ICIs is ineffective in EGFR-mutated NSCLC.

Pre-clinical studies, involving co-culture of tumor cells and peripheral blood mononuclear cells, show that combined EGFR-TKI and anti-PD-1 antibody therapies do not produce synergistic tumor cell killing effects (42). Multiple clinical studies of EGFR-TKIs combined with ICIs were terminated due to poor efficacy or severe toxicity (43). As a target antibody of vascular endothelial growth factor (VEGF), bevacizumab not only has the effect of anti-angiogenesis, but promotes T cell activation and invasion in tumor tissues (44). Combined with other immunoregulatory drugs, ICIs could be more efficient for the treatment of EGFR-TKI resistance in patients with EGFR mutation. OPN act as an important chemokine and contributes to immune suppression in human colon cancer and other cancers (14, 30). CIBERSORT analysis indicated a significant relationship between SPP1 expression and

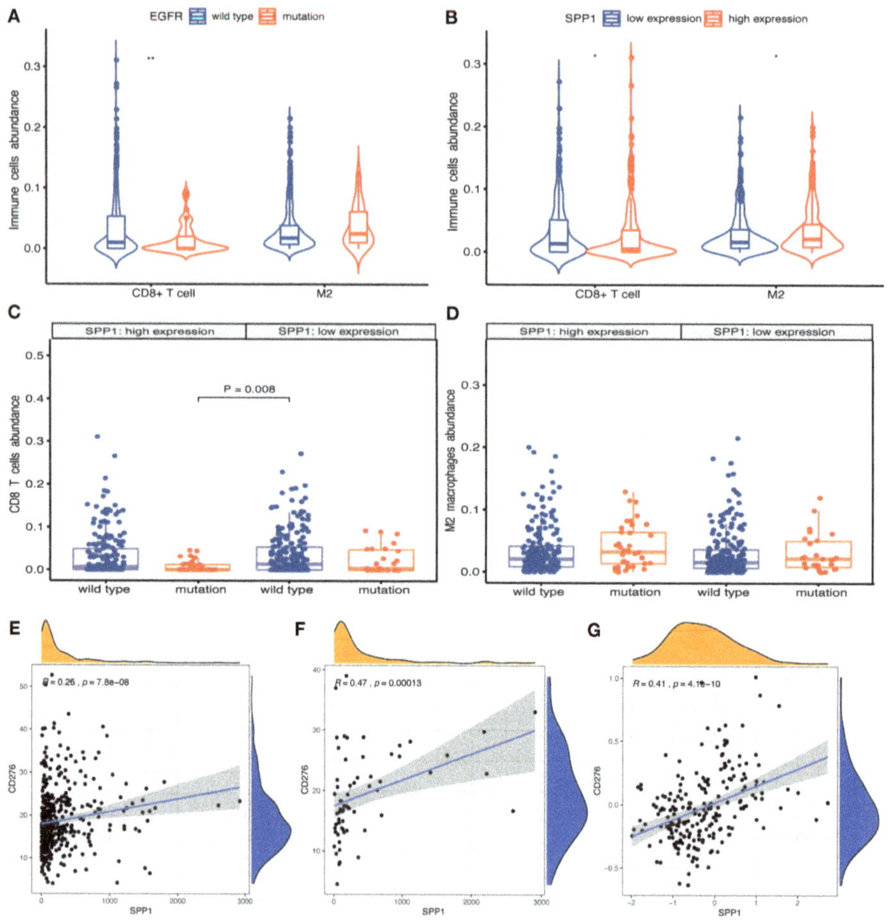

FIGURE 6 | SPP1 promotes immunosuppressive microenvironment in patients with EGFR mutation. **(A)** xCell calculated the abundance of CD8+ T cells and M2 macrophages in EGFR wild-type and mutant samples. **(B)** The abundance of CD8+ T cells and M2 macrophages in different SPP1 expression groups were evaluated by xCell. **(C)** Differences in CD8+ T cells abundance between EGFR mutation and wild-type patients with SPP1 high- or low-expression group. **(D)** Differences in M2 macrophages abundance between EGFR mutation and wild-type patients with SPP1 high- or low-expression group. **(E)** The expression of SPP1 was correlated with CD276 in EGFR wild-type patients at mRNA level. **(F)** The expression of SPP1 was correlated with CD276 in EGFR mutation patients at mRNA level. **(G)** The expression of SPP1 was correlated with CD276 at the protein level. *P < 0.05, **P < 0.01.

increased levels of M2 macrophages infiltration, and reduced CD8 + T cell, activated NK cell and activated dendritic cell infiltration. Furthermore, the similarities between CD276 and other immune checkpoints (PD-1/PD-L1, CTLA4) have led to the targeting of CD276 in novel immunotherapy strategy (16, 17). We propose that a combination regimen using anti-OPN and ICIs may be a promising treatment option for LUAD with EGFR mutation, especially with high expression of SPP1. However, further studies should be conducted.

In summary, differences in TICs in patients with EGFR mutation and those with wild-type LUAD may affect the efficacy of ICIs. We observed that LUAD with EGFR mutated have less infiltration of anti-tumor immune cells, including CD8+ T cells, activated CD4+ T cells and M1 macrophages, and increased M2 macrophages infiltration. However, SPP1 likely has an essential influence on TICs, though combined with anti-OPN therapy, has the potential to reverse immune resistance in LUAD with EGFR mutation.

AUTHOR CONTRIBUTIONS

YaZ and SH found the clinical problem and proposed the research direction. YiZ made use of the public databases for bioinformatics analysis. CX and YH searched literatures and analyzed data results. YS and QZ contributed to the original writing of the manuscript and data consolidation. YYZ and MZ undertook the task of modifying the manuscript. All authors contributed to the article and approved the submitted version.

SUPPLEMENTARY MATERIAL

Supplementary Figure 1 | Effects of EGFR mutation and wild-type on prognosis of LUAD in different SPP1 expression groups in TCGA database. **(A)** Prognosis comparison of EGFR wild-type and mutant patients in SPP1 high expression group. **(B)** Prognosis comparison of EGFR wild-type and mutant patients in SPP1 low expression group.

Supplementary Figure 2 | CD8+ T cells and M2 macrophage differed between groups with high SPP1 expression and EGFR mutation and those with low SPP1 expression and wild-type EGFR. **(A)** Differences in CD8+ T cells infiltration calculated by CIBERSORT between SPP1 high-expression with EGFR mutation and SPP1 low-expression with EGFR wild type. **(B)** Differences in M2 macrophages infiltration calculated by CIBERSORT between SPP1 high-expression with EGFR mutation and SPP1 low-expression with EGFR wild type. **(C)** The difference in CD8+ T cells abundance assessed by xCell was compared between the group of SPP1 high-expression with EGFR mutation and SPP1 low-expression with EGFR wild type samples. **(D)** The difference in M2 macrophage abundance assessed by xCell was compared between the group of SPP1 high-expression with EGFR mutation and SPP1 low-expression with EGFR wild type samples.

REFERENCES

1. Bray F, Ferlay J, Soerjomataram I, Siegel RL, Torre LA, Jemal A. Global Cancer Statistics 2018: GLOBOCAN Estimates of Incidence and Mortality Worldwide for 36 Cancers in 185 Countries. *CA Cancer J Clin* (2018) 68:394–424. doi: 10.3322/caac.21492
2. Han JY, Park K, Kim SW, Lee DH, Kim HY, Kim HT, et al. First-SIGNAL: First-Line Single-Agent Iressa Versus Gemcitabine and Cisplatin Trial in Never-Smokers With Adenocarcinoma of the Lung. *J Clin Oncol* (2012) 30:1122–8. doi: 10.1200/JCO.2011.36.8456
3. Shi YK, Wang L, Han BH, Li W, Yu P, Liu YP, et al. First-Line Icotinib Versus Cisplatin/Pemetrexed Plus Pemetrexed Maintenance Therapy for Patients With Advanced EGFR Mutation-Positive Lung Adenocarcinoma (CONVINCE): A Phase 3, Open-Label, Randomized Study. *Ann Oncol* (2017) 28:2443–50. doi: 10.1093/annonc/mdx359
4. Lu X, Yu L, Zhang Z, Ren X, Smaill JB, Ding K. Targeting EGFR(L858R/T790M) and EGFR(L858R/T790M/C797S) Resistance Mutations in NSCLC: Current Developments in Medicinal Chemistry. *Med Res Rev* (2018) 38:1550–81. doi: 10.1002/med.21488
5. Reck M, Rodriguez-Abreu D, Robinson AG, Hui R, Csoszi T, Fulop A, et al. Pembrolizumab Versus Chemotherapy for PD-L1-Positive Non-Small-Cell Lung Cancer. *N Engl J Med* (2016) 375:1823–33. doi: 10.1056/NEJMoa1606774
6. Tomasini P, Greillier L, Boyer A, Jeanson A, Barlesi F. Durvalumab After Chemoradiotherapy in Stage III Non-Small Cell Lung Cancer. *J Thorac Dis* (2018) 10:S1032–S36. doi: 10.21037/jtd.2018.04.61
7. Ribas A, Wolchok JD. Cancer Immunotherapy Using Checkpoint Blockade. *Science* (2018) 359:1350–55. doi: 10.1126/science.aar4060
8. Garassino MC, Cho BC, Kim JH, Mazieres J, Vansteenkiste J, Lena H, et al. Durvalumab as Third-Line or Later Treatment for Advanced non-Small-Cell Lung Cancer (ATLANTIC): An Open-Label, Single-Arm, Phase 2 Study. *Lancet Oncol* (2018) 19:521–36. doi: 10.1016/S1470-2045(18)30144-X
9. Gainor JF, Shaw AT, Sequist LV, Fu X, Azzoli CG, Piotrowska Z, et al. Egfr Mutations and ALK Rearrangements Are Associated With Low Response Rates to PD-1 Pathway Blockade in Non-Small Cell Lung Cancer: A Retrospective Analysis. *Clin Cancer Res* (2016) 22:4585–93. doi: 10.1158/1078-0432.CCR-15-3101
10. Haratani K, Hayashi H, Tanaka T, Kaneda H, Togashi Y, Sakai K, et al. Tumor Immune Microenvironment and Nivolumab Efficacy in EGFR Mutation-Positive Non-Small-Cell Lung Cancer Based on T790M Status After Disease Progression During EGFR-TKI Treatment. *Ann Oncol* (2017) 28:1532–39. doi: 10.1093/annonc/mdx183
11. Socinski MA, Jotte RM, Cappuzzo F, Orlandi F, Stroyakovskiy D, Nogami N, et al. Atezolizumab for First-Line Treatment of Metastatic Nonsquamous Nsclc. *N Engl J Med* (2018) 378:2288–301. doi: 10.1056/NEJMoa1716948
12. Sugiyama E, Togashi Y, Takeuchi Y, Shinya S, Tada Y, Kataoka K, et al. Blockade of EGFR Improves Responsiveness to PD-1 Blockade in EGFR-mutated Non-Small Cell Lung Cancer. *Sci Immunol* (2020) 5:eaav3937. doi: 10.1126/sciimmunol.aav3937
13. Lamort AS, Giopanou I, Psallidas I, Stathopoulos GT. Osteopontin as a Link Between Inflammation and Cancer: The Thorax in the Spotlight. *Cells* (2019) 8:815. doi: 10.3390/cells8080815
14. Anborgh PH, Mutrie JC, Tuck AB, Chambers AF. Role of the Metastasis-Promoting Protein Osteopontin in the Tumour Microenvironment. *J Cell Mol Med* (2010) 14:2037–44. doi: 10.1111/j.1582-4934.2010.01115.x
15. Zhang Y, Du W, Chen Z, Xiang C. Upregulation of PD-L1 by SPP1 Mediates Macrophage Polarization and Facilitates Immune Escape in Lung Adenocarcinoma. *Exp Cell Res* (2017) 359:449–57. doi: 10.1016/j.yexcr.2017.08.028
16. Castellanos JR, Purvis IJ, Labak CM, Guda MR, Tsung AJ, Velpula KK, et al. B7-H3 Role in the Immune Landscape of Cancer. *Am J Clin Exp Immunol* (2017) 6:66–75.
17. Picarda E, Ohaegbulam KC, Zang X. Molecular Pathways: Targeting B7-H3 (CD276) for Human Cancer Immunotherapy. *Clin Cancer Res* (2016) 22:3425–31. doi: 10.1158/1078-0432.CCR-15-2428
18. Kontos F, Michelakos T, Kurokawa T, Sadagopan A, Schwab JH, Ferrone CR, et al. B7-H3: An Attractive Target for Antibody-Based Immunotherapy. *Clin Cancer Res* (2021) 27:1227–35. doi: 10.1158/1078-0432.CCR-20-2584
19. Tomczak K, Czerwinska P, Wiznerowicz M. The Cancer Genome Atlas (TCGA): An Immeasurable Source of Knowledge. *Contemp Oncol (Pozn)* (2015) 19:A68–77. doi: 10.5114/wo.2014.47136
20. Liu J, Lichtenberg T, Hoadley KA, Poisson LM, Lazar AJ, Cherniack AD, et al. An Integrated Tcga Pan-Cancer Clinical Data Resource to Drive High-Quality Survival Outcome Analytics. *Cell* (2018) 173:400–16.e11. doi: 10.1016/j.cell.2018.02.052
21. Rudnick PA, Markey SP, Roth J, Mirokhin Y, Yan X, Tchekhovskoi DV, et al. A Description of the Clinical Proteomic Tumor Analysis Consortium (CPTAC) Common Data Analysis Pipeline. *J Proteome Res* (2016) 15:1023–32. doi: 10.1021/acs.jproteome.5b01091
22. Whiteaker JR, Halusa GN, Hoofnagle AN, Sharma V, MacLean B, Yan P, et al. Cptac Assay Portal: A Repository of Targeted Proteomic Assays. *Nat Methods* (2014) 11:703–4. doi: 10.1038/nmeth.3002
23. Goldman M, Craft B, Swatloski T, Cline M, Morozova O, Diekhans M, et al. The UCSC Cancer Genomics Browser: Update 2015. *Nucleic Acids Res* (2015) 43:D812–7. doi: 10.1093/nar/gku1073
24. Petitprez F, Vano YA, Becht E, Giraldo NA, de Reynies A, Sautes-Fridman C, et al. Transcriptomic Analysis of the Tumor Microenvironment to Guide Prognosis and Immunotherapies. *Cancer Immunol Immunother* (2018) 67:981–88. doi: 10.1007/s00262-017-2058-z
25. Chen B, Khodadoust MS, Liu CL, Newman AM, Alizadeh AA. Profiling Tumor Infiltrating Immune Cells With CIBERSORT. *Methods Mol Biol* (2018) 1711:243–59. doi: 10.1007/978-1-4939-7493-1_12
26. Aran D, Hu Z, Butte AJ. xCell: Digitally Portraying the Tissue Cellular Heterogeneity Landscape. *Genome Biol* (2017) 18:220. doi: 10.1186/s13059-017-1349-1
27. Li T, Fan J, Wang B, Traugh N, Chen Q, Liu JS, et al. Timer: A Web Server for Comprehensive Analysis of Tumor-Infiltrating Immune Cells. *Cancer Res* (2017) 77:e108–e10. doi: 10.1158/0008-5472.CAN-17-0307
28. Klauschen F, Muller KR, Binder A, Bockmayr M, Hagele M, Seegerer P, et al. Scoring of Tumor-Infiltrating Lymphocytes: From Visual Estimation to Machine Learning. *Semin Cancer Biol* (2018) 52:151–57. doi: 10.1016/j.semcancer.2018.07.001
29. Dong ZY, Zhang JT, Liu SY, Su J, Zhang C, Xie Z, et al. EGFR Mutation Correlates With Uninflamed Phenotype and Weak Immunogenicity, Causing Impaired Response to PD-1 Blockade in Non-Small Cell Lung Cancer. *Oncoimmunology* (2017) 6:e1356145. doi: 10.1080/2162402X.2017.1356145
30. Li HY, McSharry M, Bullock B, Nguyen TT, Kwak J, Poczobutt JM, et al. The Tumor Microenvironment Regulates Sensitivity of Murine Lung Tumors to PD-1/PD-L1 Antibody Blockade. *Cancer Immunol Res* (2017) 5:767–77. doi: 10.1158/2326-6066.CIR-16-0365
31. Jia Y, Li X, Jiang T, Zhao S, Zhao C, Zhang L, et al. EGFR-Targeted Therapy Alters the Tumor Microenvironment in EGFR-Driven Lung Tumors: Implications for Combination Therapies. *Int J Cancer* (2019) 145:1432–44. doi: 10.1002/ijc.32191
32. Klement JD, Paschall AV, Redd PS, Ibrahim ML, Lu C, Yang D, et al. An Osteopontin/CD44 Immune Checkpoint Controls CD8+ T Cell Activation and Tumor Immune Evasion. *J Clin Invest* (2018) 128:5549–60. doi: 10.1172/JCI123360

33. Wei J, Marisetty A, Schrand B, Gabrusiewicz K, Hashimoto Y, Ott M, et al. Osteopontin Mediates Glioblastoma-Associated Macrophage Infiltration and is a Potential Therapeutic Target. *J Clin Invest* (2019) 129:137–49. doi: 10.1172/JCI121266
34. Denhardt DT, Noda M, O'Regan AW, Pavlin D, Berman JS. Osteopontin as a Means to Cope With Environmental Insults: Regulation of Inflammation, Tissue Remodeling, and Cell Survival. *J Clin Invest* (2001) 107(9):1055–61. doi: 10.1172/JCI12980
35. Pang X, Gong K, Zhang X, Wu S, Cui Y, Qian BZ. Osteopontin as a Multifaceted Driver of Bone Metastasis and Drug Resistance. *Pharmacol Res* (2019) 144:235–44. doi: 10.1016/j.phrs.2019.04.030
36. Maeda N, Maenaka K. The Roles of Matricellular Proteins in Oncogenic Virus-Induced Cancers and Their Potential Utilities as Therapeutic Targets. *Int J Mol Sci* (2017) 18:2198. doi: 10.3390/ijms18102198
37. Salvi V, Scutera S, Rossi S, Zucca M, Alessandria M, Greco D, et al. Dual Regulation of Osteopontin Production by TLR Stimulation in Dendritic Cells. *J Leukoc Biol* (2013) 94:147–58. doi: 10.1189/jlb.0412194
38. Friedmann-Morvinski D, Narasimamurthy R, Xia Y, Myskiw C, Soda Y, Verma IM. Targeting NF-kappaB in Glioblastoma: A Therapeutic Approach. *Sci Adv* (2016) 2:e1501292. doi: 10.1126/sciadv.1501292
39. Tanaka T, Narazaki M, Kishimoto T. IL-6 in Inflammation, Immunity, and Disease. *Cold Spring Harb Perspect Biol* (2014) 6:a016295. doi: 10.1101/cshperspect.a016295
40. Yu H, Pardoll D, Jove R. Stats in Cancer Inflammation and Immunity: A Leading Role for STAT3. *Nat Rev Cancer* (2009) 9:798–809. doi: 10.1038/nrc2734
41. Gao SP, Mark KG, Leslie K, Pao W, Motoi N, Gerald WL, et al. Mutations in the EGFR Kinase Domain Mediate STAT3 Activation Via IL-6 Production in Human Lung Adenocarcinomas. *J Clin Invest* (2007) 117:3846–56. doi: 10.1172/JCI31871
42. Chen N, Fang W, Zhan J, Hong S, Tang Y, Kang S, et al. Upregulation of PD-L1 by EGFR Activation Mediates the Immune Escape in EGFR-Driven NSCLC: Implication for Optional Immune Targeted Therapy for NSCLC Patients With EGFR Mutation. *J Thorac Oncol* (2015) 10:910–23. doi: 10.1097/JTO.0000000000000500
43. Ahn MJ, Sun JM, Lee SH, Ahn JS, Park K. Egfr TKI Combination With Immunotherapy in Non-Small Cell Lung Cancer. *Expert Opin Drug Saf* (2017) 16:465–69. doi: 10.1080/14740338.2017.1300656
44. Voron T, Marcheteau E, Pernot S, Colussi O, Tartour E, Taieb J, et al. Control of the Immune Response by Pro-Angiogenic Factors. *Front Oncol* (2014) 4:70. doi: 10.3389/fonc.2014.00070

Overall Survival in Heart Disease–Related Death in Non-Small Cell Lung Cancer Patients: Nonimmunotherapy Versus Immunotherapy Era

Mohammed Safi[1], Ravindran Kanesvaran[2], Mohammed Alradhi[3†], Abdullah Al-Danakh[1†], Feng Ping[1], Najeeb Al-Sabai[4], Xiu Shan[1] and Jiwei Liu[1*]*

[1] Department of Oncology, First Affiliated Hospital of Dalian Medical University, Dalian, China, [2] National Cancer Center Singapore, Singapore General Hospital, Singapore, Singapore, [3] Department of Urology, Second Affiliated Hospital of Dalian Medical University, Dalian, China, [4] Dalian Medical University, Medical School, Dalian, China

***Correspondence:**
Jiwei Liu
liujiwei@dmu.edu.cn
Xiu Shan
shanxiudl@163.com

† These authors have contributed equally to this work and share first authorship

The cardiotoxicity during immunotherapy administration leads to mortality by more than 42% and heart disease–related mortality among immunotherapy-linked cancers is still considered to be underestimated. In this study, the advanced stage of non-small cell lung cancer (NSCLC) with heart disease–related death was selected in accordance with immunotherapy approval time. NSCLC was searched on the Surveillance, Epidemiology, and End Results (SEER) program. Results show that 538 advanced NSCLC cases, those dominated by men and elderly people aged more than 70 years, had a high percentage of heart disease–related death in both eras. The difference between contemporary groups was fairly nonsignificant ($P = > 0.05$). The overall survival (OS) of all-cause mortality difference showed improved survival in the immunotherapy group ($P = 0.0001$). In the study of heart disease–related death survival with adjusted data, the NSCLC patients show significant lower survival in the immunotherapy era compared with the nonimmunotherapy era ($P = 0.003$; hazard ratio [HR] = 1.31; 95% CI = 1.099–1.57). In the multivariate analysis of NSCLC-related immunotherapy, histology revealed that the non-squamous cell type had an independent risk for lower OS than the squamous cell type ($P = 0.04$; HR= 0.74; CI = 0, 55- 0.99). The results demonstrate the survival benefits for NSCLC in immunotherapy; however, in heart disease–related death, immunotherapy in patients with NSCLC shows decreased OS. This study highlights that NSCLC patients should be highly monitored during immunotherapy administration, and further assessment is needed.

Keywords: non-small cell lung cancer, immunotherapy, SEER database, cardiotoxicity, heart diseases

INTRODUCTION

The U.S. Food and Drug Administration (FDA) has approved several immunotherapeutic drugs for cancer since 2010, and many more are still being evaluated in other clinical studies to remarkably increase the response and survival rates of patients with advanced cancer (1). Unfortunately, cancer immunotherapies possess potential toxicity that is distinctive from other types of care, mostly due to their etiology. The occurrence of cardiovascular adverse events is particularly challenging to cancer management and has led to various clinical outcomes, ranging from cardiogenic shock to death (2).

Improving clinical effectiveness should be weighed against potentially dangerous adverse events when selecting immunotherapy plans and comparatively evaluating each related adverse event separately. Even though the incidence of cardiotoxicity-linked immunotherapy is rare, recent studies have implied its underestimation and needs to be reconsidered. In addition, an urgent intervention must be planned to reduce the mortality rate associated with adverse effects (3, 4). More studies that aim to create thorough risk and etiological stratification models and identify pathways that specify this toxicity clause are needed to improve the early prevention, detection, and treatment approach (5).

Recent studies suggest a particular increased incidence of cardiovascular toxicity in lung cancer patients among all based immunotherapies cancers (6), and the evidence of OS of heart disease–related death for NSCLC patients is still lacking. In addition to the nonimmunotherapy era, this study explains the survival variability of the differences in cardiac-related death among NSCLC patients by using the SEER database.

PATIENT AND METHODS

Study Cohorts

Patient data were collected from the latest 2018 registry with additional treatment fields on SEER Stat software (version 8.3.6). Using the sixth edition of AJCC, the appropriate codes for advanced lung cancer (IIIB, IV) were selected as labeled site codes (C34/1, 2, 3, and C61.6, respectively). In addition to the period's equality, the same era of the major targeted therapy of tyrosine kinase inhibitors, 2007, was selected as a year of insurance availability in the database when studying the effects of variables in patients with advanced NSCLC compared with 2015 (7). All patients were designated based on the type of follow-up (active follow-up), and only microscopically confirmed cases (positive histology and positive exfoliative cytology, positive histology and immunophenotyping and/or postgenetic studies, and positive microscopic nonspecified method) were included. The following variables were selected: age (20 years or more), COD to site rec KM, year of diagnosis according to contemporary intervals, ICD-0-3 hist/behav, all survival months, grade (I–II, III–IV, or others), sex (male or female), race (white, black, or others), radiation (radiation or others), chemotherapy (yes or no), vital status record, laterality (right, left, or others), ID patients, marital and insurance statuses (yes or others). The detailed inclusion and exclusion criteria are summarized in **Figure 1**.

In addition to excluding small cell types in advanced lung cancer, patients with heart diseases as the cause of death were included with known survival of 20 months as the cutoff value. The baseline demographics of patients were compared using the x^2 test, and the follow-up cutoff value was limited to 20 months,

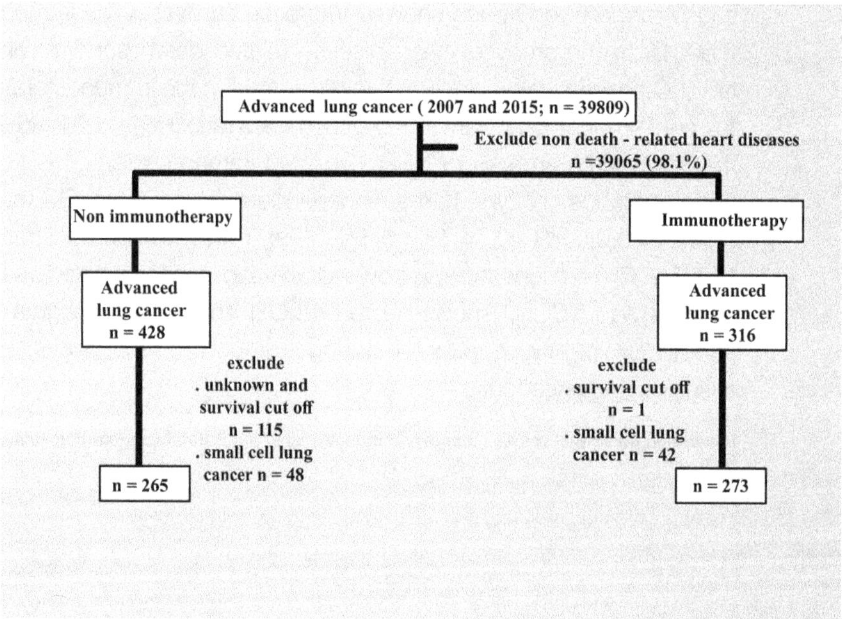

FIGURE 1 | Diagram of exclusion and inclusion criteria.

TABLE 1 | Characteristics of heart disease–related death NSCLC patients.

Parameters	Nonimmunotherapy n = 265(%)	Immunotherapy n = 273(%)	P value
Age			0.6
20-69	98 (37)	107(39.2)	
>70	167(63)	166(60.8)	
Sex			0.7
Male	170(64.5)	179(65.6)	
Female	95(35.8)	94(34.4)	
Race			0.3
White	213(80.4)	205(75.1)	
Black	37(14)	47(17.2)	
Others	15(5.7)	21(7.7)	
Marital status			0.3
Yes	130(49.1)	122(44.7)	
Others	135(50.9)	151(55.3)	
Grade			0.3
I-II	59(22.3)	45(16.5)	
III - IV	67(25.3)	94(34.4)	
Unknown	139(52.5)	134(49.1	
Origin			0.5
Left	116(43.8)	113(41.4)	
Right	149(56.2)	160(58.6)	
Others		1	
Histology			0.002
Adenocarcinoma	96(36.2)	134(49.1)	
Squamous cell cancer	79(29.8)	80((29.3)	
others	90(34)	59(21.6)	
Radiation status			0.8
Yes	97(36.6)	98(35.9)	
No	168(63.4)	175(64.1)	
Chemotherapy			0.8
Yes	105(39.6)	106(38.8)	
No	160(60.4)	167(61.2)	
Insurance			0.8
yes	161(60.8)	168(61.5)	
others	104(39.2)	105(38.5)	

depending on the time of advanced NSCLC. Median OS was analyzed using the Kaplan–Meier (KM) method *via* the log-rank test and Cox proportional hazard model for multivariate analysis. Statistical significance was considered at a p value less than 0.05 and limits of 0.0001.

RESULTS

The database contained 538 advanced NSCLC (265 in nonimmunotherapy era vs. 273 in immunotherapy era). The age of over 70 years (e.g., 52% between 75 and 79 years in lung cancer) and male predominance were high in all cases of heart disease–related death in advanced NSCLC, and the distribution of variables was reasonably uniform in both eras ($p > 0.05$). The details of all characteristics are explained in **Table 1**.

The OS difference between the nonimmunotherapy era and the immunotherapy era for advanced NSCLC was statistically significant with the improvement in median survival of the immunotherapy groups (P = 0.0001; median survival: 4 vs. 6 months) (**Figure 2A**). By contrast, when considering only heart disease–related death, the OS in the nonimmunotherapy era was significantly better in advanced NSCLC than that in the immunotherapy era (5 months OS 42% vs. 0.33%; 10 months OS months 21% vs. 13% and median survival 4 vs. 3 months; P = 0.0001), indicating the negative effect of immunotherapy (**Figure 2B**).

In the KM study of NSCLC difference in OS between the variables of nonimmunotherapy and immunotherapy eras, older age and III–IV grades showed a significant difference in median OS (4 vs. 3 months, 4 vs. 2 months, respectively). In addition, a difference was observed among most other variables with survival

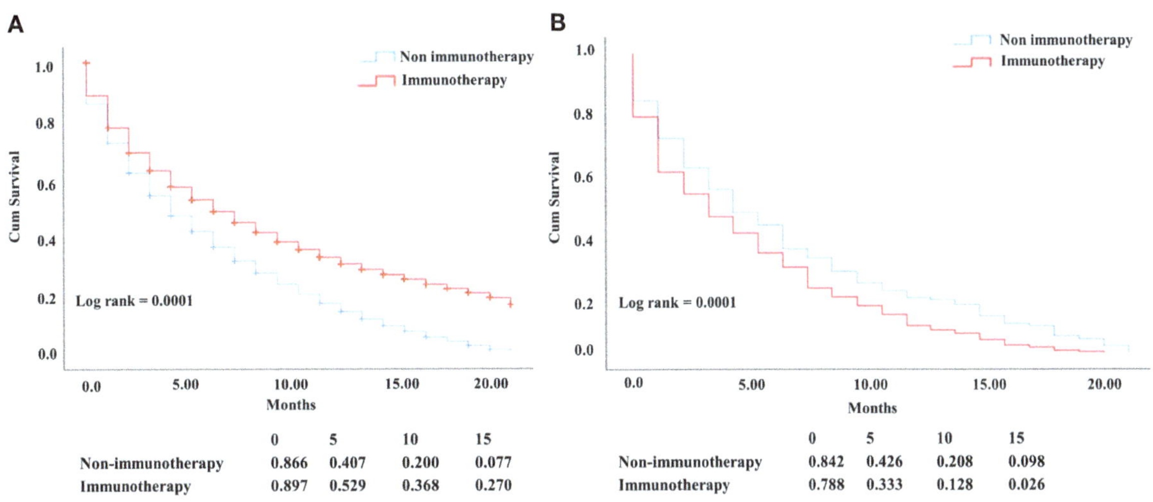

FIGURE 2 | **(A)** KM NSCLC curve comparing OS of all-cause mortality (P= 0.0001). **(B)** OS difference in patients who died from heart diseases with negative OS in the NSCLC immunotherapy era (P = 0.0001).

benefits restricted to patients in the nonimmunotherapy era (e.g., male, female, white, black, laterality, chemotherapy, and radiotherapy status) (**Figure 3**, **Table 2**). The OS in the immunotherapy era was studied, and the results reveal that chemotherapy and radiotherapy use had beneficial significance to OS (P= 0.0001, P = 0.001, respectively) with no preferences of each on other (P = 0.392). In addition, evidence of OS difference was not found in grade, histology, or laterality (P = 0.39, 0.08, 0.49, respectively) (**Figure 4A**). The negative OS of heart disease-related death in the immunotherapy era was still significantly evident after adjusting the data for age, sex, marital status, race, chemotherapy and radiation status, grade, laterality, histology, and insurance status by using Cox regression multivariate analysis (P = 0.003; hazard ratio [HR] = 1.31; 95% CI = 1.099–1.57) (**Figure 4B**).

The multivariate analysis of advanced lung cancer in the immunotherapy era revealed that the nonsquamous type was significant and showed worse survival of cardiac disease-related death patients than the squamous type (HR = 0.74; 95% CI = 0.55–0.99; P = 0.04). Chemotherapy use was not associated with poor OS in cardiac disease-related death (P = < 0.0001; HR= 1.812; CI = 1.37-2.38). Radiotherapy use in advanced lung cancer improved the OS in the nonimmunotherapy era but did not predict the OS in the immunotherapy era, mostly because of the large effect of chemotherapy use in this group, as shown in a separate model (P = 0.005; HR = 1.47; 95% CI = 1.12–1.93 vs. P = 0.06; HR = 1.29; 95% CI = 0.98–1.70) (**Table 3**).

DISCUSSION

The presence of baseline organ dysfunction in patients on immune check inhibitors demonstrates general immune

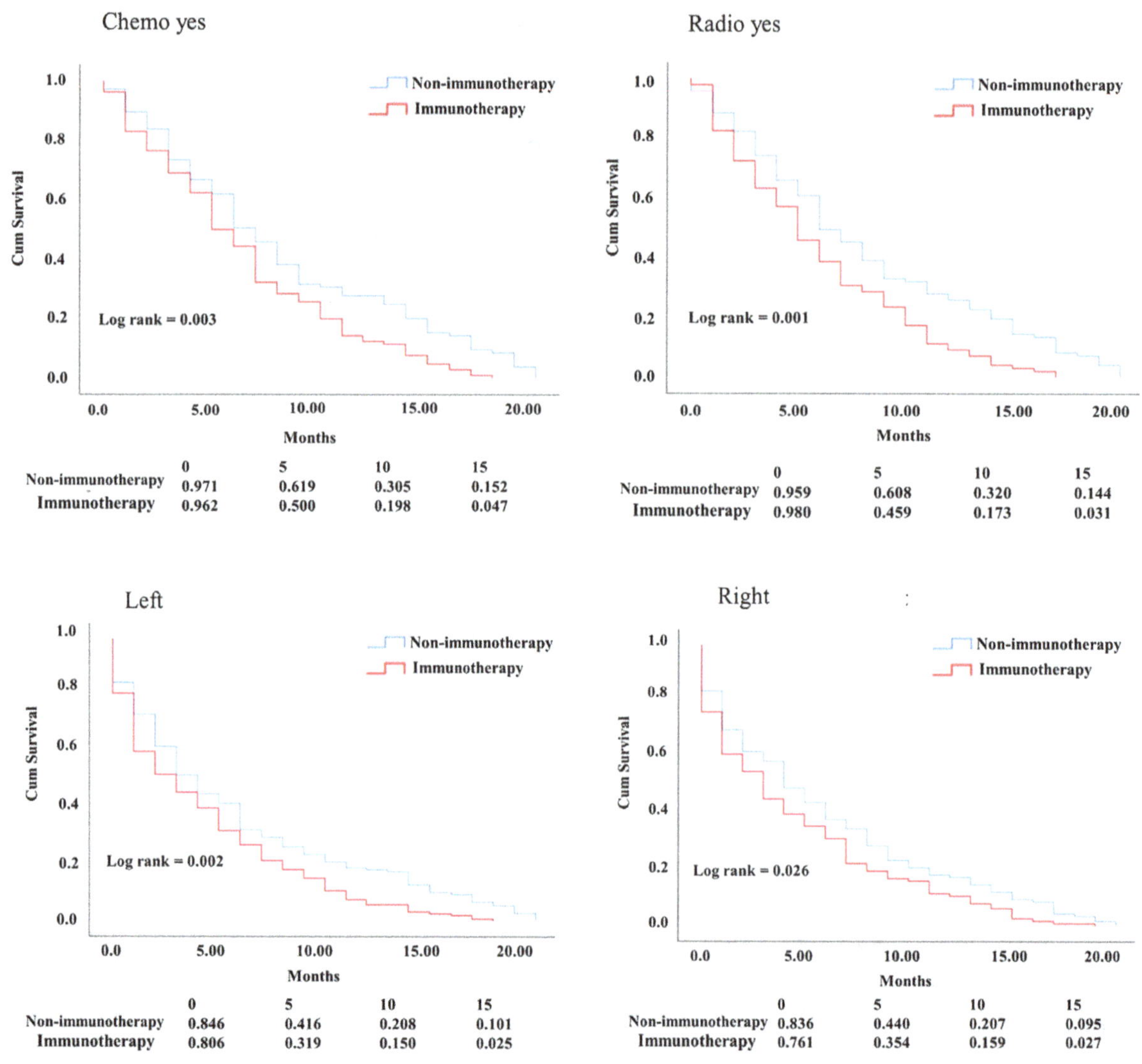

FIGURE 3 | KM curve comparing OS. Factors difference between NSCLC nonimmunotherapy versus immunotherapy era.

TABLE 2 | Survival pattern in heart disease–related death NSCLC patients.

Parameters	Nonimmunotherapy	Immunotherapy	*P* value bylog rank test
Age	median OS (months)	median OS (months)	
20-69	4	4	0.08
>70	4	3	0.001
Sex			
Male	4	3	0.007
Female	5	3	0.007
Race			
White	4	3	0.004
Black	5	3	0.03
Others	4	3	0.1
Marital status			
Yes	4	3	0.002
Others	4	3	0.02
Grade			
I-II	5	3	0.06
III-IV	4	2	0.006
Others	4	3	0.07
Unknown			
Left	4	3	0.02
Right	4	3	0.002
Missed 1			
Histology/ behave			
Adenocarcinoma	3	2	0.2
Squamous cell cancer	4	5	0.1
Others	6	3	0.0002
Radiation status			
Yes	6	5	0.001
No	2	1	0.01
Chemotherapy			
Yes	7	5	0.003
No	2	1	0.006
Insurance status			
Yes	5	3	0.003
No/unknown/ others	4	2	0.01

adverse events similar to those in previous clinical trials that included patients without organ dysfunction (8). Although it is representative of less than 1% of adverse immune events, immune inhibitor-caused myocarditis is a potentially fatal condition associated with 42% mortality (9). However, in general immunotherapy-related cardiotoxicity symptoms, several studies suggest an increase in patients with end organ failure compared with those without organ dysfunction (in both cases of myocarditis or controls without myocarditis) (10). The median time to the presentation of cardiotoxicity-related immunotherapy ranged from 2 to 454 days (23 months), and the majority occurred within the first four cycles of immunotherapy (1st month) (11). To the best knowledge of the authors, the present study was a large unique study that detected the OS of patients who died from heart diseases in the contemporary eras of immunotherapy and nonimmunotherapy NSCLC.

In this decade, many reported clinical trials for immunotherapy in various solid cancer types, including earlier challenging cancers, revealed an increase in OS and considerable strength in the treatment of NSCLC, in either combination or monotherapy (12, 13). The present study, which is a population-based study that used the SEER database, reveals good survival benefits in advanced NSCLC, which were largely attributable to the introduction of immunotherapeutic drugs to therapeutic regimens. Where the median OS increased from 4 to 6 months, this improvement was distinctly lower than those reported by related approved studies (14), However, the latter was predominantly related to the cutoff value for survival with only 20 months in all age groups regardless of their performance status and other comorbidities.

In the study of OS in patients with heart disease–related death, the OS was significantly decreased in the NSCLC immunotherapy era compared with the nonimmunotherapy era. The remaining patients in the first 5 months of survival from NSCLC were markedly lower in the treatment-based immunity era than in the nonimmunity-based era (33% vs. 42%). This finding could be explained by the following: 1) An association between high cardiotoxicity-related mortality rate and immunotherapy exists (15). 2) Regarding the relationship of cardiotoxicity and immunotherapy, most patients present their symptoms shortly after treatment (16). 3) The risk of incidence of major cardiac adverse events is increased in thoracic tumors (17). Except for adenocarcinomas and squamous cell histology of lung cancer, most variables demonstrate significant negative OS in the NSCLC immunotherapy era. In addition, aging is significantly linked to negative OS in patients with NSCLC who died from heart diseases; this finding was also recently shown in a SEER-Medicare study by Bora et al., who report that comorbidities and negative OS are related to old age in NSCLC patients who were started with immune checkpoint inhibitors (18). Recently, several reports indicate that the combining of chemoradiotherapy with immunotherapy has superior efficacy in producing improved anticancer activity (19). In the immunotherapy group of heart disease–related death, chemotherapy and radiotherapy use as monotherapy in advanced NSCLC exhibit improved OS compared with nonuse. In the study difference between radiotherapy and chemotherapy use, no survival significance has been seen. Thereby, the risk of decreased OS in this group was more independently associated with the use of immunotherapy than the synergetic negative effect of other interventions.

Cox multivariate analysis confirms that immunotherapy is a risk predictor for OS in patients who died from heart diseases in the NSCLC immunotherapy era (HR= 1.314; P = 0.003). Even though it was significant in older age based on KM, the difference in age groups demonstrated by the Cox model in the new era of NSCLC did not provide any benefits of survival. In a multicenter retrospective study of the association between age with immune-related events and OS in NSCLC, age was not an independent risk factor of survival (20). Chemotherapy and radiotherapy use was significantly observed in the nonimmunotherapy era as a high predictor of increased OS. By contrast, the use of chemotherapy significantly decreased the risk of heart disease–related death. Radiotherapy use was not a risk factor for survival

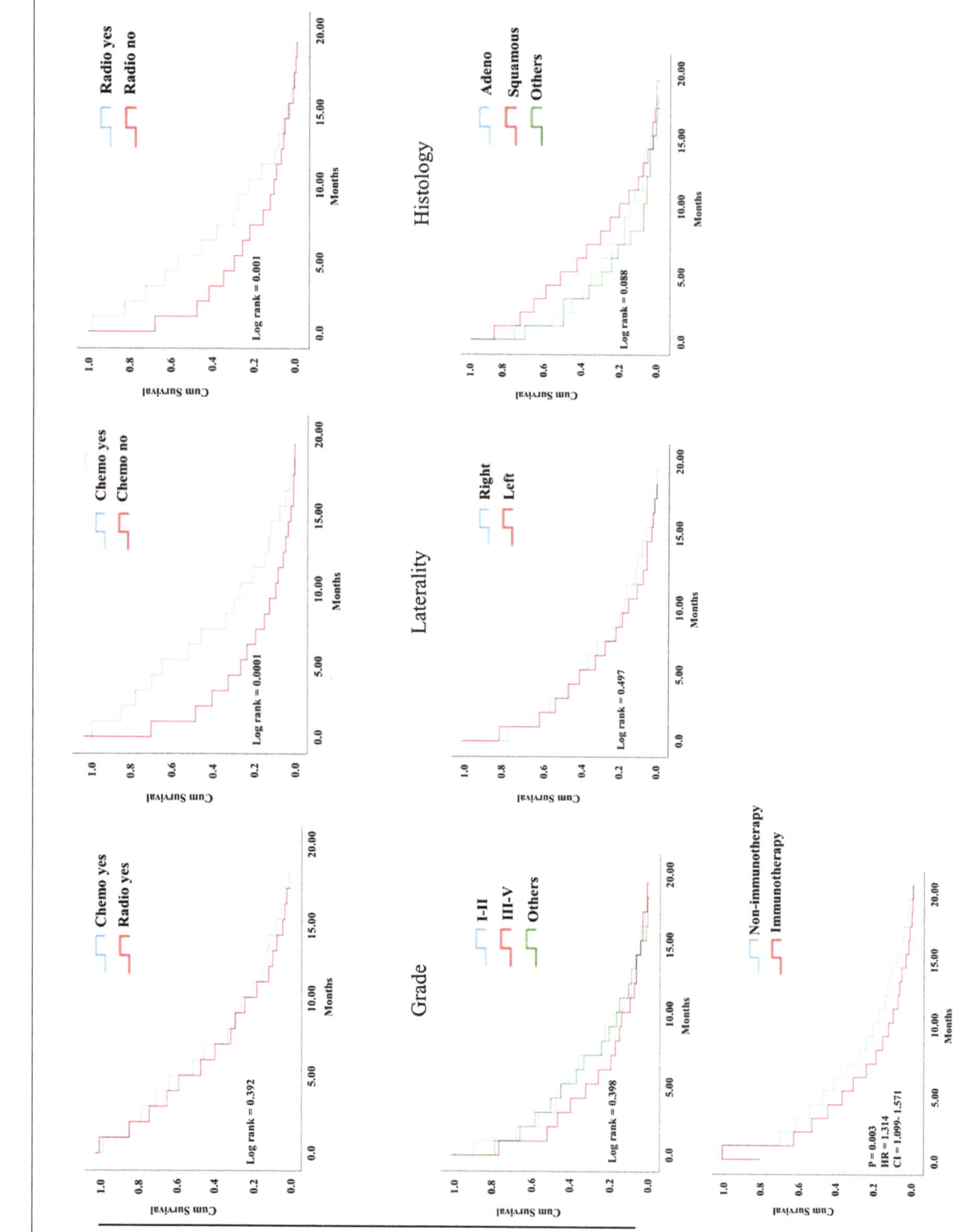

FIGURE 4 | (A) KM curve showing OS difference among factors in the NSCLC immunotherapy group of hear related- death patients. **(B)** Cox multivariate analysis difference survival of heart related death patients between NSCLC nonimmunotherapy group and immunotherapy group.

TABLE 3 | Univariate and multivariate analysis of factors affecting the survival in heart disease–related death NSCLC patients.

Parameters	Nonimmunotherapy				Immunotherapy			
	Univariate HR/CI	**P value**	**Multivariate HR/CI**	**P value**	**Univariate HR/CI**	**P value**	**Multivariate HR(95% CI)**	**P value**
Age (20-69 vs. >70)	1.06(0.82-1.36)	0.6	0.76(0.58-1.00)	0.05	0.92(0.72-1.17)	0.5	1.00(0.77-1.29	0.9
Sex Male vs. Female	1.07(0.83-1.38)	0.5	0.87(0.57-1.22)	0.3	1.03(0.80-1.33)	0.7	0.88 (0.67-1.16	0.3
Marital Yes - Others	0.84(0.66-1.07)	0.1	1.06(0.81-1.38)	0.6	0.93(0.73-1.18)	0.5	0.96(0.75-1.26)	0.8
Race								
White	Reference		Reference		Reference		Reference	
Black	0.81(0.57-1.15)	0.2	0.83(0.57-1.22)	0.3	0.97(0.70-1.34)	0.8	0.85(0.60-1.19)	0.3
Others	0.56(0.32-0.98)	0.04	0.51(0.28-0.91)	0.02	0.99(0.63-1.55)	0.9	0.82(0.51-1.30)	0.4
Chemotherapy yes vs. no	0.57(45-74)	<0.0001	1.72(1.31-2.25)	0.0001	1.76(1.38-2.26)	0.0001	1.81(1.37-2.38)	0.0001
Radiotherapy yes vs. no	0.61(48-0.79)	0.0001	1.47(1.12-1.93	0.005	1.46(1.13-1.87	0.003	1.29(0.98-1.70)	0.06
Grade								
I-II	Reference		Reference				Reference	
III-IV	1.14(0.80-1.62)	0.4	1.28(0.89-1.84	0.1	1.20(0.84-1.71)	0.3	1.24(0.86-1.79)	0.2
Unknown	1.30(0.95-1.77		1.23(0.88-1.72)	0.2	1.04(0.74-1.46)	0.8	1.05(0.73-1.49)	0.7
Laterality	0.99(0.77-1.26)	0.9	1.02(0.79-1.32)	0.8	0.93(0.73-1.18)	0.5	1.21(0.93-1.57)	0.1
Left vs. Right								
Histology/Behav								
Adenocarcinoma	Reference						Reference	
Squamous	0.77(0.57-1.04)	0.094	0.78(0.56-108)	0.1	0.80 (0.61-1.06)	0.133	0.74(0.55-0.99)	0.04
Others	0.71(0.053-0.09)	0.022	0.70(0.52-0.95)	0.02	1.12 (0.82-1.52)	0.474	0.96 (0.69-1.35)	0.8
Insurance yes vs. others	0.85(0.66-1.10)	0.228	1.07(0.81-1.41	0,6	1.21 (0.95-1.55)	0.114	1.25(0.96-1.61)	0.08

differences in the immunotherapy era, mostly due to the substantial effect of newly developed targeted therapies in recent years. The histology of squamous cancers demonstrated a prominent significance with positive survival benefits compared with nonsquamous cancers, indicating that histology could be a protective factor. Another explanation considers it could be the mortality from cancer and its poor prognosis compared with other types of histology (21, 22).

This study has several limitations. First, the SEER database did not provide an explanation about heart disease as the cause of death in patients as either real incidents before or newly related immunotherapeutic events. Second was the short median OS associated with the 20-month follow-up, the comorbidities, and the lack of performance status information. Third, the study lacked a detailed description of immunotherapy for patients.

CONCLUSION

This study demonstrates the OS benefits for NSCLC patients in the immunotherapy era compared with that in the nonimmunotherapy era that was primarily attributed to the immunotherapy. In heart disease–related death, immunotherapy in patients with NSCLC demonstrated decreased OS. Chemotherapy use increased the OS in patients with lung cancer who died from cardiac diseases, whereas no OS difference was found in radiotherapy use. Also, recognition of histology during immunotherapy, especially for nonsquamous types, could be considered as another predictor of OS reduction in patients who died from heart disease during immunotherapy. Although the incidence of cardiac toxicity is less than 1%, the risks must be assessed in all elderly patients with NSCLC. This study strongly highlighted effective clinical and preclinical studies to enhance the results.

AUTHOR CONTRIBUTIONS

Conceptualization: MS. Validation: MS and XS. Formal Analysis: MS, JL, MA, and AA-D. Investigation, writing, original draft preparation: MS. Visualization: FP, MA, AA-D and NA-S. Supervision: JL, and RK. Project administration: MS and JL. All authors contributed to the article and approved the submitted version.

REFERENCES

1. Eduati F, Lapuente-Santana Ó. Towards systems biomarkers of response to immune checkpoint blockers. *Front Oncol* (2020) 10:1027. doi: 10.3389/fonc.2020.01027
2. Salem J-E, Manouchehri A, Moey M, Lebrun-Vignes B., Bastarache L, Pariente A, et al. Cardiovascular toxicities associated with immune checkpoint inhibitors: an observational, retrospective, pharmacovigilance study. *Lancet Oncol* (2018) 19(12):1579–89. doi: 10.1016/S1470-2045(18)30608-9
3. Herrmann J. Adverse cardiac effects of cancer therapies: cardiotoxicity and arrhythmia. *Nat Rev Cardiol* (2020) 17(8):1–29. doi: 10.1038/s41569-020-0348-1
4. Dores GM, Bryant-Genevier M, Perez-Vilar S. Adverse events associated with the use of sipuleucel-T reported to the US Food and Drug Administration's Adverse Event Reporting System, 2010-2017. *JAMA Netw Open* (2019) 2(8): e199249–e199249. doi: 10.1001/jamanetworkopen.2019.9249
5. Kennedy LB, Salama AKS. A review of cancer immunotherapy toxicity. *CA: Cancer J Clin* (2020) 70(2):86–104. doi: 10.3322/caac.21596
6. Atkins KM, Rawal B, Chaunzwa TL, Lamba N, Bitterman DS, Williams CL, et al. Cardiac radiation dose, cardiac disease, and mortality in patients with

lung cancer. *J Am Coll Cardiol* (2019) 73(23):2976–87. doi: 10.1016/j.jacc.2019.03.500

7. US Food and Drug Administration. *Protecting and Promoting Your health. FDA News Release.* Available at: http://www.fda.gov/NewsEvents/Newsroom/PressAnnouncements (Accessed January 2020).
8. Kanz BA, Pollack MH, Johnpulle R, Puzanov I, Horn L, Morgans A, et al. Safety and efficacy of anti-PD-1 in patients with baseline cardiac, renal, or hepatic dysfunction. *J Immunother Cancer* (2016) 4(1):60. doi: 10.1186/s40425-016-0166-5
9. Esfahani K, Buhlaiga N, Thébault P, Lapointe R, Johnson NA, Miller WH Jr. Alemtuzumab for immune-related myocarditis due to PD-1 therapy. *New Engl J Med* (2019) 380(24):2375–6. doi: 10.1056/NEJMc1903064
10. Mahmood SS, Fradley MG, Cohen JV, Nohria A, Reynolds KL, Heinzerling LM, et al. Myocarditis in patients treated with immune checkpoint inhibitors. *J Am Coll Cardiol* (2018) 71(16):1755–64. doi: 10.1016/S0735-1097(18)31240-3
11. Safi M, Ahmed H, Al-Azab M, Xia Y-l, Shan X, Al-radhi M, et al. PD-1/PDL-1 Inhibitors and Cardiotoxicity; Molecular, Etiological and Management Outlines. *J Adv Res* (2020). doi: 10.1016/j.jare.2020.09.006
12. Ribas A, Wolchok JD. Cancer immunotherapy using checkpoint blockade. *Science* (2018) 359(6382):1350–5. doi: 10.1126/science.aar4060
13. Duan J, Cui L, Zhao X, Bai H, Cai S, Wang G, et al. Use of immunotherapy with programmed cell death 1 vs programmed cell death ligand 1 inhibitors in patients with Cancer: a systematic review and meta-analysis. *JAMA Oncol* (2020) 6(3):375–84. doi: 10.1001/jamaoncol.2019.5367
14. Chiang AC, Herbst RS. Frontline immunotherapy for NSCLC-the tale of the tail. *Nat Rev Clin Oncol* (2020) 17(2):1–2. doi: 10.1038/s41571-019-0317-y
15. Ball S, Ghosh RK, Wongsaengsak S, Bandyopadhyay D, Ghosh GC, Aronow WS, et al. Cardiovascular Toxicities of Immune Checkpoint Inhibitors: JACC Review Topic of the Week. *J Am Coll Cardiol* (2019) 74(13):1714–27. doi: 10.1016/j.jacc.2019.07.079
16. Moslehi JJ, Salem J-E, Sosman JA, Lebrun-Vignes B, Johnson DB. Increased reporting of fatal immune checkpoint inhibitor-associated myocarditis. *Lancet* (2018) 391(10124):933. doi: 10.1016/S0140-6736(18)30533-6
17. Fillon M. Lung cancer radiation may increase the risk of major adverse cardiac events. *CA: Cancer J Clin* (2019) 69(6):435–7. doi: 10.3322/caac.21581
18. Youn B, Trikalinos NA, Mor V, Wilson IB, Dahabreh IJ. Real-world use and survival outcomes of immune checkpoint inhibitors in older adults with non-small cell lung cancer. *Cancer* (2020) 126(5):978–85. doi: 10.1002/cncr.32624
19. Lazzari C, Karachaliou N, Bulotta A, Viganó M, Mirabile A, Brioschi E, et al. Combination of immunotherapy with chemotherapy and radiotherapy in lung cancer: is this the beginning of the end for cancer? *Ther Adv Med Oncol* (2018) 10:1758835918762094. doi: 10.1177/1758835918762094
20. Ksienski D, Wai ES, Croteau NS, Freeman AT, Chan A, Fiorino L, et al. Association of age with differences in immune related adverse events and survival of patients with advanced nonsmall cell lung cancer receiving pembrolizumab or nivolumab. *J Geriatr Oncol* (2020) 11(5):807–13. doi: 10.1016/j.jgo.2020.01.006
21. Wang B-Y, Huang J-Y, Chen H-C, Lin C-H, Lin S-H, Hung W-H, et al. The comparison between adenocarcinoma and squamous cell carcinoma in lung cancer patients. *J Cancer Res Clin Oncol* (2020) 146(1):43–52. doi: 10.1007/s00432-019-03079-8
22. Borghaei H, Paz-Ares L, Horn L, Spigel DR, Steins M, Ready NE, et al. Nivolumab versus docetaxel in advanced nonsquamous non-small-cell lung cancer. *New Engl J Med* (2015) 373(17):1627–39. doi: 10.1056/NEJMoa1507643

17

Aumolertinib as Neoadjuvant Therapy for Patients with Unresectable Stage III Non-Small Cell Lung Cancer with Activated EGFR Mutation

Shao Feng[1†], Zhang Qiang[1†], Cheng Wanwan[2], Zeng Zhaozhun[3], Xie Yuewu[3] and Fang Shencun[2]*

[1] Department of Thoracic Surgery, Nanjing Chest Hospital, The Affiliated Brain Hospital of Nanjing Medical University, Nanjing, China, [2] Department of Respiratory Medicine, Nanjing Chest Hospital, The Affiliated Brain Hospital of Nanjing Medical University, Nanjing, China, [3] Medical Oncology Scientific Group of the Central Medical Department, Jiangsu Hansoh Pharmaceutical Group Co., Ltd., Shanghai, China

***Correspondence:**
Fang Shencun
fang1984@aliyun.com

†These authors have contributed equally to this work

Background: There is no standard treatment for stage III lung cancer due to its low surgical resection rate, and improving PFS and survival of patients with III NSCLC has become an urgent challenge in clinical treatment. For EGFR mutation-positive patients, targeted therapy has the remarkable feature of high efficiency and low toxicity compared with first-line standard chemotherapy, and targeted neoadjuvant therapy needs to be further explored.

Method: We report 3 diagnosed cases of locally advanced unresectable NSCLC with EGFR-sensitive mutations who first received 1–2 cycles of preoperative chemotherapy neoadjuvant therapy and were treated with 110 mg daily of 3rd-generation EGFR-TKI aumolertinib instead because of poor efficacy or safety intolerance.

Result: After 2 cycles of aumolertinib treatment, all 3 patients achieved symptomatic remission and significant tumor size reduction and achieved downstaging to allow surgical treatment. No additional operative difficulties were added during the surgery. They continued to receive adjuvant therapy with the original dose of aumolertinib after surgical treatment, and no evidence of tumor recurrence was found until the most recent imaging examination. In addition, the course of neoadjuvant and adjuvant therapy was free of serious adverse effects.

Conclusion: Perioperative treatment of these three cases of locally advanced unresectable NSCLC with EGFR-sensitive mutations with the third-generation EGFR-TKI aumolertinib showed significant efficacy and excellent safety and may be a new option for targeted therapy in the perioperative period.

Keywords: aumolertinib, NSCLC, neoadjuvant, EGFR, adjuvant

INTRODUCTION

Patients with stage III non-small cell lung cancer (NSCLC) have considerable disease heterogeneity (1, 2). Treatment options include neoadjuvant therapy followed by surgical resection, adjuvant chemotherapy after surgery, or radical radiotherapy. A large meta-analysis confirmed the survival benefit of preoperative chemotherapy (3). However, the lung damage caused by preoperative chemotherapy may also make subsequent surgical resection more difficult (4, 5). No consensus exists with regard to optimal treatment approaches, particularly for unresectable advanced NSCLC characterized by single-site or multisite lymph node metastases identified by preoperative staging; the role of surgical resection after preoperative therapy remains controversial (6–8).

Epidermal growth factor receptor (EGFR) tyrosine kinase inhibitors (TKI) significantly prolong progression-free survival (PFS) in patients with advanced EGFR mutation-positive (EGFRm) NSCLC compared to chemotherapy as first-line therapy (9–11). Aumolertinib (HS-10296), a third-generation EGFR-TKI, has attracted much attention due to its reliable antitumor activity and favorable safety profile (12–14).

Although EGFR-TKI was established as an effective first-line therapy for advanced EGFRm NSCLC (9–11), the efficacy and tolerability of EGFR-TKI preoperative induction therapy remain uncertain. We report three cases of stage III NSCLC with confirmed EGFR mutations, who reached a descending stage after preoperative neoadjuvant treatment with aumolertinib and had successful surgical resection of the malignant tumor.

PRESENTATION

Case 1

A 64-year-old Chinese male, a 40-year smoker and hypertension, presented to a local hospital in January 2021 with an irritating cough and sputum with blood in the sputum, and a computed tomography chest (CT) scan showed a 7.8 × 4.9-cm left upper lung space. Lung puncture biopsy showed squamous carcinoma, and immunohistochemistry showed high PD-L1 expression, TPS ≥ 90%, EGFR mutation (exon 19 deletion) by NGS, and clinical stage IIIC (T3N3M0). PET/CT showed left lung cancer with obstructive pneumonia, enlarged lymph nodes in the left clavicular region, posterior to the anterior vena cava, aortic window, left paratracheal area, and both hila, and increased FDG metabolism. Magnetic resonance imaging (MRI) of the brain showed no evidence of central nervous system (CNS) involvement, which made her malignancy compatible. **Figure 1** shows the imaging findings of case 1.

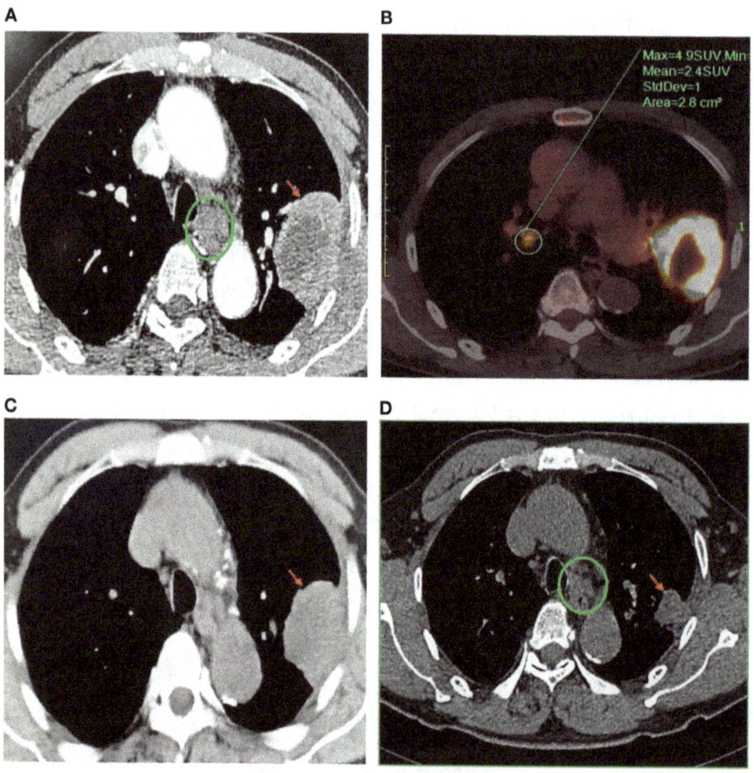

FIGURE 1 | Disease status before and after neoadjuvant chemotherapy and aumolertinib treatment. Computed tomography chest (CT) scan showed **(A)** pulmonary nodule in the left upper lobe of the lung, size 7.8 × 4.9 cm before chemotherapy. PET/CT showed **(B)** lymph node enlargement in the right hilar and pulmonary nodule in the left upper lobe before chemotherapy. **(C)** Stable disease (SD) based on imaging findings after 2 cycles of chemotherapy. **(D)** Pulmonary nodule in the left upper lobe of the lung, size 2.2 × 2.0× 1.8 cm after almost 2 months of aumolertinib treatment, with tumor remission reaching partial remission (PR).

Systemic chemotherapy was started in January 2021 with an initial dose of albumin-bound paclitaxel 400 mg and carboplatin 0.4 mg. Rash and pruritus developed during the second chemotherapy infusion of carboplatin, so treatment with carboplatin was discontinued. After 2 cycles of chemotherapy, objective tumor remission was evaluated as disease stabilization (SD) by RECIST 1.1 (efficacy evaluation criteria for solid tumors). After nearly 8 weeks of oral administration of the third-generation EGFR-TKI aumolertinib (110 mg/day) started in February 2021, imaging showed significant tumor regression, lesion volume reduction to 2.2 × 2.0 × 1.8 cm, partial remission (PR), and clinical stage reduction to stage IB (T2N0M0). After evaluation by the surgeon, the patient was eligible for surgery and underwent VATS left upper lung lobectomy + lymph node dissection with the patient's consent in April 2021. Postoperative pathology showed interstitial fibrous lung tissue with numerous lymphocytic infiltrates, with large necrotic tissue and <10% residual tumor cells (major pathological response, MPR), which was considered as posttreatment changes of squamous carcinoma. There was no metastasis of cancer tissue in any of the lymph nodes examined. After discussion with the patient, he was willing to receive adjuvant therapy with aumolertinib, and the disease was judged to be stable by imaging results in February 2022.

Case 2

A 68-year-old Chinese male with grade 3 hypertension was admitted to the hospital in December 2020 with a 1-week history of pulmonary occupancy found on physical examination. Chest CT revealed a left lingual lobe occupancy with obstructive pneumonia and enlarged mediastinal and left axillary lymph nodes; the size of the tumor was 4.0 × 3.8 × 2.3 cm, and cranial MRI, abdominal ultrasound, and bone scan was unremarkable. Lung puncture biopsy was diagnosed as adenocarcinoma, and immunohistochemistry showed a negative PD-L1 expression with TMB: 6.38 mut/bp; NGS revealed that the patient had EGFR exon 21 L858R point mutation, combined with HEBB2 amplification, EGFR amplification, and TP53 mutation; and the clinical stage was IIIA (T2N2M0). The patient's enlarged lymph node in the left hilum was completely fused with the left pulmonary artery trunk and could not be completely removed surgically, which was an unresectable stage III lung cancer. After 2 cycles of pemetrexed combined with carboplatin chemotherapy in December 2020, the tumor did not shrink significantly according to chest CT. Considering that the patient had EGFR 21 exon L858R mutation, she was treated with oral aumolertinib 110 mg/day in January 2021, and after nearly 2 months of treatment, chest CT indicated significant regression of the left hilar lymph nodes, and the mass volume was reduced to 1.2 × 1.0 × 1.5 cm, achieving PR; clinical stage was reduced to stage IB (T2N0M0); and the tumor was clearly demarcated from the left pulmonary artery trunk, which could be considered for surgical radical treatment. **Figure 2** shows the imaging findings of case 2.

Therefore, VATS left upper lung lobectomy and lymphatic dissection were performed on February 22, 2021. Postoperative pathology showed moderately differentiated adenocarcinoma with elastic plaque formation, tumor involvement in 0/10 lymph nodes, and residual tumor cells <10% (MPR). The postoperative pathological stage was stage IA (T1N0M0). After surgery, the patient had been receiving adjuvant therapy with aumolertinib for 11 months, and no evidence of malignancy recurrence was seen on spiral CT of the chest.

Case 3

A 60-year-old Chinese female with grade 2 hypertension was admitted with cough for 1 month. Chest CT showed a left lower

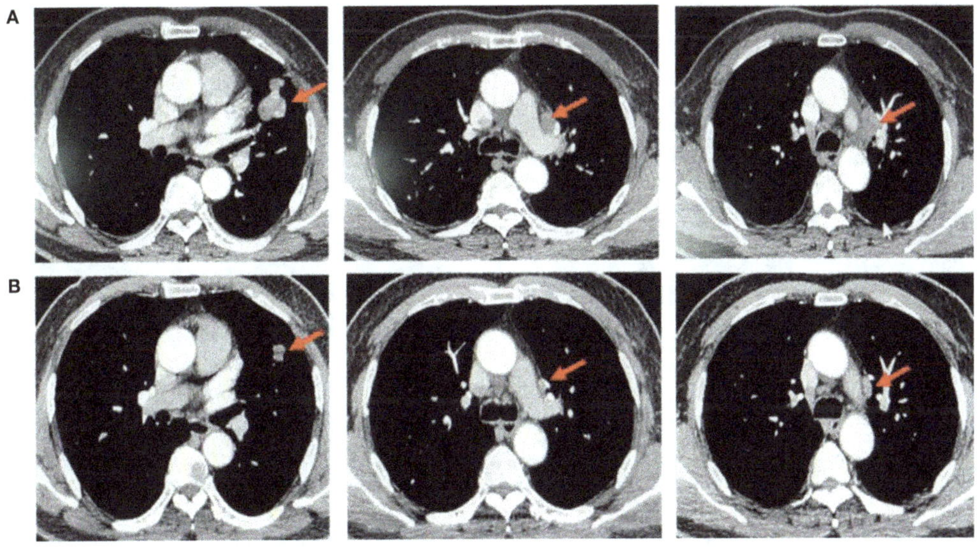

FIGURE 2 | Disease status before and after neoadjuvant almonertinib therapy. Computed tomography chest (CT) scan showed **(A)** left lingual lobe occupancy with a size of 4.0 × 3.8 × 2.3 cm, and subaortic lymph nodes before aumolertinib treatment. **(B)** Left lingual lobe occupancy with a size of 1.2 × 1 × 1.5 cm, and subaortic lymph nodes after aumolertinib treatment.

lung occupancy with pulmonary atelectasis; PET/CT showed a left lower lung soft tissue mass (10.9 × 8.9 × 6.5 cm), left lower lobe bronchial truncation, aortic window, and multiple lymph node enlargement in the left hilar, and left lung cancer with obstructive pneumonia was considered. Lung puncture biopsy and immunohistochemistry diagnosed squamous carcinoma; immunohistochemistry results showed negative PD-L1 expression, and NGS test results were EGFR L858R mutation combined with TP53 mutation, clinical stage IIIB (T4N2M0). Thoracic surgery specialists consulted and judged that there was no indication for surgery for the time being and recommended medical treatment. **Figure 3** shows the imaging findings of case 3.

The patient was treated with a chemotherapy regimen of albumin paclitaxel combined with carboplatin for two cycles in November 2020, and a chest CT review showed that the lesion was still stable, but the tumor did not shrink significantly. Therefore, the patient received oral aumolertinib (110 mg/day) for 2 cycles from January 2021, and the tumor shrank significantly from before to 3.0 × 4.0 × 4.0 cm, reaching PR and clinical stage down to stage IB (T2N0M0), which was eligible for surgery. Therefore, the patient requested surgical treatment and underwent VTAS left lower lung lobectomy, lymph node dissection, and pleural adhesion release in March 2021. Postoperative pathology showed focal fibrous tissue hyperplasia with inflammatory cell infiltration in lung tissue, focal bronchial epithelial adenoid formation, and mild alveolar epithelial cell hyperplasia; some multinucleated giant cell reaction was seen; posttreatment changes were considered; no tumor residual was seen; and the status of pathological complete response (pCR) was achieved. 0/10 lymph nodes had tumor involvement, and the postoperative pathological stage was stage 0 (T0N0M0). After surgery, the patient was treated with aumolertinib for adjuvant therapy, and the disease was judged to be stable on the chest CT findings in January 2022.

DISCUSSION

Three patients with unresectable stage III non-small-cell lung cancer were first treated with chemotherapy and were switched to aumolertinib for 2 cycles due to poor efficacy, and all achieved downstaging and met resectability criteria after neoadjuvant aumolertinib treatment. Postoperative pathology showed MPR in the first two cases and pCR in the last case. In addition, the safety profile of aumolertinib in neoadjuvant attempts was satisfactory, with no events that delayed surgery or increased surgical complications. Patient characteristics and treatment response before and after surgery are shown in **Table 1**.

In this case series report, the first patient who received chemotherapy had a more severe rash and pruritus, which the physician judged to be a hypersensitivity reaction caused by carboplatin, which has been shown to predispose patients treated with carboplatin in combination with paclitaxel (15). Symptomatic treatment was replaced with oral aumolertinib

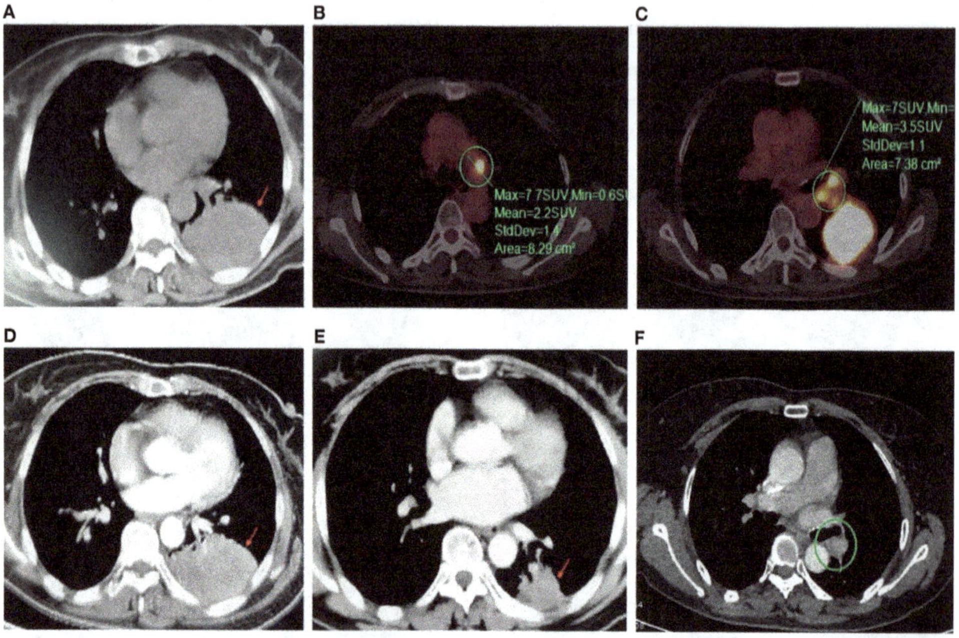

FIGURE 3 | Disease status before and after neoadjuvant chemotherapy and aumolertinib treatment. Computed tomography chest (CT) scan showed that **(A)** before chemotherapy, the size of the left lower lung soft tissue mass was 10.9 × 8.9 × 6.5 cm. PET/CT showed **(B)** mediastinal lymph node enlargement before chemotherapy. **(C)** Multiple lymph node enlargement in the left hilar before chemotherapy. CT scan showed that **(D)** after 2 cycles of chemotherapy, the disease was judged to be stable based on imaging findings. **(E)** After 2 cycles of aumolertinib treatment, the size of the left lower lung soft tissue mass was 3.0 × 4.0 × 4.0 cm, and the tumor achieved partial remission. **(F)** After 2 cycles of aumolertinib treatment, multiple lymph nodes disappeared in the left hilar.

TABLE 1 | Patient characteristics and response to treatment before and after surgery (N = 3).

Patient	Gender/ age	Histological types	EGFR mutation subtypes	PD-LI expression status	First-line treatment		Second-line treatment		Pathologicalassessment
					Treatment	Response	Treatment	Response	
1	M/64	Squamous carcinoma	exon19 deletion	Positive	Chemotherapy	SD	Aumolertinib	PR	MPR
2	M/68	Adenocarcinoma	L858R mutation	Negative	Chemotherapy	SD	Aumolertinib	PR	MPR
3	F/60	Squamous carcinoma	L858R mutation	Negative	Chemotherapy	SD	Aumolertinib	PR	pCR

SD, stable disease; PR, partial response; MPR, major pathological response; pCR, pathological complete response.

and continued for 8 weeks, with imaging showing partial remission and no serious adverse events.

The second and third cases also received 2 cycles of preoperative chemotherapy without significant tumor remission. After chemotherapy and switching to oral aumolertinib treatment for 4–8 weeks with the patient's consent, imaging showed that both patients responded well to treatment, with significant tumor volume reduction to a descending stage that allowed them to undergo surgery.

This may indicate an efficacy advantage of aumolertinib in the neoadjuvant phase of therapy. Similarly, results from the EMERGING-CTONG 1103 study showed a trend toward improved ORR, lymph node step-down, MPR, and R0 resection rates with neoadjuvant erlotinib compared to neoadjuvant chemotherapy for patients with EGFRm NSCLC, and significantly prolonged PFS (16). Evidence from case reports and small non-randomized clinical trials reported suggests that neoadjuvant EGFR-TKI therapy is potentially efficacious in patients with resectable NSCLC (17–21). This suggests that neoadjuvant-targeted therapy modalities are potentially clinically applicable and may be a viable option for patients who are not optimal chemotherapy candidates due to medical comorbidities or who refuse chemotherapy.

Finally, overall oncologic outcomes may be influenced by the timing of surgical intervention after neoadjuvant therapy. A large retrospective study found that in patients with stage IIIa NSCLC, 1- and 3-year survival rates were significantly lower in the short-delayed group after preoperative neoadjuvant therapy compared with the long-delayed group (22). Due to the significant safety advantage of targeted agents over chemotherapy, preoperative EGFR-TKI neoadjuvant therapy may reduce lung injury and make surgery less difficult. Therefore, it may shorten the time between the end of neoadjuvant therapy and surgery, thus affecting prognostic survival. Currently, the optimal duration of preoperative induction-targeted therapy is unclear, and whether 6 weeks of EGFR-TKI induction therapy is sufficient has yet to be verified, so there may be a problem of insufficient induction-targeted therapy.

Aumolertinib has demonstrated excellent tumor remission and a favorable safety profile in the neoadjuvant and adjuvant phases of these three phase III NSCLC cases, which has implications in guiding targeted therapy in the perioperative setting of NSCLC. However, its ability to be a firm choice for neoadjuvant and adjuvant treatment of NSCLC still needs to be validated by large randomized controlled studies.

AUTHOR CONTRIBUTIONS

All authors contributed toward data analysis, drafting, and critically revising of the paper, gave final approval of the version to be published, and agree to be accountable for all aspects of the work.

ACKNOWLEDGMENTS

The authors thank the patients for their participation in the study and agreeing to the publishing of the report.

REFERENCES

1. van Meerbeeck JP, Surmont VF. Stage IIIA-N2 NSCLC: A Review of its Treatment Approaches and Future Developments. *Lung Cancer* (2009) 65:257–67. doi: 10.1016/j.lungcan.2009.02.007
2. Pang Z, Yang Y, Ding N, Huang C, Zhang T, Ni Y, et al. Optimal Managements of Stage IIIA (N2) Non-Small Cell Lung Cancer Patients: A Population-Based Survival Analysis. *J Thorac Dis* (2017) 9(10):4046–56. doi: 10.21037/jtd.2017.10.47
3. NSCLC Meta-analysis Collaborative Group. Preoperative Chemotherapy for Non-Small-Cell Lung Cancer: A Systematic Review and Meta-Analysis of Individual Participant Data. *Lancet* (2014) 383(9928):1561–71. doi: 10.1016/S0140-6736(13)62159-5
4. Pisters KMW, Vallières E, Crowley JJ, Franklin WA, Bunn PA Jr, Ginsberg RJ, et al. Surgery With or Without Preoperative Paclitaxel and Carboplatin in Early-Stage Non-Small-Cell Lung Cancer: Southwest Oncology Group Trial S9900, an Intergroup, Randomized, Phase III Trial. *J Clin Oncol* (2010) 28 (11):1843–9. doi: 10.1200/JCO.2009.26.1685
5. Depierre A, Westeel V. Preoperative Chemotherapy in Non-Small Cell Lung Cancer: Advantages, Disadvantages, Level of Evidence. *Rev Mal Respir* (2007) 24:6S59–63. doi: 10.1019/200720130
6. Rusch VW, Giroux DJ, Kraut MJ, Crowley J, Hazuka M, Winton T, et al. Induction Chemoradiation and Surgical Resection for Superior Sulcus Non-Small-Cell Lung Carcinomas: Long-Term Results of Southwest Oncology Group Trial 9416 (Intergroup Trial 0160). *J Clin Oncol* (2007) 25:313–8. doi: 10.1200/JCO.2006.08.2826
7. Darling GE, Li F, Patsios D, Massey C, Wallis AG, Coate L, et al. Neoadjuvant Chemoradiation and Surgery Improves Survival Outcomes Compared With Definitive Chemoradiation in the Treatment of Stage IIIA N2 Non-Small-Cell Lung Cancer. *Eur J Cardiothorac Surg* (2015) 48:684–90. doi: 10.1093/ejcts/ezu504
8. Uy KL, Darling G, Xu W, Yi Q-L, De Perrot M, Pierre AF, et al. Improved Results of Induction Chemoradiation Before Surgical Intervention for Selected Patients With Stage IIIA-N2 Non-Small Cell Lung Cancer. *J Thorac Cardiovasc Surg* (2007) 134:188–93. doi: 10.1016/j.jtcvs.2007.01.078

9. Fukuoka M, Wu Y-L, Thongprasert S, Sunpaweravong P, Leong S-S, Sriuranpong V, et al. Biomarker Analyses and Final Overall Survival Results From a Phase III, Randomized, Open-Label, First-Line Study of Gefitinib Versus Carboplatin/Paclitaxel in Clinically Selected Patients With Advanced non-Small-Cell Lung Cancer in Asia (IPASS). *J Clin Oncol* (2011) 29:2866–74. doi: 10.1200/JCO.2010.33.4235
10. Wu Y-L, Zhou C, Hu C-P, Feng J, Lu S, Huang Y, et al. Afatinib Versus Cisplatin Plus Gemcitabine for First-Line Treatment of Asian Patients With Advanced Non-Small-Cell Lung Cancer Harbouring EGFR Mutations (LUX-Lung 6): An Open-Label, Randomised Phase 3 Trial. *Lancet Oncol* (2014) 15:213–22. doi: 10.1016/S1470-2045(13)70604-1
11. Cheng Y, He Y, Li W, Zhang H-l, Zhou Q, Wang B, et al. Osimertinib Versus Comparator EGFR TKI as First-Line Treatment for EGFR-Mutated Advanced NSCLC: FLAURA China, A Randomized Study. *Target Oncol* (2021) 16 (2):165–76. doi: 10.1007/s11523-021-00794-6
12. Lu S, Wang Q, Zhang G, Dong X, Yang CT, Song Y, et al. Efficacy of Aumolertinib (HS-10296) in Patients With Advanced EGFR T790M+ NSCLC: Updated Post-National Medical Products Administration Approval Results From the APOLLO Registrational Trial. *J Thorac Oncol* (2022) 17 (3):411–22. doi: 10.1016/j.jtho.2021.10.024
13. Romero D. Aumolertinib Is Effective in NSCLC. *Nat Rev Clin Oncol* (2022) 19 (1):6. doi: 10.1038/s41571-021-00586-x
14. Lu S, Dong X, Jian H, Chen J, Chen G, Sun Y, et al. Randomized Phase III Trial of Aumolertinib (HS-10296, Au) Versus Gefitinib (G) as First-Line Treatment of Patients With Locally Advanced or Metastatic Non-Small Cell Lung Cancer (NSCLC) and EGFR Exon 19 Del or L858R Mutations (EGFRm). *J Clin Oncol* (2021) 39. doi: 10.1200/JCO.2021.39.15_suppl.9013
15. Pujade-Lauraine E, Wagner U, Aavall-Lundqvist E, Gebski V, Heywood M, Vasey PA, et al. Pegylated Liposomal Doxorubicin and Carboplatin Compared With Paclitaxel and Carboplatin for Patients With Platinum-Sensitive Ovarian Cancer in Late Relapse. *J Clin Oncol* (2010) 28(20):3323–9. doi: 10.1200/JCO.2009.25.7519
16. Zhong WZ, Chen KN, Chen C, Gu CD, Wang J, Yang XN, et al. Erlotinib Versus Gemcitabine Plus Cisplatin as Neoadjuvant Treatment of Stage IIIA-N2 EGFR-Mutant Non-Small-Cell Lung Cancer (EMERGING-CTONG 1103): A Randomized Phase II Study. *J Clin Oncol* (2019) 37(25):2235–45. doi: 10.1200/JCO.19.00075
17. Zhong W, Yang X, Yan H, Zhang X, Su J, Chen Z, et al. Phase II Study of Biomarker-Guided Neoadjuvant Treatment Strategy for IIIA-N2 Non-Small Cell Lung Cancer Based on Epidermal Growth Factor Receptor Mutation Status. *J Hematol Oncol* (2015) 8:54. doi: 10.1186/s13045-015-0151-3
18. Lara-Guerra H, Chung CT, Schwock J, Pintilie M, Hwang DM, Leighl NB, et al. Histopathological and Immunohistochemical Features Associated With Clinical Response to Neoadjuvant Gefitinib Therapy in Early Stage Non-Small Cell Lung Cancer. *Lung Cancer* (2012) 76:235–41. doi: 10.1016/j.lungcan.2011.10.020
19. Lara-Guerra H, Waddell TK, Salvarrey MA, Joshua AM, Chung CT, Paul N, et al. Phase II Study of Preoperative Gefitinib in Clinical Stage I Non-Small-Cell Lung Cancer. *J Clin Oncol* (2009) 27:6229–36. doi: 10.1200/JCO.2009.22.3370
20. Hishida T, Nagai K, Mitsudomi T, Yokoi K, Kondo H, Horinouchi H, et al. Salvage Surgery for Advanced Non-Small Cell Lung Cancer After Response to Gefitinib. *J Thorac Cardiovasc Surg* (2010) 140:e69-e71. doi: 10.1016/j.jtcvs.2010.06.035
21. Schaake EE, Kappers I, Codrington HE, Valdes Olmos RA, Teertstra HJ, van Pel R, et al. Tumor Response and Toxicity of Neoadjuvant Erlotinib in Patients With Early-Stage non-Small-Cell Lung Cancer. *J Clin Oncol* (2012) 30:2731–8. doi: 10.1200/JCO.2011.39.4882
22. Rice JD, Heidel J, Trivedi JR, van Berkel VH. Optimal Surgical Timing After Neoadjuvant Therapy for Stage IIIa Non-Small Cell Lung Cancer. *Ann Thorac Surg* (2020) 109(3):842–7. doi: 10.1016/j.athoracsur.2019.09.076

18

A 5-Genomic Mutation Signature can Predict the Survival for Patients with NSCLC Receiving Atezolizumab

Jiamao Lin[1†], Xiaohui Wang[2†], Chenyue Zhang[3†], Shuai Bu[4], Chenglong Zhao[5] and Haiyong Wang[1]*

[1] Department of Internal Medicine Oncology, Shandong Cancer Hospital and Institute, Shandong First Medical University and Shandong Academy of Medical Sciences, Jinan, China, [2] Research Service Office, Shandong Liaocheng People's Hospital, Liaocheng, China, [3] Department of Integrated Oncology, Fudan University Shanghai Cancer Center, Shanghai, China, [4] Research Department, The Second Affiliated Hospital of Shandong University of Traditional Chinese Medicine, Jinan, China, [5] Department of Pathology, Shandong Cancer Hospital and Institute, Shandong First Medical University and Shandong Academy of Medical Sciences, Jinan, China

***Correspondence:**
Haiyong Wang
wanghaiyong6688@126.com

[†]These authors have contributed equally to this work and share first authorship

Background: At present, there is a lack of studies focusing on the survival prediction of patients with non-small cell lung cancer (NSCLC) receiving atezolizumab in light of gene mutation characteristic.

Methods: Patients with NSCLC receiving atezolizumab from the OAK study were defined as the training group. LASSO Cox regressions were applied to establish the gene mutation signature model to predict the overall survival (OS) rate of the training group. NSCLC patients receiving atezolizumab from the POPLAR study were defined as the testing group to validate the gene mutation signature model. In addition, we compared the OS rate between patients receiving atezolizumab and docetaxel classified according to their risk score based on our gene mutation signature model.

Results: We successfully established a 5-genomic mutation signature that included *CREBBP*, *KEAP1*, *RAF1*, *STK11* and *TP53* mutations. We found it was superior to the blood tumor mutation burden (bTMB) score and programmed death ligand 1 (PDL1) expression in the prediction of the OS rate for patients receiving atezolizumab. High-risk patients receiving atezolizumab had a worse OS rate compared with low-risk patients in the training (P = 0.0004) and testing (P = 0.0001) groups. In addition, low-risk patients using atezolizumab had a better OS rate compared with those in use of docetaxel for the training (P <0.0001) and testing groups (P = 0.0095). High-risk patients of the training group (P = 0.0265) using atezolizumab had a better OS rate compared with those using docetaxel. However, the OS difference between atezolizumab and docetaxel was not found in high-risk patients from the testing group (P = 0.6403). Multivariate Cox regression analysis showed that the risk model in light of 5-genomic mutation signature was an independent prognostic factor on OS for patients receiving atezolizumab (P <0.0001). In addition, significant OS benefit could only be found in low-risk patients receiving atezolizumab compared with docetaxel (P <0.0001).

Conclusions: The 5-genomic mutation signature could predict OS benefit for patients with NSCLC receiving atezolizumab. Therefore, the establishment of the 5-genomic mutation panel will guide clinicians to identify optimal patients who could benefit from atezolizumab treatment.

Keywords: atezolizumab, gene mutation, non-small cell lung cancer, survival, PD-L1 inhibitor

INTRODUCTION

Atezolizumab, an immune checkpoint inhibitor, is an immunoglobulin G1 monoclonal antibody that binds to programmed death ligand 1 (PD-L1) and blocks its interactions with programmed death 1 and B7.1 receptor (1). At present, atezolizumab plays an important role in the treatment of non-small cell lung cancer (NSCLC) patients, gradually shifting from the second to the first line of treatment. Importantly, the tumor mutational burden (TMB) score and PDL1 expression have become key markers of the clinical benefits of patients receiving atezolizumab. Indeed, TMB in blood (bTMB) was identified as a biomarker for patients that improve upon atezolizumab treatment (2). The POPLAR study also found that improvements in the survival rates were associated with PDL1 expression on tumor cells and tumor-infiltrating immune cells, suggesting that PDL1 expression is can predict benefits derived from atezolizumab treatment (3). However, it is worth noting that the benefits of atezolizumab are comparable with those of chemotherapy based on these markers. In fact, increased overall survival (OS) rates were not obtained for patients receiving atezolizumab with a high bTMB score compared with those with low bTMB score from both the OAK and POPLAR studies (2, 4). A recent study even showed that advanced NSCLC patients with low TMB might have better OS than those with medium TMB (5). Therefore, it is very important to identify markers for the prediction of patients with NSCLC that could benefit from atezolizumab treatment.

Several studies have focused on the relationship between specific gene mutations and the effect of immunotherapy. A series of gene mutations such as *STK11*, *KEAP1*, *POLD1/POLE*, and *TERT* were found to influence the outcomes of patients receiving immunotherapy (6–10). Thus, we speculated that the establishment of a specific gene mutation signature could distinguish survival differences for patients receiving atezolizumab. In our study, we first established the gene mutation signature model able to predict OS rate based on the OAK study. Then, the gene mutation signature model was validated using data from the POPLAR study. Our study would be beneficial to guide the treatment of NSCLC patients receiving atezolizumab. It would also render the treatment strategy more individual-oriented.

METHODS

Patient Data

The data of our study was obtained from a previous study (2). Our study was based on POPLAR and OAK studies, the two independent clinical trials. The POPLAR study is a multicentre, open-label, phase 2 randomized controlled trial to compare atezolizumab with docetaxel for patients with previously treated NSCLC (3). The OAK study is the first randomized phase 3 study reporting results of atezolizumab treatment, which resulted in a clinically relevant improvement of OS versus docetaxel in previously treated NSCLC (11). These relevant studies and data have been published, thus informed consent and ethical committee approval were not warranted.

Study Design

This study was divided into the training group and the testing group as shown in **Figure 1**. Patients with synonymous mutations, which are that sometimes a mutation of a base pair in a DNA fragment does not change the encoded amino acid, were excluded. The synonymous mutations have been defined in published data (2). A total of 321 patients receiving atezolizumab were included from the training group (OAK study) and 105 patients were included from the testing group (POPLAR study). LASSO Cox regression model was used to predict prognosis-related markers from the training group. Then leave one out cross validation was applied to select five optimal gene mutation types to construct a risk sore evaluation model. The risk score was calculated according to the formula: $\Sigma_i\ \omega_i\ \chi_i$ where ω_i is the coefficient and χ_i is the expression value of each respective gene. The optimal cutoff to distinct high- and low-risk was estimated through time-dependent ROC curves. OS was regarded as the main endpoint of our study.

Statistical Analysis

The Kaplan–Meier curve was constructed to compare the OS difference, and the log-rank was used to perform the statistical analysis. Multivariate Cox regression analysis was applied to develop the subgroup analysis based on clinical variables. The construction of the risk score model was based on R 3.4.2. The figures were drawn using GraphPad Prism version 6.0. All *P*-values were two-tailed, and $P < 0.05$ was considered statistically significant.

RESULTS

Construction of a Genetic Mutation Signature to Predict the Survival of Patients Receiving Atezolizumab

A total of 321 NSCLC patients receiving atezolizumab from the OAK study were included in the analysis to establish the gene mutation signature. To achieve better stability and accuracy, we constructed the trend diagram of the lasso coefficient, and found a 5-genomic mutation signature obtained from 10 cross validations that could predict survival (**Figures 2A, B**). In addition, the time-dependent receiver operating characteristic (ROC) curve was

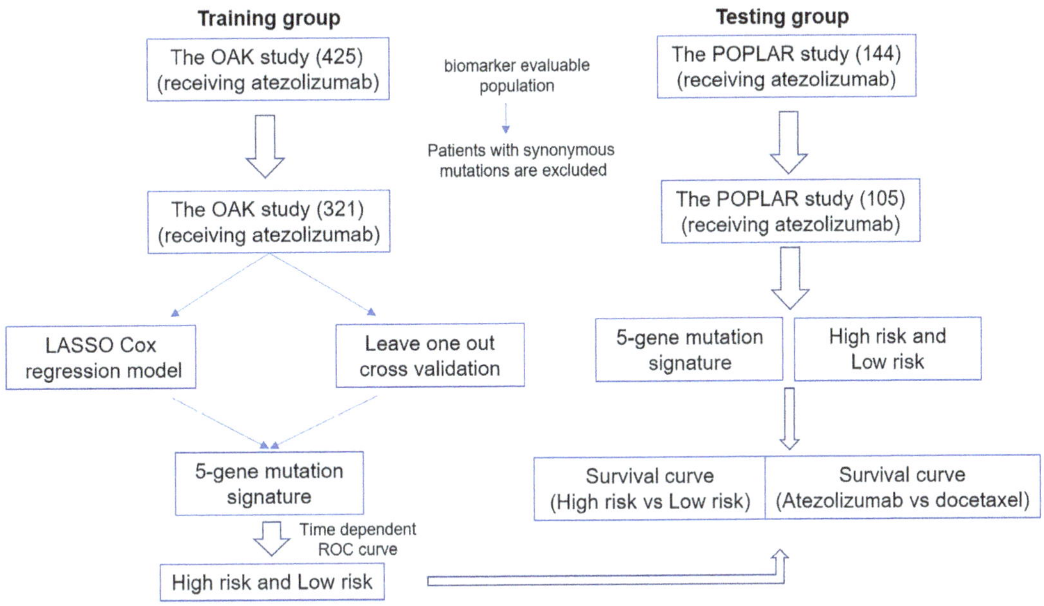

FIGURE 1 | Research and design flow chart.

applied to confirm the optimal cutoff value (0.08990467) to divide patients in high- and low-risk (**Figure 2C**). Based on the above screening, the five optimal gene mutations were: *CREBBP*, *KEAP1*, *RAF1*, *STK11* and *TP53* (**Figure 2D**). The detailed risk score is presented in **Supplementary Material 1**.

Difference in bTMB Score and PDL1 Expression High- and Low-Risk Patients Based on Our Prediction Model

Markers such as bTMB and PDL1 are vital to predict the efficacy of atezolizumab. In our study, we found that high-risk patients in the training group had a higher bTMB score compared with low-risk (high-risk 17.600 ± 1.805 *vs* low-risk 9.762 ± 0.595; *P* <0.0001) (**Figure 3A**). In addition, the PDL1 expression was divided into low (tumor cell (TC) <1%/immune cell (IC) <1%), medium (TC = 1–50%%/IC = 1–5%) and high (TC ≥50%/IC ≥5%) according to a previous study (3). The results showed that the PDL1 expression of high-risk patients was low in 35.29%, medium in 49.02% and high in 15.69% of patients, while for low-risk patients the PDL1 expression was low in 44.03%, medium in 36.94% and high in 19.03% of patients (**Figure 3B**).

The Survival Analysis for the Training Group Based on the Gene Mutation Signature

The survival analysis was used to compare the OS rate of high- and low-risk patients receiving atezolizumab. The results showed that low-risk patients had a better OS rate with a median survival of 15.343 months compared with high-risk patients that had a median survival of 6.308 months (*P* = 0.0004) (**Figure 4A**). In fact, the OS benefit of low-risk patients was demonstrated in patients receiving docetaxel from the OAK study (*P* <0.0001) (**Supplementary Figure 1A** and **Supplementary Material 2**). Importantly, bTMB was not a predictor of OS of patients receiving atezolizumab (*P* = 0.647) (**Supplementary Figure 2A**). Patients receiving atezolizumab with PDL1 ≥1% also did not present differences in OS compared with those with PDL1 <1% (*P* = 0.479) (**Supplementary Figure 2B**). Patients receiving atezolizumab with PDL1 ≥50% showed a 10.5 months median OS benefit compared with those with PDL1 <50% (*P* = 0.0058) (**Supplementary Figure 2C**). Importantly, compared with PDL1 and bTMB, our risk model had a higher Hazard Ratio (HR) and C-index to predict the OS of patients receiving atezolizumab (**Supplementary Table 1**).

Next, we analyzed the OS difference for patients receiving atezolizumab compared with those subjected to docetaxel. The results showed the high-risk patients receiving atezolizumab had a better OS benefit with a median survival of 6.308 months compared with patients receiving docetaxel that presented a 5.355 months survival (*P* = 0.0265) (**Figure 4B**). Importantly, the OS benefit of atezolizumab *vs* docetaxel was more obvious for low-risk patients (*P* <0.0001) (**Figure 4C**).

The Survival Analysis for Testing Group Patients Based on the Gene Mutation Signature

We attempted to further verify the feasibility of our prediction model using patients from the POPLAR study as our testing group. First, we screened patients receiving atezolizumab based on the same criteria (**Supplementary Material 3**). As expected, the results showed that low-risk patients receiving atezolizumab had a better OS (14.817 months) compared with high-risk

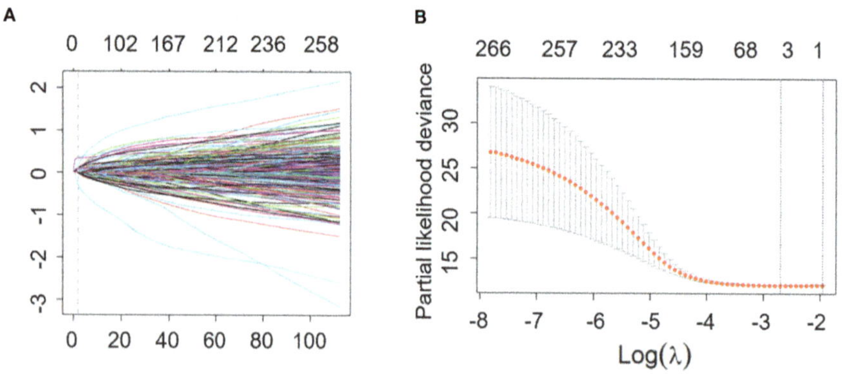

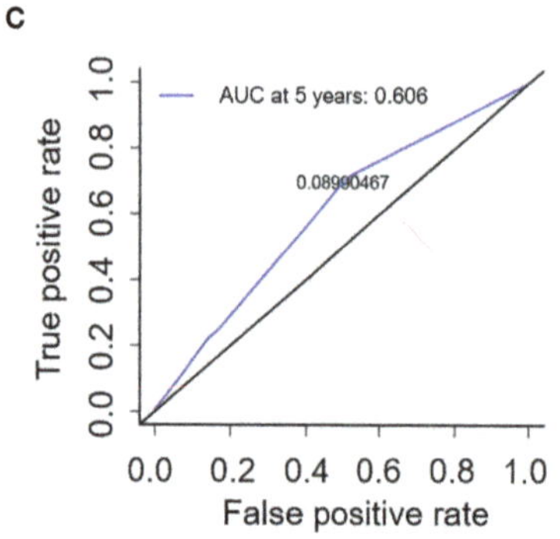

D

Gene	Coefficient
CREBBP	0.292711
KEAP1	0.306608
RAF1	-0.05406
STK11	0.023995
TP53	0.065909

FIGURE 2 | Construction of gene mutation signature to predict survival. **(A)** Trend graph of LASSO coefficients. **(B)** Partial likelihood deviation map. **(C)** Time dependent ROC curve. **(D)** 5 gene mutation types and matched coefficient.

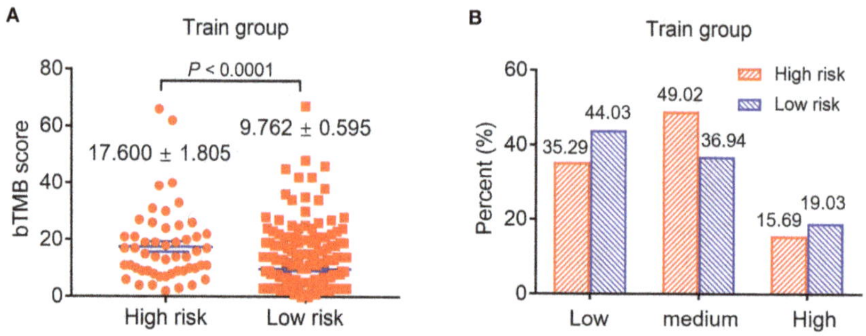

FIGURE 3 | The difference of bTMB score and PDL1 expression of patients with high and low risk. **(A)** The difference of bTMB score of patients with high and low risk ($P < 0.0001$). **(B)** The difference of PDL1 expression of patients with high and low risk.

patients (OS 6.078 months) ($P = 0.0001$) (**Figure 5A**). We also screened the patients receiving docetaxel from the POPLAR study (**Supplementary Material 4**). High-risk patients receiving docetaxel showed no OS benefits when compared to those in use of atezolizumab (median survival: 6.078 months *vs* 6.242 months, respectively) ($P = 0.6403$) (**Figure 5B**). However, low-risk patients receiving atezolizumab showed a better OS benefit with a median survival of 14.817 months compared with low-risk patients receiving docetaxel (median survival of 10.053 months) ($P = 0.0095$) (**Figure 5C**). In addition, the OS benefit of low-risk patients was also demonstrated in patients receiving docetaxel ($P = 0.0063$) (**Supplementary Figure 1B**).

Subgroup Analysis on OS After Adjusting Clinical Variables for Patients Receiving Atezolizumab Based on Training and Testing Group

Importantly, we conducted multivariate Cox analysis by adjusting clinical variables including age, race, sex, ECOG,

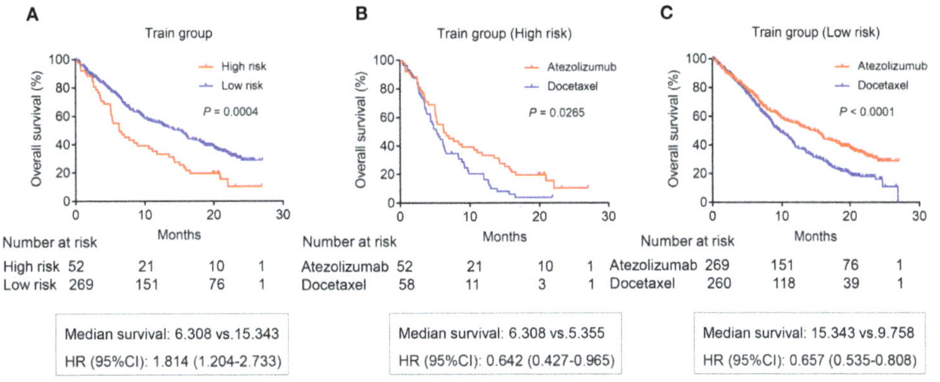

FIGURE 4 | The OS analysis for patients in the training group from OAK study. **(A)** The OS difference between the high risk and low risk patients receiving atezolizumab ($P = 0.0004$). **(B)** The OS difference of high-risk patients between atezolizumab and docetaxel ($P = 0.0265$). **(C)** The OS difference of low-risk patients between atezolizumab and docetaxel ($P < 0.0001$).

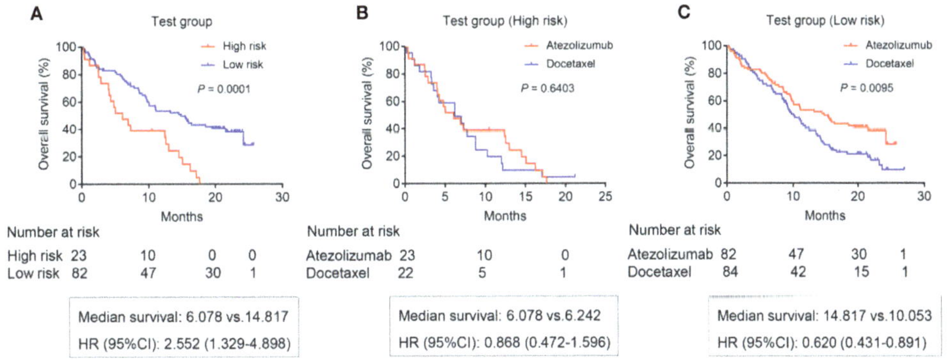

FIGURE 5 | The OS analysis for patients in the testing group from POPLAR study. **(A)** The OS difference between the high risk and low risk patients receiving atezolizumab ($P = 0.0001$). **(B)** The OS difference of high-risk patients between atezolizumab and docetaxel ($P = 0.6403$). **(C)** The OS difference of low-risk patients between atezolizumab and docetaxel ($P = 0.0095$).

Histopathology and smoking history based on the training and testing group. The results showed that risk model based on the 5-genomic mutation signature was an independent prognostic factor for patients receiving atezolizumab (HR: 95%CI: 2.031 (1.528–2.700; P <0.0001) (**Table 1**). Likewise, we also analyzed the prognostic factors for patients receiving docetaxel, the result also demonstrated that risk model based on the 5-genomic mutation signature was also an independent prognostic factor for these patients (HR:95%CI: 1.995 (1.528–2.604; P <0.0001) (**Supplementary Table 2**). Importantly, the results of multivariate Cox regression analysis showed that atezolizumab had better OS benefit compared with docetaxel in the low-risk patients (HR:95%CI: 1.572 (1.312–1.883; P <0.0001) (**Table 2**). However, the positive connection between treatment and OS was not found in high-risk patients in light of same analysis (HR:95%CI: 1.387 (0.980–1.962; P = 0.065) (**Table 3**). Interestingly, we found there is an obvious interaction between smoking history and treatment in low-risk patients based on training and testing group (P = 0.024) (**Table 2**).

DISCUSSION

The efficacy rate of immunotherapy is relatively low, which has made it imperative to explore markers to predict the efficacy of immunotherapy. It has been commonly acknowledged that high TMB and PD-L1 is associated with improved prognosis. However, there have been some limitations in their prediction of immunotherapy responses. Recently, a growing number of studies have focused on the role of genetic mutations in the prediction of immunotherapy. To explore the impact of genetic mutation on ICI prediction, we therefore developed a risk score model based on gene mutations to predict the OS of patients receiving atezolizumab. The clinical significance of our findings

TABLE 1 | Univariate and multivariate Cox regression analysis of clinical variables affecting OS for patients receiving atezolizumab based on training and testing group.

Variables	Univariate analysis		Multivariate analysis		Interaction*
	Wald	***P***	**HR (95% CI)**	***P***	***P***
Age	0.005	0.944	NI		0.692
<65					
≥65					
Race	1.656	0.198	NI		0.107
White					
Asian					
Others					
Sex	3.163	0.075	NI		0.496
Female					
Male					
Histopathology	7.668	0.006		0.005	0.806
Squamous			Reference		
Non-squamous			0.694 (0.537–0.896)	0.005	
ECOG	17.591	<0.0001		<0.0001	0.242
0			Reference		
1			1.757 (1.353–2.281)	<0.0001	
Smoking	4.242	0.039		0.180	0.098
Current			Reference		
Never			1.011 (0.649–1.576)		
Previous			1.285 (0.918–1.799)		
Risk model	25.125	<0.0001		<0.0001	
Low risk			Reference		
High risk			2.031 (1.528–2.700)	<0.0001	

*NI, not included; *Interaction between variables and risk model.*

could be seen in three aspects: First, our 5-genomic mutation signature was demonstrated to be a better predictor than PDL1 and bTMB to screen patients who would benefit from atezolizumab; It is also very convenient and economical to detect; More importantly, our 5-genomic mutation signature was able to predict OS rates of patients receiving atezolizumab, which may help clinicians select patients who could benefit more from such therapy.

The 5-genomic mutation signature of our risk score model consisted of mutations in *CREBBP*, *KEAP1*, *RAF1*, *STK11* and *TP53*. *CREBBP*, which encodes an acetyltransferase, has been frequently found to develop mutations in many tumor types (12–14). At present, there is no literature focusing on the relationship between the *CREBBP* mutation and immunotherapy outcomes. Only one previous study showed that loss of function of *CREBBP* resulted in focal depletion of enhancer *H3K27* acetylation and aberrant transcriptional silencing of genes that regulate B-cell signaling and immune responses, such as class II MHC (15). *HDAC3* inhibition represents a novel mechanism-based immune epigenetic therapy for lymphomas caused by *CREBBP* mutation (16). *KEAP1* is located at 19p13.2, and its protein has three major domains: an N-terminal broad complex, tram track, and the bric-a-brac (BTB) domain; a central intervening region (IVR); and a series of six C-terminal Kelch repeats (17). High-frequency mutations in *KEAP1* have been identified in Chinese patients with lung squamous cell carcinoma, while the somatic nonsynonymous mutation of *KEAP1* in patients with lung cancer is likely to promote tumorigenesis *via* activation of the *KEAP1/NRF2* antioxidant stress response pathway (18). Our previously study revealed that *KEAP1*-mutant NSCLC is associated with higher TMB, and also found that the OS was prolonged in NSCLC patients receiving immunotherapy with wild-type *KEAP1* compared with a mutant (6). Another study has demonstrated that *STK11/KEAP1* mutations may help identify bTMB-high patients unlikely to respond to pembrolizumab (19). Indeed, *STK11/KEAP1* mutations are prognostic, not predictive, biomarkers for anti-PD-1/anti-PDL1 therapy (20). Interestingly, we previously analyzed the relationship between *STK11* mutation and immune-related prognostic markers and immune microenvironment. The results showed that patients with the *STK11* mutation did not benefit from immune checkpoint inhibitors (6).

At present, there are a few studies focusing on *RAF1* mutation and no literature reporting the relationship between *RAF1* mutation and immunotherapy. In parallel, *BRAF* mutation was found in lung cancer even though its association with immunotherapy efficacy is controversial (21–23). *TP53* mutation is common in patients with lung cancer. Many studies focused on the relationship between *TP53* mutation and immunotherapy efficacy. Assoun et al. reported that *TP53* mutation was associated with OS benefits in NSCLC patients with advanced non-small cell lung cancer treated with immune checkpoint inhibitor (24). A study from China also demonstrated that *TP53* and *KRAS* mutations in lung adenocarcinoma might serve as a pair of potential predictive factors to guide anti-PD-1/PDL1 immunotherapy (25).

TABLE 2 | Univariate and multivariate Cox regression analysis of clinical variables affecting OS for low-risk patients based on training and testing group.

Variables	Univariate analysis		Multivariate analysis		Interaction*
	Wald	*P*	HR (95% CI)	*P*	*P*
Age	1.991	0.158	NI		0.198
<65					
≥65					
Race	2.269	0.132	NI		0.359
White					
Asian					
Others					
Sex	2.270	0.132	NI		0.826
Female					
Male					
Histopathology	15.777	<0.0001		<0.0001	0.720
Squamous			Reference		
Non-squamous			0.697 (0.577–0.842)	<0.0001	
ECOG	35.196	<0.0001		<0.0001	0.693
0			Reference		
1			1.833 (1.503–2.235)	<0.0001	
Smoking	3.367	0.067	NI		0.024
Current					
Never					
Previous					
Treatment	22.943	<0.0001		<0.0001	
Atezolizumab			Reference		
Docetaxel			1.572 (1.312–1.883)	<0.0001	

*NI, not included; *Interaction between variables and risk model.*

Altogether, the relationship between *TP53* and immunotherapy still needs further investigation.

We have successfully established a risk model based on the five genomic mutations exposed above. And the risk of death is significantly higher in high-risk cohort compared with low-risk for those receiving atezolizumab. High-risk patients were found to be those with high bTMB and PD-L1, indicating bTMB and PD-L1 were not accurate to distinguish OS for patients receiving atezolizumab. One study led by Nie also demonstrated that advanced NSCLC patients with low tumor mutation burden might derive benefit from immunotherapy (5), as consistent with our study. In fact, we compared the HR of different OS prediction models and found that our 5-genomic mutation signature had a higher HR in both the POPLAR and OAK studies when compared to other prediction models. A higher C-index was also found for our model of 5-genomic mutation signature. These results suggest that our risk score model is a better predictor of OS rate when compared to bTMB and PDL1 expression. However, more data are needed to verify our conclusions.

Another interesting finding is that our risk model could also predict the OS of patients receiving docetaxel. This may be due to the fact that these specific gene mutations are involved in the malignant biological transformation of tumors, which may not be sensitive to treatment. High-risk patients receiving atezolizumab showed a better OS compared with those treated with docetaxel from the OAK study, however, the OS benefit was not found in the POPLAR study. Maybe this is due to the smaller sample size of the POPLAR study. Moreover, there was only a one month OS benefit for high-risk patients receiving atezolizumab compared with those using docetaxel within the OAK study, which may indicate that high-risk patients have limited benefits from atezolizumab. The follow-up multivariate Cox regression analysis further proves our conjecture when combining OAK and POPLAR studies after adjusting clinical variables.

Undeniably, it has to be noted that there are some limitations of our study that need to be addressed. First, all the gene mutation types were obtained by liquid biopsies in our study, which means some gene mutations were lost. If the 5-genomic mutation signature based on liquid biopsies could be successfully verified in the future, then it could have wider clinical applications. Second, the 5-genomic mutation signature based on the OAK and POPLAR cohorts was established only to predict OS benefit for NSCLC patients receiving atezolizumab. Due to the uniqueness of PD1/PDL1 inhibitors, it is necessary to further study whether our risk score model is suitable for other immune checkpoint inhibitors. Last but not the least, we performed a data analysis based on the published OAK and POPLAR cohorts and further verification is needed in the future. And there have been several studies focusing on the role of nutritional and inflammatory indexes in the prediction of survival for patients receiving atezolizumab (26, 27). Our study distinguished from them by centering on genetic mutations. These studies are not contradictory but rather complementary to each other. Despite these limitations, our prediction model for atezolizumab still holds clinical relevance for its superiority in ICI prediction than TMB and PD-L1, as confirmed in the present study.

In conclusion, we successfully established a 5-genomic mutation signature risk score model to predict the OS rate of patients receiving atezolizumab. Importantly, low-risk patients were more

TABLE 3 | Univariate and multivariate Cox regression analysis of clinical variables affecting OS for high-risk patients based on training and testing group.

Variables	Univariate analysis		Multivariate analysis		Interaction*
	Wald	*P*	HR (95% CI)	*P*	*P*
Age	0.339	0.560	NI		0.800
<65					
≥65					
Race	2.066	0.151#		0.326	0.063
White			Reference		
Asian			0.663 (0.384–1.146)	0.141	
Others			0.868 (0.435–1.731)	0.687	
Sex	0.623	0.430	NI		0.214
Female					
Male					
Histopathology	1.540	0.215	NI		0.542
Squamous					
Non-squamous					
ECOG	1.699	0.192#		0.207	0.673
0			Reference		
1			1.270 (0.876–1.839)	0.207	
Smoking	0.297	0.586	NI		0.542
Current					
Never					
Previous					
Treatment	4.676	0.031		0.065	
Atezolizumab			Reference		
Docetaxel			1.387 (0.980–1.962)	0.065	

*NI, not included; *Interaction between variables and treatment; #P < 0.2 was included in multivariate analysis.*

likely to benefit from atezolizumab compared with those treated with docetaxel. It would be beneficial to develop a gene mutation panel to guide the treatment of NSCLC patients receiving atezolizumab in the future.

AUTHOR CONTRIBUTIONS

Study design: HW. Date collection: JL and XW. Date analysis: CyZ. Writing: JL, SB and ClZ. Chart making: JL, XW, CyZ, SB and ClZ. Supervision and amendment: HW. All authors contributed to the article and approved the submitted version.

SUPPLEMENTARY MATERIAL

Supplementary Figure 1 | The OS analysis for patients receiving docetaxel. **(A)** The OS analysis for patients receiving docetaxel from OAK study ($P < 0.0001$). **(B)** The OS analysis for patients receiving docetaxel from POPLAR study. ($P = 0.0063$).

Supplementary Figure 2 | The OS analysis for patients based on bTMB score and PDL1 expression from OAK study. **(A)** The OS difference based on different bTMB score (Cutoff=16) ($P = 0.647$). **(B)** The OS difference based on different PDL1 expression (Cutoff=1%) ($P = 0.479$). **(C)** The OS difference based on different PDL1 expression (Cutoff=50%) ($P = 0.0058$).

REFERENCES

1. Blair HA. Atezolizumab: A Review in Previously Treated Advanced Non-Small Cell Lung Cancer. *Target Oncol* (2018) 13:399–407. doi: 10.1007/s11523-018-0570-5
2. Gandara DR, Paul SM, Kowanetz M, Schleifman E, Zou W, Li Y, et al. Blood-Based Tumor Mutational Burden as a Predictor of Clinical Benefit in Non-Small-Cell Lung Cancer Patients Treated With Atezolizumab. *Nat Med* (2018) 24:1441–8. doi: 10.1038/s41591-018-0134-3
3. Fehrenbacher L, Spira A, Ballinger M, Kowanetz M, Vansteenkiste J, Mazieres J, et al. Atezolizumab Versus Docetaxel for Patients With Previously Treated Non-Small-Cell Lung Cancer (POPLAR): A Multicentre, Open-Label, Phase 2 Randomised Controlled Trial. *Lancet* (2016) 387:1837–46. doi: 10.1016/S0140-6736(16)00587-0
4. Wang Z, Duan J, Cai S, Han M, Dong H, Zhao J, et al. Assessment of Blood Tumor Mutational Burden as a Potential Biomarker for Immunotherapy in Patients With Non–Small Cell Lung Cancer With Use of a Next-Generation Sequencing Cancer Gene Panel. *JAMA Oncol* (2019) 5:696–702. doi: 10.1001/jamaoncol.2018.7098
5. Nie W, Xu MD, Gan L, Zhang Y, Qian J, Gu K, et al. Advanced Non-Small Cell Lung Cancer Patients With Low Tumor Mutation Burden Might Derive Benefit From Immunotherapy. *J Immunother* (2020) 43:189–95. doi: 10.1097/CJI.0000000000000318
6. Wang H, Guo J, Shang X, Wang Z. Less Immune Cell Infiltration and Worse Prognosis After Immunotherapy for Patients With Lung Adenocarcinoma Who Harbored STK11 Mutation. *Int Immunopharmacol* (2020) 84:106574. doi: 10.1016/j.intimp.2020.106574
7. Zhang C, Zhang C, Li J, Wang H. Keap1-Nfe2l2-Mutant NSCLC and Immune Checkpoint Inhibitors: A Large Database Analysis. *J Thorac Oncol* (2020) 15: e85–6. doi: 10.1016/j.jtho.2020.02.027
8. Li H, Li J, Zhang C, Zhang C, Wang H. TERT Mutations Correlate With Higher TMB Value and Unique Tumor Microenvironment and May Be a Potential Biomarker for Anti-CTLA4 Treatment. *Cancer Med* (2020) 15:7151–60. doi: 10.1002/cam4.3376
9. Wang F, Zhao Q, Wang YN, Jin Y, He MM, Liu ZX, et al. Evaluation of POLE and POLD1 Mutations as Biomarkers for Immunotherapy Outcomes Across Multiple Cancer Types. *JAMA Oncol* (2019) 5:1504–6. doi: 10.1001/jamaoncol.2019.2963
10. Xu X, Yang Y, Liu X, Cao N, Zhang P, Zhao S, et al. Nfe2l2/Keap1 Mutations Correlate With Higher Tumor Mutational Burden Value/PD-L1 Expression and Potentiate Improved Clinical Outcome With Immunotherapy. *Oncologist* (2020) 25:e955–63. doi: 10.1634/theoncologist.2019-0885
11. Rittmeyer A, Barlesi F, Waterkamp D, Park K, Ciardiello F, von Pawel J, et al. Atezolizumab Versus Docetaxel in Patients With Previously Treated Non-Small-Cell Lung Cancer (OAK): A Phase 3, Open-Label, Multicentre

Randomised Controlled Trial. *Lancet* (2017) 389:255–65. doi: 10.1016/S0140-6736(16)32517-X

12. Vogelsberg A, Steinhilber J, Mankel B, Federmann B, Schmidt J, Montes-Mojarro IA, et al. Genetic Evolution of in Situ Follicular Neoplasia to Aggressive B-Cell Lymphoma of Germinal Center Subtype. *Haematologica* (2020). doi: 10.3324/haematol.2020.254854
13. Carazo F, Bértolo C, Castilla C, Cendoya X, Campuzano L, Serrano D, et al. DrugSniper, a Tool to Exploit Loss-of-Function Screens, Identifies CREBBP as a Predictive Biomarker of VOLASERTIB in Small Cell Lung Carcinoma (SCLC). *Cancers (Basel)* (2020) 12:1824. doi: 10.3390/cancers12071824
14. Massé J, Truntzer C, Boidot R, Khalifa E, Pérot G, Velasco V, et al. Solid-Type Adenoid Cystic Carcinoma of the Breast, a Distinct Molecular Entity Enriched in NOTCH and CREBBP Mutations. *Mod Pathol* (2020) 33:1041–55. doi: 10.1038/s41379-019-0425-3
15. Jiang Y, Ortega-Molina A, Geng H, Ying HY, Hatzi K, Parsa S, et al. Crebbp Inactivation Promotes the Development of HDAC3-Dependent Lymphomas. *Cancer Discovery* (2017) 7:38–53. doi: 10.1158/2159-8290.CD-16-0975
16. Mondello P, Tadros S, Teater M, Fontan L, Chang AY, Jain N, et al. Selective Inhibition of HDAC3 Targets Synthetic Vulnerabilities and Activates Immune Surveillance in Lymphoma. *Cancer Discov* (2020) 10:440–59. doi: 10.1158/2159-8290.CD-19-0116
17. Singh A, Misra V, Thimmulappa RK, Lee H, Ames S, Hoque MO, et al. Dysfunctional KEAP1-NRF2 Interaction in Non-Small-Cell Lung Cancer. *PloS Med* (2006) 3:e420. doi: 10.1371/journal.pmed.0030420
18. Gong M, Li Y, Ye X, Zhang L, Wang Z, Xu X, et al. Loss-of-Function Mutations in KEAP1 Drive Lung Cancer Progression Via KEAP1/NRF2 Pathway Activation. *Cell Commun Signal* (2020) 18:98. doi: 10.1186/s12964-020-00568-z
19. Aggarwal C, Thompson JC, Chien AL, Quinn KJ, Hwang WT, Black TA, et al. Baseline Plasma Tumor Mutation Burden Predicts Response to Pembrolizumab-Based Therapy in Patients With Metastatic Non-Small Cell Lung Cancer. *Clin Cancer Res* (2020) 26:2354–61. doi: 10.1158/1078-0432
20. Papillon-Cavanagh S, Doshi P, Dobrin R, Szustakowski J, Walsh AM. STK11 and KEAP1 Mutations as Prognostic Biomarkers in an Observational Real-World Lung Adenocarcinoma Cohort. *ESMO Open* (2020) 5:e000706. doi: 10.1136/esmoopen-2020-000706
21. Zhang C, Zhang C, Lin J, Li Z, Wang H. Patients With BRAF-Mutant NSCLC May Not Benefit From Immune Checkpoint Inhibitors: A Population-Based Study. *JTO Clin Res Rep* (2020) 1:100006. doi: 10.1016/j.jtocrr.2020.100006
22. Guisier F, Dubos-Arvis C, Viñas F, Doubre H, Ricordel C, Ropert S, et al. Efficacy and Safety of Anti-PD-1 Immunotherapy in Patients With Advanced NSCLC With Braf, HER2, or MET Mutations or RET Translocation: GFPC 01-2018. *J Thorac Oncol* (2020) 15:628–36. doi: 10.1016/j.jtho.2019.12.129
23. Dudnik E, Peled N, Nechushtan H, Wollner M, Onn A, Agbarya A, et al. Braf Mutant Lung Cancer: Programmed Death Ligand 1 Expression, Tumor Mutational Burden, Microsatellite Instability Status, and Response to Immune Check-Point Inhibitors. *J Thorac Oncol* (2018) 13:1128–37. doi: 10.1016/j.jtho.2018.04.024
24. Assoun S, Theou-Anton N, Nguenang M, Cazes A, Danel C, Abbar B, et al. Association of TP53 Mutations With Response and Longer Survival Under Immune Checkpoint Inhibitors in Advanced Non-Small-Cell Lung Cancer. *Lung Cancer* (2019) 132:65–71. doi: 10.1016/j.lungcan.2019.04.005
25. Dong ZY, Zhong WZ, Zhang XC, Su J, Xie Z, Liu SY, et al. Potential Predictive Value of TP53 and KRAS Mutation Status for Response to PD-1 Blockade Immunotherapy in Lung Adenocarcinoma. *Clin Cancer Res* (2017) 23:3012–24. doi: 10.1158/1078-0432.CCR-16-2554
26. Sorich MJ, Rowland A, Karapetis CS, Hopkins AM. Evaluation of the Lung Immune Prognostic Index for Prediction of Survival and Response in Patients Treated With Atezolizumab for NSCLC: Pooled Analysis of Clinical Trials. *J Thorac Oncol* (2019) 14(8):1440–6. doi: 10.1016/j.jtho.2019.04.006
27. Hopkins AM, Kichenadasse G, Garrett-Mayer E, Karapetis CS, Rowland A, Sorich MJ. Development and Validation of a Prognostic Model for Patients With Advanced Lung Cancer Treated With the Immune Checkpoint Inhibitor Atezolizumab. *Clin Cancer Res* (2020) 26(13):3280–6. doi: 10.1158/1078-0432.CCR-19-2968

19

Efficacy and Safety of PD-1/PD-L1 Inhibitors Plus Chemotherapy Versus PD-1/PD-L1 Inhibitors in Advanced Non-Small Cell Lung Cancer

Xiang Li[1†], Shi Yan[1†], Jichun Yang[2†], Yaqi Wang[1], Chao Lv[1], Shaolei Li[1], Jun Zhao[3], Yue Yang[1], Minglei Zhuo[3] and Nan Wu[1*]*

[1] Key Laboratory of Carcinogenesis and Translational Research (Ministry of Education), Department of Thoracic Surgery II, Peking University Cancer Hospital & Institute, Beijing, China, [2] Central Laboratory, The Second Affiliated Hospital of Kunming Medical University, Kunming, China, [3] Key Laboratory of Carcinogenesis and Translational Research (Ministry of Education), Department I of Thoracic Oncology, Peking University Cancer Hospital & Institute, Beijing, China

***Correspondence:**
Nan Wu
nanwu@bjmu.edu.cn
Minglei Zhuo
minglei1978@163.com

[†]These authors have contributed equally to this work

Immune checkpoint inhibitors (ICIs) are recommended as first-line treatment for late-stage non-small cell lung cancer (NSCLC), either as monotherapy or in combination with chemotherapy. However, efficacy and safety comparisons between ICIs as monotherapy and ICIs with chemotherapy are lacking. We searched PubMed, Embase, and Cochrane Library for randomized controlled trials published before February 29th, 2020, with the search terms "immunotherapy" and "chemotherapy". 10 eligible trials were identified with a total of 5,956 patients. Of these patients, 3,204 received immune therapy and 2,752 received chemotherapy. PD-1 inhibitors with chemotherapy improved OS (HR 0.84, 0.77–0.92), PFS (HR 0.80, 0.75–0.85), and objective response rate (ORR) (odds ratio (OR) 2.55, 1.20–5.28) compared to PD-1 inhibitors as monotherapy. In contrast, PD-L1 inhibitors plus chemotherapy showed no significant differences in OS, PFS, or ORR compared with PD-L1 inhibitors as monotherapy. When patients were stratified according to PD-L1 expression level, patients with high PD-L1 expression (≥ 50%) receiving PD-1 inhibitors plus chemotherapy had improved PFS, but not other outcomes, compared to PD-1 inhibitors as monotherapy. In these patients, PD-L1 inhibitors plus chemotherapy showed no significant difference in survival compared with PD-L1 inhibitors. In the low PD-L1 expression group (1%–49%), PD-1 inhibitors plus chemotherapy improved OS and PFS, but no advantage was observed in PD-L1 inhibitors plus chemotherapy in OS, PFS, or ORR compared with PD-L1 inhibitor monotherapy. When comparing PD-1/PD-L1 inhibitors plus chemotherapy with PD-1/PD-L1 inhibitors monotherapy, no significant differences were observed in the rate of immune-related adverse events (AEs). In summary, for treating patients with late-stage NSCLC, PD-1 inhibitors plus chemotherapy have improved efficacy compared with PD-1 inhibitor monotherapy, but PD-L1 inhibitors plus chemotherapy have similar efficacy as PD-L1 monotherapy. Survival benefits of PD-1/PD-L1 inhibitors combined with chemotherapy were particularly significant in patients with low PD-L1 expression levels.

Keywords: PD-1/PD-L1 inhibitors, late-stage non-small cell lung cancer, PD-L1 expression level, survival efficacy, safety, first line treatment

INTRODUCTION

Worldwide in 2018, 2,093,876 new lung cancer patients were diagnosed and lung cancer caused 1,761,007 deaths (1). Non-small cell lung cancer (NSCLC) accounts for 80%–85% of these cases (2). Therapeutic regimes for patients with NSCLC in stage III or beyond include radical radiotherapy, chemo-radiotherapy, gene targeted therapy, and immune checkpoint inhibitors (ICIs).

ICI therapies, targeting T-cell regulatory pathways to provide significant clinical benefits against cancers (3, 4), have been heralded as a promising treatment for lung cancer. The receptor PD-1 and its ligands PD-L1 and PD-L2 play a vital role in the maintenance of immunologic self-tolerance (5). Cancers can exploit this pathway to escape T-cell-mediated attack by the immune system. Clinical practice has attempted to enhance anti-tumor immune responses by augmenting costimulatory signals, but coinhibitory signals that block anti-tumor T-cell responses have been shown to be more effective than costimulatory signals (6).

MDX1105 (nivolumab) was the first PD-1 inhibitor used in cancer therapy. In 2010, it was reported that one patient with colorectal cancer achieved a complete response and two patients with melanoma and renal cancer achieved partial response (7). More recent data have indicated that 18% of NSCLC patients respond to treatment with MDX11105 (8).

NCCN guidelines recommend the PD-1 inhibitor pembrolizumab as first-line treatment for NSCLC with PD-L1 expression level ≥50%. KEYNOTE-024 (9) demonstrated that pembrolizumab improved median OS compared to chemotherapy, with OS of 30 months with pembrolizumab and 14.2 months with chemotherapy. Similarly, KEYNOTE-042 (10) showed that median OS was 22.3 months in patients treated with pembrolizumab and 10.5 months in patients treated with chemotherapy. KEYNOTE-407 (11) evaluated pembrolizumab plus chemotherapy in patients with stage IV squamous NSCLC. In this study, median OS was 15.9 months in patients receiving combination therapy and 11.3 months in patients receiving chemotherapy. A similar trend was observed in non-squamous NSCLC patients in IMpower 130, in which the median OS was 18.6 months in patients receiving the PD-L1 inhibitor atezolizumab plus chemotherapy and 13.9 months in patients receiving chemotherapy. Comparisons between PD-1/PD-L1 inhibitor monotherapy and chemotherapy confirmed the survival benefits of immunotherapy (9, 10, 12, 13). The NCCN NSCLC panel recommended single-agent pembrolizumab as first-line therapy for NSCLC patients with PD-L1 expression level >1%, and ICIs plus chemotherapy were recommended for patients who could tolerate adverse events (AEs) (14, 15).

Although immunotherapy has gradually become the mainstay in NSCLC therapy, optimization of the treatment plan for advanced NSCLC patients is still facing challenge. This network analysis aims to compare the efficacy and safety of PD-1/PD-L1 inhibitors plus chemotherapy with PD-1/PD-L1 monotherapy.

METHODS

Data Sources and Searches

This network analysis was conducted using Preferred Reporting Item for Systemic Reviews and Meta-Analyses guidelines (16). The review is registered on the PROSPERO website as No. CRD42020166678. PubMed, Embase, and Cochrane Library were systematically searched up to February 29th, 2020, using the search terms "non-small cell lung cancer," "immune checkpoint inhibitors," "immune checkpoint blockade," "pembrolizumab," "nivolumab," "atezolizumab," "durvalumab," and "chemotherapy." See **Supplementary Material** for more information.

Study Selection

Two reviewers (XL and SY) independently screened the study titles and abstracts based on predefined inclusion and exclusion criteria. The reviewers discussed any discrepancies or, if necessary, by seeking a decision from a third reviewer (NW).

Inclusion criteria for studies were as follows: (i) Patients had histologically confirmed previously untreated unresectable advanced (stage IIIB/IIIC/IV) NSCLC without *EGFR* or *ALK* mutations. (ii) Interventions were PD-1/PD-L1 inhibitor plus platinum-based chemotherapy or PD-1/PD-L1 inhibitor alone. (iii) Comparators were platinum-based chemotherapy. (iv) Outcomes were efficacy outcomes, including OS, PFS, ORR; and safety outcomes, including AEs. OS was defined as the time from when patients enrolled into trials to death with any cause. PFS was defined as the time from randomization until progression for any cause. ORR was defined as the proportion of patients achieving partial or complete remission. AEs were defined and graded according to the common terminology criteria from the National Cancer Institute (17). (v) Only randomized controlled trials (RCTs) were included.

Studies were excluded according to the following exclusion criteria: (i) Patients had cytologically or histologically confirmed small cell lung cancer or other kinds of lung cancer. Patients with driver gene-mutations were excluded. Patients who had received previous systemic treatment were excluded. (ii) Patients who received spontaneous anti-CTLA-4 were excluded. Patients who received concurrent or sequential radio-chemotherapy were excluded. (iii) Studies other than RCTs were excluded.

Data Extraction and Risk of Bias Assessment

Data were extracted using ADDIS 16.7 software. Two investigators independently reviewed the full text of included studies and extracted information, including first author, year of publication, patient characteristics, inclusion and exclusion criteria, treatment protocol, outcomes, HR for OS, HR for PFS, OR for ORR, and OR for AEs. We concentrated on treatment-related severe AEs, defined as grades 3–5. The included trials were performed at multiple sites worldwide over long periods, so we extracted data from the most recent published articles or conference reports possible. Risk of bias of trials was assessed independently by two investigators using the Cochrane risk of bias tool (18). Differences in data extraction were mediated by Prof. N.W.

Data Synthesis and Statistical Analysis

Direct Comparison

Pooled HRs with 95% confidence intervals (95% CI) were calculated for OS and PFS and pooled ORs with 95% CI were calculated for ORR and the rate of AEs using the random-effects model in REVMAN 5.3 (Cochrane). The quantity I^2 was used to describe heterogeneity between studies. We included only low risk of bias in the sensitivity analysis.

Indirect and Mixed Comparisons

A random-effects network meta-analysis (NMA) within a Bayesian framework was then performed using OpenBUGS version 3.2.3. Pooled HRs and ORs with 95% CI were also summarized. Each treatment was ranked using the surface under the cumulative ranking curve (SUCRA) and a treatment hierarchy was generated. A treatment ranked as 100% is certain to be the best and a treatment ranked as 0% is certain to be the worst in terms of efficacy and safety outcomes. We also used the contribution plot to measure the percent contribution of each direct comparison to the mixed estimates, the indirect estimates, and the entire network, as shown in the **Supplementary Material**.

Examination of Assumptions in Network Meta-Analysis

To check the consistency of the NMA, we used the node-splitting model to assess inconsistencies between direct and indirect treatment effects. A predictive interval plot was used to estimate heterogeneity for all comparisons.

Additional Analyses

We used the comparison-adjusted funnel plot to assess small-study effects. The synthesized endpoints included OS, PFS, ORR, and treatment-related grade 3–5 AEs. HRs of OS and PFS were preferentially reported and were adjusted for confounders in individual studies (19). HR could also be estimated according to the method described by Tierney and colleagues (20). Consistency was assessed by comparing synthesized HR of NMA with pairwise head-to-head meta-analyses. The ORs of ORR and AEs were calculated using Bayesian statistics.

Bayesian NMA was done using a Markov Chain Monte Carlo simulation technique in OpenBUGS version 3.2.3. We used non-informative uniform and normal prior distributions (21) and three different sets of initial values to fit the model. For OS and PFS, 30,000 sample iterations were generated with 5,000 burn-ins and a thinning interval of 10. For ORR and AE, 50,000 sample iterations were generated with 20,000 burn-ins and a thinning interval of 10.

Transitivity was estimated by assessing studies that compared two treatments and evaluating direct and indirect comparisons (22). All included studies were RCTs that compared experimental treatments with platinum-based chemotherapy, providing convincing and stable transitivity.

Patients were stratified according to PD-L1 expression (≥ 50% or 1%–49%). PD-1 inhibitors and PD-L1 inhibitors were evaluated to determine their effect on the NMA.

RESULTS

Systematic Review and Characteristics

We screened 1,426 records (**Figure 1**) and identified 24 studies for full-text reads. Ten eligible RCTs were included in this NMA (**Table 1**), with a total of 5,956 patients receiving one of six treatment strategies as first-line therapy for advanced unresectable lung cancer. Of these patients, 3,204 patients received immune therapy and 2,752 patients received chemotherapy. Most of the included trials were published with low bias (see **Supplementary Material**).

The included trials (9–13, 23–27) reported HRs for OS and PFS. Four of the trials (9, 10, 12, 13) evaluated a PD-1 or PD-L1 inhibitor as monotherapy while six of the trials (11, 23–27) evaluated a PD-1 or PD-L1 inhibitor in combination with chemotherapy. Six trials (9, 12, 13, 23, 24, 26) used a platinum-based chemotherapy plus pemetrexed or gemcitabine, three trials (11, 25, 27) used a platinum-based chemotherapy plus paclitaxel, and one trial (10) used a platinum-based chemotherapy plus pemetrexed/paclitaxel (**Table 1**). Some studies reported efficacy outcomes stratified according to PD-L1 expression; eight trials (9–13, 23, 25, 27) reported survival data in patients with high PD-L1 expression (≥ 50%) and five trials (10, 11, 23, 25, 27) reported survival data in patients with low PD-L1 expression (1-49%) (**Figure 2**).

Results of Pairwise Meta-Analysis

Head-to-head comparisons revealed that compared with chemotherapy, OS was improved in patients treated with PD-1 inhibitors (HR 0.85, 0.76–0.95), PD-1 inhibitors plus chemotherapy (HR 0.57, 0.48–0.69), and PD-L1 inhibitors plus chemotherapy (HR 0.83, 0.74–0.94). PFS was also improved in patients treated with PD-L1 inhibitors (HR 0.77, 0.63–0.94), PD-1 inhibitors plus chemotherapy (HR 0.54, 0.47–0.62), and PD-L1 inhibitors plus chemotherapy (HR 0.65, 0.59–0.72). No significant difference in PFS was observed when comparing

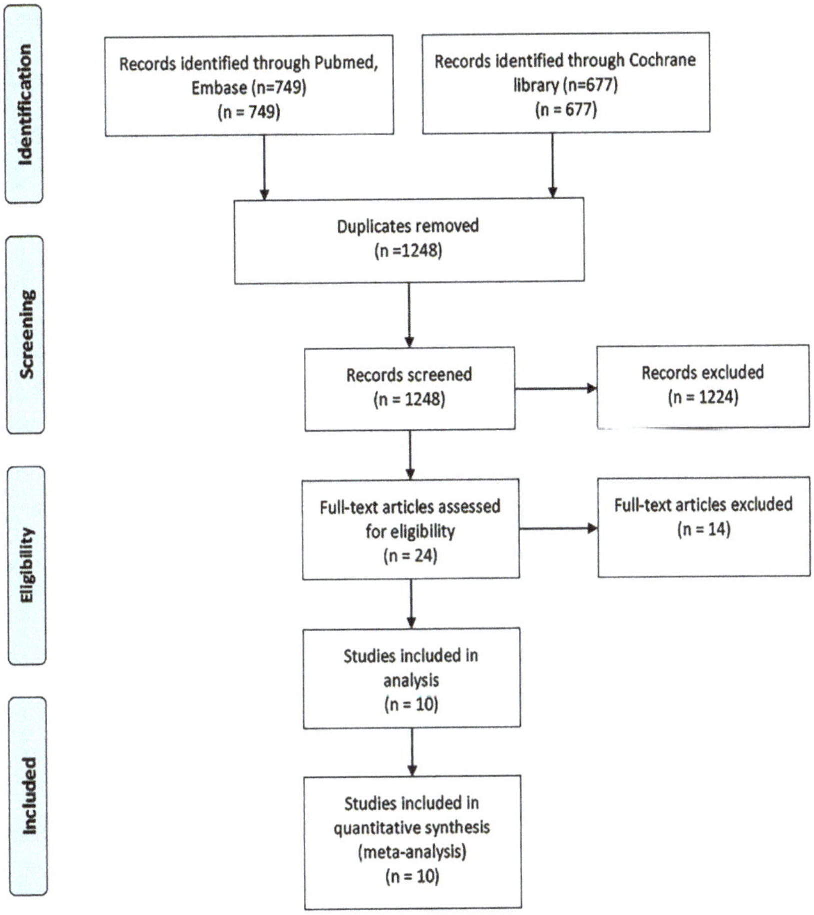

FIGURE 1 | The flow diagram of studies selection.

PD-1 inhibitors as monotherapy with chemotherapy (HR 1.0, 0.91–1.1).

Efficacy Outcomes

Compared with PD-1/PD-L1 inhibitors as monotherapy, PD-1 and PD-L1 inhibitors combined with chemotherapy did not significantly improve OS (HR 0.94, 0.90–1.01), but the combination therapy did significantly improve PFS (HR 0.82, 0.78–0.87).

Compared with PD-1 inhibitor monotherapy, PD-1 inhibitors plus chemotherapy significantly improved OS (HR 0.84, 0.77–0.92), PFS (HR 0.80, 0.75–0.85), and ORR (OR 2.55, 1.20–5.28).

Compared with PD-L1 inhibitor monotherapy, PD-L1 inhibitors plus chemotherapy showed no significant difference in OS (HR 1.01, 0.89–1.13), PFS (0.91, 0.82–1.01), and ORR (OR 2.02, 0.68–5.80) (**Figure 3**).

Compared with PD-L1 inhibitor plus chemotherapy, PD-1 inhibitor plus chemotherapy significantly improved OS (HR 0.85, 0.76–0.93) but not PFS (HR 0.99, 0.92–1.06) (**Figure 4**).

High PD-L1 Expression Level

In patients with high PD-L1 expression levels (≥ 50%), PD-1/PD-L1 inhibitors plus chemotherapy did not significantly improve OS compared to PD-1/PD-L1 inhibitors as monotherapy (HR 0.94, 0.82–1.07), but did significantly improve PFS (HR 0.78, 0.70–0.86). PD-1 inhibitors plus chemotherapy did not significantly improve OS compared with PD-1 inhibitors (HR 0.86, 0.73–1.03), but did significantly improve PFS (HR 0.72, 0.63–0.83). PD-L1 inhibitors plus chemotherapy did not significantly improve OS (HR 1.08, 0.85–1.37) or PFS (HR 0.89, 0.73–1.08) compared with PD-L1 inhibitors as monotherapy. PD-1 inhibitors plus chemotherapy significantly improved OS (HR 0.85, 0.76–0.93), but not PFS (HR 0.99, 0.92–1.06) compared with PD-L1 inhibitors plus chemotherapy.

Low PD-L1 Expression Level

In patients with low PD-L1 expression levels (1%–49%), PD-1/PD-L1 inhibitors plus chemotherapy significantly improved OS (HR 0.84, 0.73–0.96) and PFS (HR 0.79, 0.73–0.85) compared

TABLE 1 | Characteristics and results of included trials.

Patient Numbers		HR (95% CI)		ORR (%)	AEs	
		OS	PFS		All	Severe
IMpower-110	572					
Atezolizumab 1200 mg Q3W	286	0.83	0.77	29.2	258	91
Cisplatin 75 mg/m² or carboplatin AUC 6, pemetrexed 500 mg/m² IV Q3W; cisplatin 75 mg/m² + gemcitabine 1,250 mg/m² or carboplatin AUC 5 + gemcitabine 1,000 mg/m² IV Q3W	286	(0.65–1.07)	(0.63–0.94)	31.8	249	144
IMpower-130	705					
Atezolizumab 1,200 mg Q3W, then carboplatin 6 mg/ml Q3W plus nab-paclitaxel 100 mg/m2 QW	473	0.79	0.64	49.2	455	354
Carboplatin 6 mg/mL Q3W + nab-paclitaxel 100 mg/m2 QW	232	(0.64–0.98)	(0.54–0.77)	31.9	215	141
IMpower-131	683					
Atezolizumab 1,200 mg IV Q3W, then carboplatin AUC 6 IV Q3W, nab-paclitaxel 100 mg/m² IV QW	343	0.96	0.61	49	332	274
Carboplatin AUC 6 IV Q3W, nab-paclitaxel 100 mg/m² IV QW	340	(0.78–1.18)	(0.48–0.77)	41	324	234
IMpower-132	578					
Atezolizumab 1,200 mg IV Q3W, then carboplatin AUC 6 mg/ml/min IV Q3W or cisplatin 75 mg/m² IV Q3W, pemetrexed 500 mg/m² IV Q3W	292	0.81	0.60	47	286	202
Carboplatin AUC 6 mg/ml/min IV Q3W or cisplatin 75 mg/m² IV Q3W, pemetrexed 500 mg/m² IV Q3W	286	(0.64–1.03)	(0.49–0.72)	32	266	161
CheckMate-026	541					
Nivolumab 3 mg/kg Q2W	271	1.02	1.15	26	190	47
Cisplatin 75 mg/m² + gemcitabine 1,250 mg/m² or carboplatin AUC 5 + gemcitabine 1,000 mg/m² or carboplatin AUC 6 + paclitaxel 2,000 mg/m²; cisplatin 75 mg/m² or carboplatin AUC 6 + pemetrexed 500 mg/m²	270	(0.8–1.3)	(0.91–1.45)	33	243	133
KEYNOTE-021	123					
Pembrolizumab 200 mg + carboplatin AUC 5 + pemetrexed 500 mg/m² IV Q3W	60	0.90	1.17	42.7	55	23
Carboplatin AUC 5 + pemetrexed 500 mg/m² IV Q3W	63	(0.42–1.91)	(0.95–1.43)	18.4	56	16
KEYNOTE-024	305					
Pembrolizumab 200 mg Q3W, 35 cycles	154	0.60	0.50	44.8	113	41
Carboplatin AUC 5/6 Q3W or cisplatin 75 mg/m² + pemetrexed 500 mg/m² Q3W; cisplatin 75 mg/m² or carboplatin AUC 5/6 + gemcitabine 1,250 mg/m² Q3W or paclitaxel 200 mg/m² Q3W	151	(0.41–0.89)	(0.37–0.68)	41.98	135	80
KEYNOTE-042	1274					
Pembrolizumab 200 mg Q3W, 35 cycles	637	0.79	0.64	27	399	113
Carboplatin AUC 5/6 Q3W + paclitaxel 200 mg/m² Q3W or carboplatin AUC 5/6 Q3W + pemetrexed 500 mg/m² Q3W, 6 cycles	637	(0.64–0.98)	(0.54–0.77)	27	553	252
KEYNOTE-189	616					
Pembrolizumab 200 mg + pemetrexed 500 mg/m² + carboplatin AUC 5 or cisplatin 75 mg/m² Q3W, 4 cycles	410	0.79	0.64	47.6	404	272
Placebo (saline) + pemetrexed 500 mg/m² + carboplatin AUC 5 or cisplatin 75 mg/m² Q3W, 4 cycles	206	(0.64–0.98)	(0.54–0.77)	18.9	200	133
KEYNOTE-407	559					
Pembrolizumab 200 mg Q3W + carboplatin AUC 6 + paclitaxel 200 mg/m² or nab-paclitaxel 100 mg/m² Q3W, then pembrolizumab 200 mg Q3W	278	0.64	0.56	57.4 58.7	273	194
Carboplatin AUC 6 + paclitaxel 200 mg/m² or nab-paclitaxel 100 mg/m² Q3W, then pembrolizumab 200 mg Q3W	281	(0.49–0.85)	(0.45–0.70)	37.7 39.5	274	191

OS = overall survival; PFS = progression-free survival; ORR = objective response rate; AEs = adverse events; all = all AEs; severe = grade3-5 AEs.

with PD-1/PD-L1 inhibitors as monotherapy. PD-1 inhibitors combined with chemotherapy significantly improved OS (HR 0.81, 0.68–0.95) and PFS (HR 0.75, 0.67–0.85) compared with PD-1 inhibitors as monotherapy. No significant differences were observed in OS (HR 0.91, 0.71–1.15) or PFS (HR 0.93, 0.80–1.07) when comparing PD-1 inhibitors plus chemotherapy with PD-L1 inhibitors plus chemotherapy (**Figure 5**).

Safety Outcomes

In this network analysis, PD-1/PD-L1 inhibitors combined with chemotherapy were more likely to cause AEs, and especially severe AEs (grade 3–5) than PD-1/PD-L1 inhibitors as monotherapy (**Figure 6**). PD-1 inhibitors plus chemotherapy caused more AEs than PD-1 inhibitors as monotherapy when considering any AEs (OR 7.73, 2.99–19.88) and also when considering only severe AEs (OR 4.55, 2.94–7.69). Compared with PD-L1 inhibitor monotherapy, PD-L1 inhibitor plus chemotherapy caused more AEs overall (OR 4.96, 1.39–20.34) and more severe AEs (OR 4.76, 2.27–10.0). Compared with PD-1 inhibitor plus chemotherapy, PD-L1 inhibitor plus chemotherapy caused more AEs overall (OR 1.60, 0.51–5.20) and more severe AEs (OR 1.52, 0.88–2.56), but no significant differences were observed. Compared with PD-L1 inhibitors as monotherapy, PD-1 inhibitors as monotherapy did not cause significantly more overall AEs (OR 0.69, 0.14–1.35) or severe AEs (grade 3–5) (OR 0.41, 0.14–1.33) (**Figure 7**).

When comparing PD-1 inhibitors plus chemotherapy with PD-1 inhibitors as monotherapy, no significant differences were observed in the rate of immune-related AEs, including hypothyroidism (OR 0.41, 0.12–1.46), hyperthyroidism (OR

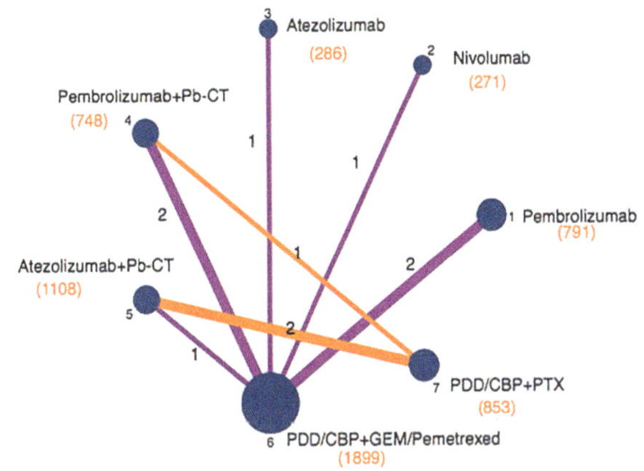

FIGURE 2 | Net plot of included trials.

0.38, 0.04–3.75), pneumonia (OR 0.18, 0.03–1.41), and skin reactions (OR 0.10, 0.00–1.45). When comparing PD-L1 plus chemotherapy with PD-1 plus chemotherapy, no significant differences were observed in the rate of immune-related AEs, including hypothyroidism (OR 3.57, 0.68–24.47), hyperthyroidism (OR 4.82, 0.19–291.1), and pneumonia (OR 1.17, 0.17–13.44).

Rank Probabilities

Ranking probabilities of the six treatments were summarized for OS, PFS, ORR, and AEs (**Supplementary Material**). PD-1 inhibitor plus chemotherapy provided the most favorable balance between efficacy and safety. For ORR, PD-1 inhibitor plus chemotherapy ranked first (89%) and PD-L1 inhibitor plus chemotherapy ranked second (77%). Similarly, PD-1 inhibitor plus chemotherapy had the highest SUCRA ranking. Nivolumab had the highest SUCRA ranking for AEs, causing the fewest severe AEs (98.9%) and overall AEs (90.5%). Pembrolizumab plus chemotherapy ranked first in OS (98.9%) and PFS (98.4%), pembrolizumab ranked second in OS (52.5%), and atezolizumab plus chemotherapy ranked second (91.2%) in PFS.

Assessment of Heterogeneity

Heterogeneity estimates were calculated in four sub-group pairwise analyses (see **Supplementary Figures 8, 9, 40**). During analysis, no heterogeneity (I^2 = 0%) or low heterogeneity (I^2<50%) was used to assess comparisons. Notably, the I^2 values of "PD-1 inhibitors versus platinum-based chemotherapy" were 75% for OS, 91% for PFS, and 33% for severe AEs. Meanwhile, the I^2 value of "PD-1 inhibitors plus platinum-based chemotherapy versus platinum-based chemotherapy" showed moderated heterogeneity (41%). Other comparisons showed minimal heterogeneity (I^2 = 0%).

Node-split plots for ORR and AEs were listed (see **Supplementary Material**) and consistency was confirmed for p-values > 0.05. Forest plots of direct and indirect comparisons were generated for OS (**Figure 8**), PFS (**Figure 9**), ORR (**Supplementary Material**), and AEs (**Supplementary Material**). Funnel plots indicated little report bias among trials (**Supplementary Material**).

DISCUSSION

Immunotherapy has been proved to be an effective treatment in NSCLC and its use has gradually increased in clinical practice. The appropriate choice of ICI and treatment regime requires solid evidence. ICIs monotherapy and ICIs with chemotherapy are both recommended in NCCN guidelines. ICIs target T-cell

PD-1	0.80 (0.28 to 2.31)	2.55 (1.20 to 5.28)	1.62 (0.75 to 3.51)	0.90 (0.51 to 1.55)
1.25 (0.43 to 3.56)	**PD-L1**	3.18 (1.08 to 8.80)	2.02 (0.68 to 5.80)	1.12 (0.43 to 2.80)
0.39 (0.19 to 0.84)	0.31 (0.11 to 0.93)	**PD-1+Pb-CT**	0.63 (0.31 to 1.36)	0.35 (0.22 to 0.59)
0.62 (0.29 to 1.34)	0.50 (0.17 to 1.48)	1.58 (0.73 to 3.21)	**PD-L1+Pb-CT**	0.56 (0.33 to 0.96)
1.11 (0.65 to 1.95)	0.89 (0.36 to 2.31)	2.82 (1.71 to 4.58)	1.79 (1.05 to 3.07)	**Pb-CT**

FIGURE 3 | Network meta-analysis of objective response rate in all patients.

Overall survival (upper right); Progression-free survival (lower left)

PD-1	0.99 (0.88 to 1.11)	0.84 (0.77 to 0.92)	0.99 (0.92 to 1.07)	1.07 (1.02 to 1.13)
1.12 (1.02 to 1.24)	PD-L1	0.85 (0.74 to 0.97)	1.01 (0.89 to 1.13)	1.08 (0.97 to 1.21)
1.25 (1.17 to 1.33)	1.11 (1.01 to 1.23)	PD-1+Pb-CT	1.18 (1.07 to 1.31)	1.28 (1.18 to 1.38)
1.23 (1.15 to 1.32)	1.10 (0.99 to 1.22)	0.99 (0.92 to 1.06)	PD-L1+Pb-CT	1.08 (1.03 to 1.14)
1.002 (0.96 to 1.05)	0.89 (0.82 to 0.97)	0.80 (0.76 to 0.84)	0.81 (0.77 to 0.86)	Pb-CT

FIGURE 4 | Network meta-analysis of all patients.

Overall survival (upper right); Progression-free survival (lower left)

PD-1	0.81 (0.68 to 0.95)	0.89 (0.72 to 1.09)	1.04 (0.96 to 1.12)
1.33 (1.18 to 1.50)	PD-1+Pb-CT	1.10 (0.87 to 1.40)	1.29 (1.11 to 1.49)
1.23 (1.12 to 1.36)	0.93 (0.80 to 1.07)	PD-L1+Pb-CT	1.17 (0.96 to 1.41)
1.03 (1.01 to 1.05)	0.77 (0.69 to 0.87)	0.84 (0.76 to 0.92)	Pb-CT

FIGURE 5 | Network meta-analysis of patients with PD-L1 expression level 1% to 49%.

regulatory pathways to enhance the anti-tumor immune response, providing significant benefit in cancer therapy (3, 4). Further, ICIs as monotherapy have performed better than chemotherapy alone in several large multicenter trials (9, 10, 13). The NCCN NSCLC panel has recommended single-agent pembrolizumab as first-line treatment for eligible patients with metastatic advanced NSCLC regardless of histology for patients with PD-L1 expression levels greater than 50% and without EGFR, ALK, ROS1, and BRAF V600E mutations. Pembrolizumab is also recommended as monotherapy in patients with low PD-L1 expression (1%–49%) (15), and recent research has suggested that patients with PD-L1 expression levels just below and just above 50% are likely to have a similar response (28). Combining ICIs and chemotherapy sometimes performed better than ICIs as monotherapy, but there is not consistent clinical evidence to support this treatment approach. This study was designed to

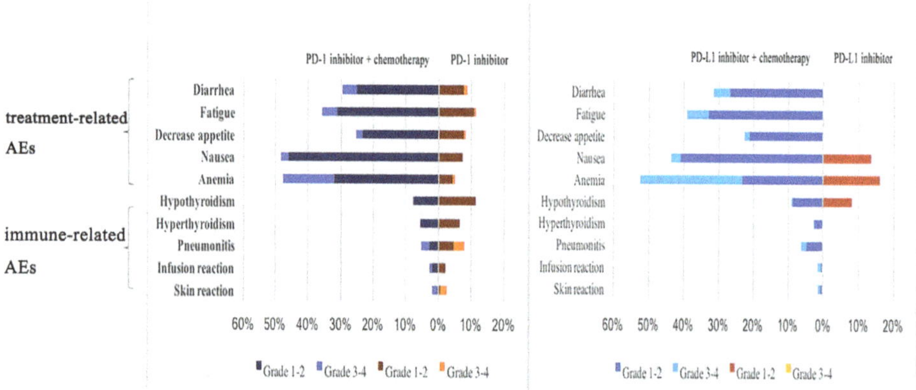

FIGURE 6 | Proportion of adverse events in all patients.

All adverse events (upper right); Grade 3-5 adverse events (lower left)

PD-1	2.47 (0.75 to 7.32)	7.73 (2.99 to 19.88)	12.22 (4.69 to 34.36)	4.77 (2.68 to 7.75)
0.69 (0.14 to 1.35)	**PD-L1**	3.15 (0.90 to 11.63)	4.96 (1.39 to 20.34)	1.94 (0.72 to 5.44)
0.22 (0.13 to 0.34)	0.32 (0.16 to 0.62)	**PD-1+Pb-CT**	1.60 (0.51 to 5.20)	0.62 (0.27 to 1.35)
0.14 (0.08 to 0.24)	0.21 (0.10 to 0.44)	0.66 (0.39 to 1.14)	**PD-L1+Pb-CT**	0.39 (0.15 to 0.88)
0.28 (0.19 to 0.39)	0.40 (0.22 to 0.74)	1.28 (0.93 to 1.80)	1.93 (1.28 to 2.97)	**Pb-CT**

FIGURE 7 | Network meta-analysis of adverse events in all patients.

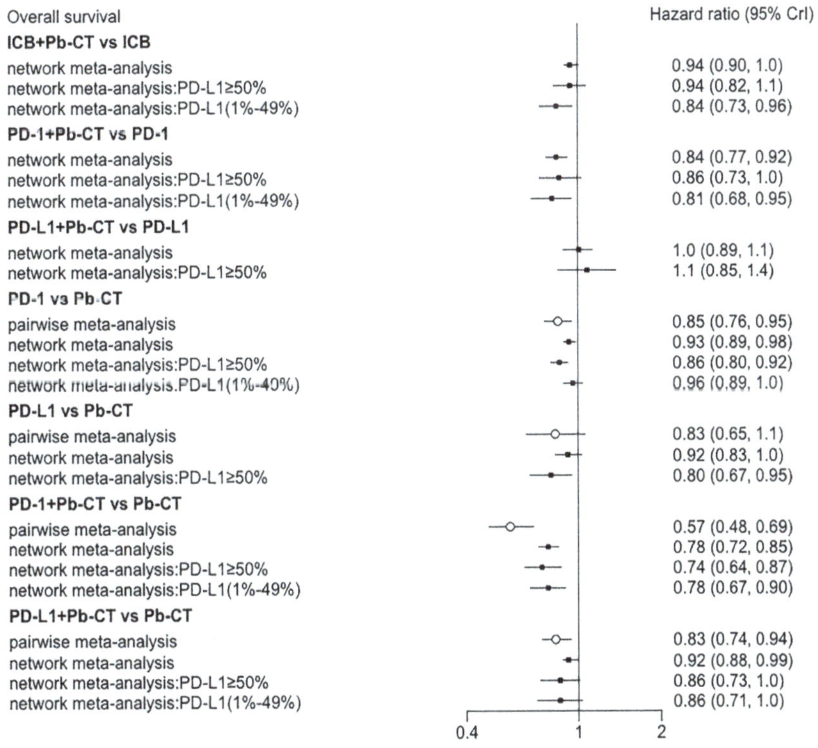

FIGURE 8 | Consistency analysis for overall survival.

provide additional guidance on choosing the optimal treatment plan for NSCLC patients with different PD-L1 expression levels.

10 trials evaluating PD-1/PD-L1 inhibitors were included in this analysis. We considered efficacy outcomes (OS, PFS, and ORR) and safety outcomes (AEs) to compare treatment with PD-1/PD-L1 inhibitor plus chemotherapy with PD-1/PD-L1 inhibitors as monotherapy. The trial results were also examined for effect modifiers. Consistency analysis indicated well-behaved data with robust stability.

Our results demonstrated: (i) PD-1/PD-L1 inhibitors plus chemotherapy performed better than PD-1/PD-L1 inhibitors as monotherapy, particularly in patients with low PD-L1 expression levels (1-49%). (ii) PD-1 inhibitors plus chemotherapy improved OS compared with PD-L1 inhibitors plus chemotherapy. (iii) PD-1/PD-L1 inhibitors plus chemotherapy caused more AEs than PD-1/PD-L1 inhibitors as monotherapy.

PD-1/PD-L1 inhibitors plus chemotherapy improved PFS compared with PD-1/PD-L1 inhibitors as monotherapy, but no

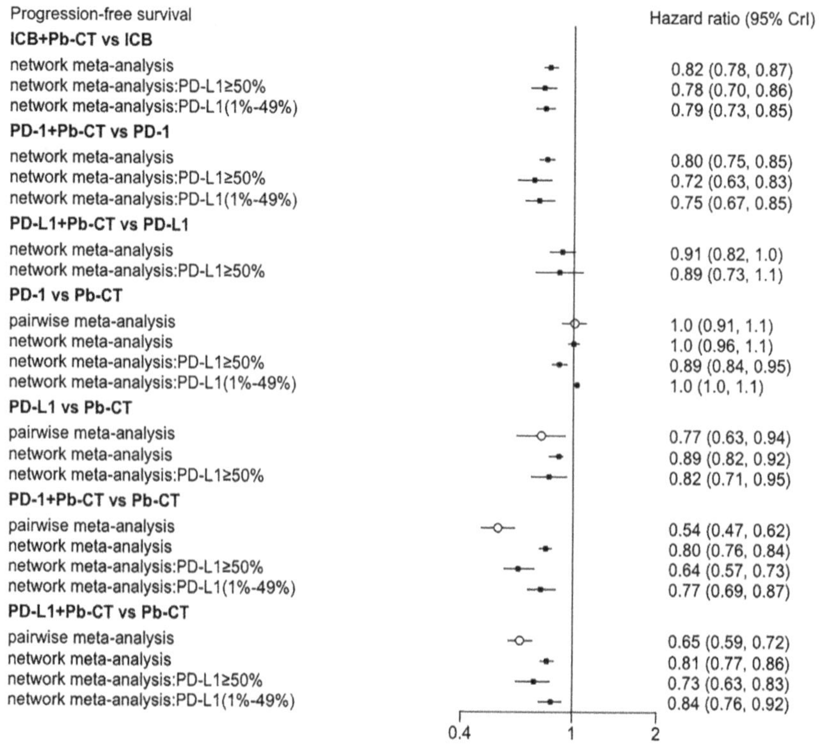

FIGURE 9 | Consistency analysis for progression-free survival.

significant differences were observed for OS. Nonsynonymous mutations and neo-antigens in tumors are associated with improved efficacy, durable clinical benefits, and PFS (5). Stratifying patients based on PD-L1 expression demonstrated that patients with lower PD-L1 expression level (1%–49%) may obtain better OS and PFS benefits from immunotherapy plus chemotherapy compared to immunotherapy alone. Likewise, patients receiving PD-1 inhibitors plus chemotherapy had improved OS and PFS compared with patients receiving PD-1 inhibitors as monotherapy, regardless of PD-L1 expression level. Multiple factors may impact the clinical efficacy of immunotherapy (29). In such cases, ICIs plus chemotherapy may be a better option for patients (30) than platinum-based chemotherapy (11, 23–25, 27).

Basic research has revealed that synergistic anti-tumor effects of immunotherapy and chemotherapy could be mediated through several pathways. First, cytotoxic T lymphocyte (CTL) could generate an immune response to kill tumor cells by releasing perforin or cytokines or through FasL-mediated apoptosis. Chemotherapy increased the expression level of mannose-6-phosphate receptors, with more Granzyme B expressed on CTLs allowing them to enter tumor cells (31). Second, chemotherapy can enhance tumor cell immunogenicity by increasing HSP 70/90 expression on the surface of tumor cells or increasing DNA cross-linking. Tumors with high autophagy would release more adenosine triphosphate than those lacking autophagy, as the latter cannot adequately stimulate T lymphocytes or recruit CD4 and CD8, while the former could raise more dendritic cells (DC) and T lymphocytes (32). Third, chemotherapy causes immunogenic cell death in tumors, causing calreticulin/HSP exposure and adenosine triphosphate/HMGB1 (high-mobility group box 1) release (33). Fourth, chemotherapy could help clear immune-suppressing cells. Along with decreased lymphocytes, immunosuppressive CD4+, CD25+, Foxp3+ regulatory T cells, and myeloid derived suppressor cells could also be cleared (34). Finally, chemotherapy could change the tumor micro-environment to promote antigen presentation and anti-tumor immune response, causing tumor cells to release HMGB1. This could recruit and activate DC as well as induce DC maturation. The combination of HMGB1 and toll-like receptor 4 on DC may also prevent degradation of tumor antigens (35).

PD-L1 expression level may serve as a biomarker to predict ICI efficacy. In this study, patients with lower PD-L1 expression levels (1%–49%) obtained improved survival benefits from PD-1/PD-L1 inhibitors plus chemotherapy compared with PD-1/PD-L1 inhibitors as monotherapy. Meanwhile, PD-1/PD-L1 inhibitors plus chemotherapy showed no survival advantage for patients with high PD-L1 expression level (≥ 50%). Recent research has revealed that T cells secrete cytokines, inducing multiple positive feedback loops. Chemokines promote T cell infiltration, and the altered antigen presentation could help T cells recognize tumor cells. Accordingly, the activation of the PD-1 or PD-L1 pathway is more important than PD-L1 expression level (36).

Interestingly, when PD-1 inhibitors plus chemotherapy were compared with PD-L1 inhibitors plus chemotherapy, the former improved OS, but no significant difference was observed for PFS.

Patient stratification according to PD-L1 expression level removed any advantage for OS, PFS, and ORR. Pembrolizumab plus chemotherapy did have a significant advantage compared with atezolizumab plus chemotherapy in terms of OS and PFS.

AEs caused by ICIs may be enhanced by chemotherapy as these treatments cause different kinds of toxicities. Other studies have shown that severe AEs after immune therapy, and especially immune-related AEs, hinder the efficacy of immune treatments. Previous studies have revealed several mechanisms causing AEs (37). Immune therapy increases T-cell activity against antigens present on both tumors and healthy tissue, and immune therapy causes increased levels of preexisting autoantibodies. In addition, immune therapy increases the level of inflammatory cytokines and enhances complement-mediated inflammation due to direct binding of an anti-CTLA-4 antibody to CTLA-4 expressed by normal tissue (38).

Compared with PD-L1 inhibitor monotherapy, PD-1 inhibitor monotherapy improved treatment outcomes in multiple tumor types (39). In treating NSCLC, no significant differences were observed between monotherapy with these two ICIs. PD-1 inhibitors block the interaction between PD-1 and B7.1/PD-L1, while PD-L1 inhibitors block the interaction between PD-L1 and PD-1/RGMB. Once the PD-1-PD-L1 pathway is suppressed, T cells can kill tumor cells. This may explain the similar efficacy of PD-1 inhibitor monotherapy and PD-L1 inhibitor monotherapy in terms of OS, PFS, ORR, and AEs.

IMPLICATION

This network analysis provides new evidence which helps clinician to choose optimal treatments for previously untreated advanced NSCLC patients. PD-1/PD-L1 inhibitors plus chemotherapy did not significantly improve survival compared to PD-1/PD-L1 monotherapy. However, PD-1 inhibitors plus chemotherapy did significantly improve OS, PFS, and ORR, compared to PD-1 inhibitor monotherapy, but also caused increased AEs. PD-L1 inhibitors plus chemotherapy showed no significant improvement in OS, PFS, or ORR compared with PD-L1 inhibitor monotherapy. In addition, patients were stratified according to their PD-L1 expression level. Our results suggest that patients with high PD-L1 expression level (≥ 50%) might be optimally treated with PD-1/PD-L1 inhibitor monotherapy, while patients with low PD-L1 expression level (1-49%) may obtain more benefits from PD-L1 inhibitors plus chemotherapy compared with PD-1 inhibitors as monotherapy, as long as patients could tolerate increased immune-related AEs. Consistent with the comparison between PD-1 inhibitors and PD-L1 inhibitors given as monotherapy, no significant differences in PFS, ORR, or AEs were observed between PD-1 inhibitors plus chemotherapy and PD-L1 inhibitors plus chemotherapy.

LIMITATIONS

This study has several limitations. Due to the essence of network analysis, this research provides a starting point for clinical practice. Several of the multicenter RCTs included in this study are ongoing and this research will need to be updated as more data are available. In addition, patients were not stratified according to histology (adenocarcinoma or squamous cell cancer) for analysis. Another limitation was the high heterogeneity observed when comparing PD-1 to platinum-based chemotherapy, both in OS (I^2 = 75%) and PFS (I^2 = 91%). In subgroup analysis, we did not show efficiency in patients with negative PD-L1 expression (<1%), because data within these patients were not available in enrolled published studies, which needs further exploration. Furthermore, this study only included trials evaluating the PD-L1 inhibitor atezolizumab as trials with durvalumab did not meet inclusion criteria. Finally, the KEYNOTE studies measured PD-L1 expression level with 22C3 pharmDx assays and IMpower trials used SP142 assays. These difference in detection methods could potentially cause patients to be misclassified (38).

CONCLUSIONS

PD-1 inhibitors combined with chemotherapy improved outcomes for patients with late-stage NSCLC compared with PD-1 inhibitor monotherapy, while PD-L1 inhibitors combined with chemotherapy had similar outcomes as PD-L1 monotherapy. The survival benefits of PD-1/PD-L1 inhibitors combined with chemotherapy were particularly striking in patients with low PD-L1 expression levels.

AUTHOR CONTRIBUTIONS

NW, MZ, and XL conceptualized and designed the study, collected and organized the data, and drafted the initial manuscript. XL, SY, YW, and SL collected and organized the data, review the included articles, and conducted the analyses. XL, JY, CL, and JZ collected and organized the data and reviewed the included articles. NW and MZ conceptualized and designed the study, coordinated and supervised data collected, and critically reviewed and revised the manuscript. YY critically reviewed and revised the manuscript. All authors contributed to the article and approved the submitted version.

REFERENCES

1. Bray F, Ferlay J, Soerjomataram I, Siegel RL, Torre LA, Jemal A. Global cancer statistics 2018: GLOBOCAN estimates of incidence and mortality worldwide for 36 cancers in 185 countries. *CA Cancer J Clin* (2018) 68(6):394–424. doi: 10.3322/caac.21492
2. Research UK. *Lung Cancer Risk Factors*. [Available from: http://www.cancerresearchuk.org/health-professional/cancer-statistics/statistics-by-cancer-type/lung-cancer/incidence - collapseFour.
3. Gubin MM, Zhang X, Schuster H, Caron E, Ward JP, Noguchi T, et al. Checkpoint blockade cancer immunotherapy targets tumour-specific mutant antigens. *Nature* (2014) 515(7528):577–81. doi: 10.1038/nature13988

4. La-Beck NM, Jean GW, Huynh C, Alzghari SK, Lowe DB. Immune Checkpoint Inhibitors: New Insights and Current Place in Cancer Therapy. *Pharmacotherapy* (2015) 35(10):963–76. doi: 10.1002/phar.1643
5. Boussiotis VA. Molecular and Biochemical Aspects of the PD-1 Checkpoint Pathway. *New Engl J Med* (2016) 375(18):1767–78. doi: 10.1056/NEJMra1514296
6. Allison JP, Hurwitz AA, Leach DR. Manipulation of costimulatory signals to enhance antitumor T-cell responses. *Curr Opin Immunol* (1995) 7(5):682–6. doi: 10.1016/0952-7915(95)80077-8
7. Brahmer JR, Drake CG, Wollner I, Powderly JD, Picus J, Sharfman WH, et al. Phase I study of single-agent anti-programmed death-1 (MDX-1106) in refractory solid tumors: safety, clinical activity, pharmacodynamics, and immunologic correlates. *J Clin Oncol Off J Am Soc Clin Oncol* (2010) 28 (19):3167–75. doi: 10.1200/JCO.2009.26.7609
8. Topalian SL, Hodi FS, Brahmer JR, Gettinger SN, Smith DC, McDermott DF, et al. Safety, activity, and immune correlates of anti-PD-1 antibody in cancer. *New Engl J Med* (2012) 366(26):2443–54. doi: 10.1056/NEJMoa1200690
9. Reck M, Rodríguez-Abreu D, Robinson AG, Hui R, Csőszi T, Fülöp A, et al. Pembrolizumab versus Chemotherapy for PD-L1-Positive Non-Small-Cell Lung Cancer. *New Engl J Med* (2016) 375(19):1823–33. doi: 10.1056/NEJMoa1606774
10. Mok TSK, Wu YL, Kudaba I, Kowalski DM, Cho BC, Turna HZ, et al. Pembrolizumab versus chemotherapy for previously untreated, PD-L1-expressing, locally advanced or metastatic non-small-cell lung cancer (KEYNOTE-042): a randomised, open-label, controlled, phase 3 trial. *Lancet (London England)* (2019) 393(10183):1819–30. doi: 10.1016/S0140-6736(18)32409-7
11. Paz-Ares L, Luft A, Vicente D, Tafreshi A, Gumus M, Mazieres J, et al. Pembrolizumab plus Chemotherapy for Squamous Non-Small-Cell Lung Cancer. *New Engl J Med* (2018) 379(21):2040–51. doi: 10.1056/NEJMoa1810865
12. Carbone DP, Reck M, Paz-Ares L, Creelan B, Horn L, Steins M, et al. First-Line Nivolumab in Stage IV or Recurrent Non-Small-Cell Lung Cancer. *New Engl J Med* (2017) 376(25):2415–26. doi: 10.1056/NEJMoa1613493
13. Spigel DR, De Marinis F, Giaccone G, Reinmuth N, Vergnenegre A, Barrios CH, et al. IMpower110: Interim OS Analysis of a Phase III Study of Atezolizumab (atezo) vs Platinum-Based Chemotherapy (chemo) as 1L Treatment (tx) in PD-L1–selected NSCLC. *ESMO* (2019) 379:v915. doi: 10.1093/annonc/mdz293
14. Zhou C, Wang J, Bu H, Wang B, Han B, Lu Y, et al. Chinese Experts Consensus on Immune Checkpoint Inhibitors for Non-small Cell Lung Cancer (2019 version). *Zhongguo Fei Ai Za Zhi Chin J Lung Cancer* (2020) 23(2):65–76. doi: 10.3779/j.issn.1009-3419.2020.02.01
15. Pai-Scherf L, Blumenthal GM, Li H, Subramaniam S, Mishra-Kalyani PS, He K, et al. FDA Approval Summary: Pembrolizumab for Treatment of Metastatic Non-Small Cell Lung Cancer: First-Line Therapy and Beyond. *Oncol* (2017) 22(11):1392–9. doi: 10.1634/theoncologist.2017-0078
16. Moher D, Liberati A, Tetzlaff J, Altman DG, Group P. Preferred reporting items for systematic reviews and meta-analyses: the PRISMA statement. *J Clin Epidemiol* (2009) 62(10):1006–12. doi: 10.1016/j.jclinepi.2009.06.005
17. Basch E, Iasonos A, Mcdonough T, Barz A, Schrag D. Patient versus clinician symptom reporting using the National Cancer Institute Common Terminology Criteria for Adverse Events: Results of a questionnaire-based study. *Lancet Oncol* (2006) 7(11):903–9. doi: 10.1016/S1470-2045(06)70910-X
18. Higgins JPT, Altman DG. *Assessing Risk of Bias in Included Studies.* Chichester, West Sussex, United Kingdom: John Wiley & Sons, Ltd (2008).
19. Woods BS, Hawkins N, Scott DA. Network meta-analysis on the log-hazard scale, combining count and hazard ratio statistics accounting for multi-arm trials: a tutorial. *BMC Med Res Methodol* (2010) 10:54. doi: 10.1186/1471-2288-10-54
20. Tierney JF, Stewart LA, Ghersi D, Burdett S, Sydes MR. Practical methods for incorporating summary time-to-event data into meta-analysis. *Trials* (2007) 8:16. doi: 10.1186/1745-6215-8-16
21. Sutton A, Ades AE, Cooper N, Abrams K. Use of indirect and mixed treatment comparisons for technology assessment. *Pharmacoeconomics* (2008) 26(9):753–67. doi: 10.2165/00019053-200826090-00006
22. Cipriani A, Higgins JP, Geddes JR, Salanti G. Conceptual and technical challenges in network meta-analysis. *Ann Internal Med* (2013) 159(2):130–7. doi: 10.7326/0003-4819-159-2-201307160-00008
23. Gandhi L, Rodriguez-Abreu D, Gadgeel S, Esteban E, Felip E, De Angelis F, et al. Pembrolizumab plus Chemotherapy in Metastatic Non-Small-Cell Lung Cancer. *New Engl J Med* (2018) 378(22):2078–92. doi: 10.1056/NEJMoa1801005
24. Langer CJ, Gadgeel SM, Borghaei H, Papadimitrakopoulou VA, Patnaik A, Powell SF, et al. Carboplatin and pemetrexed with or without pembrolizumab for advanced, non-squamous non-small-cell lung cancer: a randomised, phase 2 cohort of the open-label KEYNOTE-021 study. *Lancet Oncol* (2016) 17 (11):1497–508. doi: 10.1016/S1470-2045(16)30498-3
25. West H, McCleod M, Hussein M, Morabito A, Rittmeyer A, Conter HJ, et al. Atezolizumab in combination with carboplatin plus nab-paclitaxel chemotherapy compared with chemotherapy alone as first-line treatment for metastatic non-squamous non-small-cell lung cancer (IMpower130): a multicentre, randomised, open-label, phase 3 trial. *Lancet Oncol* (2019) 20 (7):924–37. doi: 10.1016/S1470-2045(19)30167-6
26. Papadimitrakopoulou V. IMpower132: Atezolizumab Plus Carboplatin and Pemetrexed in Stage IV Nonsquamous NSCLC. *WCLC* (2018).
27. Jotte RM. IMpower131 Study: Atezolizumab Plus Chemotherapy in Advanced Squamous NSCLC. *ASCO* (2018).
28. Kerr KM, Nicolson MC. Non-Small Cell Lung Cancer, PD-L1, and the Pathologist. *Arch Pathol Lab Med* (2016) 140(3):249–54. doi: 10.5858/arpa.2015-0303-SA
29. Liu Q, Zhu H, Tiruthani K, Shen L, Chen F, Gao K, et al. Nanoparticle-Mediated Trapping of Wnt Family Member 5A in Tumor Microenvironments Enhances Immunotherapy for B-Raf Proto-Oncogene Mutant Melanoma. *ACS Nano* (2018) 12(2):1250–61. doi: 10.1021/acsnano.7b07384
30. Sharma P, Allison JP. The future of immune checkpoint therapy. *Science* (2015) 348(6230):56–61. doi: 10.1126/science.aaa8172
31. Motyka B, Korbutt G, Pinkoski MJ, Heibein JA, Caputo A, Hobman M, et al. Mannose 6-phosphate/insulin-like growth factor II receptor is a death receptor for granzyme B during cytotoxic T cell-induced apoptosis. *Cell* (2000) 103(3):491–500. doi: 10.1016/S0092-8674(00)00140-9
32. Michaud M, Martins I, Sukkurwala AQ, Adjemian S, Ma Y, Pellegatti P, et al. Autophagy-Dependent Anticancer Immune Responses Induced by Chemotherapeutic Agents in Mice. *Autophagy* (2012) 334(3):1573–7. doi: 10.1126/science.1208347
33. Vacchelli E, Senovilla L, Eggermont A, Fridman WH, Galon J, Zitvogel L, et al. Trial watch: Chemotherapy with immunogenic cell death inducers. *Oncoimmunology* (2013) 2(3):e23510. doi: 10.4161/onci.23510
34. Muranski P, Boni A, Wrzesinski C, Citrin DE, Rosenberg SA, Childs R, et al. Increased intensity lymphodepletion and adoptive immunotherapy–how far can we go? *Nat Clin Pract Oncol* (2006) 3(12):668–81. doi: 10.1038/ncponc0666
35. Liu Y, Cao X. Synergistic antitumor effects of immunotherapy and chemotherapy and the underlying mechanism. *Chin J Cancer Biother* (2014) 21(1):98–103. doi: 10.3872/j.issn.1007-385X.2014.1.017
36. Shen X, Zhao B. Efficacy of PD-1 or PD-L1 inhibitors and PD-L1 expression status in cancer: meta-analysis. *BMJ* (2018) 362:v3529. doi: 10.1136/bmj.k3529
37. Postow MA, Sidlow R, Hellmann MD. Immune-Related Adverse Events Associated with Immune Checkpoint Blockade. *New Engl J Med* (2018) 378 (2):158–68. doi: 10.1056/NEJMra1703481
38. Zhou Y, Huang D, Paris PL, Sauter CS, Prock KA, Hoffman GS. An analysis of CTLA-4 and proinflammatory cytokine genes in Wegener's granulomatosis. *Arthritis Rheumatol* (2004) 50(8):2645–50. doi: 10.1002/art.20385
39. Duan J, Cui L, Zhao X, Bai H, Cai S, Wang G, et al. Use of Immunotherapy With Programmed Cell Death 1 vs Programmed Cell Death Ligand 1 Inhibitors in Patients With Cancer: A Systematic Review and Meta-analysis. *JAMA Oncol* (2019) 6(3):375–84. doi: 10.1001/jamaoncol.2019.5367

20

The Evolution of BRAF Activation in Non-Small-Cell Lung Cancer

Longyao Zhang[1]*, Linpeng Zheng*[1]*, Qiao Yang*[2] *and Jianguo Sun*[1*]

[1] Cancer Institute, Xinqiao Hospital, Army Medical University, Chongqing, China, [2] Department of Ultrasound, The 941Hospital of the Chinese People's Liberation Army (PLA) Joint Logistic Support Force, Xining, China

***Correspondence:**
Jianguo Sun
sunjg09@aliyun.com*

Non-small-cell lung cancer (NSCLC) is the most common subtype of lung cancer, of which approximate 4% had BRAF activation, with an option for targeted therapy. BRAF activation comprises of V600 and non-V600 mutations, fusion, rearrangement, in-frame deletions, insertions, and co-mutations. In addition, BRAF primary activation and secondary activation presents with different biological phenotypes, medical senses and subsequent treatments. BRAF primary activation plays a critical role in proliferation and metastasis as a driver gene of NSCLC, while secondary activation mediates acquired resistance to other targeted therapy, especially for epidermal growth factor tyrosine kinase inhibitor (EGFR-TKI). Treatment options for different activation of BRAF are diverse. Targeted therapy, especially two-drug combination therapy, is an important option. Besides, immune checkpoint inhibitors (ICIs) would be another option since BRAF activation would be a positive biomarker of tumor response of ICIs therapy. To date, no high level evidences support targeted therapy or immunotherapy as prioritized recommendation. After targeted therapy, the evolution of BRAF includes the activation of the upstream, downstream and bypass pathways of BRAF. In this review, therapeutic modalities and post-therapeutic evolutionary pathways of BRAF are discussed, and future research directions are also provided.

Keywords: BRAF activation, EGFR mutation, non-small cell lung cancer, targeted therapy, acquired resistance, immune checkpoint inhibitors

INTRODUCTION

Lung cancer is the leading reason of cancer death worldwide, accounting for 18% of all and non-small-cell lung cancer (NSCLC) is the most common subtype of lung cancer (1). With the development of precision medicine, especially next-generation sequencing (NGS) technology and circulating tumor DNA (ctDNA) technology, targeted therapy has replaced platinum-based chemotherapy as the first-line treatment for NSCLC patients with driver gene mutations (2, 3). More and more driver genes have been found in NSCLC, among which activated BRAF proto-oncogene accounts for approximate 4% (4, 5). BRAF mutant tumors are characterized as an aggressive histologic pattern with micropapillary features, and indicates a poor prognosis.

This review provides a comprehensive overview of characteristics, treatment modalities, and outcomes for NSCLC patients with different BRAF mutations. The pathways of activation and evolution of BRAF are divided into primary and secondary mutations. And different BRAF types have different clinical, biological and pathological features. The mechanism of acquired resistance and subsequent evolution of BRAF activation and the strategies after resistance are also discussed.

A BRIEF HISTORY OF BRAF SIGNALING

The RAF kinase has been closely and inextricably linked to cancer since 1983, when v-raf was first described by Ulf Rapp et al. (6) This is a murine retroviral oncogene with a mammalian cell homolog, called CRAF. And in 1984-1985, two CRAF-related genes were identified in studies in mice and humans: ARAF and BRAF (7, 8). In 2002, following the pioneering work of Davies et al. (9) on the BRAF gene, a number of studies have clarified the specific implications of BRAF mutations in lung cancer (10, 11). In 2011, following the results of a phase III trial (BRIM-3), the FDA approved the first drug targeting BRAF-mutated cancers, PLX4032 (vemurafenib) (12). Two years later, based on the results of the Phase III trial (NCT01227889), another targeted agent against BRAF mutations, Dabrafenib (GSK21188436), was also approved by the FDA for the treatment of advanced melanoma (13). In the same year, Trametinib (GSK1120212) was also approved for the treatment of patients with advanced melanoma with the BRAF V600E mutation (14). In 2017, dabrafenib and trametinib received FDA approval for the treatment of metastatic non-small cell lung cancer carrying the BRAF V600E mutation (15). The next year, the FDA approved encorafenib in combination with binimetinib which is an anti-MEK1/2 protein kinase inhibitor for the treatment of unresectable or metastatic melanoma patients with mutations in BRAF V600E or BRAF V600K based on a Phase III randomized, active-controlled, open-label, multicenter trial (COLUMBUS) (16). (**Figure 1**).

THE ACTIVATION OF BRAF

The Primary Activation of BRAF

BRAF is a mammalian cytosolic serine/threonine kinase that belongs to the rapidly accelerated fibrosarcoma (RAF) kinase family (ARAF, BRAF, CRAF), which uses the mitogen-activated protein kinase (MAPK) pathway to transmit signals downstream of RAS (17). The primary activation of BRAF comprises of BRAF classic mutations, BRAF rare mutations, BRAF fusion and amino acid insertion, etc. (17, 18). Different types of BRAF classical mutations have different clinical, pathological and biological characteristics. Studies have found that the occurrences of BRAF V600E mutations were not associated with age, tumor size, lymph node status, tumor stage and BRAF V600E mutation is more common in female lung adenocarcinoma, but very rare in male or squamous cell carcinoma (19). Besides, BRAF non-V600E mutations were prone to be found in smokers. Their occurrences were not associated with clinicopathological parameters or had no impact on prognosis. When treated with platinum-based chemotherapy, NSCLC patients with BRAF V600E mutation had a tendency of shorter progression-free survival (PFS) than those with BRAF non-V600E mutations, and the clinical outcomes between patients with BRAF mutation-positive and wild-types were similar, suggesting that BRAF mutations were not sensitive to chemotherapy.

The BRAF primary classic mutations process that leads to tumors can be broadly divided into three categories. Compared to wild-type, Class I (BRAF V600 mutation) increases 500-700 times kinase activity and activates downstream MAPK cascade pathways through activating monomers in a non-RAS dependent form and transcription factors. Class II and class III are mainly BRAF non-V600 mutations. Class II mutants have moderate kinase activity and can transmit signals through RAS independent constituent dimer to activate MEK1, which in turn activate ERK1/2, ultimately promote cell growth and infinite reproduction. Unlike class II mutants, class III mutants have no or little kinase activity, relying on RAS generates upstream signals that induce class III mutants to signal in the form of dimers (17, 20, 21). In general, class I and class II BRAF mutants can be independent of RAS signals and inhibit the negative feedback of ERK signals. In addition, class I BRAF mutants transmit signals in the form of active monomer, while class II

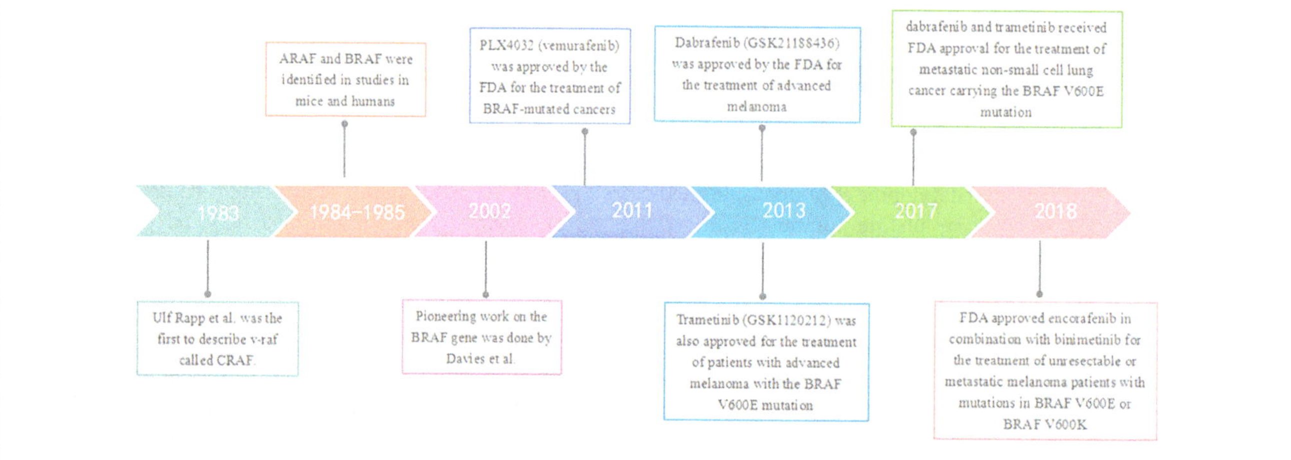

FIGURE 1 | Timeline of key events in BRAF signaling research.

and III BRAF mutants in the form of dimer, and the final signal transduction leads to the continuous activation of MAPK.

In addition to the three types of BRAF mutations, there are other forms of mutations that lead to over-activation of the pathway and ultimately the development of tumors. For example, BRAF in-frame deletions are mutually exclusive with RAS mutations, and these mutations can continuously transmit signals to activate the MAPK pathway by forming BRAF homologous dimers (22). Another study has also demonstrated that BRAF internal deletion is a mechanism of acquired drug resistance to BRAF/MEK inhibitors (23).

BRAF fusion has also been reported to be associated with tumorigenesis and progress. It was reported that BRAF fusion could cause the deletion of n-terminal inhibitory domain and activate downstream MAP kinase signal through recruiting CRAF protein to form a dimer (24, 25). In addition, a study reported that two melanoma cases whose pathogenesis was similar to BRAF fusion leading to tumorigenesis, but different from BRAF fusion, these two cases leaded to the over-activation of the pathway through the loss of BRAF inhibitory domain caused by chromosomal translocations of BRAF oncogene (26).

Amino acid insertions were found at position 599 of the BRAF codon, which is rare in the BRAF primary gene alteration. It is speculated that this may be related to the increase of kinase activity caused by changes in the spatial structure of the P ring (18).

NGS technology has revealed better comprehensive understanding of the gene mutations in various tumors. For BRAF, more and more co-mutations have been found between BRAF and other genes, which also indicates that the branching cloning process occurs at the early stage of tumor evolution, which leads to the generation of BRAF co-mutations. According to literature reports, BRAF can co-occur with KRAS mutation (27, 28), NRAS mutation (29), PTEN mutation (30, 31), MEK2 mutation (32), PIK3CA mutation (33) and other gene mutations. And most of these BRAF co-mutations occur in melanoma and lung cancer, but also found in other tumors.

The Secondary Activation of BRAF

The secondary activation of BRAF includes BRAF classic mutations, BRAF fusion and rearrangement, which are mainly acquired resistance to EGFR-TKI (25). Osimertinib has been prior recommended to the resistance caused by first- and second-generation EGFR-TKIs (34). But it will inevitably cause acquired resistance. It has been reported that the underlying mechanisms of acquired resistance to third-generation EGFR-TKIs include activation of parallel pathways, such as mutations of BRAF or other genes, and rearrangement of resistant genes, such as fusions of BRAF or other genes (25). The mutation and fusion mechanism of BRAF induced by EGFR-TKI resistance constitute an important part of BRAF gene evolution, and different treatment schemes have been explored for different types of BRAF evolution. BRAF rearrangement accounts for 4.4% of BRAF changes in NSCLC, and BRAF fusion is a form of BRAF rearrangement. Four cases were reported that BRAF fusion was a mechanism of EGFR-TKI acquired resistance in EGFR mutant lung adenocarcinoma (25).

Three cases revealed BRAF V600E mutation may be the mechanism for acquired crizotinib resistance after ROS1 rearrangement in NSCLC, two of them had acquired ROS1 rearrangement co-existing with BRAF V600E (35, 36). In another patient, ROS1 rearrangement was lost during treatment, leaving only the BRAF V600E mutation (37). Through single circulating tumor cell (CTC) sequencing, researchers found that patients with ALK mutation developed acquired drug resistance after ALK-TKIs therapy (27). And the mechanism of ALK-TKIs resistance mainly included mutations of RTK-KRAS pathway and TP53 pathway independent of ALK pathway. In the RTK-KRAS pathway, BRAF mutations accounted for 6.2% of the RTK-KRAS pathway (38). In addition, studies showed that BRAF mutation and BRAF fusion were secondary to adagrasib therapy in patients with KRAS G12C mutation (39).

THE THERAPY OF BRAF ACTIVATION

The treatment of BRAF mutation is mainly divided into two types, one is BRAF V600 mutation and the other is BRAF non-V600 mutation. BRAF V600 accounts for approximately 50% of BRAF mutation, and is more aggressive, and it occurs by mutation of glutamate into valine at position 600 of exon 15 (40). BRAF V600 develops by the previously described Class I mutation that activates the pathway in RAS independent monomer form. The other type of BRAF non-V600 mutation is mainly the previously described Class II and III BRAF mutations, which develop from signaling to downstream molecules in the form of dimers (17). The class II BRAF mutant is divided into class IIa within the activation segment and class IIb within the glycine-rich p-loop (20). The different structure, mechanism of occurrence and development leads to different treatment modalities for BRAF V600 and BRAF non-V600 mutations. On the other hand, current targeted drugs are mainly targeted at BRAF V600E, while there is no specific treatment modality for BRAF non-V600E.

Targeting BRAF V600 Mutation

BRAF V600 mutations including V600E, V600K, V600D and other subtypes, among which V600E is the most common subtype. The initial treatment for BRAF V600 mutation was monotherapy and FDA approved the first successful therapy targeting BRAF mutant melanoma called vemurafenib, an oral small molecule inhibitor of BRAF V600 mutations in 2011 (41). The evidence came from a histology-independent, flexible, early phase II "basket" study of vemurafenib in patients with non-melanoma cancers harboring BRAF (42). In this study, the objective response rate (ORR) was 42% (95% confidence interval [CI], 20 to 67%) and the median PFS was 7.3 months (95% CI, 3.5 to 10.8 months). The 12-month rate of PFS was 23% (95% CI, 6 to 46%) and the preliminary 12-month overall survival (OS) rate was 66% (95% CI, 36 to 85%). The most common adverse event was nausea. Vivek Subbiah et al. (43) explored whether BRAF V600E mutations in NSCLC were sensitive to vemurafenib or not. The results turned out that among sixty-two NSCLC patients with BRAF V600 mutation, the overall ORR was 37.1% (95% CI, 25.2 to 50.3%), and 37.5% (95% CI, 8.5 to 75.5%) in previously untreated patients, and 37.0% (95% CI, 24.3 to 51.3%) in previously treated patients. The median PFS was 6.5 months (95% CI, 5.2 to 9.0 months), and the median OS was 15.4 months (95% CI, 9.6 to 22.8 months). Vemurafenib had a similar safety profile in studies focused on melanoma patients. Furthermore, the French National Cancer Institute (INCA) conducted a trial to assess the efficacy and safety of vemurafenib in cancers with various BRAF mutations (44). Among 118 NSCLC patients, 101 of them presented with a BRAF V600E mutation and 17 with BRAF non-V600 mutations. In the BRAF V600 cohort, the ORR was 44.9%, the median PFS was 5.2monthes (95% CI: 3.8 to 6.8%), and the OS was 10 months (95% CI, 6.8 to 15.7 months). The results indicated that vemurafenib is beneficial to NSCLC patients with BRAF V600E mutation.

By inhibiting BRAF V600E kinase activity, dabrafenib resulted in decreased phosphorylation of MEK and ERK, inhibition of cell proliferation, and ultimately G1 cell cycle arrest and cell death (45). In a phase II, multicenter, nonrandomized, open-label study, 84 advanced NSCLC patients with BRAF V600E mutation showed dabrafenib had some active killing effect, though the effect was limited. The adverse events were mainly skin-related, but these adverse events were tolerable (46).

A study had demonstrated that the acquire resistance to BRAF inhibitors was largely caused by reactivating the MAPK signaling pathway (47). Trametinib is a MEK1/2 inhibitor which blocks MEK1/2 kinase activity and prevents RAF-dependent MEK phosphorylation (48). A phase II, multicenter, non-randomized, open-label study assessed the efficacy of the combination of trametinib and dabrafenib, among previously treated or untreated metastatic NSCLC patients with BRAF V600E mutation. All patients were divided into three cohorts. In cohort B, 57 patients were enrolled and resulted in an ORR of 63.2%, disease control rate (DCR) of 79%, median PFS of 9.7 months (95%CI: 6.9-19.6) and 37 patients (65% [95% CI 51–76]) achieved 6-month PFS and median duration of response was 9·0 months ([95% CI 6·9–18·3]. The median OS data are immature, but 47 (82%) of 57 patients were alive at 6 months. The most common adverse event is pyrexia in 26 patients (46%) (49). The results of cohort C of this phase II study demonstrated promising results with ORR of 64% and DCR of 75%,the median PFS of OS 10.9 months and OS of 24.6 months, which was slightly better than in the previously treated cohort (cohort B) of this trial (50). In addition, the side effect profile was mostly similar to that of cohort B, BRAF-MEK combination therapy (dabrafenib plus trametinib) demonstrated tolerability and efficacy in a recent phase II clinical trial and in light of these promising results, combination dabrafenib and trametinib was approved by the US FDA for patients with metastatic melanoma and BRAF V600E mutation. Moreover, a real-life cohort of patients with BRAF mutant advanced NSCLC shows that treatment with BRAF inhibitors and MEK inhibitors in BRAF V600E tumors is associated with ORR of 67%, median PFS of 5.5 months, and median OS since treatment initiation of 9.5 months, which indicate the combination of BRAF inhibitors and MEK inhibitors is clearly superior to monotherapy with a BRAF inhibitors (51). In addition, the incidences of pyrexia and myelosuppression are higher with combination therapy than with monotherapy.

NSCLC patients with EGFR mutation could develop BRAF V600E mutation after acquiring resistance to targeted therapy. Given the secondary activation of BRAF, Huang et al. (52) proposed a strategy of combination of dabrafenib, trametinib and osimertinib, and the patient achieved long-term control of the disease. Another study also demonstrated that the combination of dabrafenib, trametinib and osimertinib was effective to NSCLC patient who developed a BRAF V600 mutation after EGFR-TKI resistance. In addition, the adverse events could be controlled by reducing the dose (53). In another experiment, the treatment of patient also demonstrated that the BRAF inhibitor encorafenib inhibited MEK signaling but had no significant effect on ERK phosphorylation, while the combination of encorafenib and osimertinib significantly reduced MEK and ERK phosphorylation and cell growth (54). In addition, in the review of 7 additional patients who were also reported to be treated with combined therapy of dabrafenib, trametinib and osimertinib, all patients obtained extended PFS and clinical benefit (54–57). In summary, NSCLC patients harbored secondary BRAF V600E mutations because of acquired resistance to EGFR-TKI could benefit from the combination with EGFR-TKI (e.g., osimertinib) and FDA-approved two-drug therapy (e.g., dabrafenib, trametinib).

In 3 patients with secondary activation of BRAF V600E, two patients had both ROS1 rearrangement and BRAF V600E mutations and one of them died 15 days after taking dabrafenib, while the other one died 11 days after taking dabrafenib and trametinib (35, 36). The third patient who developed BRAF V600E secondary to ROS1 rearrangement loss on crizotinib received a partial response of more than 6 months with dabrafenib and trametinib (37).

To date, two-drug therapy is only approved in NSCLC with BRAF V600E for FDA indication and recommended by the NCCN guideline. However, some studies showed that the treatment mode and clinical characteristics of BRAF V600E were similar with other subtypes, such as BRAF V600K (58). In light of guidelines for BRAF V600 mutated melanoma, dual-targeted therapy is also recommended. Therefore, this review recommends that dual-targeted therapy (dabrafenib and trametinib) could be initiated in BRAF V600 mutated patients, as a congener disease as well. Now that we know the treatment for BRAF V600, and then we talk about how to treat BRAF non-V600?

Targeting BRAF Non-V600

The most patients of BRAF non-V600 mutation has less aggressive phenotype and significantly superior survival compared to those with BRAF V600 mutation, suggesting the potential need of different therapeutic strategies (59). A retrospective multicenter cohort study concluded that patients with BRAF non-V600E mutations located outside of the activation segment of the BRAF kinase domain were resistant to BRAF therapy (60). Another trial recommended chemotherapy as the dominant strategy for non-V600 mutation patients in the first-line treatment (61).

Recent experiences *in vitro* and *in vivo* show that class IIa BRAF mutant cells were sensitive to single-agent BRAF inhibitors, whereas class IIb BRAF mutant cells were not (62). Moreover, dual MAPK pathway inhibition (dMAPKi) effectively impaired the growth of subsets of non-V600 (62). *In vitro*, other trials have also demonstrated that BRAF non-V600 (L597, K601E) had significant response to MEK inhibitors (63).

Instead, research about class III mutant that have impaired kinase activity or are kinase-dead and linked with high RAS levels suggest Class III BRAF mutants may be treated with MEK inhibitors which co-existing with mutations in *RAS* and NF1 in melanomas, but in epithelial tumors, the great majority of class III mutations are not associated with RAS/NF1 alterations and may be treated with receptor tyrosine kinase (RTK) inhibitors that block the RAS pathway (20). Another study came to similar conclusions (64). A case report have also shown that dMPAKi is also benefit for patients harboring a dual G469A and W604C BRAF mutations and the response is more than 15 months (65). However, other studies found vemurafenib is not effective in NSCLC patients with BRAF non-V600 mutation (44, 66).

There is no evidence for patients resisted to EGFR-TKI yet, which could result in BRAF non-V600 mutations. A basic research demonstrated that, in osimertinib resistant PC9 cells transfected with BRAF G469A mutant plasmid, the combination of osimertinib, selumetinib (MEK 1/2 inhibitor) and trametinib (MEK 1/2 inhibitor) or dabrafenib reversed osimertinib resistance (67). Except for the two classical mutations of BRAF V600 and non-V600, there are also co-mutations of BRAF, and we will continue to discuss the treatment of BRAF co-mutations.

Treatment Recommendations for BRAF Co-Mutations

There is no high-level clinical trial for primary BRAF co-mutations to date. Since BRAF co-mutations were a clinical problem, we provide some recommendations for reference. Based on the studies on EGFR/ALK co-mutations, the phosphorylation level of the mutant genes would be a rational treatment option, and the abundance of gene mutations was also a positive biomarker for clinical decision (68). Besides, the treatment of primary BRAF co-mutation can refer to the treatment of secondary BRAF activation with EGFR/ALK/ROS1 mutation and adopt double or triple targeted therapy (53, 69). Considering the cost effectiveness and adverse events, immunotherapy, specifically immune checkpoint inhibitors (ICIs) would be a choice for BRAF co-mutations, which is introduced in detail as follows. We have solutions for all three of BRAF mutation patterns. And in recent years, the rise of immunotherapy has also brought new solutions to BRAF mutations.

Immunotherapy

Studies have reported BRAF mutant NSCLC patients have high expression of programmed cell death ligand 1 (PD-L1), which means that patients with BRAF mutation have great potential for ICIs (4). A retrospective cohort study conducted in 31 NSCLC patients with BRAF mutations showed that there was no statistically significant difference in OS among BRAF classic mutant patients who received first-line chemotherapy or immunotherapy (70). In a multi-institution retrospective chart review of 39 patients with BRAF mutated NSCLC, 22 of whom received ICIs, the ORR for V600E and non-V600E were 25% and 33%, respectively (P =1.0); PFS was similar in patients received ICIs treatment; median OS was equal for patients who received or did not receive ICIs (71). Another study collecting 4178 patients and 4462 samples from a cBioPortal database showed that BRAF wild-type mutants had a longer OS than BRAF mutants. Unlike previous study, this study showed that non-V600E had a longer OS than V600E under ICIs treatment (72). A BRAF G469A mutant NSCLC case obtained a deep and durable response after ICIs treatment, which suggested that BRAF non-V600 mutation may benefit more from immunotherapy than EGFR/ALK-driven mutation in NSCLC (73). However, in a retrospective, multicenter and real world analysis, 44 of 107 patients with BRAF mutations (V600:26, non-V600:18) received ICIs, with the response rates of 26% in BRAF V600 cohort and 35% in the non-V600 cohort. Besides, BRAF V600 cohort have longer PFS and OS than non-V600 cohort (74).

The above studies demonstrate the survival in various types of BRAF mutations treated with ICIs immunotherapy or targeted therapy are different. However, there is a lack of high-level evidence to prove which is better. Further prospective clinical trials are necessary to prove which is the optimal first line strategy. We have solutions for all three of BRAF mutation patterns. In recent years, the rise of immunotherapy has also brought new solutions to BRAF mutations.

Strategies for Resistance to BRAF Inhibitors

BRAF mutant tumors might initially respond to treatment with BRAF inhibitors, but eventually developed drug resistance. For acquired resistance to BRAF inhibitors caused by BRAF fusion, clinical trials have demonstrated the efficacy of pan-RAF inhibitors in patients with BRAF fusion (75). Evidence suggests that BRAF proteins undergo homodimerization and heterodimerization, therefore BRAF rearrangement is very insensitive to BRAF inhibitors. And RAF inhibitors could bind and inhibit all RAF isomers, so they are effective for BRAF fusion (76, 77). Evidence is also provided that a combination of MEK inhibitors and EGFR inhibitors is effective in patients with BRAF fusion (25, 77). As for acquired drug resistance, a series of post-resistance measures were reported. Intermittent dosing would be a choice. A melanoma case with vemurafenib showed the accelerated growth of RAS-mutant leukemia, and intermittent dosing of vemurafenib relieved the disease and reduced the disease burden (78). Subsequent studies showed that intermittent dosing of BRAF inhibitors and RAF inhibitors may delay the progression of resistant tumors and make it sensitive to inhibitors again (79, 80). An international team of 180 scientists proposed the concept of a low toxicity "broad-spectrum" treatment based on the sequencing of the cancer's genome, which targeted multiple key tumorigenesis pathways and mechanisms to prevent cancer growth (81). What's more, for resistant mutations at different gene target, different drug combinations could be adopt. For example, FDA has approved the combination of BRAF inhibitors (Vemurafenib and Dabrafenib) and MEK inhibitor trametinib for the treatment of BRAF inhibition resistance. And clinical studies of PI3K/AKT inhibitor plus MAPK inhibitor, everolimus (RAD001) plus bevacizumab, everolimus (RAD001) plus temozolomide (TMZ), and targeted therapy plus immunotherapy have also been conducted, but there is a lack of more data to support these therapies, so further exploration is needed (82). The strategies for resistance to BRAF inhibitors were listed in **Table 1**.

THE EVOLUTION OF BRAF ACTIVATION

The Pathways of BRAF Evolution

As reported, the evolution of BRAF comes from the changes of various genes mainly in the following three ways after targeted therapy (**Figure 2**). First, the changes of BRAF itself and BRAF downstream molecules which lead to resistance to BRAF targeted inhibitors mainly come from the following aspects. BRAF splice variants are the most common situation. Studies has demonstrated that AGK-BRAF fusion leads to loss of the CR1 region of BRAF, thereby eliminating the inhibitory RAS-binding domain, and results in RAS-independent constitutive activation of the kinase (83). A research has found that the loss of the inhibitory RAS binding domain resulting from the loss of the internal BRAF leads to the reactivation of RAS-RAF-MEK-ERK signaling and mediates resistance to BRAF inhibitors (23). Besides, BRAF copy number amplification also can lead to resistance to BRAF targeted inhibitors. Hubing Shi et al. (84) proved that BRAF V600E amplification was the mechanism of acquired resistance of BRAF inhibitors, providing evidence for drug target changes leading to clinical relapse. Moreover, Montagut et al. (85) found that CRAF overexpression to increased ERK1/2 level indicating some BRAF mutant tumor cells were primary insensitive to RAF inhibition in the experiment, which was related to a switch from BRAF to CRAF dependency in tumor cells. And Lu et al. (86) found p21-activated kinases phosphorylate CRAF and MEK to reactivate ERK, which drive acquired drug resistance to MAPK inhibitors in BRAF mutants. Furthermore, MEK1 mutation can also lead to reactivation of the MAPK pathway. MEK is downstream of RAS signaling MEK reactivation caused by MEK mutation does not require stimulation of BRAF signaling, so BRAF inhibitors are ineffective against MEK1/2 mutation. Therefore, MEK1 mutation can promotes ERK phosphorylation, and MEK2 can also heterodimerize with MEK1, ultimately leading to the reactivation of EKR (87).

Second, changes in upstream molecules of BRAF lead to the evolution of BRAF mainly from the following aspects. First of all, studies have shown that NRAS upregulation is another resistance mechanism of BRAF inhibitors and NRAS upregulation may promote the dimerization of RAF, which will cause insensitivity of ERK signaling to drugs, leading to tumor drug resistance (88–90). And the mutation of RAS gene may lead to the reactivation of MAPK pathway. On the one hand, the mutant RAS protein will not dissociate after binding to GTP but become permanently activated. On the other hand, overactivated RAS may lead to overactivation of ARAF and CRAF, and thus cell proliferation. These two aspects jointly promote signal transduction of MAPK pathway (89, 91, 92). And ERK protein is a negative regulator of RAS protein, BRAF inhibitors can inhibit ERK pathway, thereby inducing part of RAS activity and leading to the activation of MAPK pathway (93, 94). And as well as RTKs alteration, overexpression of platelet derived growth factor receptor (PDGFR)-β or siRNA knockdown of PDGFRβ demonstrates the potential role of PDGFRβ signaling in drug resistance, and the introduction of PDGFRβ into untreated cells reduces sensitivity to vemurafenib (89). In addition, up-regulation of EGFR expression was found in BRAF inhibitor resistant cell lines and resistant tumor biopsies (95). EGFR activation binds to specific tyrosine residues on the receptor and results in a conformation change of Sos protein, thereby recruiting and activating RAS-GDP, and finally ERK activation induces cell proliferation (96). Besides, the upregulation of IGF1R/IR in BRAF and MEK inhibitor resistant cells and the maintenance of P-ERK and P-Akt suggest that IGF1R/IR may mediate resistance to inhibitors through the reactivation of MAPK (97).

Third, activation of bypass pathways leads to overactivation of the BRAF signaling pathway mainly come from the following aspects. At first, elevate expression of COT, like CRAF, activates ERK through MEK-dependent mechanisms that do not require RAF signals, thus driving resistance to RAF inhibition (98). Besides, studies have shown that loss of STAG2 or STAG3 inhibits CCCTC-binding factor (CTCF) mediated dual

TABLE 1 | Strategies for resistance to BRAF inhibitors.

Situation	Strategies	Ref.
BRAF fusion	pan-RAF inhibitors	(75)
	BRAF inhibitors and RAF inhibitors	(76, 77)
	combination of MEK inhibitors and EGFR inhibitors	(25, 77)
Acquired drug resistance to vemurafenib	intermittent dosing	(78–80)
Changes in multiple key tumorigenesis pathways and mechanisms	low toxicity "broad-spectrum" treatment	(81)
Resistant mutations at different gene target	different drug combinations	(82)

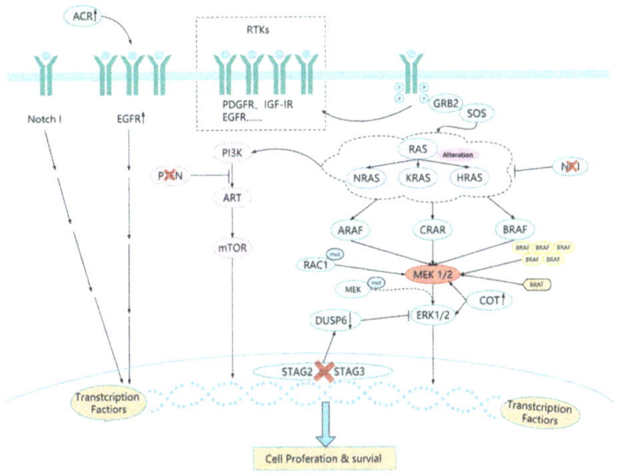

FIGURE 2 | The resistance pathways of BRAF inhibitor. BRAF mutated tumor cells evolve different drug resistance pathways to maintain cell growth after chronic inhibition by BRAF inhibitors. These evolutionary mechanisms (**Table 2**) include BRAF splice variants, BRAF copy number amplification, CRAF overexpression, MEK1 mutations, and other mechanisms. Different pathways of BRAF evolution can tell us how to overcome the problem of resistance to BRAF inhibitors and how to develop more rational protocols to address the resistance problem.

specificity phosphatase 6 (DUSP6) expression, leading to a significant decrease in DUSP6 protein levels and ultimately reactivation of MEK-ERK signaling in BRAF-inhibitor treated melanoma cells (99). What's more, RAC1 is a GTP-binding protein that modulates cytoskeletal rearrangement by signaling g-protein-coupled receptors and other molecules and RAC1 P29S mutations may mediate resistance to vemurafenib and dabrafenib by maintaining MAPK signaling (100). Additionally, NF1 is a tumor suppressor that inhibits RAS activity. Experiments have proved that loss of NF1 can re-drive MAPK pathway by activating RAS activity and increasing CRAF, thus mediating resistance to RAF inhibitors (101). Moreover, studies have found that ACK1 can inhibit the expression of EGFR, so the loss of ACK1 induces the increase of EGFR protein, thus increasing cell signal transduction to mediate the generation of drug resistance (102). Furthermore, it has been confirmed that increased Notch signaling results in increased expression of markers associated with cell dedifferentiation and increased cell migration and does not reactivate ERK in the presence of drug therapy to mediate acquired resistance to MAPK inhibitors (103). Finally, the study of Hubing Shi et al. (56) named the PI3K-PTEN-AKT pathway as the second core resistance pathway, and it has been reported that upregulation of the PI3K pathway accounts for approximately 22% of BRAF inhibitor acquired resistance melanoma. PTEN is an important tumor suppressor, which acts to counteract the effect of PI3K and when PTEN is lost, mutant or methylated, the activity of PI3K pathway will increase, and cells can finally survive by adopting PI3K signal (104). The evolution and pathways of BRAF activation were listed in **Table 2** and **Figure 2**. We have collected several paths of BRAF evolution. In addition, we hope to find certain rules from the evolutionary pathway, so we need to study the pathway of BRAF evolution through some methodologies.

Methodology to Track the BRAF Evolution

Due to the diversity and randomness of gene evolution, we need to use various emerging technologies and methods to find certain rules from dynamic evolution, so as to obtain certain therapeutic effects, and also to find effective therapeutic strategies. With the advent of cancer genomics and the development of multi-region sequencing, single-cell correlation sequencing and cloning techniques, it has become possible to describe gene phylogeny and evolution (105–107). In recent years, studies have been carried out on clonal phylogeny using single time point snapshot, multi-region sampling and spatio-temporal modeling to analyze diseases. In addition, mathematical models and other methods can be used to explore new evolutionary methods. At the same time, it also puts forward the direction and challenge to bioinformatics and computer science (108). In addition, it has been proposed that the development of single-cell multi-omics technology is crucial for a comprehensive understanding of the evolutionary mechanism. For example, multiple sampling methods can be used to analyze the evolutionary mechanism of tumors by different sampling methods (such as multiple regions or multiple times). And examples include *in vivo* and *in vitro* modeling of tumor evolution through optical or sequencing barcodes (109). Furthermore, deep sequencing of multiple regions of a tumor directly to detect evolutionary mutations is another way (110).

UNDERGOING STUDIES FOR BRAF ACTIVATION

The efficacy and safety of BRAF inhibitors are being explored in several clinical studies (e.g., NCT03915951, NCT04543188 etc.). In addition, more treatment options for patients with BRAF mutations can be explored, for example, BRAF inhibitors as adjuvant/neoadjuvant therapy for patients with NSCLC; BRAF inhibitor combined with MEK inhibitor and EGFR-TKI as three-target combination therapy; BRAF inhibitors combined with immunotherapy, anti-angiogenic drugs and other drug combinations. With the success of the ADAURA study, a new direction of targeted therapy in the adjuvant treatment for NSCLC patients has been opened. Therefore, we believe that the use of dabrafenib in combination with trametinib in neoadjuvant/adjuvant therapy for early-stage NSCLC patients is worthy of further exploration (111). Besides, for patients with acquired resistance to BRAF inhibitors, re-biopsy and NGS test to find new targeted drugs or new combination therapy are necessary. Finally, we still want to know if the strategy of dual-targeted or triple-targeted therapy could be re-challenged. Small-sample case reports suggest that sequential therapy with targeted therapy and immunotherapy, combined with the "rechallenge"

TABLE 2 | The evolution and pathways of BRAF activation.

Cancer types	Evolutionary types	Evolutionary pathways	Ref.
Melanoma	changes in BRAF itself	BRAF splice variants	(23, 83)
Melanoma	-	BRAF copy number amplification	(84)
Melanoma	downstream of the BRAF	CRAF overexpression	(85, 86)
Melanoma	-	MEK1 mutations	(87)
Melanoma	upstream of the BRAF	RAS alteration	(88, 94)
Melanoma	–	RTKs alteration	(89, 95, 97)
Melanoma	activation of bypass pathways	Elevated expression levels of COT	(98)
Melanoma	–	Loss of stromal antigen 2 (STAG2) or STAG3	(99)
Melanoma	–	RAC1 mutation	(100)
Melanoma	–	Loss of NF1	(101)
Melanoma	–	Loss of ACK1	(102)
Breast cancer and melanoma	–	Activation of the Notch1 pathway	(103)
Melanoma	–	Phosphoinositide 3-kinase (PI3K)/AKT pathway dysregulation	(56, 104)

TABLE 3 | Selected ongoing trials with BRAF Inhibitors for NSCLC.

Clinical Trial Identifier	Study Design	Intervention/s	Setting	Primary Endpoint	Phase	Status
NCT03915951	90 participants Open-label, Multicenter, Non-randomized, Phase 2 study	Encorafenib plus Binimetinib	First line	ORR	Phase 2	Recruiting
NCT04543188	225 participants two-part, phase 1A/B, open-label, multicenter trial evaluating pharmacokinetics	PF-07284890 plus Binimetinib plus Midazolam	First line	DLTs, AEs, Overall response	Phase 1	Recruiting
NCT04526782	119 participants Open-label, Multicenter, multi-cohort Phase 2 study	encorafenib plus binimetinib	First line	ORR	Phase 2	Recruiting
NCT05003622	6 participants Multicenter, Open-label, Phase 1 Study	Encorafenib	First line	DLTs	Phase 1	Active, not recruiting
NCT05065398	20 participants Open Label, Multicenter Phase II Clinical Trial	HLX208	First line	ORR	Phase 2	Recruiting
NCT05275374	221 participants Dose-escalation and Expansion Phase I/IIa Study	XP-102 or XP-102 plus Trametinib or	First line	Characterize the safety of XP-102, Evaluate the pharmacokinetics of XP-102, Establish maximum tolerated dose of XP-102	Phase 1 Phase 2	Not yet recruiting
NCT05195632	55 participants Multicenter, Open-label, phase 2 study	Encorafenib plus Binimetinib	First line	DLTs, ORR	Phase 2	Not yet recruiting
NCT02974725	331 participants Phase Ib, Open-label, Multicenter Study	LXH254 plus LTT462 or LXH254 plus Trametinib or LXH254 plus Ribociclib	First line	DLTs, AEs, Tolerability	Phase 1	Recruiting
NCT04620330	100 participants Multicenter, Non-randomized, Open-label Phase 1b/2 study	VS-6766 or VS-6766 plus Defactinib	First line	the optimal regimen, the efficacy of the optimal regimen	Phase 2	Recruiting

of dabrafenib and trametinib, may benefit patients with V600E mutation and positive PD-L1 (112). Among the 2 patients in the prospective match-R study, 1 patient was switched to chemotherapy and then dual-target therapy after double-target drug resistance. Another patient, after double-target drug resistance, was first switched to immunotherapy, followed by chemotherapy, and then sequential double-target therapy, all of which achieved disease stability in the "re-challenge" of double-target therapy (113). These explorations are expected to become hot research directions in the future, and we eagerly look forward to more effective drugs or treatments. The undergoing studies for BRAF activation were listed in **Table 3**.

CONCLUSIONS

There are many forms of activation of BRAF in primary and secondary activation, including classical mutations (BRAF V600 and non-V600), other mutations, BRAF fusion, rearrangement, in-frame deletions, insertions, co-mutations, etc. with different biological phenotypes, medical senses and different subsequent treatments. Currently, the FDA recommends dual targeted drug combination for BRAF V600, while there is no unified treatment regimen for other types of BRAF mutations. As for the treatment of primary BRAF co-mutations, it could base on a comprehensive consideration of the phosphorylation level and abundance of the mutant genes, cost effectiveness and adverse events of combined targeted therapy. Immunotherapy can also benefit for patients with BRAF mutations with high PD-L1 expression in small sample size studies. After resistance of BRAF inhibitors, the evolution of BRAF mainly evolves through activation of upstream, downstream and bypass pathways of BRAF. The evolutionary pathway can be tracked by various emerging technologies including genomics, next-generation sequencing, single-cell sequencing and cloning techniques, which may find a solution for the resistance of BRAF inhibitors.

In the future, it's necessary to explore head to head clinical trials to compare targeted therapy with immunotherapy, to develop drugs for other BRAF mutations except V600, to find new strategies for the resistance of BRAF inhibitors. Furthermore, whether BRAF inhibitors can be used as adjuvant/neoadjuvant therapy or re-challenged treatment are likely to be hot topics.

AUTHOR CONTRIBUTIONS

LYZ and JS researched the data, wrote the review, and designed the figure. JGS, LPZ, and QY reviewed and revised the manuscript. All authors contributed to the article and approved the submitted version.

REFERENCES

1. Arbour KC, Riely GJ. Systemic Therapy for Locally Advanced and Metastatic Non-Small Cell Lung Cancer: A Review. *JAMA* (2019) 322:764–74. doi: 10.1001/jama.2019.11058
2. Frisone D, Friedlaender A, Malapelle U, Banna G, Addeo A. A BRAF New World. *Crit Rev Oncol Hematol* (2020) 152:103008. doi: 10.1016/j.critrevonc.2020.103008
3. Baik CS, Myall NJ, Wakelee HA. Targeting BRAF-Mutant Non-Small Cell Lung Cancer: From Molecular Profiling to Rationally Designed Therapy. *Oncologist* (2017) 22(7):786–96. doi: 10.1634/theoncologist.2016-0458
4. O'Leary CG, Andelkovic V, Ladwa R, Pavlakis N, Zhou CC, Hirsch F, et al. ung Cancer. *Transl Lung Cancer Res* (2019) 8(6):1119–24. doi: 10.21037/tlcr.2019.10.22
5. Dhillon AS, Hagan S, Rath O, Kolch W. MAP Kinase Signalling Pathways in Cancer. *Oncogene.*(2007) 26(22):3279–90. doi: 10.1038/sj.onc.1210421
6. Rapp UR, Goldsborough MD, Mark GE, Bonner TI, Groffen J, Reynolds FH, et al. Structure and Biological Activity of V-Raf, a Unique Oncogene Transduced by a Retrovirus. *Proc Natl Acad Sci* (1983) 80:4218–22. doi: 10.1073/pnas.80.14.4218
7. Bonner T, O'Brien SJ, Nash WG, Rapp UR, Morton CC, Leder P. The Human Homologs of the *Raf* (*Mil*) Oncogene Are Located on Human Chromosomes 3 and 4. *Science* (1984) 223:71–4. doi: 10.1126/science.6691137
8. Bonner TI, Kerby SB, Sutrave P, Gunnell MA, Mark G, Rapp UR. Structure and Biological Activity of Human Homologs of the Raf/Mil Oncogene. *Mol Cell Biol* (1985) 5:1400–7. doi: 10.1128/MCB.5.6.1400
9. Davies H, Bignell GR, Cox C, Stephens P, Edkins S, Clegg S, et al. Mutations of the BRAF Gene in Human Cancer. *Nature* (2002) 417:949–54. doi: 10.1038/nature00766
10. Dankort D, Filenova E, Collado M, Serrano M, Jones K, McMahon M. A New Mouse Model to Explore the Initiation, Progression, and Therapy of *BRAF* ^{V600E}-Induced Lung Tumors. *Genes Dev* (2007) 21:379–84. doi: 10.1101/gad.1516407
11. Ji H, Wang Z, Perera SA, Li D, Liang M-C, Zaghlul S, et al. Mutations in BRAF and KRAS Converge on Activation of the Mitogen-Activated Protein Kinase Pathway in Lung Cancer Mouse Models. *Cancer Res* (2007) 67:4933–9. doi: 10.1158/0008-5472.CAN-06-4592
12. Kim G, Mckee AE, Ning Y-M, Hazarika M, Theoret M, Johnson JR, et al. FDA Approval Summary: Vemurafenib for Treatment of Unresectable or Metastatic Melanoma With the BRAF(V600E) Mutation. *Clin Cancer Res* (2014) 20:4994–5000. doi: 10.1158/1078-0432.CCR-14-0776
13. Hauschild A, Grob J-J, Demidov LV, Jouary T, Gutzmer R, Millward M, et al. Dabrafenib in BRAF-Mutated Metastatic Melanoma: A Multicentre, Open-Label, Phase 3 Randomised Controlled Trial. *Lancet* (2012) 380:358 65. doi: 10.1016/S0140-6736(12)60868-X
14. Abe H, Kikuchi S, Hayakawa K, Iida T, Nagahashi N, Maeda K, et al. Discovery of a Highly Potent and Selective MEK Inhibitor: GSK1120212 (JTP-74057 DMSO Solvate). *ACS Med Chem Lett* (2011) 2:320–4. doi: 10.1021/ml200004g
15. Odogwu L, Mathieu L, Blumenthal G, Larkins E, Goldberg KB, Griffin N, et al. FDA Approval Summary: Dabrafenib and Trametinib for the Treatment of Metastatic Non-Small Cell Lung Cancers Harboring *BRAF V600E* Mutations. *Oncologist* (2018) 23:740–5. doi: 10.1634/theoncologist.2017-0642
16. Dummer R, Ascierto PA, Gogas HJ, Arance A, Mandala M, Liszkay G, et al. Encorafenib Plus Binimetinib Versus Vemurafenib or Encorafenib in Patients With BRAF -Mutant Melanoma (COLUMBUS). A Multicentre, Open-Label, Randomised Phase 3 Trial. *Lancet Oncol* (2018) 19:603–15. doi: 10.1016/S1470-2045(18)30142-6
17. Dankner M, Rose AAN, Rajkumar S, Siegel PM, Watson IR. Classifying BRAF Alterations in Cancer: New Rational Therapeutic Strategies for Actionable Mutations. *Oncogene* (2018) 37(24):3183–99. doi: 10.1038/s41388-018-0171-x
18. Trubini S, Ubiali A, Paties CT, Cavanna L. Novel BRAF Mutation in Melanoma: A Case Report. *Mol Clin Oncol* (2018) 8(3):460–2. doi: 10.3892/mco.2018.1555
19. Cardarella S, Ogino A, Nishino M, Butaney M, Shen J, Lydon C, et al. Clinical, Pathologic, and Biologic Features Associated With BRAF Mutations in Non-Small Cell Lung Cancer. *Clin Cancer Res* (2013) 19 (16):4532–40. doi: 10.1158/1078-0432.CCR-13-0657
20. Yao Z, Yaeger R, Rodrik-Outmezguine VS. Et alTumours With Class 3 BRAF Mutants Are Sensitive to the Inhibition of Activated RAS. *Nature* (2017) 548(7666):234–8. doi: 10.1038/nature23291
21. Yao Z, Torres NM, Tao A, Gao Y, Luo L, Li Q, et al. BRAF Mutants Evade ERK-Dependent Feedback by Different Mechanisms That Determine Their Sensitivity to Pharmacologic Inhibition. *Cancer Cell* (2015) 28:370–83. doi: 10.1016/j.ccell.2015.08.001
22. Chen SH, Zhang Y, Van Horn RD, Yin TG, Buchanan S, Yadav V, et al. Oncogenic BRAF Deletions That Function as Homodimers and Are Sensitive to Inhibition by RAF Dimer Inhibitor Ly3009120. *Cancer Discov* (2016) 6(3):300–15. doi: 10.1158/2159-8290.CD-15-0896
23. Johnson DB, Childress MA, Chalmers ZR, Frampton GM, Ali SM, Rubinstein SM, et al. BRAF Internal Deletions and Resistance to BRAF/

MEK Inhibitor Therapy. *Pigment Cell Melanoma Res* (2018) 31:432–6. doi: 10.1111/pcmr.12674

24. Kim HS, Jung M, Kang HN, Kim H, Park CW, Kim SM, et al. Oncogenic BRAF Fusions in Mucosal Melanomas Activate the MAPK Pathway and Are Sensitive to MEK/PI3K Inhibition or MEK/CDK4/6 Inhibition. *Oncogene* (2017) 36(23):3334–45. doi: 10.1038/onc.2016.486
25. Vojnic M, Kubota D, Kurzatkowski C, Offin M, Suzawa K, Benayed R, et al. Acquired BRAF Rearrangements Induce Secondary Resistance to EGFR Therapy in EGFR-Mutated Lung Cancers. *J Thorac Oncol* (2019) 14:802–15. doi: 10.1016/j.jtho.2018.12.038
26. Dessars B, De Raeve LE, Housni HE, Debouck CJ, Sidon PJ, Morandini R, et al. Chromosomal Translocations as a Mechanism of BRAF Activation in Two Cases of Large Congenital Melanocytic Nevi. *J Invest. Dermatol* (2007) 127:1468–70. doi: 10.1038/sj.jid.5700725
27. Bourhis Amélie, Remoué A, Uguen A. KRAS and BRAF Double Mutations and Functional Classes of BRAF Mutations in Non-Small-Cell Lung Cancers. *Clin Lung Cancer* (2020) 21(4):e240–2. doi: 10.1016/j.cllc.2020.02.018
28. Deshwar A, Margonis GA, Andreatos N, Barbon C, Wang J, Buettner S, et al. Double KRAS and BRAF Mutations in Surgically Treated Colorectal Cancer Liver Metastases: An International, Multi-Institutional Case Series. *Anticancer Res* (2018) 38:2891–5. doi: 10.21873/anticanres.12535.
29. del Regno L, Louveau B, Battistella M, Sadoux A, Baroudjian B, Delyon J, et al. Clinical Significance of BRAF/NRAS Concurrent Mutations in a Clinic-Based Metastatic Melanoma Cohort. *Br J Dermatol* (2020) 182:1281–3. doi: 10.1111/bjd.18641
30. Agosto-Arroyo E, Rosa M, Chau A, Khazai L. Concurrent BRAF and PTEN Mutations in Melanoma of Unknown Origin Presenting as a Breast Mass. *SAGE Open Med Case Rep* (2017) 5:2050313X17711064. doi: 10.1177/2050313X17711064
31. Dantis K, Gupta AKDr., Kashyap NKDr., Kashyap Y, Ranganath TGDr., Pati SKDr., et al. Pulmonary Sclerosing Pneumocytoma Masquerading Adenocarcinoma With Co-Existing BRAF V600E and PTEN Mutation. *Cancer Treat Res Commun* (2021) 28:100429. doi: 10.1016/j.ctarc.2021.100429
32. Villanueva J, Infante JR, Krepler C, Reyes-Uribe P, Samanta M, Chen H-Y, et al. Concurrent MEK2 Mutation and BRAF Amplification Confer Resistance to BRAF and MEK Inhibitors in Melanoma. *Cell Rep* (2013) 4:1090–9. doi: 10.1016/j.celrep.2013.08.023
33. Li W, Qiu T, Dong L, Zhang F, Guo L, Ying J. Prevalence and Characteristics of PIK3CA Mutation in Mismatch Repair-Deficient Colorectal Cancer. *J Cancer* (2020) 11:3827–33. doi: 10.7150/jca.37437
34. Ding H, Zhuang Z, Xie J, Huang H, Tao Z, Liu Z. Durable Clinical Response of Advanced Lung Adenocarcinoma Harboring EGFR-19del/T790M/BRAFV600E Mutations After Treating With Osimertinib and Dabrafenib Plus Trametinib: A Case Report. *OncoTar. Ther* (2020) 13:7933–9. doi: 10.1016/j.celrep.2013.08.023
35. Watanabe J, Furuya N, Fujiwara Y. Appearance of a BRAF Mutation Conferring Resistance to Crizotinib in Non-Small Cell Lung Cancer Harboring Oncogenic ROS1 Fusion. *J Thorac Oncol* (2018) 13(4):e66–9. doi: 10.1016/j.jtho.2017.11.125
36. Ren S, Huang S, Ye X, Feng L, Lu Y, Zhou C, et al. Crizotinib Resistance Conferred by BRAF V600E Mutation in Non–Small Cell Lung Cancer Harboring an Oncogenic ROS1 Fusion. *Cancer Treat Res Commun* (2021) 27:100377. doi: 10.1016/j.ctarc.2021.100377
37. Li J, Wang Q, Ge J, Tian Y, Yao W. BRAF V600E Mediates Crizotinib Resistance and Responds to Dabrafenib and Trametinib in a ROS1-Rearranged Non-Small Cell Lung Cancer: A Case Report. *Oncologist* (2021) 26:e2115–9. doi: 10.1002/onco.13979
38. Pailler E, Faugeroux V, Oulhen M, Mezquita L, Laporte M, Honoré A, et al. Acquired Resistance Mutations to ALK Inhibitors Identified by Single Circulating Tumor Cell Sequencing in ALK-Rearranged Non–Small-Cell Lung Cancer. *Clin Cancer Res* (2019) 25:6671–82. doi: 10.1158/1078-0432.CCR-19-1176
39. Awad MM, Liu S, Rybkin II, Arbour KC, Dilly J, Zhu VW, et al. Acquired Resistance to KRASG12C Inhibition in Cancer. *N Engl J Med* (2021) 384 (25):2382–93. doi: 10.1056/NEJMoa2105281
40. Negrao MV, Raymond VM, Lanman RB, Robichaux JP, He J, Nilsson MB, et al. Molecular Landscape of BRAF-Mutant NSCLC Reveals an Association Between Clonality and Driver Mutations and Identifies Targetable Non-V600 Driver Mutations. *J Thorac Oncol* (2020) 15:1611–23. doi: 10.1016/j.jtho.2020.05.021
41. Halle BR, Johnson DB. Defining and Targeting BRAF Mutations in Solid Tumors. *Curr Treat Options Oncol* (2021) 22:30. doi: 10.1007/s11864-021-00827-2
42. Hyman DM, Puzanov I, Subbiah V, Faris JE, Chau I, Blay JY, et al. Vemurafenib in Multiple Nonmelanoma Cancers With BRAF V600 Mutations. *N Engl J Med* (2015) 373:726–36:8. doi: 10.1056/NEJMoa1502309
43. Subbiah V, Gervais R, Riely G, Hollebecque A, Blay J-Y, Felip E, et al. Efficacy of Vemurafenib in Patients With Non–Small-Cell Lung Cancer With *BRAF* V600 Mutation: An Open-Label, Single-Arm Cohort of the Histology-Independent VE-BASKET Study. *JCO Precis. Oncol* (2019) 3:1–9. doi: 10.1200/PO.18.00266
44. Mazieres J, Cropet C, Montané L, Barlesi F, Souquet PJ, Quantin X, et al. Vemurafenib in Non-Small-Cell Lung Cancer Patients With BRAFV600 and BRAFnonV600 Mutations. *Ann Oncol* (2020) 31:289–94. doi: 10.1016/j.annonc.2019.10.022
45. King AJ, Arnone MR, Bleam MR, Moss KG, Yang JS, Fedorowicz KE, et al. Dabrafenib; Preclinical Characterization, Increased Efficacy When Combined With Trametinib, While BRAF/MEK Tool Combination Reduced Skin Lesions. *PloS One* (2013) 8(7):e67583. doi: 10.1371/journal.pone.0067583
46. Planchard D, Kim TM, Mazieres J, Quoix E, Riely G, Barlesi F, et al. Dabrafenib in Patients With BRAFV600E-Positive Advanced Non-Small-Cell Lung Cancer: A Single-Arm, Multicentre, Open-Label, Phase 2 Trial. *Lancet Oncol* (2016) 17:642–50. doi: 10.1016/S1470-2045(16)00077-2
47. Rissmann R, Hessel MHM, Cohen AF. Vemurafenib/dabrafenib and Trametinib. *Br J Clin Pharmacol* (2015) 80(4):765–7. doi: 10.1111/bcp.12651
48. Khunger A, Khunger M, Velcheti V. Dabrafenib in Combination With Trametinib in the Treatment of Patients With BRAF V600-Positive Advanced or Metastatic non-Small Cell Lung Cancer: Clinical Evidence and Experience. *Ther Adv Respir Dis* (2019) 12:1753466618767611. doi: 10.1177/1753466618767611
49. Planchard D, Besse B, Groen HJM, Souquet P-J, Quoix E, Baik CS, et al. Dabrafenib Plus Trametinib in Patients With Previously Treated BRAF (V600E)-Mutant Metastatic Non-Small Cell Lung Cancer: An Open-Label, Multicentre Phase 2 Trial. *Lancet Oncol* (2016) 17:984–93. doi: 10.1016/S1470-2045(16)30146-2
50. Planchard D, Smit EF, Groen HJM, Mazieres J, Besse B, Helland Å., et al. Dabrafenib Plus Trametinib in Patients With Previously Untreated BRAFV600E-Mutant Metastatic Non-Small-Cell Lung Cancer: An Open-Label, Phase 2 Trial. *Lancet Oncol* (2017) 18:1307–16. doi: 10.1016/S1470-2045(17)30679-4
51. Dudnik E, Bar J, Peled N, Bshara E, Kuznetsov T, Cohen AY, et al. Efficacy and Safety of BRAF Inhibitors With or Without MEK Inhibitors in BRAF-Mutant Advanced Non-Small-Cell Lung Cancer: Findings From a Real-Life Cohort. *Clin Lung Cancer* (2019) 20:278–286.e1. doi: 10.1016/j.cllc.2019.03.007
52. Huang Y, Gan JD, Guo KB, Deng YY, Fang WF. Acquired BRAF V600E Mutation Mediated Resistance to Osimertinib and Responded to Osimertinib, Dabrafenib, and Trametinib Combination Therapy. *J Thorac Oncol* (2019) 14:10. doi: 10.1016/j.jtho.2019.05.040
53. Mauclet C, Collard P, Ghaye B, Hoton D, Nana FA. Tumor Response to EGFR/BRAF/MEK Co-Inhibition in a Patient With EGFR Mutated Lung Adenocarcinoma Developing a BRAFV600 Mutation as an Acquired Resistance Mechanism. *Lung Cancer* (2021) 159:42–4. doi: 10.1016/j.lungcan.2021.06.025
54. Ho C-C, Liao W-Y, Lin C-A, Shih J-Y, Yu C-J, Chih-Hsin YJ. Acquired BRAF V600E Mutation as Resistant Mechanism After Treatment With Osimertinib. *J Thorac Oncol* (2017) 12:567–72. doi: 10.1016/j.jtho.2016.11.2231
55. Zhou F, Zhao W, Chen X, Zhang J, Zhou CC. Response to the Combination of Dabrafenib, Trametinib and Osimertinib in a Patient With EGFR-Mutant

NSCLC Harboring an Acquired BRAFV600E Mutation. *Lung Cancer* (2019) 139:219–20. doi: 10.1016/j.lungcan.2019.10.014
56. Shi H, Hugo W, Kong X, Hong A, Koya RC, Moriceau G, et al. Acquired Resistance and Clonal Evolution in Melanoma During BRAF Inhibitor Therapy. *Cancer Discovery* (2014) 4:80–93. doi: 10.1158/2159-8290.CD-13-0642
57. Solassol J, Vendrell JA, Senal R, Audran P, Leenhardt F, Quantin X. Challenging BRAF/EGFR Co-Inhibition in NSCLC Using Sequential Liquid Biopsies. *Lung Cancer* (2019) 133:45–7. doi: 10.1016/j.lungcan.2019.05.003
58. Zengarini C, Mussi M, Veronesi G, Alessandrini A, Lambertini M, Dika E. BRAF V600K vs BRAF V600E: A Clinical, Dermoscopic, and Response to Immunotherapies and Targeted Therapies Comparison. *Clin Exp Dermatol* (2022). doi: 10.1111/ced.15113
59. Fontana E, Valeri N. Class(y) Dissection of BRAF Heterogeneity: Beyond Non-V600. *Clin Cancer Res* (2019) 25:6896–8. doi: 10.1158/1078-0432.CCR-19-2732
60. Gautschi O, Milia J, Cabarrou B, Bluthgen M-V, Besse B, Smit EF, et al. Targeted Therapy for Patients With BRAF-Mutant Lung Cancer Results From the European EURAF Cohort. *J Thorac Oncol* (2015) 10:1451–7. doi: 10.1097/JTO.0000000000000625
61. Mu Y, Yang K, Hao X, Wang Y, Wang L, Liu Y, et al. Clinical Characteristics and Treatment Outcomes of 65 Patients With BRAF-Mutated Non-Small Cell Lung Cancer. *Front Oncol* (2020) 10:603. doi: 10.3389/fonc.2020.00603
62. Dankner M, Lajoie M, Moldoveanu D, Nguyen T-T, Savage P, Rajkumar S, et al. Dual MAPK Inhibition Is an Effective Therapeutic Strategy for a Subset of Class II BRAF Mutant Melanomas. *Clin Cancer Res* (2018) 24:6483–94. doi: 10.1158/1078-0432.CCR-17-3384
63. Dahlman KB, Xia J, Hutchinson K, Ng C, Hucks D, Jia P, et al. BRAF(L597) Mutations in Melanoma Are Associated With Sensitivity to MEK Inhibitors. *Cancer Discov* (2012) 2:791–7. doi: 10.1158/2159-8290.CD-12-0097
64. Kotani H, Adachi Y, Kitai H, Tomida S, Bando H, Faber AC, et al. Distinct Dependencies on Receptor Tyrosine Kinases in the Regulation of MAPK Signaling Between BRAF V600E and Non-V600E Mutant Lung Cancers. *Oncogene* (2018) 37:1775–87. doi: 10.1038/s41388-017-0035-9
65. Reyes R, Mayo-de-las-Casas C, Teixidó C, Cabrera C, Marín E, Vollmer I, et al. Clinical Benefit From BRAF/MEK Inhibition in a Double Non-V600E BRAF Mutant Lung Adenocarcinoma: A Case Report. *Clin Lung Cancer* (2019) 20:e219–23. doi: 10.1016/j.cllc.2019.02.022
66. Mazieres J, Montané L, Barlesi F, Coudert B, Souquet PJ, Otto J, et al. OA12.05 Vemurafenib in Patients Harboring V600 and Non V600 BRAF Mutations: Final Results of the NSCLC Cohort From the AcSé Trial. *J Thorac Oncol* (2018) 13:S348–9. doi: 10.1016/j.jtho.2018.08.302
67. La Monica S, Minari R, Cretella D, Bonelli M, Fumarola C, Cavazzoni A, et al. Acquired BRAF G469A Mutation as a Resistance Mechanism to First-Line Osimertinib Treatment in NSCLC Cell Lines Harboring an EGFR Exon 19 Deletion. *Targeting Oncol* (2019) 14:619–26. doi: 10.1007/s11523-019-00669-x
68. Lou N-N, Zhang X-C, Chen H-J, Zhou Q, Yan L-X, Xie Z, et al. Clinical Outcomes of Advanced Non-Small-Cell Lung Cancer Patients With EGFR Mutation, ALK Rearrangement and EGFR / ALK Co-Alterations. *Oncotarget* (2016) 7:65185–95. doi: 10.18632/oncotarget.11218
69. Meng P, Koopman B, Kok K, ter Elst A, Schuuring E, van Kempen LC, et al. Combined Osimertinib, Dabrafenib and Trametinib Treatment for Advanced Non-Small-Cell Lung Cancer Patients With an Osimertinib-Induced BRAF V600E Mutation. *Lung Cancer* (2020) 146:358–61. doi: 10.1016/j.lungcan.2020.05.036
70. Tan I, Stinchcombe TE, Ready NE, Crawford J, Datto MB, Nagy RJ, et al. Therapeutic Outcomes in Non-Small Cell Lung Cancer With BRAF Mutations: A Single Institution, Retrospective Cohort Study. *Transl Lung Cancer Res* (2020) 8(3):258–67. doi: 10.21037/tlcr.2019.04.03
71. Dudnik E, Peled N, Nechushtan H, Wollner M, Onn A, Agbarya A, et al. BRAF Mutant Lung Cancer: Programmed Death Ligand 1 Expression, Tumor Mutational Burden, Microsatellite Instability Status, and Response to Immune Check-Point Inhibitors. *J Thorac Oncol* (2018) 13:1128–37. doi: 10.1016/j.jtho.2018.04.024
72. Zhang C, Zhang C, Lin J, Li Z, Wang H. Patients With BRAF-Mutant NSCLC May Not Benefit From Immune Checkpoint Inhibitors: A Population-Based Study. *JTO Clin Res Rep* (2020) 1(1):100006. doi: 10.1016/j.jtocrr.2020.100006
73. Rittberg R, Banerji S, Green S, Qing G, Dawe DE. Immunotherapy Benefit in a Patient With Non-Small Cell Lung Cancer and a Rare BRAF Mutation. *Cureus.* (2020) 12(10):e11224. doi: 10.7759/cureus.11224
74. Guisier F, Dubos-Arvis C, Viñas F, Doubre H, Ricordel C, Ropert S, et al. Efficacy and Safety of Anti-PD-1 Immunotherapy in Patients With Advanced NSCLC With BRAF, HER2, or MET Mutations or RET Translocation: GFPC 01-2018. *J Thorac Oncol* (2020) 15:628–36. doi: 10.1016/j.jtho.2019.12.129
75. Wang L, Zhang Y, Zhang Q, Zhu G, Zhang Z, Duan C, et al. Discovery of Potent Pan-Raf Inhibitors With Increased Solubility to Overcome Drug Resistance. *Eur J Med Chem* (2019) 163:243–55. doi: 10.1016/j.ejmech.2018.11.033
76. Peng S-B, Henry JR, Kaufman MD, Lu W-P, Smith BD, Vogeti S, et al. Inhibition of RAF Isoforms and Active Dimers by LY3009120 Leads to Anti-Tumor Activities in RAS or BRAF Mutant Cancers. *Cancer Cell* (2015) 28:384–98. doi: 10.1016/j.ccell.2015.08.002
77. Dagogo-Jack I, Piotrowska Z, Cobb R, Banwait M, Lennerz JK, Hata AN, et al. Response to the Combination of Osimertinib and Trametinib in a Patient With EGFR-Mutant NSCLC Harboring an Acquired BRAF Fusion. *J Thorac Oncol* (2019) 14:e226–8. doi: 10.1016/j.jtho.2019.05.046
78. Callahan MK, Rampal R, Harding JJ, Klimek VM, Chung YR, Merghoub T, et al. Progression of RAS-Mutant Leukemia During RAF Inhibitor Treatment. *N ENG J OF MED* (2012) 367(24):2316–21. doi: 10.1056/NEJMoa1208958
79. Das Thakur M, Stuart DD. The Evolution of Melanoma Resistance Reveals Therapeutic Opportunities. *Cancer Res* (2013) 73:6106–10. doi: 10.1158/0008-5472.CAN-13-1633
80. Seghers AC, Wilgenhof S, Lebbé C, Neyns B. Successful Rechallenge in Two Patients With BRAF-V600-Mutant Melanoma Who Experienced Previous Progression During Treatment With a Selective BRAF Inhibitor. *Melanoma Res* (2012) 22(6):466–72. doi: 10.1097/CMR.0b013e3283541541
81. Block KI, Gyllenhaal C, Lowe L, Amedei A, Amin ARMR, Amin A, et al. Designing a Broad-Spectrum Integrative Approach for Cancer Prevention and Treatment. *Semin Cancer Biol* (2015) 35:S276–304. doi: 10.1016/j.semcancer.2015.09.007
82. Li QS, Shen BN, Xu HJ, Ruan BF. Promising Strategies for Overcoming BRAF Inhibitor Resistance Based on Known Resistance Mechanisms. *Anticancer Agents Med Chem* (2020) 20(12):1415–30. doi: 10.2174/1871520620666200422073622
83. Botton T, Yeh I, Nelson T, Vemula SS, Sparatta A, Garrido MC, et al. Recurrent BRAF Kinase Fusions in Melanocytic Tumors Offer an Opportunity for Targeted Therapy. *Pigment Cell Melanoma Res* (2013) 26:845–51. doi: 10.1111/pcmr.12148
84. Shi H, Moriceau G, Kong X, Lee M-K, Lee H, Koya RC, et al. Melanoma Whole-Exome Sequencing Identifies V600EB-RAF Amplification-Mediated Acquired B-RAF Inhibitor Resistance. *Nat Commun* (2012) 3:724. doi: 10.1038/ncomms1727
85. Montagut C, Sharma SV, Shioda T, McDermott U, Ulman M, Ulkus LE, et al. Elevated CRAF as a Potential Mechanism of Acquired Resistance to BRAF Inhibition in Melanoma. *Cancer Res* (2008) 68:4853–61. doi: 10.1158/0008-5472.CAN-07-6787
86. Lu H, Liu S, Zhang G, Wu B, Zhu Y, Frederick DT, et al. PAK Signalling Drives Acquired Drug Resistance to MAPK Inhibitors in BRAF-Mutant Melanomas. *Nature* (2017) 550:133–6. doi: 10.1038/nature24040
87. Emery CM, Vijayendran KG, Zipser MC, Sawyer AM, Niu L, Kim JJ, et al. MEK1 Mutations Confer Resistance to MEK and B-RAF Inhibition. *Proc Natl Acad Sci USA* (2009) 106:20411–6. doi: 10.1073/pnas.0905833106
88. Poulikakos PI, Rosen N. Mutant BRAF Melanomas—Dependence and Resistance. *Cancer Cell* (2011) 19:11–5. doi: 10.1016/j.ccr.2011.01.008
89. Nazarian R, Shi H, Wang Q, Kong X, Koya RC, Lee H, et al. Melanomas Acquire Resistance to B-RAF(V600E) Inhibition by RTK or N-RAS Upregulation. *Nature* (2010) 468:973–7. doi: 10.1038/nature09626
90. Johnson DB, Menzies AM, Zimmer L, Eroglu Z, Ye F, Zhao S, et al. Acquired BRAF Inhibitor Resistance: A Multicenter Meta-Analysis of the Spectrum and Frequencies, Clinical Behaviour, and Phenotypic Associations of Resistance Mechanisms. *Eur J Cancer Oxf. Engl 1990* (2015) 51(18):2792–99. doi: 10.1016/j.ejca.2015.08.022

91. Romano E, Pradervand S, Paillusson A, Weber J, Harshman K, Muehlethaler K, et al. Identification of Multiple Mechanisms of Resistance to Vemurafenib in a Patient With BRAFV600E-Mutated Cutaneous Melanoma Successfully Rechallenged After Progression. *Clin Cancer Res* (2013) 19:5749–57. doi: 10.1158/1078-0432.CCR-13-0661
92. Corcoran RB, Settleman J, Engelman JA. Potential Therapeutic Strategies to Overcome Acquired Resistance to BRAF or MEK Inhibitors in BRAF Mutant Cancers. *Oncotarget* (2011) 2(4):336–46. doi: 10.18632/oncotarget.262
93. Villanueva J, Vultur A, Lee JT, Somasundaram R, Fukunaga-Kalabis M, Cipolla AK, et al. Acquired Resistance to BRAF Inhibitors Mediated by a RAF Kinase Switch in Melanoma Can Be Overcome by Cotargeting MEK and IGF-1r/PI3K. *Cancer Cell* (2010) 18:683–95. doi: 10.1016/j.ccr.2010.11.023
94. Spagnolo F, Ghiorzo P, Orgiano L, Pastorino L, Picasso V, Tornari E, et al. BRAF-Mutant Melanoma: Treatment Approaches, Resistance Mechanisms, and Diagnostic Strategies. *OncoTar. Ther* (2015) 8:157–68. doi: 10.2147/OTT.S39096
95. Staibano S, Pepe S, Soyer P, Argenziano G, Somma P, Mansueto G, et al. Epidermal Growth Factor Receptor (EGFR) Expression in Cutaneous Melanoma: A Possible Role as Prognostic Marker. *Melanoma Res* (2004) 14(2):S26. doi: 10.1097/00008390-200404000-00030
96. Seshacharyulu P, Ponnusamy MP, Haridas D, Jain M, Ganti AK, Batra SK. Targeting the EGFR Signaling Pathway in Cancer Therapy. *Expert Opin Ther Targets* (2012) 16:15–31. doi: 10.1517/14728222.2011.648617
97. Patel H, Mishra R, Yacoub N, Alanazi S, Kilroy MK, Garrett JT. IGF1R/IR Mediates Resistance to BRAF and MEK Inhibitors in BRAF-Mutant Melanoma. *Cancers* (2021) 13:5863. doi: 10.3390/cancers13225863
98. Johannessen CM, Boehm JS, Kim SY, Thomas SR, Wardwell L, Johnson LA, et al. COT Drives Resistance to RAF Inhibition Through MAP Kinase Pathway Reactivation. *Nature* (2010) 468:968–72. doi: 10.1038/nature09627
99. Shen C-H, Kim SH, Trousil S, Frederick DT, Piris A, Yuan P, et al. Loss of Cohesin Complex Components STAG2 or STAG3 Confers Resistance to BRAF Inhibition in Melanoma. *Nat Med* (2016) 22:1056–61. doi: 10.1038/nm.4155
100. Watson IR, Li L, Cabeceiras PK, Mahdavi M, Gutschner T, Genovese G, et al. The RAC1 P29S Hotspot Mutation in Melanoma Confers Resistance to Pharmacological Inhibition of RAF. *Cancer Res* (2014) 74:4845–52. doi: 10.1158/0008-5472.CAN-14-1232-T
101. Whittaker SR, Theurillat J-P, Allen EV, Wagle N, Hsiao J, Cowley GS, et al. A Genome-Scale RNA Interference Screen Implicates NF1 Loss in Resistance to RAF Inhibition. *Cancer Discov* (2013) 3:350–62. doi: 10.1158/2159-8290.CD-12-0470
102. Ji Z, Njauw C-N, Guhan S, Kumar R, Reddy B, Rajadurai A, et al. Loss of ACK1 Upregulates EGFR and Mediates Resistance to BRAF Inhibition. *J Invest. Dermatol* (2021) 141:1317–1324.e1. doi: 10.1016/j.jid.2020.06.041
103. Martz CA, Ottina KA, Singleton KR, Jasper JS, Wardell SE, Peraza-Penton A, et al. Systematic Identification of Signaling Pathways With Potential to Confer Anticancer Drug Resistance. *Sci Signal* (2014) 7(357): ra121.doi: 10.1126/scisignal.aaa1877
104. Aguissa-Touré A-H, Li G. Genetic Alterations of PTEN in Human Melanoma. *Cell Mol Life Sci* (2012) 69:1475–91. doi: 10.1007/s00018-011-0878-0
105. Podlaha O, Riester M, De S, Michor F. Evolution of the Cancer Genome. *Trends Genet* (2012) 28(4):155–63. doi: 10.1016/j.tig.2012.01.003
106. Navin N, Kendall J, Troge J, Andrews P, Rodgers L, McIndoo J, et al. Tumour Evolution Inferred by Single-Cell Sequencing. *Nature* (2011) 472:90–U119. doi: 10.1038/nature09807
107. Gerlinger M, Horswell S, Larkin J, Rowan AJ, Salm MP, Varela I, et al. Genomic Architecture and Evolution of Clear Cell Renal Cell Carcinomas Defined by Multiregion Sequencing. *Nat Genet* (2014) 46:225–33. doi: 10.1038/ng.2891
108. Greaves M. Evolutionary Determinants of Cancer. *Cancer Discov* (2015) 5:806–20. doi: 10.1158/2159-8290.CD-15-0439
109. Nam AS, Chaligne R, Landau DA. Integrating Genetic and Non-Genetic Determinants of Cancer Evolution by Single-Cell Multi-Omics. *Nat Rev Genet* (2021) 22:3–18. doi: 10.1038/s41576-020-0265-5
110. Mroz EA, Rocco JW. The Challenges of Tumor Genetic Diversity. *Cancer* (2017) 123:917–27. doi: 10.1002/cncr.30430
111. Wu Y-L, Tsuboi M, He J, John T, Grohe C, Majem M, et al. Osimertinib in Resected EGFR-Mutated Non–Small-Cell Lung Cancer. *N Engl J Med* (2020) 383:1711–23. doi: 10.1056/NEJMoa2027071
112. Li SD, Martial A, Schrock AB, Liu JJ. Extraordinary Clinical Benefit to Sequential Treatment With Targeted Therapy and Immunotherapy of a BRAF V600E and PD-L1 Positive Metastatic Lung Adenocarcinoma. *Exp Hematol Oncol* (2017) 6:29. doi: 10.1186/s40164-017-0089-y
113. Facchinetti F, Lacroix L, Mezquita L, Scoazec J-Y, Loriot Y, Tselikas L, et al. Molecular Mechanisms of Resistance to BRAF and MEK Inhibitors in BRAFV600E non–Small Cell Lung Cancer. *Eur J Cancer* (2020) 132:211–23. doi: 10.1016/j.ejca.2020.03.025

21

The Resistance Mechanisms of Lung Cancer Immunotherapy

*Fen Wang[1,2], Shubin Wang[2] and Qing Zhou[1]**

[1] Guangdong Provincial Key Laboratory of Translational Medicine in Lung Cancer, Guangdong Provincial People's Hospital, Guangdong Academy of Medical Sciences, School of Medicine, Guangdong Lung Cancer Institute, South China University of Technology, Guangzhou, China, [2] Shenzhen Key Laboratory of Gastrointestinal Cancer Translational Research, Department of Oncology, Cancer Institute of Shenzhen-PKU-HKUST Medical Center, Peking University Shenzhen Hospital, Shenzhen, China

***Correspondence:**
Qing Zhou
gzzhouqing@126.com

Immunotherapy has revolutionized lung cancer treatment in the past decade. By reactivating the host's immune system, immunotherapy significantly prolongs survival in some advanced lung cancer patients. However, resistance to immunotherapy is frequent, which manifests as a lack of initial response or clinical benefit to therapy (primary resistance) or tumor progression after the initial period of response (acquired resistance). Overcoming immunotherapy resistance is challenging owing to the complex and dynamic interplay among malignant cells and the defense system. This review aims to discuss the mechanisms that drive immunotherapy resistance and the innovative strategies implemented to overcome it in lung cancer.

Keywords: resistance mechanism, immunotherapy, PD-1/PD-L1, Immune check Inhibitor, lung cance

INTRODUCTION

The discovery of the immune checkpoint inhibitors (ICIs), represented by the monoclonal antibodies that block cytotoxic T–lymphocyte–associated protein 4 (CTLA-4), programmed death protein 1 (PD-1), and programmed death protein ligand 1 (PD-L1), has revolutionized the therapeutic landscape of lung cancer. The significant survival benefit derived from ICI-containing treatment has established it as the mainstay first-line therapy in patients with advanced or locally advanced non-small cell lung cancer (NSCLC) and extensive small-cell lung cancer (SCLC). Unprecedented long-term clinical benefit or even, in some cases, a complete recovery has been witnessed in lung cancer, particularly in patients with high PD-L1-expressing tumors (1–3). Currently, investigations are under way aimed at integrating immunotherapy in the treatment of early-stage lung cancer.

However, most patients with NSCLC develop primary resistance during ICI monotherapy and only 15 to 20% achieve partial or complete response (3). Acquired resistance also occurs in initially responding patients with advanced NSCLC treated with ICIs, after a median progression-free survival (PFS) of 4–10 months (4–9). The mechanisms of resistance to immunotherapy are not yet fully understood, and methods to overcome them must be developed. Herein, we discuss the pathways driving resistance to immunotherapy in lung cancer to help clinicians in their current practice, as well as identify future research priorities and treatment strategies.

DIFFERENT SCHEMAS OF RESISTANCE TO IMMUNOTHERAPY

Unlike molecular targeted therapy and chemotherapy targeting tumor cells, immunotherapy targets the immune system of the host by mobilizing the immune cells to recognize and eventually eliminate tumor cells. This mechanism of action determines the complexity of the resistance mechanisms in immunotherapy. Different mechanisms of immunotherapy resistance are listed in **Table 1**.

In accordance with the timing of development, resistance can be considered as either primary, when no initial response or clinical benefit to the therapy is observed, or acquired, as disease progression occurs after an initial period of clinical benefit (10). Clinically, 6-month treatment duration is adopted as a cutoff value (11). This classification schema correlates with real-time observations by clinicians and contributes to the clinical decision-making process in the absence of other information such as immune characteristics and tumor genetics.

Resistance is additionally classified as intrinsic or extrinsic to cancer cells. The former occurs in the tumor cell itself and encompasses the inherent characteristics related to gene expression, cell signaling, immune recognition, and DNA damage response, whereas the latter is seen in the microenvironment or systemic circulation throughout the T-cell bioactivation process (12, 13).

The cancer–immunity cycle is linked to immunotherapy resistance in another related schema (14). This classification divides resistance from an immunological perspective into immune desert (tumor fails to evoke an immune reaction), immune inflamed (tumor inhibits immune activities notwithstanding abundant immune cells infiltration), or excluded (tumor prevents immune cells infiltration in spite of adequate immunogenicity) (13).

It is noteworthy that the immune response is a continuous and dynamic process rather than categorical (binary). Multiple complex interactions, including immunologic, genomic, and host characteristics and treatment interventions, rather than a single, dominant determinant are involved in the resistance to immunotherapy. The fs can be overlapping or parallel in some cases despite the different timing of occurrence (11).

TABLE 1 | Different schemas of resistance to immunotherapy.

Schemas	Classifications	Description
Temporal perspective	Primary	Lack of initial response or clinical benefit to therapy
	Acquired	Disease progression after an initial period (6 months) of clinical benefit
Spatial perspective	Intrinsic	Tumor-related resistance
	Extrinsic	Factors involved in microenvironment or tumor-immunity cycle
Immunological perspective	Immune inflamed	Tumor inhibits immune activities notwithstanding abundant immune cells infiltration
	Immune desert	Tumor fails to evoke an immunoreaction
	Immune excluded	Tumor prevents immune cells infiltration in spite of adequate immunogenicity

RESISTANCE MECHANISMS TO IMMUNOTHERAPY

Underlying mechanisms of primary resistance span an extensive range from tumor factors including genomic features, transcriptomic signatures, and immune landscape, to host factors. The potential mechanisms of acquired resistance at least partly overlap with those involved in primary resistance and mainly include loss of neoantigen and deficiency in presentation, loss of T-cell effector function, and up-regulation of alternate immune checkpoint receptors (10). Here, we will discuss the mechanisms of resistance to immunotherapy from tumor aspects (intrinsic and extrinsic mechanisms) and host-related characteristics in order to avoid confusion and repetition (**Figure 1**).

Tumor Cell-Intrinsic Mechanisms

Genomic Features

Low tumor mutation burden and neoantigen load

Tumor-specific antigens are the key to activate T cells to recognize tumor as foreign, which is the first step of tumor-induced adaptive immune responses and immune-mediated tumor killing (15). These neoantigens, interestingly, are derived from somatic mutations and contain new epitopes, and subsequently lead to tumor immunogenicity. Preclinical and clinical studies have revealed that the response of neoantigen-specific effector T cell (Teff) paralleled tumor shrinkage (16–20).

With the improvement of sequencing techniques, it was found that nonsynonymous mutations can generate neoantigens that trigger cytotoxic responses against tumors (21, 22). Nonsynonymous mutation burden, rather than total mutation burden of exons, was demonstrated to be more closely associated with the clinical advantage of anti-PD-1 treatment, validating the importance of neoantigens in dictating response (23). Tumor mutation burden (TMB) is calculated as the total number of nonsynonymous mutations per DNA Megabase (Mb) (21, 24, 25). Low TMB, or low numbers of clonal neoantigens, presenting reduced tumor immunogenicity, is considered as a primary resistance marker to immunotherapy (15, 26).

Clinically, low TMB or neoantigen load has correlated with inferior response and poor PFS to monotherapy of anti–PD1/PD-L1 antibodies in NSCLC (25, 27–30). However, it fails to predict the clinical outcomes, in regard to overall survival (OS) and combination regimens (31, 32). The influence on the OS by subsequent treatments and the additional complexities to the study of immunotherapy resistance added by combinations may partly explain these controversial findings. Recently, a corrected TMB (cTMB) approach based on the adjustment of tumor purity was developed by Anagnostou and colleagues, which was identified on abundant tumor samples mined from The Cancer Genome Atlas (TCGA) and then confirmed in a patient cohort received ICIs therapy. This cTMB more accurately predicted the outcomes of immunotherapy, suggesting that the TMB in samples with low tumor purity was mistakenly underestimated, which was especially important for metastatic NSCLC, because

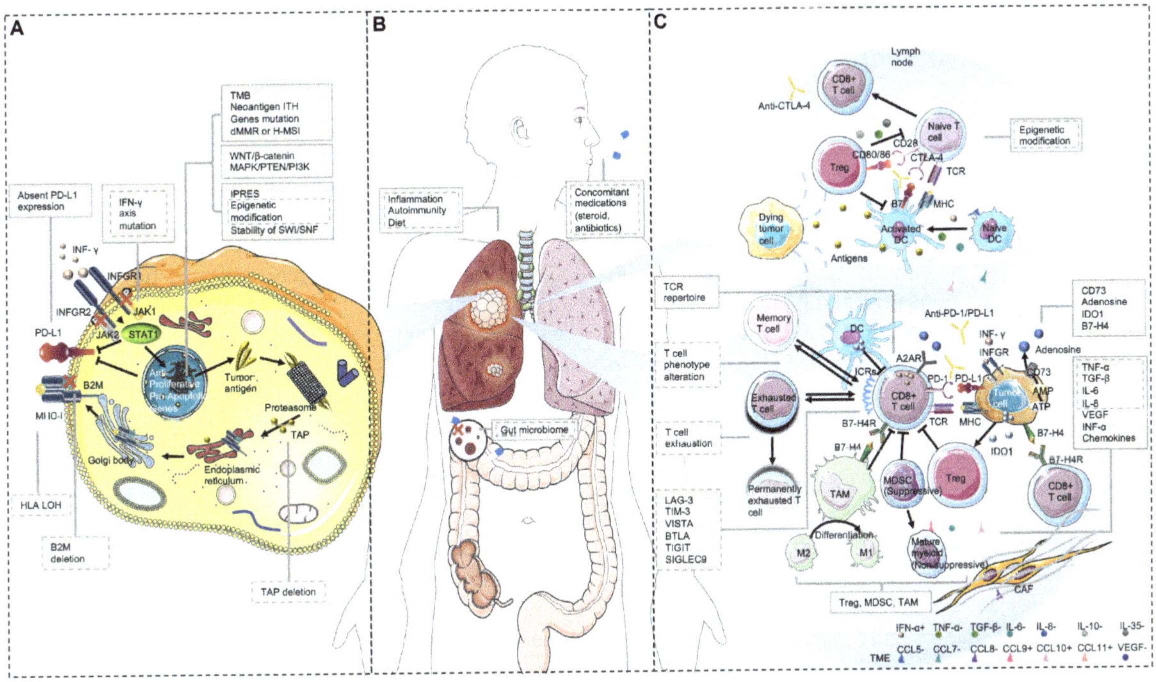

FIGURE 1 | Mechanisms of resistance to immunotherapy. **(A)** Tumor intrinsic mechanisms that are associated with resistance to immunotherapy include lack of tumor immunogenicity (low TMB, heterogenous antigens, mutation of certain genes, and IPRES transcriptional signatures), deficiency in antigen presentation (alterations in INF-γ signaling pathway, HLA LOH, B2M, and TAP deletion), aberrations in several signaling pathways (MAPK, PI3K, WNT, and IFN), and absent PD-L1 expression. **(B)** Host-related characteristics that lead to primary or secondary resistance include the gut microbiome, diet, concomitant medications, inflammation state, and autoimmunity. **(C)** Tumor extrinsic mechanisms involved in resistance to immunotherapy include T cell-related factors (alternative immune checkpoints, T cell exhaustion and phenotype alteration, TCR repertoire, and epigenetic modification), immunosuppressive cells (Treg, MDSC, and M2-TAM), and cytokines and metabolites (e.g., TGF-β, adenosine) released into the tumor microenvironment. Factors in the solid text boxes are involved in primary resistance, whereas those in the dotted text boxes are involved in secondary or acquired resistance. Factors with solid and dotted dual text boxes are involved in both. Cytokines with "+" and "-" represent positive and negative modulators to antitumor immune response, respectively. Abbreviations: TME, tumor microenvironment; MHC, major histocompatibility complex; TCR, T cell receptor; Treg, regulatory T cell; MDSC, myeloid-derived suppressor cell; M2-TAM, type II tumor-associated macrophage; ICR, immune checkpoint receptor; CAF, cancer-associated fibroblast; and IPRES, innate anti-PD-1 resistance.

the tumor purity of tissue samples obtained by bronchoscopy or puncture biopsy was often limited (33).

The dilemma of insufficient tissue sample for TMB assessment in a considerable number of patients with NSCLC has given rise to the employment of peripheral blood TMB (bTMB) as a substitute predictor of response or resistance to ICIs in NSCLC (34). In keeping with what was previously reported in tissue, low bTMB evaluated by different plasma sequencing assays was significantly correlated with poor survival or response to immunotherapy in several retrospective and prospective studies (35–37).

Increased neoantigen intratumor heterogeneity

In addition to the TMB or the numbers of clonal neoantigens, increased neoantigen intratumor heterogeneity (ITH, defined as relative fraction of subclonal neoantigens) can also impair the sensitivity to ICIs by elevating the likelihood of selection of subclones with poor immunogenicity (25, 38). The considerable variation of neoantigen heterogeneity was demonstrated by McGranahan and colleagues in seven primary NSCLCs (25). On average, 44% of heterogeneous neoantigens were reported only in a subset of tumor regions. They conducted neoantigen and clonality analysis in lung cancer data from TCGA and then validated the approach in a cohort of NSCLC patients treated with ICIs. Compared with high TMB alone, the combination of high TMB with low ITH seems to have a stronger association with clinical benefit to ICIs in this population.

Aberrations in certain oncogene/tumor suppressor genes

Aberrations in oncogenes and tumor suppressor genes can regulate immune response by amending cytokine profile and immune cell composition and thus render tumor cells resistant or sensitive to ICIs.

Generally, alterations in oncogenic driver genes are characterized as resistant markers to immunotherapy. Although epidermal growth factor receptor (EGFR) mutations and anaplastic lymphoma kinase (ALK) rearrangement tend to have high PD-L1 expression due to the activation of signaling pathways (39, 40), the low mutation or neoantigen load (41), along with the following mechanisms, impairs the immunotherapy sensitivity in this group of patients with lung cancer. First, EGFR mutations have the potential to shape an inert immune environment by up-modulating a series of immune suppressors including inhibitory immune checkpoints (e.g., PD-1 and CTLA-4), immunosuppressive cells (macrophages and regulatory T cells), and cytokines (like TGF-β, IL-6, and IL-10) (42, 43). It has been reported that activated EGFR cascade was associated with elevated T-cell exhaustion and reduced cytotoxic T lymphocytes (CTLs) in a lung adenocarcinoma model (40). Second, downstream pathways of EGFR mutation, such as MAPK, PI3K/AKT, and Janus kinase (JAK)/STAT pathway, negatively affect immunoregulation. Other oncogenic driver-genes that frequently have high PD-L1 expression in lung cancer include ROS1 rearrangements (44), MET exon 14 skipping mutations (45), and BRAF mutations (44, 46). In contrast, RET rearrangements (47) and HER2 mutations (44) have been reported recently to exhibit low PD-L1 expression. None of these oncogenotypes demonstrated favorable clinical responses to ICIs monotherapy except for BRAF mutations, either V600E or non-V600E.

STK11 gene inactivation either by mutational or non-mutational machinery is linked to an indolent immune microenvironment with lower Tumor-infiltrating lymphocyte (TILs; CD3+, CD4+, and CD8+ cells) and PD-L1 expression in spite of the existence of moderate to high TMB (48). Inactivated STK11 gene was recently reported to weaken the innate immune responses by epigenetic inhibition of stimulator of IFN genes (STING), suggesting epigenetic silencing is likely to mediate the promotion of T-cell exclusion by the loss of STK11 (49). In line with these findings, it has been observed in several studies that compared with the wild-type gene, STK11 mutation predicted poorer clinical outcomes of immunotherapy in advanced NSLCL (50, 51). The tumor suppressor TP53 mutation, a well-known negative prognostic factor in lung cancer, is found to be associated with increased PD-L1 expression and higher TMB in non-squamous NSCLC (30) and KRAS-mutated lung adenocarcinoma (51).

KRAS-mutated lung cancer presents distinct immune profiles, biology, and therapeutic vulnerabilities in different subsets classified by co-occurring genetic events (50). Generally, KRAS/TP53 co-mutation predicts sensitivity while KRAS/STK11 co-mutation predicts resistance to immunotherapy in NSCLC. Dong et al. identified TP53/KRAS co-mutated subclass exhibited the highest percentage of PD-L1+/CD8A+ and particular increased PD-L1 expression. They further confirmed a remarkable clinical benefit from pembrolizumab in this population (52). Co-mutation of STK11 was shown to cause the accrual of neutrophils with T-cell-suppressive effects, accompanied with an analogous elevation in the production of T-cell depletion biosignatures and tumor-promoting cytokines (50, 53). TIL numbers and the expression of PD-L1 were also decreased (53). Consistent with these preclinical predictions, patients with KRAS/STK11 co-mutation or single mutation of STK11 had poor response and survival compared with those with wild-type when treated with ICIs (51, 54).

The Kelch-like ECG-associated protein 1 (KEAP1) gene, regulating the cellular antioxidant and cytoprotective transcriptional programs, plays a key role in mediating immune evasion in NSCLC. Depletion of KEAP1 is associated with reduced leukocyte infiltration, increased PD-L1 expression and might also influence other immune cells such as NK cell recruitment and function (55, 56). Co-occurring KEAP1 and phosphatase and tensin homolog (PTEN) inactivation represent an immunologically "cold" tumor while concurrent mutations in KEAP1 and STK11 leads to absence of pro-cancerogenic M2 macrophages (57). However, there are conflicting data on the role of KEAP1 mutation and its co-mutation with STK11 in immunotherapy resistance in NSCLC. KEAP1/STK11 co-mutations were verified to correlate with resistance to ICIs in patients with NSCLC despite high TMB (58). Similarly, STK11, and/or KEAP1 genomic variations posited lack of clinical advantages from combination of immunotherapy with chemotherapy in patients with NSCLC (59). However, inconsistent results were reported recently that clinical benefit from pembrolizumab compared to chemotherapy was poorer in the patients with STK11 and KEAP1 mutation compared with those in wild type in Keynote 042 trial, but the response and survival to immunotherapy were not significantly different between mutant and wild subgroups (60).

The WNT/β-catenin pathway is an additional immunotherapy resistance mechanism. A negative relationship was demonstrated between the level of β-catenin and TILs, which was modulated by deficiency in the recruitment of CD103+ dendritic cells (DCs) essential to T-cell priming and reduced expression of the cytokine CCL4, suggesting WNT/β-catenin signaling pathway is likely to mediate ICIs resistance through T-cell exclusion (61).

Similarly, the MAPK/PTEN/PI3K signaling pathway has been identified to be involved in immunotherapy resistance. Loss of PTEN and the bioactivation of the phosphatidylinositol 3-kinase (PI3K) signaling pathway in tumors decrease the activity of CTLs through the recruitment of inhibitory cells to the microenvironment and Vascular endothelial growth factor (VEGF) expression (62, 63), so that they promote resistance to ICIs (63, 64). The association of PTEN deletions or *PIK3CA/AKT* mutations with increased PD-L1 expression and immune resistance was also found in glioma (65). It was shown in preclinical models that a PI3K-γ inhibitor decreased myeloid-derived suppressor cells (MDSCs) and improved response to ICIs (66).

DNA repair and replication gene alterations

Genetic instability caused by alterations in DNA replication and repair genes can augment immunogenicity via a high-TMB neoantigen load (67–69). Correspondingly, deficient DNA mismatch repair (dMMR) or high microsatellite instability (H-MSI) are suggested as sensitive predictors to ICI immunotherapy in many tumor types. Beyond high TMB, increased CD8+ TILs were also reported to be associated with alterations in mismatch repair genes (70), *BRCA2* (71), and *POLE* (72) in different tumors. However, the role of these genes in immunoregulation in NSCLC remains to be elucidated.

Interferon-gamma signaling mutation

The interferon-gamma (INF-γ) signaling cascade is a crucial component of immunotherapy and tends to serve a critical function in primary, adaptive, and acquired resistance to ICI treatment (73–75). IFN-γ is a critical cytokine secreted by activated T cells, natural killer (NK) T cells, in the cancer microenvironment, and it moderates the immune reaction via the downstream enzymes JAK 1/2 and the signal transducer and activators of transcription (STATs) (76). The INF-γ axis exerts both positive and negative impacts on antitumor immune reactions (77). On one hand, it activates an functional antitumor immune reactive via (1) intensifying antigen presentation by up-modulated secretion of MHC-I; (2) recruiting other immune cells by up-regulation of the expression of chemokines (CXCL9, CXCL10, and CXCL11) with effective chemoattractant impacts on T cells (78); and (3) exerting direct anti-proliferative and pro-apoptotic impacts on cancer cells (79). On the other hand, IFN-γ acts in a negative-feedback axis to elevate PD-L1 expression as well as other crucial immune inhibitory components, including IDO1, down-modulating the cytotoxic reaction and adaptive resistance to cancer cells (80, 81) (**Figure 1A**).

Additionally, copy-number alterations (CNAs) linked to DNA damage response and regulation of DNA editing/repair gene expression were shown to emanate from the malignant exposure to IFN-γ-secreting antigen-specific CTLs *in vivo*, implying that intensified genetic instability could be among the mechanisms through which CTLs and IFN-γ immunoedits cancers, changing their immune resistance due to genetic evolution (82).

Tumors neutralize the impact of IFN-γ by mutating or down-regulating the molecules involved in the IFN-γ signaling pathway, including IFN-γ receptor chains, regulatory factors, JAK1/2, and STATs upon continuous IFN-γ exposure (73, 83). Multiple studies have demonstrated that mutations of IFN-γ axis and consequent loss of JAK/STAT contribute to immune escape of tumor cells and by that leads to primary or acquired resistance to ICI therapy via incapacity of up-regulating the expression of PD-L1 and MHC-I (73, 78, 84). Any deficiencies in IFN-γ, JAK1/2, or STATs including gene mutations, loss of protein expression, negative regulator presence, or epigenetic silencing would prevent signaling in response to IFN-γ and thereby end up to the up-regulated tumor growth and apoptosis inhibition and down-regulated T-cell infiltration and expression of PD-L1 and MHC-I (74, 78, 85, 86). Correspondingly, genomic changes disturbing IFN-γ pathway genes, including the amplification of suppressor genes PIAS4 and SOCS1 and the deletion of IFNGR1, IFNGR2, IFIT1, IFIT2, IFIT3, IRF1, MTAP, and miR31, have been described as possible machinery of primary resistance to various ICI therapies (73). An IFN-γ-related mRNA profile that contains 10 genes (CCR5, CXCL9, CXCL10, CXCL11, GZMA, HLA-DRA, IDO1, IFNG, PRF1, and STAT1) was additionally identified to predict the response to anti-PD-1 therapy in melanoma (87).

Transcriptomic Signatures

In a recent publication, transcriptional signatures, referred to as innate anti-PD-1 resistance (IPRES) with inflammatory and mesenchymal tumor phenotypes, were shown to manifest poor response to anti-PD-1 therapy in metastatic melanoma (88). Approximately 700 differentially expressed genes (DEGs) were identified between the responsive and non-responsive pretreated tumors. Compared with those of responsive tumors, the transcriptomes of non-responsive tumors were dominated by gene up-regulation events. The up-regulated DEGs in non-responsive tumors, considered as T cell suppressive, are involved in mesenchymal transition (*TWIST2, TAGLN, FAP, AXL, ROR2, WNT5A,* and *LOXL2*), monocyte/macrophage chemotaxis (*CCL2, CCL7, CCL8,* and *CCL13*), immunosuppression (*IL10, VEGFA,* and *VEGFC*), and angiogenesis and wound healing (89–91). By contrast, down-regulated gene *CDH1* (which is typically down-regulated by mesenchymal tumor cells) was also detected in non-responsive pretreated tumors. Interestingly, there was no difference in the expression of INF-γ pathway signatures, other T-cell-related genes (e.g., *CD8A/B, PD-L1,* and *LAG3*), and the genes that presumably modulate immune checkpoint sensitivity between responsive and non-responsive groups, suggesting that T-cell-suppressive inflammatory and mesenchymal phenotypes of tumor are associated with primary resistance to anti-PD-1 therapy.

Epigenetic Modification

Emerging evidence has suggested that epigenetic modification may mediate primary resistance and contribute to acquired resistance during ICI therapy through the profound effect on many aspects of antitumor immunity: neoantigen presentation and processing; T-cell functions, differentiation, and proliferation; memory T-cell phenotype acquisition; interfering with T-cell migration; and mediating T-cell exhaustion (10, 92–94).

Epigenetic targeting agents, including those targeting histone deacetylation or methylation as well as targeting DNA methylation, have exhibited encouraging antitumor activity either as monotherapy or in combination with immunotherapy in preclinical studies (94, 95). Clinical trials investigating the performance of these agents combined with adaptive T-cell transfer (ACT) in patients with acquired resistance to prior immunotherapy are ongoing (96).

Stability of Chromatin Remodeling Complexes

Stability of chromatin remodeling complexes within tumor cells can also contribute to immunotherapy resistance by multiple mechanisms. It was found that tumor cells were more sensitive to CTL killing, which leads to increased response to anti-PD-1/PD-L1 therapy, due to the deficiency in chromatin remodeling complex SWI/SNF (97, 98). BRG1-associated factor (BAF) and polybromo-associated BAF (PBAF), as the mammalian analogs of the SWI/SNF complex, are essential tumor suppressors and loss of function (LOF) mutations of them were shown to sensitize tumor cells to ICI therapy (98). The inactivated PBAF subunits exhibited elevated CXCL9/CXCL10 expression and TILs recruitment as a result of increase of chromatin accessibility to transcriptional regulators of IFN-γ-inducible genes (97). ARID1A/B subunits are unique to BAF, while other subunits (ARID2, BRD7, and PBRM1) are exclusively contained by PBAF, despite the high similarity of these complexes (99). In another study, loss of ARID1A was found to elevate MSI by defective recruitment of mismatch repair genes and thus increase TMB, which eventual sensitize tumor cells to PD-L1 inhibitor (100).

Absent Tumor PD-L1 Expression

The PD-1/PD-L1 axis represents one of the foremost mechanisms of modulation of peripheral immune tolerance as well as T-cell activation. Up-regulation of PD-L1 by cancer cells and antigen-presenting cells (APCs) is one approach through which tumors avoid immunosurveillance and constitutes the principle behind PD-1/PD-L1 blockade therapies (101). Absent PD-L expression of tumors has been found to be generally associated with less responses and inferior survival benefits to anti-PD-1/PD-L1 therapies compared with higher expression (102) and may serve as a resistant marker. However, up to 20% of PD−L1−negative malignancies showed responses to PD−1 inhibitors in some cohorts (103), as PD-L1 expression can be up-regulated by other factors including activated IFN-γ cascade (will be discussed in a separated part), suggesting tumor PD-L1 expression alone is not dependable at predicting outcomes of PD-1/PD-L1 inhibitors.

Any factors that affect the PD-L1 expression of tumor cells may lead to resistance to immunotherapy. Beyond encoding genes, PD-L1 expression can be affected by the mutational features of tumor although it is not paralleled with TMB in most of the tumors (104–106). The inherent mechanisms, which have been shown to result in constitutive expression of PD-L1 by tumor cells, consist of alterations in the PTEN/PI3K/AKT pathway (65, 107), MYC overexpression (108), EGFR mutations (40), CDK5 truncation (109), and elevated PD-L1 transcripts stabilized by disruption of the 3-untranslated region (UTR) of this gene (110). Tumor-specific immune response may also be affected by constitutive expression of PD-L1 caused by these oncogenic signaling processes on tumor cell surface. Although it is still unclear whether it causes an increased or decreased possibility of responding to anti-PD-1/PD-L1 therapies, the constitutive PD-L1 expression could result into inadequate response to other immunotherapeutic approaches by suppressing antitumor effect of T cells. The other transcriptional factors constituting HIF1, NFkB, and STAT3, as well as epigenetic factors, additionally participate in the modulation of PD-L1 expression (111).

Inflammatory and hypoxic tumor microenvironment (TME) can also lead to PD-L1 expression on many cell types including tumor cells by Toll-like receptor (TLR) ligands. The recruitment of activated T cells can increase the inflammatory mediators and successively induce the PD-L1 expression on the surface of tumor cells. These tumor cells specifically locate at the invasive periphery where T cells are often abundant (112, 113).

Besides, PD-L1 is stabilized through N-glycosylation and palmitoylation (114, 115). This is crucial for its interaction with PD-1. The resistance to anti-PD-1/PD-L1 treatment could moreover be attributed to the degree of generation and secretion of soluble forms of PD-L1. These variants without the transmembrane domain because of alternative splicing have been reported in recurrent NSCLC incidences that re-occurred after anti-PD-L1 antibody therapy with the ability to act as soluble imitates for anti-PD-L1 antibodies (116).

Deficiency in Antigen Presentation

Loss of neoantigen

Loss of neoantigens in the context of immune-mediated pressure is postulated to be another mechanism leading to resistance. In the concept of immunoediting, the constant interactions between tumor cells and the immune system trigger the production of subclones that do not express neoantigens, consequently conferring poor immunogenicity and resistance to ICIs (117). It was demonstrated by Anagnostou and colleagues that seven to eight putative neoantigens were lost in the recurrent NSCLC after ICI treatment, suggesting that immunoediting plays a role in acquired resistance to immunotherapy (118). T-cell-mediated neoantigen immunoediting can be induced by the dynamic interactions between T cells and tumor cells, consequently causing partial or total loss of neoantigen (119). Consistently, deficiency in genes that encode target tumor antigens was demonstrated to be associated with acquired resistance in a murine model treated with adoptive T-cell therapy (ACT) in melanoma (120). However, this relationship between acquired resistance and loss of target neoantigens was not observed in a single patient case who achieved a complete response to ACT in a separate study (121), suggesting that down-regulation/loss of neoantigens may occur during immunotherapy, but should be taken as a canonical mechanism of acquired immune resistance.

Proinflammatory cytokines are likely to contribute to immune escape by inducing loss of antigen expression, resulting in acquired resistance too. The process of Tumor necrosis factor-α (TNF-α)-induced epithelial-to-mesenchymal de-differentiation was shown to lead to a loss of neoantigens causing transformation to a tumor phenotype that is less immunogenic and can more readily evade immune surveillance in the ACT-treated mouse model in melanoma (122). Other TIL generated cytokines, such as IL-6 or TGF-β, are also shown to be involved in the induction of epithelial-to-mesenchymal transition in mouse models across numerous types of tumors, indicating that acquired resistance can be promoted by inflammation.

Defective neoantigen presentation

Defective neoantigen presentation serves a crucial function in ICI acquired resistance. The alterations in this process could happen in beta-2-microglobulin (B2M), transporters associated with antigen processing (TAP), or MHC itself (123, 124) (**Figure 1A**).

As part of the MHC class I (MHC-I), B2M is crucial during antigen presentation and its genetic deficiency, including loss of heterozygosity (LOH) and deletions or point mutations, was identified to be an important route for primary and acquired resistance to ICIs (125, 126). Other defects that would affect neoantigen presentation include T-cell receptor (TCR) binding domain mutations of MHC-I (127), loss of tapasin (a MHC-I antigen processing molecule), selective epigenetic silencing of the human leukocyte antigen (HLA) A3 antigen, loss of one HLA haplotype (128, 129), and LOH in HLA (130). Homozygosity in one or more of the three highly variable genes (HLA-A, HLA-B, and HLA-C) that encode MHC-I, which are likely to restrict neoantigen presentation to CTLs, was identified to have a significant association between resistance to ICI therapy in a large cohort of cancer patients (131). In contrast to anti-CTLA-4, the expression of MHC-II (but not MHC-I) proteins by tumor and the presence of IFN-γ-mediated gene signatures were found to be associated with the positive responses to anti-PD-1 therapy in melanoma (132).

Defective neoantigen presentation may be mediated by IFN-γ signaling pathway through JAK1/2 and the STATs, by down-regulating the expression of MHC-I (133). Actually, the IFN-γ pathway has both unfavorable and favorable impacts on antitumor immune responses and plays a key role in acquired and primary resistance to ICI therapy (as discussed above).

Tumor Cell-Extrinsic Immune Landscape

T-Cell-Related Factors Involved in Tumor-Cancer Immune Cycle

Tumor-infiltrating lymphocytes

Tumor-infiltrating lymphocytes constitute a complex group of immune cells with distinct functions and different clinical impacts. Among them, tumor-specific CD8+ T cells can execute anti-cancer activities by killing tumor cells directly and has a strong prognostic effect in NSCLC (134, 135). CD4+ cells are composed of a group of lymphocytes (Tregs CD4+, Th1, Th2, and Th17) secreting diverse cytokine to activate and suppress CD8+ cells. Th1 secretes IFN-γ and IL2, while Th2 secretes IL-4, IL-5, IL-9, IL-10, IL-13, and IL-25 (136, 137). CD45RO+ T cells, also known as memory T lymphocytes, are another subclass of TILs. Regulator and memory T lymphocytes will be discussed in *section* "Suppressive tumor microenvironment."

Low CD8+ TIL density was correlated with impaired efficacy and survival in NSCLC patients treated with ICIs (138), suggesting that immunotherapy resistance was mediated by low TILs but was then positively modulated by PD-L1. TILs can be assessed by immunohistochemistry or standard hematoxylin and eosin (H&E) staining; however, no consensus has been reached hitherto in the various scoring models using H&E staining in NSCLC (139–142). A radiomic fingerprint of CD8+ TIL derived via computerized tomography was developed recently and showed promising efficacy in predicting response to ICI therapies but requires further validation (143).

Thus, tumors can be described as three main immune organization profiles (hot, altered, and cold) as per the presence of TILs and correlated proinflammatory cytokines (144). The "cold" immune tumor is characterized as absence of TIL within and at the edges of tumor, manifesting resistance to immunotherapy either due to absent immune stimulation (as with low neoantigen cancer's poor antigen presentation) or because of failed T-cell priming (as with intrinsic insensitivity to T-cell killing). The "altered" immune tumor is characterized as low TIL within the tumor ("immunosuppressed") or high TIL at the edges of the tumor ("excluded"), whereas "hot" is high degree of TIL (144). Recently, intratumorally geospatial heterogeneity of TIL was revealed in NSCLC. Tumor subclones from "cold" immune regions were related to mutation space more closely and diversifying more recently compared with those from "hot" immune regions. Higher risk of recurrence was observed in tumors with more than one "cold" immune region (145).

Impaired T-cell priming and infiltration

Reduced proliferation and inadequate diversification of T cells possibly contribute to ICI resistance. Impeded priming of naive T cells by blocked DCs recruitment was demonstrated in melanoma to be correlated to the lack of TILs and ICIs resistance (146). The function of DCs can be potentially influenced by the cytokines in the TME through (1) impaired migratory capacity as well as decreased synthesis of costimulatory components (CD86/80) by TGF-β (147, 148); (2) prevented DCs maturation by IL-6-gp130-STAT3 axis; and (3) inhibited activity by Indoleamine 2,3-dioxygenase 1 (IDO, will be discussed in *Section* "Suppressive tumor microenvironment"). IFN-α signaling pathway is important to the priming of T cells by DCs. It was found that TME with remarkable insufficient IFN-α-producing DCs naturally led to lessened antitumor T-cell priming and thus resistance to ICIs (149, 150). Activated IFN-α stimulated production of the chemokine CXCL10 to recruit TILs to tumor beds and in turn initiate spontaneous antitumor T-cell response (149–151). Preliminary trials combining IFN-α 2b therapy with anti-CTLA-4 inhibitors have indicated clinical activity, which could be caused by diminished populations of MDSC (152, 153). Combinations of other ICIs and IFN-α 2b are currently investigated (154).

Immune resistance also occurs if the tumors evolve the ability to prevent infiltration even if tumor-specific Teffs are formed. Mechanisms that lead to impaired T-cell infiltration involve components in the epigenetic silencing of immune cells (155) and the modification of secreted chemokines (156, 157). Transcriptional program that is associated with T-cell exclusion and thereby predictive resistance to anti-PD-1 therapy was identified in melanoma (158). Stromal cells surrounding tumors within TME can develop the capacity to obstruct effector T-cell entry, and the TGF-β cascade appears to serve a crucial role in promoting T-cell exclusion features in peritumoral fibroblasts (123, 159).

T-cell receptor clonality

T-cell receptor clonality is emerging as a new biomarker to predict the resistance and immune-related adverse events to ICIs therapy. Since baseline CD8+ T-cell density was found to overlap between respondents and non-respondents to ICI therapy (160–162), it led to the speculation that a constrict TCR arsenal possessed by the baseline T cells concentrated on the antitumor immune reaction and is associated with response to ICI therapies. T-cell clones can be identified by detecting TCR rearrangements constituting genes in the variable (V)-diversity (D)-joining (J) region, which generate the antigen-specific complementarity-determining region 3 (CDR3). The responsivity of TCRs generated by TILs determines their potential to interplay with tumor antigens that are presented on APCs. Thus, the assessment of T-cell clonality divulges the extent of T-cell expansions caused by tumor antigens and contributes to explore the mechanisms underlying T-cell toleration to tumor antigens.

A lower baseline clonal T-cell arsenal has been shown to be linked to worse clinical benefits to ICIs and survival in cancer patients (162, 163). Besides, a remarkable increase in T-cell clones was reported in responders during anti-PD-1 therapy compared to non-responders, implying a cancer-specific reaction to immunotherapy for these patients. Moreover, baseline TCR clonality did not strongly associate with TIL density, implying that low-TIL density tumors could still respond to anti-PD-1 treatment if TIL has a narrow TCR clonality specific to the tumor antigen (164). Inconsistently, it was recently found that T-cell clonality had a positive relationship with T-cell density, PD-L1 expression, and TMB, and a negative relationship with EGFR mutation in NSCLC (165). A corresponding relationship was found between the number of TCR sequences and the number of nonsynonymous mutations, spatial heterogeneity in expanded TCR repertoire, and spatial mutational heterogeneity within tumors in NSCLC, respectively. This intratumorally spatial heterogeneity of TCR repertoire maps the neoantigen landscape, sculptured by focal antigen processing defects or HLA loss (166). Thereby, further investigations to identify the role of TCR clonality in immunotherapy are required.

Alternate immune checkpoint receptor up-regulation

Compensatory up-regulation of numerous alternate immune checkpoint receptors during ICI therapy as a result of the activation of diverse cellular signals and IFN-γ signaling pathway were observed across multiple studies and have been characterized to be linked to ICI adaptive resistance in NSCLC (84, 167, 168). The expression of CD8+ T cells harboring receptors showed serious flaws in proliferation, migration, and cytokine secretion, indicating their immunosuppressive capacity. In addition, progressive T-cell exhaustion was found in the tumors with highly expressive or co-expressive receptors and different receptor displayed different exhausted phenotype (167).

Among these receptors, lymphocyte activation gene 3 (LAG-3) has great potentiality in cancer immunotherapy because co-expression of PD-1 and LAG-3 was often found in T-cell-depleted immune microenvironment, and PD-1 inhibitors combined with LAG-3 blockades showed strong synergic antitumor responses in preliminary models (169). LAG-3 is a co-inhibitory receptor extensively expressed in TILs in various tumors and serves a crucial function in mediating immune escape by suppressing T-cell antitumor functions. It exerts immunosuppression via binding to MHC-II molecules and other ligands such as galectin-3 and fibrinogen-like protein 1 (FGL1) (170). Thus, blocking LAG-3 can restore antitumor immunity and the combined LAG-3 inhibitors therapy may accordingly overcome immunotherapy resistance. In addition, the expression of these ligands, on the basis of the receptor–ligand interactions, may serve as important biomarkers to predict the efficacy of LAG-3 blockades in lung cancer (167).

The other alternative immune checkpoint receptors, e.g., T-cell immunoglobulin and mucin-3 (TIM-3), V-domain immunoglobulin-containing suppressor of T-cell activation (VISTA), B and T lymphocyte attenuator (BTLA; also referred to as CD272), T-cell immunoreceptor tyrosine-based inhibition motif domain (TIGIT), and sialic acid-binding Ig-like lectin 9 (SIGLEC9), have been discovered (144). Thus, these alternate immune checkpoints are likely to be combined with existing ICI therapy to conquer the resistance. Increased efficacy of PD-1 inhibitors combined with anti-TIM-3 or anti-LAG-3 regimens has been observed in either pre-clinical models or phase I clinical trials (171, 172). Currently, numerous clinical trials evaluating the therapeutic impact of alternate immune checkpoint blockade applied on its own or in combination with PD-1/PD-L1 inhibitors in multiple malignances are ongoing.

T-cell exhaustion and phenotype alteration

T-cell exhaustion is another factor involved in the primary and acquired resistance to ICI therapy (**Figure 1C**). Exhausted T cells exhibit impaired activity with progressive LOF and antigen persistence compared with Teffs and can be induced by the PD-1/PD-L1 interactions (173). Chronic exposure to cognate antigen triggers increased expression of PD-1, which results in the accumulation of T-cell exhaustion and thus T-cell dysfunction (174). The presence of PD-1 high expression can either exist prior to PD-1 inhibitors, which is associated with primary resistance partially depending on tumor-associated regulatory T cells (Tregs), or develop after the anti-PD-1 therapy, which leads to acquired resistance by severe T-cell exhaustion. In contrast, studies showed that the exhausted T cells with PD-1 low to intermediate phenotype retain the capacity to be reinvigorated by ICIs (158, 175). Epigenetic alterations were found to be associated with T-cell exhaustion too recently. Exhausted T cell displayed a unique chromatin landscape, which alters the transcriptional state, limits its effect function, and determines its capacity to be reprogrammed after therapeutic intervention (176–178).

The formation of memory T cells is crucial to the avoidance of tumor relapse and therapy resistance following drug withdrawal, especially in the long-lasting duration of responses to ICI therapy. Research evidence shows that patients with resistance to anti-PD-1 treatment have fewer tumor-correlated memory T cells relative to sensitive patients (179). Memory T cells remain dormant until antigen re-challenge (180, 181) and if precursor memory T cells are exhausted under chronic antigen exposure, it will lead to memory T-cell deletion and lack of formation (173, 177).

Acquired resistance can be mediated by the alteration from cytotoxic activity to inactivity phenotype of antitumor T cells during TCR-engineered ACT. The original highly cytolytic profile when administrated to patients, which showed strong efficacy initially, was reported to change to a phenotype with impaired cytotoxic functions and Th2-related cytokine release when tumor relapses within months (182, 183).

Suppressive Tumor Microenvironment

Increased immunosuppressive cells

The TME is a complex net consisting of a variety of immune and stromal cells, cytokines, extracellular matrix, and vasculature, which affect response to immunotherapy. Immune-suppressive cells, including Tregs, MDSCs, M2 macrophages, along with inhibitory cytokines in the TME, can contribute to the inhibition to immune responses (136, 184) (**Figure 1C**).

Tregs can inhibit Teff reactions by secreting certain inhibitory cytokines (IL-10, IL-35, and TGF-β) or by direct cell contact (185–187). The cytokine IL-10 influences antigen presentation by down-regulating the expression of MHC-II and co-stimulatory components on DCs, thus intercepting the Teff activation (187). The ratio of Teffs to Tregs was shown to be related to the responses to ICIs in mouse models, in that incapacity of either increasing Teffs or decreasing Tregs may cause resistance to immunotherapy (188, 189). Factors that affect Tregs activity, at the same time, are putative biomarkers of resistance. For instance, soluble CD25, an IL-2 receptor whose binding is assumed to stimulate Treg proliferation, was established as a negative predictor of OS for patients treated with anti-CTLA−4 (190). However, tumor-infiltrating Tregs might likely coexist with multiple immune cells, insinuating a potential immunoreactivity. It was reported that a high baseline expression of FoxP3+ Tregs in the tumor is positively associated with better survival in a retrospective study involving patients under the treatment of anti-CTLA-4 antibodies (161).

Myeloid-derived suppressor cells promote immune evasion and tumor growth and have emerged as critical modulators of immune responses in cancer. Studies have suggested the existence of MDSCs in TME correlates with reduced efficacy of immunotherapies, including ICIs therapy (191), ACT (192), and DC vaccination (193). Therefore, reprogramming or eradicating MDSCs might improve clinical response to immunotherapy.

Tumor-associated macrophages (TAMs) can be classified into M1 and M2 macrophages according to disparities in surface molecules, expression of transcription factors, cytokine profiles, and metabolism (194, 195). They promote antitumor immunity effects (mediated by M1) and pro-tumorigenic properties (mediated by M2) that modify the TME (196). The role of TAMs in mediating immunotherapeutic resistance in tumor has been discussed in several reports (197, 198). It was indicated to directly inhibit T-cell responses through PD-L1 in preclinical studies of liver (199) and ovarian cancer (200). The inhibitor of CSF-1R, a receptor for macrophage colony-stimulating growth factor, was investigated in mouse models of pancreatic cancer where it decreased the frequencies of TAMs, while increasing IFN production and delaying tumor progression (201, 202). Similarly, CSF-1R inhibitor was found to synergize ACT therapy in a melanoma model (203). These data suggest that CSF-1R inhibitor may overcome the resistance to immunotherapy.

Specific chemokines, such as CCL5, CCL7, and CXCL8, play an important role in the recruitment of Tregs and MDSCs to the TME, consequently boosting an immunosuppressive climate (204). Alternately, chemokines CXCL9 and CXCL10 recruit CTLs to the TME (205) and the epigenetic silencing of the genes encoding them can reduce TILs and consequently promote resistance to ICIs (205). Epigenetic modulators of these chemokine receptors relieved the suppression of these Th1-cell-type chemokines and increased TILs leading to improved therapeutic efficacy of PD-L1 inhibitor in a model for ovarian cancer (155).

Elevated immunosuppressive cytokines

The cytokine milieu is critical to the recruitment, activation, and proliferation of immune cell, performing both immune stimulatory and suppressive effects (206). Transforming growth factor-β (TGF-β) is a cytokine playing key roles in angiogenesis and immunosuppression by stimulating Tregs (207) and excluding T cell in peritumoral fibroblasts (123, 159). Up-regulated TGF-β signaling was correlated with poorly immunogenic tumors and restrained response to ICIs in a colorectal cancer model, indicating resistance to therapy (159). Consequently, enhanced antitumor response to ICIs was observed following application of TGF-β inhibitor either alone or in combination with anti-CTLA-4 or radiation therapy (208, 209). Bintrafusp alfa, a bifunctional fusion protein composed of the extracellular domain of TGF-β receptor II (a TGF-β "trap") fused to a human immunoglobulin G1 antibody blocking PD-L1, demonstrated favorable efficacy in patients with advanced NSCLC. Ongoing phase III trial is expected to validate the efficacy of bintrafusp alfa vs. pembrolizumab in the first-line setting in advanced NSCLC (NCT03631706).

Tumor necrosis factor-α pathway is postulated to be another immune evasion machinery conferring resistance to PD1 blockade. The expression of TNFα in an inflamed TME positively correlates with the expression of PD-L1 and TIM-3, along with impaired accumulation and increased activation-induced death of CD8+ TILs in melanoma models treated with anti-PD1 therapy. Accordingly, inhibition of TNF-α prevents the expression of PD-L1 and TIM3 and hampers anti-PD1-induced TIL death (210). Therefore, this study offers a rationale for the combination of PD-1/PD-L1 inhibitors with TNFα blockade as a novel immunotherapeutic strategy to overcome resistance in lung cancer, and the phase I clinical trial testing the combination is ongoing (NCT03293784).

Vascular endothelial growth factor has been linked to both decreased T−cell infiltration and immunosuppressive effects in addition to promoting angiogenesis and thus is associated with resistance to ICIs (211). Multiple mechanisms are involved in the interaction of VEGF with antitumor immunity: (1) VEGF prevented the commitment of lymphoid progenitors, decreasing progression to the T-cell lineage (212); (2) VEGF signaling promotes the infiltration of Tregs through a selective endothelium and reduces trafficking and extravasation of CTLs into the TME (213); and (3) VEGF increases expression of inhibitory receptors, contributing to CTL exhaustion (214). Higher levels of VEGF were found in anti-PD-1-resistant patients than sensitive ones (160). Based on these findings and the synergy between angiogenesis blockade and ICI therapies observed in preliminary studies, multiple trials of combination therapy are underway, including bevacizumab and VEGFR-TKI with anti-PD-1 therapy.

Higher levels of interleukin 6 (IL-6) and interleukin 8 (IL-8) have been found recently to be linked to reduced responses and worse clinical outcomes to ICI therapies across multiple types of cancers (215–217). IL-6 is a proinflammatory cytokine generated by T cells and macrophages and is usually involved in the immunoregulation connected to the IFN-γ signaling pathway. It can reduce the expression of PD-L1 and MHC-I, and result in tumor escape and resistance to ICI therapy (218). IL-8 is a proinflammatory chemokine and a chemoattractant for myeloid leukocytes expressed in multiple cancers (219, 220). It potently regulates the chemotaxis of neutrophils (221, 222) and exerts direct pro-tumorigenic effects (223). High levels of IL-8 are regarded to be associated with more neutrophil and monocyte infiltration, defective T-cell functions, and impaired antigen presentation, which subsequently result in resistance to ICI therapy (216, 217).

Additional immunoregulative molecules

Contributions from inflammatory processes could participate in quashing the desired impacts of ICIs (**Figure 1C**). Adenosine can be produced under the condition of hypoxia and ischemia caused by tumor inflammation. It was reported to inhibit the cytotoxic function and proliferation of T cells via the A2A receptor on T cells (224). CD73, which mediates the generation of adenosine through dephosphorylation of adenosine monophosphate, was also demonstrated to suppress immune function (225). CD73 overexpression promotes T-cell exhaustion and is linked to the resistance to ICIs (226, 227).

IDO1 expressed in myeloid cells and cancer cells is a rate-limiting enzyme that converts tryptophan to its immunosuppressive metabolite kynurenine. This enzyme can induce T-cell anergy and apoptosis by gathering kynurenines and consuming the essential amino acid tryptophan and prevent the T-cell clonal expansion (228). It is particularly activated in DCs after binding with CTLA−4 and can be unregulated by CTLA−4 during adaptive immune resistance (229). Reduced expression of IDO at baseline was noted to be associated with poor response to ipilimumab in a phase II study in melanoma (161). Low level of IDO is likely to manifest insufficiency of suppressed TILs feasible to be reactivated by immunotherapy. Correspondingly, IDO-knockout mice exhibited improved OS with ICI compared with wild-type mice, and ICI therapy combined with IDO inhibitors showed both increased numbers and functions of TILs in the TME in an experimental setting (230, 231). However, despite encouraging results observed in preclinical and early-phase clinical studies in different types of tumors, no difference was shown in pembrolizumab combined with IDO1-selective inhibitor vs with placebo in a phase III study in metastatic melanoma (232).

B7-H4 has been proposed as another resistance marker to ICIs recently due to its negative modulation of T cells. B7-H4 constitutes a type I transmembrane protein of the B7 immunoglobulin superfamily and is encoded by the V-set domain containing T-cell activation inhibitor 1 (VTCN 1) gene. It is induced by activated T lymphocytes and down-regulates T-cell function by inhibiting proliferation, cytotoxicity activity, and interleukin secretion, after binding with T cells (233–235). Positive B7-H4 protein expression in patients with advanced NSCLC treated with nivolumab was recently reported to have an enhanced risk of tumor progression and tumor-related death compared with negative expression (236).

Host-Related Characteristics

Host-related characteristics, including gut microbiome, diet, and antibiotic exposure that adversely affect the gut microbiome, diet, steroid use, vaccine exposure, inflammation state, and autoimmunity, have been shown to relate to primary and acquired resistance to ICI therapy in lung cancer (237, 238) (**Figure 1B**).

Gut Microbiome

Evidence is arising to support the vigorous impact of the gut microbiome on immunotherapy resistance. Multiple studies have demonstrated that less bacterial diversity and lack of enrichment of specific species showed a significant correlation with resistance to ICI therapies. Relative abundance of *Bacteroidales* was found in non-responders, while responders were more likely to have *Faecalibacterium* and *Ruminococcaceae* (239, 240). Furthermore, transplanting the responder's feces into aseptic mice exhibited improvement in the treatment of PD-L1 inhibitor (241). Certain species can be altered by the antibiotic's exposure, which partly explained modified response to ICI therapy either in a good or in a bad way (242–244).

The alteration tendency of gut microbiome structure or dominant bacteria may differentially affect the T-cell immune response. It may be due to the cross-reactivity between intestinal microbiota and tumor-associated antigens, enhancing the inflammatory cytokine production, activation of DCs, and antigen presentation (245, 246). IFN-γ-producing CD8+ T cells were successfully induced from a consortium of 11 bacteria in the intestine, and colonization with this 11-bacterial mixture resulted in enhanced efficacy of ICIs in mouse models (247). Consistently, "good" bacteria introduction was reported to significantly increase IFN-γ production in spleen and tumor-draining lymph nodes (TDLN) (246) and induce DCs to secrete IL-12, resulting in increased recruitment of CCR9+CXCR3+CD4+ T cells into tumor beds (244). The activation of DCs was reported to be modulated by the gut microbiome in animal models and cancer patients. The resistance to anti-CTLA-4 therapy can be reversed by oral administration of *Bacteroides fragilis*, which induced Th1 immune response in TDLN and promoted DCs maturation (243). *Bifidobacterium*-feeding mouse presented higher expression of MHC-II in DCs within tumors (248). It remains controversial whether intestinal microbes lead to immunotherapy resistance by affecting the production of Tregs. A higher level of peripheral Tregs was found in patients with "bad" bacteria and was associated with poor response to ipilimumab in metastatic melanoma patients (249). *B. fragilis* can produce a microbial molecule, polysaccharide A, which can promote the formation of the inducible population of CD4+Foxp3+Tregs (a subset of Tregs), thereby negatively regulating the immune system (250), whereas the other two studies reported no differences in Treg differentiation between pancreatic duct adenosarcoma-bearing mice and control, and the number of Foxp3+ T cells between *Bifidobacterium*- and PBS-feeding mice (251, 252). The majority of chemokine genes were reported to be up-regulated by specific species of gut microbiome including *Fusobacterium nucleatum*, *B. fragilis*, and *Escherichia coli* in colorectal cancer cells. Additionally, the gut microbiota-derived microbial load was associated with increased chemokine production (251).

The gut microbiome also acts as an instructive modulator of mutant TP53, which ultimately affects tumor proliferation and the immune system. Kadoshi et al. recently found that mutant TP53 presented contrasting effects in different segments of the gut in a mouse model: a remarkable tumor-suppressive effect in proximal gut and the expected oncogenic effect in distal gut (253). The gut microbiome and its single metabolite gallic acid turned mutant TP53 from a tumor-suppressive effect to an oncogenic one, suggesting that the function of mutant TP53 is plastic and under the control of microbiome and microbiota-derived metabolites.

Concomitant Medications

Antibiotics exposure has been reported to be associated with inferior clinical outcomes during ICIs therapy in NSCLC (244, 254). However, it remains debated if antibiotics exposure represents an independent predictive biomarker of ICIs therapy or it is a surrogate for patients with worse prognosis (e.g., poorer performance status, higher comorbidities). The use of antibiotics has an unfavorable impact on the recolonization and subsequent alterations in microbiota composition, which eventually leads to a decline in microbial symbiotic diversity (255). The antibiotics-induced dysbiosis destroys the gut homeostasis and extends from childhood to adulthood, with long-lasting adverse effects on the immune system as well as body metabolism (256–258). The antitumor immune response-induced cyclophosphamide was impaired by antibiotics exposure in the fibrosarcoma model, which was associated with an improvement in the Teff-to-Treg ratio and the loss of *Enterococcus hirae*-elicited helper T cell in tumor immune infiltrate (259, 260). Correspondingly, the absolute numbers of neutrophils and monocytes decreased after oral administration of imipenem, vancomycin, and neomycin before tumor inoculation in lymphoma and colon models treated with oxaliplatin or IL-10 inhibitor (261). On the contrary, the growth of *Fusobacterium* spp.-containing tumor was slowed down after the administration of metronidazole in the mouse model of colon cancer, suggesting such bacteria promote tumor progression (262).

Long-term use of steroids adversely impacts the efficacy of ICIs because of their supposed anti-inflammatory and immunosuppressive effects that potentially hamper the mode of ICI action (263), whereas a transient use of steroids aimed at management of ir-AEs did not negatively affect patients' survival outcomes (264, 265). Beyond affecting gut microbiome, steroids are known to prevent the activation of T lymphocytes, inhibit the amplification of T helper subsets, recruit Tregs, and promote M2 macrophage polarization (266, 267). Hence, early use of steroids on ICI treatment may prevent this phase of T-cell recruitment and thus impair effective antitumor immune response. The increment of neutrophil-to-lymphocyte ratio (NLR), derived NLR (dNLR), and absolute neutrophil count (ANC) after steroids has been shown to be associated with unfavorable clinical outcome in NSCLC patients treated with ICIs (268). Steroids-induced imbalance of immune cells in TME, especially increased MDSCs resulting in elevated ANC and NLR, is the intermediate of immunotherapy resistance in NSCLC (269).

Diet

Diet can affect tumor growth within TME through systemic or local effects in multiple ways. First, it may alter the composition and diversity of gut microbiome, which in turn exerts drastically different effects on host immune function. Second, specific ingredients (e.g., vitamins) may be regulated by dietary patterns and then have an impact on immune status. It is well-known that the general metabolic status determining deviations from ideal body weight, as well as the metabolic factors (e.g., low-level arginine and tryptophan, high-level lactate, and the adenosine pathway induced by increased glucose metabolism), highly influences the immune activity (270–272). An appropriate diet can maintain the homeostatic equilibrium between the inflammatory cascade triggered by Th17 cells and the anti-inflammatory pathway mainly based on the activity of Treg (273).

Additional Factors

Chronic accumulation and production of inflammatory molecules in the chronic inflammatory status lead to an immunosuppressant state, which is linked to immunotherapy resistance. Proinflammatory and carcinogenic mediators such as IL-6, TNF-α, and chemokines are released in the TME and tend to trigger a variety of molecular signaling cascades including PI3K/MAPK, JAK/STAT, and WNT/B-catenin, which are involved in the resistance to immunotherapy as mentioned previously. The components of immune cells are also altered to be more immunosuppressive with more TAMs, Tregs, and tumor-associated neutrophils within TME (274). Therefore, blocking inflammation might be an effective strategy to improve the outcome of immunotherapy in NSCLC (275).

Tumor development and autoimmunity are two opposite results of imbalanced immune homeostasis in controlling tumor cell growth (low immune responses) and regulating autoreactive responses (immune overreaction). The host autoimmunity affects the efficacy of immunotherapy in bringing more ir-AEs when too strong or incapacity to prime and activate immune cells when too weak (276). In addition, autoimmunity has an inextricable link with host gut microbiome and anti-microbial immunity, as effector responses that lead to inflammatory tissue damage are the same as those that mediate effective host defense (277).

The relationship between smoking and the efficacy of ICIs remains controversial (278–281). Smoking is associated with high TMB, especially nonsynonymous mutations, subsequently enhances the immunogenicity of tumor, and improves the outcome of ICIs therapy (23, 282). Additionally, PD-L1 expression can be up-regulated by smoking through oxidative stress-dependent mechanism (283) and induced by cigarette smoke and the carcinogen benzopyrene (BaP) via aryl hydrocarbon receptor (AhR) (284). Moreover, smoking may also have an impact on the status of TILs (285) and other immune modulators such as B7-H3 (CD276) (286) and in turn affect the efficacy of ICIs therapy.

THERAPEUTIC APPROACHES TO CONQUER IMMUNOTHERAPY RESISTANCE

Research and design of therapies to conquer immunotherapy resistance has been advancing along with mechanistic investigations. Combinatory treatments, either via combinations of diverse immunotherapeutic agents or through combinations with traditional treatments, developed to revitalize the defense system with complementing/synergetic mechanisms, have been introduced to serve as alternative approaches for NSCLC therapy. Diverse targets discussed herein have the potential to serve as both biomarkers of resistance and combination therapy targets. In view of the different resistance mechanisms, the combinatory therapy strategies are mainly manifested in the following aspects (the examples of ongoing studies trying to reverse resistance are summarized in **Supplementary Table 1**):

Enhance Tumor Immunogenicity

1. Emerging evidence has indicated the positive immunologic effects of chemotherapy (287). On one hand, it regulates the composition and function of immune cells such as CTLs (288), MDSCs, and Tregs (289) in the TME and the molecules expressed on tumor cells; on the other hand, it restores the recognition of immune system to tumor through enhancing tumor antigen presentation via up-regulating the expression of MHC-I and through boosting antitumor immune responses via chemo-induced tumor cell apoptosis (290–292). Multiple randomized phase III clinical trials have compared the combination of chemotherapy and ICIs with chemotherapy alone in treatment-naïve advanced lung cancer (4, 9, 293). The results consistently showed that the combination strategies are superior to chemotherapy alone in the first-line setting, regardless of PD-L1 expression, suggesting that the synergistic activity between chemotherapy and ICIs may offset the insensitivity due to low PD-L1 expression.
2. Similar to the effects induced by chemotherapy, radiation therapy combined with ICIs leads to long-lasting tumor regression through escalating antigen exposure secondary to cancer cell apoptosis, enhancing an inflamed TME (294), raising DCs activation and up-regulating proinflammatory cytokines, causing elevated TILs (295), and facilitating cancer relapsing by non-redundant immune mechanisms (296, 297). Consolidative PD-L1 inhibition after concurrent chemo-radiation significantly improved survival in unresectable stage III NSCLC in the PACIFIC study, and this approach has become the standard care of locally advanced NSCLC (298). Clinical trials evaluating the concurrent administration of radiation therapy with ICIs are ongoing.
3. Vaccines using cancer-specific peptides or DCs (237, 299, 300) and oncolytic virus therapy (301, 302) escalate the antigen presentation and priming of T cells.

Target Oncogenic Genes

1. Blocking the MAPK/PTEN/PI3K axis such as BRAF, MEK, and PI3K inhibitors contributes to Teff expansion, avoiding T-cell exhaustion and apoptosis, activating an immune-stimulatory transcriptional program, and promoting the production of proinflammatory cytokines and T-cell cytotoxicity (303, 304). BRAF and MEK inhibitors in combination with PD-1 blockade therapy showed a 73% overall response rate (ORR) and 93% stable disease in BRAF V600-mutated metastatic melanoma (305). However, cobimetinib, a MEK1/2 inhibitor, combined with atezolizumab was evaluated in a phase Ib umbrella platform MORPHEUS. The combination did not show better efficacy compared with the control arm in the NSCLC cohort of this study (306).
2. PARP inhibitors, as synergistic activating CD8+T-cell-mediated antitumor response despite up-regulating PD-L1 expression, which can be complementally inhibited by anti-PD-L1 therapy (307).
3. The combinations of nivolumab with veliparib and pembrolizumab with olaparib were tested in advanced solid tumors (308, 309). No response was observed and PFS and OS were 9.0 and 26.8 weeks, respectively, in the former trial while no results are available in the latter one.

Promote T-Cell Priming and Enhance TILs

(1) Agonists of TLRs, as contributing to the DC mutations and T-cell priming; (2) STING, as activating inflammatory reactions via IFN-α cascade upon recognition of foreign DNA; (3) dual block CTLA-4 and PD-1, as CTLA-4 inhibitor enhances the T-cell priming, Treg exhaustion, and CTL-mediated immune responses via more antigen recognition (310), while PD-1 inhibitor participates in later reactivation of Teff response; (4) adoptive T-cell transfer either alone or in combination with ICIs therapy, as increasing TILs and T-cell cytotoxicity (311, 312); and (5) bispecific monoclonal antibodies, as redirecting cytotoxic effector cells to the TME, depleting suppressive cells, and activating effector cells by targeting a cancer-specific antigen and either CD3 on CTLs or CD16A on NK cells; or targeting cancer-specific antigen and immune regulators, or targeting dual immunomodulators (313).

Reshape Immunosuppressive TME

(1) Colony-stimulating factor 1 receptor (CSF1R) blockades, as reducing tumor invasion via the MDSCs and M2 macrophages; (2) inhibition of CD73, A2A receptor, as improving TME by targeting suppressive factors; (3) dual blockade of the TGF-β and checkpoint inhibitory receptors, as facilitating tumor penetration with T cells and reversing the immune suppressive TME (208); (4) anti-CXCR2/CXCR4 antibodies, as voiding immune evasion (314); (5) VEGF inhibitors, as normalizing the immune suppressive TME and reversing ICIs resistance (315); and (6) IL-1β inhibitor canakinumab, as targeting tumor inflammatory response and reducing immunosuppression. To date, there are four clinical trials of canakinumab in various settings in the treatment of NSCLC under way, and preliminary results from two of them were released in AACR this year. Pembrolizumab plus chemotherapy combined with canakinumab was safe and well tolerated in the first-line treatment in locally advanced or advanced NSCLC, and the recommended phase III dose of canakinumab was 200 mg s.c. Q3W (316). The efficacy of canakinumab or pembrolizumab monotherapy or in combination as neoadjuvant treatment in resectable NSCLC was assessed in the CANOPY-N study and the results are not reported (317).

Target Alternate Immune Checkpoints and Immune-Stimulatory Receptors

(1) Blockade of alternate coinhibitory immune checkpoint receptors, such as LAG-3, TIM-3, TIGIT, BTLA, VISTA, and SIGLEC9; (2) costimulatory agonists, including 4-1BB, OX40, CD40, GITR, and ICOS, as enhancing T-cell expansion

and effector functions while controlling Treg cell-suppressive functions (318, 319).

Although not being widely used in clinical practice, the antibodies targeting these immune checkpoints have exhibited promising antitumor activity in early clinical trials in various malignancies. LAG-3 blockades, Relatlimab [humanized anti-LAG-3 monoclonal antibody (mAb)], and Eftilagimod alpha (a soluble LAG-3 protein) combined with PD-1 inhibitors achieved an ORR of 15% in previously treated melanoma (320) and 52.9% in treatment-naïve advanced NSCLC (321), respectively. Based on the positive preclinical results, TIGIT blockade, especially in combination with anti-PD-1/PD-L1 mAb, has been explored in various clinical settings of advanced tumors. MK-7684 (an anti-TIGIT mAb) alone or combined with pembrolizumab showed a disease control rate of 35% and 47%, respectively, in a phase I study (322). Etigilimab (a humanized anti-TIGIT mAb) also presented early signs of efficacy as a monotherapy, with a 0% ORR but 22% stabilized disease in advanced malignancies (322). Tiragolumab is a fully human IgG1/kappa TIGIT monoclonal antibody with an intact Fc region that blocks TIGIT from binding to its PVR ligand and to the co-activating receptor CD226. It improved ORR either alone or combined with atezolizumab compared to historical data in a phase I study (323). The clinically meaningful improvement in ORR and PFS was confirmed recently in the CITYSCAPE study (a phase II study of tiragolumab plus atezolizumab vs placebo plus atezolizumab as first-line treatment in patients with PD-L1-selected NSCLC) (324). Cobolimab is a novel IgG4 anti-TIM-3 mAb and showed clinical benefit with an ORR of 15% and 40% stable disease in combination with anti-PD-1 mAb in a phase I clinical trial (325). Other anti-TIM-3 mAbs including MBG453, Sym023, INCAGN2390, LY3321367, BMS-986258, and SHR1702, as well as a bispecific antibody targeting PD-1 and TIM-3 (RO7121661), have also being evaluated in phase I trials with no clinical results available.

Apart from blocking coinhibitory immune checkpoint receptors mentioned above, several costimulatory agonists are also attractive targets, a few of which have stepped into clinical studies. ATOR-1015, a CTLA-4 × OX40 bispecific antibody, was tested in a phase I study for safety and tolerability in advanced solid tumors (326). GSK998, a humanized IgG1 agonistic OX40 mAb, combined with or without pembrolizumab was also evaluated in a phase I trial of advanced solid tumors including NSCLC (327). A lipid nanoparticle encapsulated mRNA encoding human OX40L, mRNA-2416, showed good tolerability when intratumorally injected as monotherapy in advanced malignancies in a phase I/II trial, and the combination with durvalumab is ongoing (328).

Epigenetic Modulation

(1) DNA methyltransferase inhibitors, e.g., sensitizing tumors to PD-L1 blockade and elevating the secretion of the immunostimulatory chemokines CXCL10 and CXCL9 (155); (2) histone deacetylase inhibitors, as down-regulating MDSCs, increasing the expression of MHC-I and antigen presentation, and increasing tumor-infiltrating $CD8^+$ T cells (95); and (3) histone methyltransferase Ezh2 inhibitor, as reversing the effects of loss of immunogenicity and antigen presentation (94).

Gut Microbiota Modulation

Modifying the composition of gut microbiome might eliminate resistance to ICIs. Dietary modification, probiotics, and fecal microbiota transplantation have been emerging as an adjunct treatment to ICIs.

Of note, combination strategies that have been successful in preclinical models do not necessarily pass safety and performance assessments in clinical trials. In addition to considering the complementarity of immunotherapy resistance mechanisms, the timing and sequence are also important when formulating combination treatment strategies. Therefore, the preclinical model, translational study, and pharmacokinetic study of each of these agents in combination and in isolation are indispensable for the clinical success of combination strategies. Furthermore, multimodal approaches, for example, local therapy for oligo-progression after response to ICIs, should be implemented on therapeutic combinations for better clinical benefits.

CONCLUSION

It remains challenging to clarify the resistance mechanisms of immunotherapy since they are complex and dynamic, and certain mechanisms alternately overlap. Further understanding of the primary and acquired resistance mechanisms of immunotherapy will help clinicians to make reasonable combination treatment decisions to bring superior survival and avoid additional toxicity for patients with lung cancer.

AUTHOR CONTRIBUTIONS

FW conceptualized and drafted the review. QZ and SW contributed to the significant portions of the manuscript. All authors listed approved it for publication.

FUNDING

The study was supported by the National Key R&D Program of China (Grant No. 2016YFC1303800 to QZ), the High-level Hospital Construction Project (Grant No. DFJH201810 to QZ), the Key Lab System Project of Guangdong Science and Technology Department—Guangdong Provincial Key Lab of Translational Medicine in Lung Cancer (Grant No. 2017B030314120 to Yi-Long Wu), and the Research Foundation of Peking University Shenzhen Hospital (Grant No. JCYJ2018010).

REFERENCES

1. Antonia SJ, Borghaei H, Ramalingam SS, Horn L, De Castro Carpeno J, Pluzanski A, et al. Four-year survival with nivolumab in patients with previously treated advanced non-small-cell lung cancer: a pooled analysis. *Lancet Oncol.* (2019) 20:1395–408. doi: 10.1016/S1470-2045(19)30407-3
2. Garon EB, Hellmann MD, Rizvi NA, Carcereny E, Leighl NB, Ahn MJ, et al. Five-year overall survival for patients with advanced nonsmall-cell lung cancer treated with pembrolizumab: results from the phase I KEYNOTE-001 study. *J Clin Oncol.* (2019) 37:2518–27. doi: 10.1200/JCO.19.00934
3. Topalian SL, Hodi FS, Brahmer JR, Gettinger SN, Smith DC, McDermott DF, et al. Five-year survival and correlates among patients with advanced melanoma, renal cell carcinoma, or non-small cell lung cancer treated with nivolumab. *JAMA Oncol.* (2019). 5:1411–20. doi: 10.1001/jamaoncol.2019.2187
4. West H, McCleod M, Hussein M, Morabito A, Rittmeyer A, Conter HJ, et al. Atezolizumab in combination with carboplatin plus nab-paclitaxel chemotherapy compared with chemotherapy alone as first-line treatment for metastatic non-squamous non-small-cell lung cancer (IMpower130): a multicentre, randomised, open-label, phase 3 trial. *Lancet Oncol.* (2019) 20:924–37. doi: 10.1016/S1470-2045(19)30167-6
5. Socinski MA, Jotte RM, Cappuzzo F, Orlandi F, Stroyakovskiy D, Nogami N, et al. Atezolizumab for first-line treatment of metastatic nonsquamous NSCLC. *N Engl J Med.* (2018) 378:2288–301. doi: 10.1056/NEJMoa1716948
6. Reck M, Rodriguez-Abreu D, Robinson AG, Hui R, Csoszi T, Fulop A, et al. Updated analysis of KEYNOTE-024: pembrolizumab versus platinum-based chemotherapy for advanced non-small-cell lung cancer with PD-L1 tumor proportion score of 50% or greater. *J Clin Oncol.* (2019) 37:537–46. doi: 10.1200/JCO.18.00149
7. Paz-Ares L, Luft A, Vicente D, Tafreshi A, Gumus M, Mazieres J, et al. Pembrolizumab plus chemotherapy for squamous non-small-cell lung cancer. *N Engl J Med.* (2018) 379:2040–51. doi: 10.1056/NEJMoa1810865
8. Mok TSK, Wu YL, Kudaba I, Kowalski DM, Cho BC, Turna HZ, et al. Pembrolizumab versus chemotherapy for previously untreated, PD-L1-expressing, locally advanced or metastatic non-small-cell lung cancer (KEYNOTE-042): a randomised, open-label, controlled, phase 3 trial. *Lancet.* (2019) 393:1819–30.
9. Gandhi L, Rodriguez-Abreu D, Gadgeel S, Esteban E, Felip E, De Angelis F, et al. Pembrolizumab plus chemotherapy in metastatic non-small-cell lung cancer. *N Engl J Med.* (2018) 378:2078–92. doi: 10.1056/NEJMoa1801005
10. Sharma P, Hu-Lieskovan S, Wargo JA, Ribas A. Primary, adaptive, and acquired resistance to cancer immunotherapy. *Cell.* (2017) 168:707–23. doi: 10.1016/j.cell.2017.01.017
11. Remon J, Passiglia F, Ahn MJ, Barlesi F, Forde PM, Garon EB, et al. Immune checkpoint inhibitors in thoracic malignancies: review of the existing evidence by an IASLC expert panel and recommendations. *J Thorac Oncol.* (2020) 15:914–47. doi: 10.1016/j.jtho.2020.03.006
12. Fares CM, Van Allen EM, Drake CG, Allison JP, Hu-Lieskovan S. Mechanisms of resistance to immune checkpoint blockade: why does checkpoint inhibitor immunotherapy not work for all patients? *Am Soc Clin Oncol Educ Book.* (2019) 39:147–64. doi: 10.1200/EDBK_240837
13. Chae YK, Oh MS, Giles FJ. Molecular biomarkers of primary and acquired resistance to T-cell-mediated immunotherapy in cancer: landscape, clinical implications, and future directions. *Oncologist.* (2018) 23:410–21. doi: 10.1634/theoncologist.2017-0354
14. Chen DS, Mellman I. Elements of cancer immunity and the cancer-immune set point. *Nature.* (2017) 541:321–30. doi: 10.1038/nature21349
15. Schumacher TN, Schreiber RD. Neoantigens in cancer immunotherapy. *Science.* (2015) 348:69–74. doi: 10.1126/science.aaa4971
16. Linnemann C, van Buuren MM, Bies L, Verdegaal EM, Schotte R, Calis JJ, et al. High-throughput epitope discovery reveals frequent recognition of neo-antigens by CD4+ T cells in human melanoma. *Nat Med.* (2015) 21:81–5. doi: 10.1038/nm.3773
17. Matsushita H, Vesely MD, Koboldt DC, Rickert CG, Uppaluri R, Magrini VJ, et al. Cancer exome analysis reveals a T-cell-dependent mechanism of cancer immunoediting. *Nature.* (2012) 482:400–4. doi: 10.1038/nature10755
18. Matsutake T, Srivastava PK. The immunoprotective MHC II epitope of a chemically induced tumor harbors a unique mutation in a ribosomal protein. *Proc Natl Acad Sci USA.* (2001) 98:3992–7. doi: 10.1073/pnas.071523398
19. Snyder A, Makarov V, Merghoub T, Yuan J, Zaretsky JM, Desrichard A, et al. Genetic basis for clinical response to CTLA-4 blockade in melanoma. *N Engl J Med.* (2014) 371:2189–99. doi: 10.1056/NEJMoa1406498
20. Tran E, Turcotte S, Gros A, Robbins PF, Lu YC, Dudley ME, et al. Cancer immunotherapy based on mutation-specific CD4+ T cells in a patient with epithelial cancer. *Science.* (2014) 344:641–5. doi: 10.1126/science.1251102
21. Alexandrov LB, Nik-Zainal S, Wedge DC, Aparicio SA, Behjati S, Biankin AV, et al. Signatures of mutational processes in human cancer. *Nature.* (2013) 500:415–21.
22. Sjoblom T, Jones S, Wood LD, Parsons DW, Lin J, Barber TD, et al. The consensus coding sequences of human breast and colorectal cancers. *Science.* (2006) 314:268–74.
23. Rizvi NA, Hellmann MD, Snyder A, Kvistborg P, Makarov V, Havel JJ, et al. Cancer immunology. mutational landscape determines sensitivity to PD-1 blockade in non-small cell lung cancer. *Science.* (2015) 348:124–8. doi: 10.1126/science.aaa1348
24. Greillier L, Tomasini P, Barlesi F. The clinical utility of tumor mutational burden in non-small cell lung cancer. *Transl Lung Cancer Res.* (2018) 7:639–46. doi: 10.21037/tlcr.2018.10.08
25. McGranahan N, Furness AJ, Rosenthal R, Ramskov S, Lyngaa R, Saini SK, et al. Clonal neoantigens elicit T cell immunoreactivity and sensitivity to immune checkpoint blockade. *Science.* (2016) 351:1463–9.
26. Riaz N, Morris L, Havel JJ, Makarov V, Desrichard A, Chan TA. The role of neoantigens in response to immune checkpoint blockade. *Int Immunol.* (2016) 28:411–9. doi: 10.1093/intimm/dxw019
27. Carbone DP, Reck M, Paz-Ares L, Creelan B, Horn L, Steins M, et al. First-line nivolumab in stage IV or recurrent non-small-cell lung cancer. *N Engl J Med.* (2017) 376:2415–26. doi: 10.1056/NEJMoa1613493
28. Melendez B, Van Campenhout C, Rorive S, Remmelink M, Salmon I, D'Haene N. Methods of measurement for tumor mutational burden in tumor tissue. *Transl Lung Cancer Res.* (2018) 7:661–7. doi: 10.21037/tlcr.2018.08.02
29. Owada-Ozaki Y, Muto S, Takagi H, Inoue T, Watanabe Y, Fukuhara M, et al. Prognostic impact of tumor mutation burden in patients with completely resected non-small cell lung cancer: brief report. *J Thorac Oncol.* (2018) 13:1217–21. doi: 10.1016/j.jtho.2018.04.003
30. Rizvi H, Sanchez-Vega F, La K, Chatila W, Jonsson P, Halpenny D, et al. Molecular determinants of response to anti-programmed cell death (PD)-1 and Anti-programmed death-ligand 1 (PD-L1) blockade in patients with non-small-cell lung cancer profiled with targeted next-generation sequencing. *J Clin Oncol.* (2018) 36:633–41. doi: 10.1200/JCO.2017.75.3384
31. Hellmann MD, Ciuleanu TE, Pluzanski A, Lee JS, Otterson GA, Audigier-Valette C, et al. Nivolumab plus ipilimumab in lung cancer with a high tumor mutational burden. *N Engl J Med.* (2018) 378:2093–104. doi: 10.1056/NEJMoa1801946
32. Hellmann MD, Paz-Ares L, Bernabe Caro R, Zurawski B, Kim SW, Carcereny Costa E, et al. Nivolumab plus ipilimumab in advanced non-small-cell lung cancer. *N Engl J Med.* (2019) 381:2020–31. doi: 10.1056/NEJMoa1910231
33. Anagnostou V, Niknafs N, Marrone KA, Bruhm DC, White JR. Multimodal genomic features predict outcome of immune checkpoint blockade in non-small-cell lung cancer. *Nat Cancer.* (2020) 1:99–111. doi: 10.1038/s43018-019-0008-8
34. Russo A, De Miguel Perez D, Gunasekaran M, Scilla K, Lapidus R, Cooper B, et al. Liquid biopsy tracking of lung tumor evolutions over time. *Expert Rev Mol Diagn.* (2019) 19:1099–108. doi: 10.1080/14737159.2020.1680287
35. Gandara DR, Paul SM, Kowanetz M, Schleifman E, Zou W, Li Y, et al. Blood-based tumor mutational burden as a predictor of clinical benefit in non-small-cell lung cancer patients treated with atezolizumab. *Nat Med.* (2018) 24:1441–8. doi: 10.1038/s41591-018-0134-3
36. Georgiadis A, Durham JN, Keefer LA, Bartlett BR, Zielonka M, Murphy D, et al. Noninvasive detection of microsatellite instability and high tumor mutation burden in cancer patients treated with PD-1 blockade. *Clin Cancer Res.* (2019) 25:7024–34. doi: 10.1158/1078-0432.CCR-19-1372
37. Wang Z, Duan J, Cai S, Han M, Dong H, Zhao J, et al. Assessment of blood tumor mutational burden as a potential biomarker for immunotherapy in patients with non-small cell lung cancer with use of a next-generation

sequencing cancer gene panel. *JAMA Oncol.* (2019) 5:696–702. doi: 10.1001/jamaoncol.2018.7098
38. Riaz N, Havel JJ, Makarov V, Desrichard A, Urba WJ, Sims JS, et al. Tumor and microenvironment evolution during immunotherapy with nivolumab. *Cell.* (2017) 171:934–49.e16. doi: 10.1016/j.cell.2017.09.028
39. Koh J, Jang JY, Keam B, Kim S, Kim MY, Go H, et al. EML4-ALK enhances programmed cell death-ligand 1 expression in pulmonary adenocarcinoma via hypoxia-inducible factor (HIF)-1alpha and STAT3. *Oncoimmunology.* (2016) 5:e1108514. doi: 10.1080/2162402X.2015.1108514
40. Akbay EA, Koyama S, Carretero J, Altabef A, Tchaicha JH, Christensen CL, et al. Activation of the PD-1 pathway contributes to immune escape in EGFR-driven lung tumors. *Cancer Discov.* (2013) 3:1355–63. doi: 10.1158/1535-7163.TARG-13-B290
41. Offin M, Rizvi H, Tenet M, Ni A, Sanchez-Vega F, Li BT, et al. Tumor mutation burden and efficacy of EGFR-tyrosine kinase inhibitors in patients with EGFR-mutant lung cancers. *Clin Cancer Res.* (2019) 25:1063–9. doi: 10.1158/1078-0432.CCR-18-1102
42. Gainor JF, Shaw AT, Sequist LV, Fu X, Azzoli CG, Piotrowska Z, et al. EGFR mutations and ALK rearrangements are associated with low response rates to PD-1 pathway blockade in non-small cell lung cancer: a retrospective analysis. *Clin Cancer Res.* (2016) 22:4585–93. doi: 10.1158/1078-0432.CCR-15-3101
43. Busch SE, Hanke ML, Kargl J, Metz HE, MacPherson D, Houghton AM. Lung cancer subtypes generate unique immune responses. *J Immunol.* (2016) 197:4493–503. doi: 10.4049/jimmunol.1600576
44. Mazieres J, Drilon A, Lusque A, Mhanna L, Cortot AB, Mezquita L, et al. Immune checkpoint inhibitors for patients with advanced lung cancer and oncogenic driver alterations: results from the IMMUNOTARGET registry. *Ann Oncol.* (2019) 30:1321–8. doi: 10.1093/annonc/mdz167
45. Sabari JK, Leonardi GC, Shu CA, Umeton R, Montecalvo J, Ni A, et al. PD-L1 expression, tumor mutational burden, and response to immunotherapy in patients with MET exon 14 altered lung cancers. *Ann Oncol.* (2018) 29:2085–91. doi: 10.1093/annonc/mdy334
46. Dudnik E, Peled N, Nechushtan H, Wollner M, Onn A, Agbarya A, et al. BRAF mutant lung cancer: programmed death ligand 1 expression, tumor mutational burden, microsatellite instability status, and response to immune check-point inhibitors. *J Thorac Oncol.* (2018) 13:1128–37. doi: 10.1016/j.jtho.2018.04.024
47. Offin M, Guo R, Wu SL, Sabari J, Land JD, Ni A, et al. Immunophenotype and response to immunotherapy of RET-rearranged lung cancers. *JCO Precis Oncol.* (2019) 3:PO.18.00386. doi: 10.1200/PO.18.00386
48. Cerami E, Gao J, Dogrusoz U, Gross BE, Sumer SO, Aksoy BA, et al. The cBio cancer genomics portal: an open platform for exploring multidimensional cancer genomics data. *Cancer Discov.* (2012) 2:401–4. doi: 10.1158/2159-8290.CD-12-0095
49. Kitajima S, Ivanova E, Guo S, Yoshida R, Campisi M, Sundararaman SK, et al. Suppression of STING associated with LKB1 loss in KRAS-driven lung cancer. *Cancer Discov.* (2019) 9:34–45. doi: 10.1158/2159-8290.CD-18-0689
50. Skoulidis F, Byers LA, Diao L, Papadimitrakopoulou VA, Tong P, Izzo J, et al. Co-occurring genomic alterations define major subsets of KRAS-mutant lung adenocarcinoma with distinct biology, immune profiles, and therapeutic vulnerabilities. *Cancer Discov.* (2015) 5:860–77. doi: 10.1158/2159-8290.CD-14-1236
51. Skoulidis F, Goldberg ME, Greenawalt DM, Hellmann MD, Awad MM, Gainor JF, et al. STK11/LKB1 mutations and PD-1 inhibitor resistance in KRAS-mutant lung adenocarcinoma. *Cancer Discov.* (2018) 8:822–35.
52. Dong ZY, Zhong WZ, Zhang XC, Su J, Xie Z, Liu SY, et al. Potential predictive value of TP53 and KRAS mutation status for response to PD-1 blockade immunotherapy in lung adenocarcinoma. *Clin Cancer Res.* (2017) 23:3012–24. doi: 10.1016/j.jtho.2016.11.504
53. Koyama S, Akbay EA, Li YY, Aref AR, Skoulidis F, Herter-Sprie GS, et al. STK11/LKB1 deficiency promotes neutrophil recruitment and proinflammatory cytokine production to suppress T-cell activity in the lung tumor microenvironment. *Cancer Res.* (2016) 76:999–1008. doi: 10.1158/0008-5472.CAN-15-1439
54. Bange E, Marmarelis ME, Hwang WT, Yang YX, Thompson JC, Rosenbaum J, et al. Impact of KRAS and TP53 co-mutations on outcomes after first-line systemic therapy among patients with STK11-mutated advanced non-small-cell lung cancer. *JCO Precis Oncol.* (2019) 3:10.1200/PO.18.00326. doi: 10.1200/PO.18.00326
55. Best SA, Ding S, Kersbergen A, Dong X, Song JY, Xie Y, et al. Distinct initiating events underpin the immune and metabolic heterogeneity of KRAS-mutant lung adenocarcinoma. *Nat Commun.* (2019) 10:4190. doi: 10.1038/s41467-019-12164-y
56. Best SA, Sutherland KD. "Keaping" a lid on lung cancer: the Keap1-Nrf2 pathway. *Cell Cycle.* (2018) 17:1696–707. doi: 10.1080/15384101.2018.1496756
57. Kadara H, Choi M, Zhang J, Parra ER, Rodriguez-Canales J, Gaffney SG, et al. Whole-exome sequencing and immune profiling of early-stage lung adenocarcinoma with fully annotated clinical follow-up. *Ann Oncol.* (2018) 29:1072. doi: 10.1093/annonc/mdx062
58. Arbour K, Shen R, Plodkowski A, Rizvi H, Ni A, Long N, et al. Concurrent mutations in STK11 and KEAP1 is associated with resistance to PD-(L)1 blockade in patients with NSCLC despite high TMB. *J Thorac Oncol.* (2018) 13:S424. doi: 10.1016/j.jtho.2018.08.480
59. Skoulidis F, Arbour KC, Hellmann MD, Patil PD, Marmarelis ME, Awad MM, et al. STK11 and/or KEAP1 genomic alterations showed lack of clinical benefits from addition of immunotherapy to chemotherapy in NSCLC patients. *Proceedings of the ASCO Annual Meeting 2019*, Chicago. (2019).
60. Cho BC, Lopes G, Kowalski DM, Kasahara K, Wu YL, Castro G, et al. *Relationship between STK11 and KAEP1 Mutational Status and Efficacy in KEYNOTE-042: Pembrolizumab Monotherapy versus Platinum-based Chemotherapy as First-line Therapy for PD-L1-Positive advanced NSCLC.* AACR 2020, Abstract 084. (2020). doi: 10.1158/1538-7445.AM2020-CT084
61. Spranger S, Bao R, Gajewski TF. Melanoma-intrinsic beta-catenin signalling prevents anti-tumour immunity. *Nature.* (2015) 523:231–5. doi: 10.1038/nature14404
62. George S, Miao D, Demetri GD, Adeegbe D, Rodig SJ, Shukla S, et al. Loss of PTEN is associated with resistance to anti-PD-1 checkpoint blockade therapy in metastatic uterine leiomyosarcoma. *Immunity.* (2017) 46:197–204. doi: 10.1016/j.immuni.2017.02.001
63. Peng W, Chen JQ, Liu C, Malu S, Creasy C, Tetzlaff MT, et al. Loss of PTEN promotes resistance to T cell-mediated immunotherapy. *Cancer Discov.* (2016) 6:202–16. doi: 10.1158/1538-7445.AM2016-4363
64. Toso A, Revandkar A, Di Mitri D, Guccini I, Proietti M, Sarti M, et al. Enhancing chemotherapy efficacy in Pten-deficient prostate tumors by activating the senescence-associated antitumor immunity. *Cell Rep.* (2014) 9:75–89. doi: 10.1016/j.celrep.2014.08.044
65. Parsa AT, Waldron JS, Panner A, Crane CA, Parney IF, Barry JJ, et al. Loss of tumor suppressor PTEN function increases B7-H1 expression and immunoresistance in glioma. *Nat Med.* (2007) 13:84–8. doi: 10.1038/nm1517
66. De Henau O, Rausch M, Winkler D, Campesato LF, Liu C, Cymerman DH, et al. Overcoming resistance to checkpoint blockade therapy by targeting PI3Kgamma in myeloid cells. *Nature.* (2016) 539:443–7. doi: 10.1038/nature20554
67. Howitt BE, Shukla SA, Sholl LM, Ritterhouse LL, Watkins JC, Rodig S, et al. Association of polymerase e-mutated and microsatellite-instable endometrial cancers with neoantigen load, number of tumor-infiltrating lymphocytes, and expression of PD-1 and PD-L1. *JAMA Oncol.* (2015) 1:1319–23. doi: 10.1001/jamaoncol.2015.2151
68. Timmermann B, Kerick M, Roehr C, Fischer A, Isau M, Boerno ST, et al. Somatic mutation profiles of MSI and MSS colorectal cancer identified by whole exome next generation sequencing and bioinformatics analysis. *PLoS One.* (2010) 5:e15661. doi: 10.1371/journal.pone.0015661
69. Tomlinson IP, Novelli MR, Bodmer WF. The mutation rate and cancer. *Proc Natl Acad Sci USA.* (1996) 93:14800–3. doi: 10.1073/pnas.93.25.14800
70. Maby P, Tougeron D, Hamieh M, Mlecnik B, Kora H, Bindea G, et al. Correlation between density of CD8+ T-cell infiltrate in microsatellite unstable colorectal cancers and frameshift mutations: a rationale for personalized immunotherapy. *Cancer Res.* (2015) 75:3446–55. doi: 10.1158/0008-5472.CAN-14-3051
71. Wen WX, Leong CO. Association of BRCA1- and BRCA2-deficiency with mutation burden, expression of PD-L1/PD-1, immune infiltrates, and T cell-inflamed signature in breast cancer. *PLoS One.* (2019) 14:e0215381. doi: 10.1371/journal.pone.0215381

72. Mehnert JM, Panda A, Zhong H, Hirshfield K, Damare S, Lane K, et al. Immune activation and response to pembrolizumab in POLE-mutant endometrial cancer. *J Clin Invest.* (2016) 126:2334–40. doi: 10.1172/JCI84940
73. Gao J, Shi LZ, Zhao H, Chen J, Xiong L, He Q, et al. Loss of IFN-gamma pathway genes in tumor cells as a mechanism of resistance to anti-CTLA-4 therapy. *Cell.* (2016) 167:397–404.e9. doi: 10.1016/j.cell.2016.08.069
74. Zaretsky JM, Garcia-Diaz A, Shin DS, Escuin-Ordinas H, Hugo W, Hu-Lieskovan S, et al. Mutations associated with acquired resistance to PD-1 blockade in melanoma. *N Engl J Med.* (2016) 375:819–29. doi: 10.1056/NEJMoa1604958
75. Sharma P, Allison JP. The future of immune checkpoint therapy. *Science.* (2015) 348:56–61. doi: 10.1126/science.aaa8172
76. Taube JM, Anders RA, Young GD, Xu H, Sharma R, McMiller TL, et al. Colocalization of inflammatory response with B7-h1 expression in human melanocytic lesions supports an adaptive resistance mechanism of immune escape. *Sci Transl Med.* (2012) 4:127ra37. doi: 10.1126/scitranslmed.3003689
77. Ikeda H, Old LJ, Schreiber RD. The roles of IFN gamma in protection against tumor development and cancer immunoediting. *Cytokine Growth Factor Rev.* (2002) 13:95–109. doi: 10.1016/S1359-6101(01)00038-7
78. Shin DS, Zaretsky JM, Escuin-Ordinas H, Garcia-Diaz A, Hu-Lieskovan S, Kalbasi A, et al. Primary resistance to PD-1 blockade mediated by JAK1/2 mutations. *Cancer Discov.* (2017) 7:188–201. doi: 10.1158/2159-8290.CD-16-1223
79. Platanias LC. Mechanisms of type-I- and type-II-interferon-mediated signalling. *Nat Rev Immunol.* (2005) 5:375–86. doi: 10.1038/nri1604
80. Prendergast GC, Smith C, Thomas S, Mandik-Nayak L, Laury-Kleintop L, Metz R, et al. Indoleamine 2,3-dioxygenase pathways of pathogenic inflammation and immune escape in cancer. *Cancer Immunol Immunother.* (2014) 63:721–35. doi: 10.1007/s00262-014-1549-4
81. Toulmonde M, Penel N, Adam J, Chevreau C, Blay JY, Le Cesne A, et al. Use of PD-1 targeting, macrophage infiltration, and IDO pathway activation in sarcomas: a phase 2 clinical trial. *JAMA Oncol.* (2018) 4:93–7. doi: 10.1001/jamaoncol.2017.1617
82. Takeda K, Nakayama M, Hayakawa Y, Kojima Y, Ikeda H, Imai N, et al. IFN-gamma is required for cytotoxic T cell-dependent cancer genome immunoediting. *Nat Commun.* (2017) 8:14607. doi: 10.1038/ncomms14607
83. Darnell JE Jr., Kerr IM, Stark GR. Jak-STAT pathways and transcriptional activation in response to IFNs and other extracellular signaling proteins. *Science.* (1994) 264:1415–21. doi: 10.1126/science.8197455
84. Benci JL, Xu B, Qiu Y, Wu TJ, Dada H, Twyman-Saint Victor C, et al. Tumor interferon signaling regulates a multigenic resistance program to immune checkpoint blockade. *Cell.* (2016) 167:1540–54.e12. doi: 10.1016/j.cell.2016.11.022
85. Sucker A, Zhao F, Pieper N, Heeke C, Maltaner R, Stadtler N, et al. Acquired IFNgamma resistance impairs anti-tumor immunity and gives rise to T-cell-resistant melanoma lesions. *Nat Commun.* (2017) 8:15440. doi: 10.1038/ncomms15440
86. Bach EA, Aguet M, Schreiber RD. The IFN gamma receptor: a paradigm for cytokine receptor signaling. *Annu Rev Immunol.* (1997) 15:563–91. doi: 10.1146/annurev.immunol.15.1.563
87. Ayers M, Lunceford J, Nebozhyn M, Murphy E, Loboda A, Kaufman DR, et al. IFN-gamma-related mRNA profile predicts clinical response to PD-1 blockade. *J Clin Invest.* (2017) 127:2930–40. doi: 10.1172/JCI91190
88. Hugo W, Zaretsky JM, Sun L, Song C, Moreno BH, Hu-Lieskovan S, et al. Genomic and transcriptomic features of response to anti-PD-1 therapy in metastatic melanoma. *Cell.* (2016) 165:35–44. doi: 10.1016/j.cell.2016.02.065
89. Motz GT, Coukos G. The parallel lives of angiogenesis and immunosuppression: cancer and other tales. *Nat Rev Immunol.* (2011) 11:702–11. doi: 10.1038/nri3064
90. Schafer M, Werner S. Cancer as an overhealing wound: an old hypothesis revisited. *Nat Rev Mol Cell Biol.* (2008) 9:628–38. doi: 10.1038/nrm2455
91. Voron T, Marcheteau E, Pernot S, Colussi O, Tartour E, Taieb J, et al. Control of the immune response by pro-angiogenic factors. *Front Oncol.* (2014) 4:70. doi: 10.3389/fonc.2014.00070
92. Gallagher SJ, Shklovskaya E, Hersey P. Epigenetic modulation in cancer immunotherapy. *Curr Opin Pharmacol.* (2017) 35:48–56. doi: 10.1016/j.coph.2017.05.006
93. Nagarsheth N, Peng D, Kryczek I, Wu K, Li W, Zhao E, et al. PRC2 epigenetically silences Th1-type chemokines to suppress effector T-cell trafficking in colon cancer. *Cancer Res.* (2016) 76:275–82. doi: 10.1158/0008-5472.CAN-15-1938
94. Zingg D, Arenas-Ramirez N, Sahin D, Rosalia RA, Antunes AT, Haeusel J, et al. The histone methyltransferase Ezh2 controls mechanisms of adaptive resistance to tumor immunotherapy. *Cell Rep.* (2017) 20:854–67. doi: 10.1016/j.celrep.2017.07.007
95. Wang LX, Mei ZY, Zhou JH, Yao YS, Li YH, Xu YH, et al. Low dose decitabine treatment induces CD80 expression in cancer cells and stimulates tumor specific cytotoxic T lymphocyte responses. *PLoS One.* (2013) 8:e62924. doi: 10.1371/journal.pone.0062924
96. Vo DD, Prins RM, Begley JL, Donahue TR, Morris LF, Bruhn KW, et al. Enhanced antitumor activity induced by adoptive T-cell transfer and adjunctive use of the histone deacetylase inhibitor LAQ824. *Cancer Res.* (2009) 69:8693–9. doi: 10.1158/0008-5472.CAN-09-1456
97. Pan D, Kobayashi A, Jiang P, de Andrade L, Tay RE, Luoma AM, et al. A major chromatin regulator determines resistance of tumor cells to T cell-mediated killing. *Science.* (2018) 359:770–5. doi: 10.1126/science.aao1710
98. Miao D, Margolis CA, Gao W, Voss MH, Li W, Martini DJ, et al. Genomic correlates of response to immune checkpoint therapies in clear cell renal cell carcinoma. *Science.* (2018) 359:801–6. doi: 10.1126/science.aan5951
99. Kadoch C, Crabtree GR. Mammalian SWI/SNF chromatin remodeling complexes and cancer: mechanistic insights gained from human genomics. *Sci Adv.* (2015) 1:e1500447. doi: 10.1126/sciadv.1500447
100. Shen J, Ju Z, Zhao W, Wang L, Peng Y, Ge Z, et al. ARID1A deficiency promotes mutability and potentiates therapeutic antitumor immunity unleashed by immune checkpoint blockade. *Nat Med.* (2018) 24:556–62. doi: 10.1038/s41591-018-0012-z
101. Zou W, Wolchok JD, Chen L. PD-L1 (B7-H1) and PD-1 pathway blockade for cancer therapy: mechanisms, response biomarkers, and combinations. *Sci Transl Med.* (2016) 8:328rv4. doi: 10.1126/scitranslmed.aad7118
102. Martin AM, Nirschl TR, Nirschl CJ, Francica BJ, Kochel CM, van Bokhoven A, et al. Paucity of PD-L1 expression in prostate cancer: innate and adaptive immune resistance. *Prostate Cancer Prostatic Dis.* (2015) 18:325–32. doi: 10.1038/pcan.2015.39
103. Lipson EJ, Forde PM, Hammers HJ, Emens LA, Taube JM, Topalian SL. Antagonists of PD-1 and PD-L1 in cancer treatment. *Semin Oncol.* (2015) 42:587–600. doi: 10.1053/j.seminoncol.2015.05.013
104. Yarchoan M, Albacker LA, Hopkins AC, Montesion M, Murugesan K, Vithayathil TT, et al. PD-L1 expression and tumor mutational burden are independent biomarkers in most cancers. *JCI Insight.* (2019) 4:e126908. doi: 10.1172/jci.insight.126908
105. Prestipino A, Zeiser R. Clinical implications of tumor-intrinsic mechanisms regulating PD-L1. *Sci Transl Med.* (2019) 11:eaav4810. doi: 10.1126/scitranslmed.aav4810
106. Sun C, Mezzadra R, Schumacher TN. Regulation and function of the PD-L1 checkpoint. *Immunity.* (2018) 48:434–52. doi: 10.1016/j.immuni.2018.03.014
107. Lastwika KJ, Wilson W III, Li QK, Norris J, Xu H, Ghazarian SR, et al. Control of PD-L1 expression by oncogenic activation of the AKT-mTOR pathway in non-small cell lung cancer. *Cancer Res.* (2016) 76:227–38. doi: 10.1158/0008-5472.CAN-14-3362
108. Casey SC, Tong L, Li Y, Do R, Walz S, Fitzgerald KN, et al. MYC regulates the antitumor immune response through CD47 and PD-L1. *Science.* (2016) 352:227–31. doi: 10.1126/science.aac9935
109. Dorand RD, Nthale J, Myers JT, Barkauskas DS, Avril S, Chirieleison SM, et al. Cdk5 disruption attenuates tumor PD-L1 expression and promotes antitumor immunity. *Science.* (2016) 353:399–403. doi: 10.1126/science.aae0477
110. Kataoka K, Shiraishi Y, Takeda Y, Sakata S, Matsumoto M, Nagano S, et al. Aberrant PD-L1 expression through 3'-UTR disruption in multiple cancers. *Nature.* (2016) 534:402–6.
111. Chen J, Jiang CC, Jin L, Zhang XD. Regulation of PD-L1: a novel role of pro-survival signalling in cancer. *Ann Oncol.* (2016) 27:409–16. doi: 10.1093/annonc/mdv615
112. Deschoolmeester V, Baay M, Van Marck E, Weyler J, Vermeulen P, Lardon F, et al. Tumor infiltrating lymphocytes: an intriguing player in the survival of

colorectal cancer patients. *BMC Immunol.* (2010) 11:19. doi: 10.1186/1471-2172-11-19
113. He J, Hu Y, Hu M, Li B. Development of PD-1/PD-L1 pathway in tumor immune microenvironment and treatment for non-small cell lung cancer. *Sci Rep.* (2015) 5:13110. doi: 10.1038/srep13110
114. Li CW, Lim SO, Chung EM, Kim YS, Park AH, Yao J, et al. Eradication of triple-negative breast cancer cells by targeting Glycosylated PD-L1. *Cancer Cell.* (2018) 33:187–201.e10. doi: 10.1016/j.ccell.2018.01.009
115. Yao H, Lan J, Li C, Shi H, Brosseau JP, Wang H, et al. Inhibiting PD-L1 palmitoylation enhances T-cell immune responses against tumours. *Nat Biomed Eng.* (2019) 3:306–17. doi: 10.1038/s41551-019-0375-6
116. Gong B, Kiyotani K, Sakata S, Nagano S, Kumehara S, Baba S, et al. Secreted PD-L1 variants mediate resistance to PD-L1 blockade therapy in non-small cell lung cancer. *J Exp Med.* (2019) 216:982–1000. doi: 10.1084/jem.20180870
117. Dunn GP, Old LJ, Schreiber RD. The three Es of cancer immunoediting. *Annu Rev Immunol.* (2004) 22:329–60. doi: 10.1146/annurev.immunol.22.012703.104803
118. Anagnostou V, Smith KN, Forde PM, Niknafs N, Bhattacharya R, White J, et al. Evolution of neoantigen landscape during immune checkpoint blockade in non-small cell lung cancer. *Cancer Discov.* (2017) 7:264–76. doi: 10.1158/1538-7445.AM2017-NG01
119. Verdegaal EM, de Miranda NF, Visser M, Harryvan T, van Buuren MM, Andersen RS, et al. Neoantigen landscape dynamics during human melanoma-T cell interactions. *Nature.* (2016) 536:91–5. doi: 10.1038/nature18945
120. Ribas A, Hamid O, Daud A, Hodi FS, Wolchok JD, Kefford R, et al. Association of pembrolizumab with tumor response and survival among patients with advanced melanoma. *JAMA.* (2016) 315:1600–9. doi: 10.1001/jama.2016.4059
121. Kaluza KM, Thompson JM, Kottke TJ, Flynn Gilmer HC, Knutson DL, Vile RG. Adoptive T cell therapy promotes the emergence of genomically altered tumor escape variants. *Int J Cancer.* (2012) 131:844–54. doi: 10.1002/ijc.26447
122. Landsberg J, Kohlmeyer J, Renn M, Bald T, Rogava M, Cron M, et al. Melanomas resist T-cell therapy through inflammation-induced reversible dedifferentiation. *Nature.* (2012) 490:412–6. doi: 10.1038/nature11538
123. Mariathasan S, Turley SJ, Nickles D, Castiglioni A, Yuen K, Wang Y, et al. TGFbeta attenuates tumour response to PD-L1 blockade by contributing to exclusion of T cells. *Nature.* (2018) 554:544–8.
124. Sucker A, Zhao F, Real B, Heeke C, Bielefeld N, Mabetaen S, et al. Genetic evolution of T-cell resistance in the course of melanoma progression. *Clin Cancer Res.* (2014) 20:6593–604. doi: 10.1158/1078-0432.CCR-14-0567
125. Pereira C, Gimenez-Xavier P, Pros E, Pajares MJ, Moro M, Gomez A, et al. Genomic profiling of patient-derived xenografts for lung cancer identifies B2M inactivation impairing immunorecognition. *Clin Cancer Res.* (2017) 23:3203–13. doi: 10.1158/1078-0432.CCR-16-1946
126. Gettinger S, Choi J, Hastings K, Truini A, Datar I, Sowell R, et al. Impaired HLA Class I antigen processing and presentation as a mechanism of acquired resistance to immune checkpoint inhibitors in lung cancer. *Cancer Discov.* (2017) 7:1420–35. doi: 10.1158/2159-8290.CD-17-0593
127. Giannakis M, Mu XJ, Shukla SA, Qian ZR, Cohen O, Nishihara R, et al. Genomic correlates of immune-cell infiltrates in colorectal carcinoma. *Cell Rep.* (2016) 15:857–65. doi: 10.1016/j.celrep.2016.03.075
128. Chang CC, Pirozzi G, Wen SH, Chung IH, Chiu BL, Errico S, et al. Multiple structural and epigenetic defects in the human leukocyte antigen class I antigen presentation pathway in a recurrent metastatic melanoma following immunotherapy. *J Biol Chem.* (2015) 290:26562–75. doi: 10.1074/jbc.M115.676130
129. Donia M, Harbst K, van Buuren M, Kvistborg P, Lindberg MF, Andersen R, et al. Acquired immune resistance follows complete tumor regression without loss of target antigens or IFNgamma signaling. *Cancer Res.* (2017) 77:4562–6. doi: 10.1158/0008-5472.CAN-16-3172
130. McGranahan N, Rosenthal R, Hiley CT, Rowan AJ, Watkins TBK, Wilson GA, et al. Allele-specific HLA loss and immune escape in lung cancer evolution. *Cell.* (2017) 171:1259–71.e11.
131. Chowell D, Morris LGT, Grigg CM, Weber JK, Samstein RM, Makarov V, et al. Patient HLA class I genotype influences cancer response to checkpoint blockade immunotherapy. *Science.* (2018) 359:582–7. doi: 10.1126/science.aao4572
132. Rodig SJ, Gusenleitner D, Jackson DG, Gjini E, Giobbie-Hurder A, Jin C, et al. MHC proteins confer differential sensitivity to CTLA-4 and PD-1 blockade in untreated metastatic melanoma. *Sci Transl Med.* (2018) 10:eaar3342. doi: 10.1126/scitranslmed.aar3342
133. Boehm U, Klamp T, Groot M, Howard JC. Cellular responses to interferon-gamma. *Annu Rev Immunol.* (1997) 15:749–95. doi: 10.1146/annurev.immunol.15.1.749
134. Donnem T, Kilvaer TK, Andersen S, Richardsen E, Paulsen EE, Hald SM, et al. Strategies for clinical implementation of TNM-Immunoscore in resected nonsmall-cell lung cancer. *Ann Oncol.* (2016) 27:225–32. doi: 10.1093/annonc/mdv560
135. Geng Y, Shao Y, He W, Hu W, Xu Y, Chen J, et al. Prognostic role of tumor-infiltrating lymphocytes in lung cancer: a meta-analysis. *Cell Physiol Biochem.* (2015) 37:1560–71. doi: 10.1159/000438523
136. Gajewski TF, Schreiber H, Fu YX. Innate and adaptive immune cells in the tumor microenvironment. *Nat Immunol.* (2013) 14:1014–22. doi: 10.1038/ni.2703
137. Kim HJ, Cantor H. CD4 T-cell subsets and tumor immunity: the helpful and the not-so-helpful. *Cancer Immunol Res.* (2014) 2:91–8. doi: 10.1158/2326-6066.CIR-13-0216
138. Rittmeyer A, Barlesi F, Waterkamp D, Park K, Ciardiello F, von Pawel J, et al. Atezolizumab versus docetaxel in patients with previously treated non-small-cell lung cancer (OAK): a phase 3, open-label, multicentre randomised controlled trial. *Lancet.* (2017) 389:255–65. doi: 10.1016/S0140-6736(16)32517-X
139. Brambilla E, Le Teuff G, Marguet S, Lantuejoul S, Dunant A, Graziano S, et al. Prognostic effect of tumor lymphocytic infiltration in resectable non-small-cell lung cancer. *J Clin Oncol.* (2016) 34:1223–30. doi: 10.1200/JCO.2015.63.0970
140. Feng W, Li Y, Shen L, Cai XW, Zhu ZF, Chang JH, et al. Prognostic value of tumor-infiltrating lymphocytes for patients with completely resected stage IIIA(N2) non-small cell lung cancer. *Oncotarget.* (2016) 7:7227–40. doi: 10.18632/oncotarget.6979
141. Kilic A, Landreneau RJ, Luketich JD, Pennathur A, Schuchert MJ. Density of tumor-infiltrating lymphocytes correlates with disease recurrence and survival in patients with large non-small-cell lung cancer tumors. *J Surg Res.* (2011) 167:207–10. doi: 10.1016/j.jss.2009.08.029
142. Ruffini E, Asioli S, Filosso PL, Lyberis P, Bruna MC, Macri L, et al. Clinical significance of tumor-infiltrating lymphocytes in lung neoplasms. *Ann Thorac Surg.* (2009) 87:365–71. doi: 10.1016/j.athoracsur.2008.10.067
143. Sun R, Limkin EJ, Vakalopoulou M, Dercle L, Champiat S, Han SR, et al. A radiomics approach to assess tumour-infiltrating CD8 cells and response to anti-PD-1 or anti-PD-L1 immunotherapy: an imaging biomarker, retrospective multicohort study. *Lancet Oncol.* (2018) 19:1180–91. doi: 10.1016/S1470-2045(18)30413-3
144. Galon J, Bruni D. Approaches to treat immune hot, altered and cold tumours with combination immunotherapies. *Nat Rev Drug Discov.* (2019) 18:197–218. doi: 10.1038/s41573-018-0007-y
145. AbdulJabbar K, Raza SEA, Rosenthal R, Jamal-Hanjani M, Veeriah S, Akarca A, et al. Geospatial immune variability illuminates differential evolution of lung adenocarcinoma. *Nat Med.* (2020) 26:1054–62. doi: 10.1038/s41591-020-0900-x
146. Spranger S, Luke JJ, Bao R, Zha Y, Hernandez KM, Li Y, et al. Density of immunogenic antigens does not explain the presence or absence of the T-cell-inflamed tumor microenvironment in melanoma. *Proc Natl Acad Sci USA.* (2016) 113:E7759–68. doi: 10.1073/pnas.1609376113
147. Flavell RA, Sanjabi S, Wrzesinski SH, Licona-Limon P. The polarization of immune cells in the tumour environment by TGFbeta. *Nat Rev Immunol.* (2010) 10:554–67. doi: 10.1038/nri2808
148. MartIn-Fontecha A, Sebastiani S, Hopken UE, Uguccioni M, Lipp M, Lanzavecchia A, et al. Regulation of dendritic cell migration to the draining lymph node: impact on T lymphocyte traffic and priming. *J Exp Med.* (2003) 198:615–21. doi: 10.1084/jem.20030448
149. Diamond MS, Kinder M, Matsushita H, Mashayekhi M, Dunn GP, Archambault JM, et al. Type I interferon is selectively required by dendritic

cells for immune rejection of tumors. *J Exp Med.* (2011) 208:1989–2003. doi: 10.1084/jem.20101158
150. Fuertes MB, Kacha AK, Kline J, Woo SR, Kranz DM, Murphy KM, et al. Host type I IFN signals are required for antitumor CD8+ T cell responses through CD8{alpha}+ dendritic cells. *J Exp Med.* (2011) 208:2005–16. doi: 10.1084/jem.20101159
151. Sistigu A, Yamazaki T, Vacchelli E, Chaba K, Enot DP, Adam J, et al. Cancer cell-autonomous contribution of type I interferon signaling to the efficacy of chemotherapy. *Nat Med.* (2014) 20:1301–9. doi: 10.1038/nm.3708
152. Tarhini AA, Butterfield LH, Shuai Y, Gooding WE, Kalinski P, Kirkwood JM. Differing patterns of circulating regulatory T cells and myeloid-derived suppressor cells in metastatic melanoma patients receiving anti-CTLA4 antibody and interferon-alpha or TLR-9 agonist and GM-CSF with peptide vaccination. *J Immunother.* (2012) 35:702–10. doi: 10.1097/CJI.0b013e318272569b
153. Tarhini AA, Cherian J, Moschos SJ, Tawbi HA, Shuai Y, Gooding WE, et al. Safety and efficacy of combination immunotherapy with interferon alfa-2b and tremelimumab in patients with stage IV melanoma. *J Clin Oncol.* (2012) 30:322–8. doi: 10.1200/JCO.2011.37.5394
154. Buque A, Bloy N, Aranda F, Castoldi F, Eggermont A, Cremer I, et al. Trial watch: immunomodulatory monoclonal antibodies for oncological indications. *Oncoimmunology.* (2015) 4:e1008814. doi: 10.1080/2162402X.2015.1008814
155. Peng D, Kryczek I, Nagarsheth N, Zhao L, Wei S, Wang W, et al. Epigenetic silencing of TH1-type chemokines shapes tumour immunity and immunotherapy. *Nature.* (2015) 527:249–53. doi: 10.1038/nature15520
156. Molon B, Ugel S, Del Pozzo F, Soldani C, Zilio S, Avella D, et al. Chemokine nitration prevents intratumoral infiltration of antigen-specific T cells. *J Exp Med.* (2011) 208:1949–62. doi: 10.1084/jem.20101956
157. Proost P, Mortier A, Loos T, Vandercappellen J, Gouwy M, Ronsse I, et al. Proteolytic processing of CXCL11 by CD13/aminopeptidase N impairs CXCR3 and CXCR7 binding and signaling and reduces lymphocyte and endothelial cell migration. *Blood.* (2007) 110:37–44. doi: 10.1182/blood-2006-10-049072
158. Blackburn SD, Shin H, Freeman GJ, Wherry EJ. Selective expansion of a subset of exhausted CD8 T cells by alphaPD-L1 blockade. *Proc Natl Acad Sci USA.* (2008) 105:15016–21. doi: 10.1073/pnas.0801497105
159. Tauriello DVF, Palomo-Ponce S, Stork D, Berenguer-Llergo A, Badia-Ramentol J, Iglesias M, et al. TGFbeta drives immune evasion in genetically reconstituted colon cancer metastasis. *Nature.* (2018) 554:538–43. doi: 10.1038/nature25492
160. Chen PL, Roh W, Reuben A, Cooper ZA, Spencer CN, Prieto PA, et al. Analysis of immune signatures in longitudinal tumor samples yields insight into biomarkers of response and mechanisms of resistance to immune checkpoint blockade. *Cancer Discov.* (2016) 6:827–37. doi: 10.1158/2159-8290.CD-15-1545
161. Hamid O, Schmidt H, Nissan A, Ridolfi L, Aamdal S, Hansson J, et al. A prospective phase II trial exploring the association between tumor microenvironment biomarkers and clinical activity of ipilimumab in advanced melanoma. *J Transl Med.* (2011) 9:204. doi: 10.1186/1479-5876-9-204
162. Tumeh PC, Harview CL, Yearley JH, Shintaku IP, Taylor EJ, Robert L, et al. PD-1 blockade induces responses by inhibiting adaptive immune resistance. *Nature.* (2014) 515:568–71.
163. Cha E, Klinger M, Hou Y, Cummings C, Ribas A, Faham M, et al. Improved survival with T cell clonotype stability after anti-CTLA-4 treatment in cancer patients. *Sci Transl Med.* (2014) 6:238ra70. doi: 10.1126/scitranslmed.3008211
164. Hirsch FR, Scagliotti GV, Mulshine JL, Kwon R, Curran WJ Jr., Wu YL, et al. Lung cancer: current therapies and new targeted treatments. *Lancet.* (2017) 389:299–311. doi: 10.1016/S0140-6736(16)30958-8
165. Reuben A, Zhang J, Chiou SH, Gittelman RM, Li J, Lee WC, et al. Comprehensive T cell repertoire characterization of non-small cell lung cancer. *Nat Commun.* (2020) 11:603. doi: 10.1038/s41467-019-14273-0
166. Joshi K, de Massy MR, Ismail M, Reading JL, Uddin I, Woolston A, et al. Spatial heterogeneity of the T cell receptor repertoire reflects the mutational landscape in lung cancer. *Nat Med.* (2019) 25:1549–59. doi: 10.1038/s41591-019-0592-2
167. Thommen DS, Schreiner J, Muller P, Herzig P, Roller A, Belousov A, et al. Progression of lung cancer is associated with increased dysfunction of T cells defined by coexpression of multiple inhibitory receptors. *Cancer Immunol Res.* (2015) 3:1344–55. doi: 10.1158/2326-6066.CIR-15-0097
168. Topalian SL, Drake CG, Pardoll DM. Immune checkpoint blockade: a common denominator approach to cancer therapy. *Cancer Cell.* (2015) 27:450–61. doi: 10.1016/j.ccell.2015.03.001
169. Hellmann MD, Friedman CF, Wolchok JD. Combinatorial Cancer Immunotherapies. *Adv Immunol.* (2016) 130:251–77. doi: 10.1016/bs.ai.2015.12.005
170. Balko JJ, Wang D, Ericsson-Gonzalez P, Nixon M, Salgado R, Sanchez V, et al. MHC-II expression to drive a unique pattern of adaptive resistance to antitumor immunity through receptor checkpoint engagement. *J Clin Oncol.* (2018) 36:180. doi: 10.1200/JCO.2018.36.5_suppl.180
171. Du W, Yang M, Turner A, Xu C, Ferris RL, Huang J, et al. TIM-3 as a target for cancer immunotherapy and mechanisms of action. *Int J Mol Sci.* (2017) 18:645. doi: 10.3390/ijms18030645
172. Manieri NA, Chiang EY, Grogan JL. TIGIT: a key inhibitor of the cancer immunity cycle. *Trends Immunol.* (2017) 38:20–8. doi: 10.1016/j.it.2016.10.002
173. Wherry EJ, Kurachi M. Molecular and cellular insights into T cell exhaustion. *Nat Rev Immunol.* (2015) 15:486–99. doi: 10.1038/nri3862
174. Wei F, Zhong S, Ma Z, Kong H, Medvec A, Ahmed R, et al. Strength of PD-1 signaling differentially affects T-cell effector functions. *Proc Natl Acad Sci USA.* (2013) 110:E2480–9. doi: 10.1073/pnas.1305394110
175. Ngiow SF, Young A, Jacquelot N, Yamazaki T, Enot D, Zitvogel L, et al. A Threshold Level of Intratumor CD8+ T-cell PD1 Expression Dictates Therapeutic Response to Anti-PD1. *Cancer Res.* (2015) 75:3800–11. doi: 10.1158/0008-5472.CAN-15-1082
176. Pauken KE, Sammons MA, Odorizzi PM, Manne S, Godec J, Khan O, et al. Epigenetic stability of exhausted T cells limits durability of reinvigoration by PD-1 blockade. *Science.* (2016) 354:1160–5. doi: 10.1126/science.aaf2807
177. Sen DR, Kaminski J, Barnitz RA, Kurachi M, Gerdemann U, Yates KB, et al. The epigenetic landscape of T cell exhaustion. *Science.* (2016) 354:1165–9. doi: 10.1126/science.aae0491
178. Mognol GP, Spreafico R, Wong V, Scott-Browne JP, Togher S, Hoffmann A, et al. Exhaustion-associated regulatory regions in CD8(+) tumor-infiltrating T cells. *Proc Natl Acad Sci USA.* (2017) 114:E2776–85. doi: 10.1073/pnas.1620498114
179. Ribas A, Shin DS, Zaretsky J, Frederiksen J, Cornish A, Avramis E, et al. PD-1 blockade expands intratumoral memory T cells. *Cancer Immunol Res.* (2016) 4:194–203. doi: 10.1158/2326-6066.CIR-15-0210
180. Farber DL, Yudanin NA, Restifo NP. Human memory T cells: generation, compartmentalization and homeostasis. *Nat Rev Immunol.* (2014) 14:24–35. doi: 10.1038/nri3567
181. Woodland DL, Kohlmeier JE. Migration, maintenance and recall of memory T cells in peripheral tissues. *Nat Rev Immunol.* (2009) 9:153–61. doi: 10.1038/nri2496
182. Ma C, Cheung AF, Chodon T, Koya RC, Wu Z, Ng C, et al. Multifunctional T-cell analyses to study response and progression in adoptive cell transfer immunotherapy. *Cancer Discov.* (2013) 3:418–29. doi: 10.1158/2159-8290.CD-12-0383
183. Ma C, Fan R, Ahmad H, Shi Q, Comin-Anduix B, Chodon T, et al. A clinical microchip for evaluation of single immune cells reveals high functional heterogeneity in phenotypically similar T cells. *Nat Med.* (2011) 17:738–43. doi: 10.1038/nm.2375
184. Fridman WH, Zitvogel L, Sautes-Fridman C, Kroemer G. The immune contexture in cancer prognosis and treatment. *Nat Rev Clin Oncol.* (2017) 14:717–34. doi: 10.1038/nrclinonc.2017.101
185. Oida T, Zhang X, Goto M, Hachimura S, Totsuka M, Kaminogawa S, et al. CD4+CD25- T cells that express latency-associated peptide on the surface suppress CD4+CD45RBhigh-induced colitis by a TGF-beta-dependent mechanism. *J Immunol.* (2003) 170:2516–22. doi: 10.4049/jimmunol.170.5.2516
186. Sakaguchi S, Yamaguchi T, Nomura T, Ono M. Regulatory T cells and immune tolerance. *Cell.* (2008) 133:775–87. doi: 10.1016/j.cell.2008.05.009
187. Sundstedt A, O'Neill EJ, Nicolson KS, Wraith DC. Role for IL-10 in suppression mediated by peptide-induced regulatory T cells

in vivo. *J Immunol.* (2003) 170:1240–8. doi: 10.4049/jimmunol.170.3.1240
188. Simpson TR, Li F, Montalvo-Ortiz W, Sepulveda MA, Bergerhoff K, Arce F, et al. Fc-dependent depletion of tumor-infiltrating regulatory T cells co-defines the efficacy of anti-CTLA-4 therapy against melanoma. *J Exp Med.* (2013) 210:1695–710. doi: 10.1084/jem.20130579
189. Viehl CT, Moore TT, Liyanage UK, Frey DM, Ehlers JP, Eberlein TJ, et al. Depletion of CD4+CD25+ regulatory T cells promotes a tumor-specific immune response in pancreas cancer-bearing mice. *Ann Surg Oncol.* (2006) 13:1252–8. doi: 10.1245/s10434-006-9015-y
190. Hannani D, Vetizou M, Enot D, Rusakiewicz S, Chaput N, Klatzmann D, et al. Anticancer immunotherapy by CTLA-4 blockade: obligatory contribution of IL-2 receptors and negative prognostic impact of soluble CD25. *Cell Res.* (2015) 25:208–24. doi: 10.1038/cr.2015.3
191. Meyer C, Cagnon L, Costa-Nunes CM, Baumgaertner P, Montandon N, Leyvraz L, et al. Frequencies of circulating MDSC correlate with clinical outcome of melanoma patients treated with ipilimumab. *Cancer Immunol Immunother.* (2014) 63:247–57. doi: 10.1007/s00262-013-1508-5
192. Kodumudi KN, Weber A, Sarnaik AA, Pilon-Thomas S. Blockade of myeloid-derived suppressor cells after induction of lymphopenia improves adoptive T cell therapy in a murine model of melanoma. *J Immunol.* (2012) 189:5147–54. doi: 10.4049/jimmunol.1200274
193. Laborde RR, Lin Y, Gustafson MP, Bulur PA, Dietz AB. Cancer vaccines in the world of immune suppressive monocytes (CD14(+)HLA-DR(lo/neg) Cells): the gateway to improved responses. *Front Immunol.* (2014) 5:147. doi: 10.3389/fimmu.2014.00147
194. Biswas SK, Mantovani A. Macrophage plasticity and interaction with lymphocyte subsets: cancer as a paradigm. *Nat Immunol.* (2010) 11:889–96. doi: 10.1038/ni.1937
195. Hu W, Li X, Zhang C, Yang Y, Jiang J, Wu C. Tumor-associated macrophages in cancers. *Clin Transl Oncol.* (2016) 18:251–8. doi: 10.1007/s12094-015-1373-0
196. Chanmee T, Ontong P, Konno K, Itano N. Tumor-associated macrophages as major players in the tumor microenvironment. *Cancers (Basel).* (2014) 6:1670–90. doi: 10.3390/cancers6031670
197. De Palma M, Lewis CE. Macrophage regulation of tumor responses to anticancer therapies. *Cancer Cell.* (2013) 23:277–86. doi: 10.1016/j.ccr.2013.02.013
198. Ruffell B, Coussens LM. Macrophages and therapeutic resistance in cancer. *Cancer Cell.* (2015) 27:462–72. doi: 10.1016/j.ccell.2015.02.015
199. Kuang DM, Zhao Q, Peng C, Xu J, Zhang JP, Wu C, et al. Activated monocytes in peritumoral stroma of hepatocellular carcinoma foster immune privilege and disease progression through PD-L1. *J Exp Med.* (2009) 206:1327–37. doi: 10.1084/jem.20082173
200. Kryczek I, Zou L, Rodriguez P, Zhu G, Wei S, Mottram P, et al. B7-H4 expression identifies a novel suppressive macrophage population in human ovarian carcinoma. *J Exp Med.* (2006) 203:871–81. doi: 10.1084/jem.20050930
201. Le DT, Lutz E, Uram JN, Sugar EA, Onners B, Solt S, et al. Evaluation of ipilimumab in combination with allogeneic pancreatic tumor cells transfected with a GM-CSF gene in previously treated pancreatic cancer. *J Immunother.* (2013) 36:382–9. doi: 10.1097/CJI.0b013e31829fb7a2
202. Zhu Y, Knolhoff BL, Meyer MA, Nywening TM, West BL, Luo J, et al. CSF1/CSF1R blockade reprograms tumor-infiltrating macrophages and improves response to T-cell checkpoint immunotherapy in pancreatic cancer models. *Cancer Res.* (2014) 74:5057–69. doi: 10.1158/0008-5472.CAN-13-3723
203. Mok S, Koya RC, Tsui C, Xu J, Robert L, Wu L, et al. Inhibition of CSF-1 receptor improves the antitumor efficacy of adoptive cell transfer immunotherapy. *Cancer Res.* (2014) 74:153–61. doi: 10.1158/0008-5472.CAN-13-1816
204. Highfill SL, Cui Y, Giles AJ, Smith JP, Zhang H, Morse E, et al. Disruption of CXCR2-mediated MDSC tumor trafficking enhances anti-PD1 efficacy. *Sci Transl Med.* (2014) 6:237ra67. doi: 10.1126/scitranslmed.3007974
205. Rabin RL, Park MK, Liao F, Swofford R, Stephany D, Farber JM. Chemokine receptor responses on T cells are achieved through regulation of both receptor expression and signaling. *J Immunol.* (1999) 162:3840–50.
206. Joyce JA, Fearon DT. T cell exclusion, immune privilege, and the tumor microenvironment. *Science.* (2015) 348:74–80. doi: 10.1126/science.aaa6204
207. Lebrun JJ. The dual role of TGFbeta in human cancer: from tumor suppression to cancer metastasis. *ISRN Mol Biol.* (2012) 2012:381428. doi: 10.5402/2012/381428
208. Vanpouille-Box C, Diamond JM, Pilones KA, Zavadil J, Babb JS, Formenti SC, et al. TGFbeta is a master regulator of radiation therapy-induced antitumor immunity. *Cancer Res.* (2015) 75:2232–42. doi: 10.1158/0008-5472.CAN-14-3511
209. Hanks B, Holtzhausen A, Evans K, Heid M, Blobe G. Combinatorial TGF-{beta} signaling blockade and anti-CTLA-4 antibody immunotherapy in a murine BRAFV600E-PTEN-/-transgenic model of melanoma. *Paper Presented at: ASCO Annual Meeting Proceedings 2014*, Chicago. (2014). doi: 10.1200/jco.2014.32.15_suppl.3011
210. Bertrand F, Montfort A, Marcheteau E, Imbert C, Gilhodes J, Filleron T, et al. TNFalpha blockade overcomes resistance to anti-PD-1 in experimental melanoma. *Nat Commun.* (2017) 8:2256. doi: 10.1038/s41467-017-02358-7
211. Ott PA, Hodi FS, Buchbinder EI. Inhibition of immune checkpoints and vascular endothelial growth factor as combination therapy for metastatic melanoma: an overview of rationale, preclinical evidence, and initial clinical data. *Front Oncol.* (2015) 5:202. doi: 10.3389/fonc.2015.00202
212. Ohm JE, Gabrilovich DI, Sempowski GD, Kisseleva E, Parman KS, Nadaf S, et al. VEGF inhibits T-cell development and may contribute to tumor-induced immune suppression. *Blood.* (2003) 101:4878–86. doi: 10.1182/blood-2002-07-1956
213. Motz GT, Santoro SP, Wang LP, Garrabrant T, Lastra RR, Hagemann IS, et al. Tumor endothelium FasL establishes a selective immune barrier promoting tolerance in tumors. *Nat Med.* (2014) 20:607–15. doi: 10.1038/nm.3541
214. Voron T, Colussi O, Marcheteau E, Pernot S, Nizard M, Pointet AL, et al. VEGF-A modulates expression of inhibitory checkpoints on CD8+ T cells in tumors. *J Exp Med.* (2015) 212:139–48. doi: 10.1084/jem.20140559
215. Bjoern J, Juul Nitschke N, Zeeberg Iversen T, Schmidt H, Fode K, Svane IM. Immunological correlates of treatment and response in stage IV malignant melanoma patients treated with Ipilimumab. *Oncoimmunology.* (2016) 5:e1100788. doi: 10.1080/2162402X.2015.1100788
216. Schalper KA, Carleton M, Zhou M, Chen T, Feng Y, Huang SP, et al. Elevated serum interleukin-8 is associated with enhanced intratumor neutrophils and reduced clinical benefit of immune-checkpoint inhibitors. *Nat Med.* (2020) 26:688–92. doi: 10.1038/s41591-020-0856-x
217. Yuen KC, Liu LF, Gupta V, Madireddi S, Keerthivasan S, Li C, et al. High systemic and tumor-associated IL-8 correlates with reduced clinical benefit of PD-L1 blockade. *Nat Med.* (2020) 26:693–8. doi: 10.1158/1538-7445.AM2020-2000
218. Garcia-Diaz A, Shin DS, Moreno BH, Saco J, Escuin-Ordinas H, Rodriguez GA, et al. Interferon receptor signaling pathways regulating PD-L1 and PD-L2 expression. *Cell Rep.* (2017) 19:1189–201. doi: 10.1016/j.celrep.2017.04.031
219. Moore BB, Arenberg DA, Stoy K, Morgan T, Addison CL, Morris SB, et al. Distinct CXC chemokines mediate tumorigenicity of prostate cancer cells. *Am J Pathol.* (1999) 154:1503–12. doi: 10.1016/S0002-9440(10)65404-1
220. Najjar YG, Rayman P, Jia X, Pavicic PG Jr., Rini BI, Tannenbaum C, et al. Myeloid-derived suppressor cell subset accumulation in renal cell carcinoma parenchyma is associated with intratumoral expression of IL1beta, IL8, CXCL5, and Mip-1alpha. *Clin Cancer Res.* (2017) 23:2346–55. doi: 10.1158/1078-0432.CCR-15-1823
221. Baggiolini M. CXCL8–the first chemokine. *Front Immunol.* (2015) 6:285. doi: 10.3389/fimmu.2015.00285
222. Baggiolini M, Walz A, Kunkel SL. Neutrophil-activating peptide-1/interleukin 8, a novel cytokine that activates neutrophils. *J Clin Invest.* (1989) 84:1045–9. doi: 10.1172/JCI114265
223. Alfaro C, Teijeira A, Onate C, Perez G, Sanmamed MF, Andueza MP, et al. Tumor-produced interleukin-8 attracts human myeloid-derived suppressor cells and elicits extrusion of neutrophil extracellular traps (NETs). *Clin Cancer Res.* (2016) 22:3924–36. doi: 10.1158/1078-0432.CCR-15-2463
224. Zhang H, Conrad DM, Butler JJ, Zhao C, Blay J, Hoskin DW. Adenosine acts through A2 receptors to inhibit IL-2-induced tyrosine phosphorylation of STAT5 in T lymphocytes: role of cyclic adenosine 3',5'-monophosphate and phosphatases. *J Immunol.* (2004) 173:932–44. doi: 10.4049/jimmunol.173.2.932
225. Stagg J, Divisekera U, McLaughlin N, Sharkey J, Pommey S, Denoyer D, et al. Anti-CD73 antibody therapy inhibits breast tumor growth and metastasis.

Proc Natl Acad Sci USA. (2010) 107:1547–52. doi: 10.1073/pnas.0908801107
226. Allard B, Pommey S, Smyth MJ, Stagg J. Targeting CD73 enhances the antitumor activity of anti-PD-1 and anti-CTLA-4 mAbs. *Clin Cancer Res.* (2013) 19:5626–35. doi: 10.1158/1078-0432.CCR-13-0545
227. Beavis PA, Slaney CY, Milenkovski N, Henderson MA, Loi S, Stagg J, et al. CD73: a potential biomarker for anti-PD-1 therapy. *Oncoimmunology.* (2015) 4:e1046675. doi: 10.1080/2162402X.2015.1046675
228. Platten M, von Knebel Doeberitz N, Oezen I, Wick W, Ochs K. Cancer immunotherapy by targeting IDO1/TDO and their downstream effectors. *Front Immunol.* (2014) 5:673. doi: 10.3389/fimmu.2014.00673
229. Munn DH, Sharma MD, Mellor AL. Ligation of B7-1/B7-2 by human CD4+ T cells triggers indoleamine 2,3-dioxygenase activity in dendritic cells. *J Immunol.* (2004) 172:4100–10. doi: 10.4049/jimmunol.172.7.4100
230. Holmgaard RB, Zamarin D, Munn DH, Wolchok JD, Allison JP. Indoleamine 2,3-dioxygenase is a critical resistance mechanism in antitumor T cell immunotherapy targeting CTLA-4. *J Exp Med.* (2013) 210:1389–402. doi: 10.1084/jem.20130066
231. Spranger S, Koblish HK, Horton B, Scherle PA, Newton R, Gajewski TF. Mechanism of tumor rejection with doublets of CTLA-4, PD-1/PD-L1, or IDO blockade involves restored IL-2 production and proliferation of CD8(+) T cells directly within the tumor microenvironment. *J Immunother Cancer.* (2014) 2:3. doi: 10.1186/2051-1426-2-3
232. Long GV, Dummer R, Hamid O, Gajewski TF, Caglevic C, Dalle S, et al. Epacadostat plus pembrolizumab versus placebo plus pembrolizumab in patients with unresectable or metastatic melanoma (ECHO-301/KEYNOTE-252): a phase 3, randomised, double-blind study. *Lancet Oncol.* (2019) 20:1083–97. doi: 10.1016/S1470-2045(19)30274-8
233. Mott KR, Gate D, Matundan HH, Ghiasi YN, Town T, Ghiasi H. CD8+ T cells play a bystander role in mice latently infected with herpes simplex virus 1. *J Virol.* (2016) 90:5059–67. doi: 10.1128/JVI.00255-16
234. Zang X, Loke P, Kim J, Murphy K, Waitz R, Allison JP. B7x: a widely expressed B7 family member that inhibits T cell activation. *Proc Natl Acad Sci USA.* (2003) 100:10388–92. doi: 10.1073/pnas.1434299100
235. Zou W, Chen L. Inhibitory B7-family molecules in the tumour microenvironment. *Nat Rev Immunol.* (2008) 8:467–77. doi: 10.1038/nri2326
236. Genova C, Boccardo S, Mora M, Rijavec E, Biello F, Rossi G, et al. Correlation between B7-H4 and survival of non-small-cell lung cancer patients treated with nivolumab. *J Clin Med.* (2019) 8:1566. doi: 10.3390/jcm8101566
237. Ott PA, Hu Z, Keskin DB, Shukla SA, Sun J, Bozym DJ, et al. An immunogenic personal neoantigen vaccine for patients with melanoma. *Nature.* (2017) 547:217–21.
238. Son CH, Bae JH, Shin DY, Lee HR, Choi YJ, Jo WS, et al. CTLA-4 blockade enhances antitumor immunity of intratumoral injection of immature dendritic cells into irradiated tumor in a mouse colon cancer model. *J Immunother.* (2014) 37:1–7. doi: 10.1097/CJI.0000000000000007
239. Chaput N, Lepage P, Coutzac C, Soularue E, Le Roux K, Monot C, et al. Baseline gut microbiota predicts clinical response and colitis in metastatic melanoma patients treated with ipilimumab. *Ann Oncol.* (2019) 30:2012. doi: 10.1093/annonc/mdz224
240. Gopalakrishnan V, Spencer CN, Nezi L, Reuben A, Andrews MC, Karpinets TV, et al. Gut microbiome modulates response to anti-PD-1 immunotherapy in melanoma patients. *Science.* (2018) 359:97–103.
241. Matson V, Fessler J, Bao R, Chongsuwat T, Zha Y, Alegre ML, et al. The commensal microbiome is associated with anti-PD-1 efficacy in metastatic melanoma patients. *Science.* (2018) 359:104–8. doi: 10.1126/science.aao3290
242. Derosa L, Routy B, Fidelle M, Iebba V, Alla L, Pasolli E, et al. Gut bacteria composition drives primary resistance to cancer immunotherapy in renal cell carcinoma patients. *Eur Urol.* (2020) 78:195–206. doi: 10.1016/j.eururo.2020.04.044
243. Vetizou M, Pitt JM, Daillere R, Lepage P, Waldschmitt N, Flament C, et al. Anticancer immunotherapy by CTLA-4 blockade relies on the gut microbiota. *Science.* (2015) 350:1079–84. doi: 10.1126/science.aad1329
244. Routy B, Le Chatelier E, Derosa L, Duong CPM, Alou MT, Daillere R, et al. Gut microbiome influences efficacy of PD-1-based immunotherapy against epithelial tumors. *Science.* (2018) 359:91–7.
245. Pitt JM, Vetizou M, Daillere R, Roberti MP, Yamazaki T, Routy B, et al. Resistance mechanisms to immune-checkpoint blockade in cancer: tumor-intrinsic and -extrinsic factors. *Immunity.* (2016) 44:1255–69. doi: 10.1016/j.immuni.2016.06.001
246. Sivan A, Corrales L, Hubert N, Williams JB, Aquino-Michaels K, Earley ZM, et al. Commensal Bifidobacterium promotes antitumor immunity and facilitates anti-PD-L1 efficacy. *Science.* (2015) 350:1084–9. doi: 10.1126/science.aac4255
247. Tanoue T, Morita S, Plichta DR, Skelly AN, Suda W, Sugiura Y, et al. A defined commensal consortium elicits CD8 T cells and anti-cancer immunity. *Nature.* (2019) 565:600–5. doi: 10.1038/s41586-019-0878-z
248. Kim YG, Udayanga KG, Totsuka N, Weinberg JB, Nunez G, Shibuya A. Gut dysbiosis promotes M2 macrophage polarization and allergic airway inflammation via fungi-induced PGE(2). *Cell Host Microbe.* (2014) 15:95–102. doi: 10.1016/j.chom.2013.12.010
249. Chaput N, Lepage P, Coutzac C, Soularue E, Le Roux K, Monot C, et al. Baseline gut microbiota predicts clinical response and colitis in metastatic melanoma patients treated with ipilimumab. *Ann Oncol.* (2017) 28:1368–79. doi: 10.1093/annonc/mdx108
250. Round JL, Mazmanian SK. Inducible Foxp3+ regulatory T-cell development by a commensal bacterium of the intestinal microbiota. *Proc Natl Acad Sci USA.* (2010) 107:12204–9. doi: 10.1073/pnas.0909122107
251. Cremonesi E, Governa V, Garzon JFG, Mele V, Amicarella F, Muraro MG, et al. Gut microbiota modulate T cell trafficking into human colorectal cancer. *Gut.* (2018) 67:1984–94. doi: 10.1158/1538-7445.AM2018-1001
252. Pushalkar S, Hundeyin M, Daley D, Zambirinis CP, Kurz E, Mishra A, et al. The pancreatic cancer microbiome promotes oncogenesis by induction of innate and adaptive immune suppression. *Cancer Discov.* (2018) 8:403–16. doi: 10.1158/2159-8290.CD-17-1134
253. Kadosh E, Snir-Alkalay I, Venkatachalam A, May S, Lasry A, Elyada E, et al. The gut microbiome switches mutant p53 from tumour-suppressive to oncogenic. *Nature.* (2020) 586:133–38. doi: 10.1038/s41586-020-2541-0
254. Derosa L, Hellmann MD, Spaziano M, Halpenny D, Fidelle M, Rizvi H, et al. Negative association of antibiotics on clinical activity of immune checkpoint inhibitors in patients with advanced renal cell and non-small-cell lung cancer. *Ann Oncol.* (2018) 29:1437–44. doi: 10.1093/annonc/mdy103
255. Suez J, Zmora N, Zilberman-Schapira G, Mor U, Dori-Bachash M, Bashiardes S, et al. Post-antibiotic gut mucosal microbiome reconstitution is impaired by probiotics and improved by autologous FMT. *Cell.* (2018) 174:1406–23.e16. doi: 10.1016/j.cell.2018.08.047
256. Vangay P, Ward T, Gerber JS, Knights D. Antibiotics, pediatric dysbiosis, and disease. *Cell Host Microbe.* (2015) 17:553–64. doi: 10.1016/j.chom.2015.04.006
257. Tamburini S, Shen N, Wu HC, Clemente JC. The microbiome in early life: implications for health outcomes. *Nat Med.* (2016) 22:713–22. doi: 10.1038/nm.4142
258. Routy B, Gopalakrishnan V, Daillere R, Zitvogel L, Wargo JA, Kroemer G. The gut microbiota influences anticancer immunosurveillance and general health. *Nat Rev Clin Oncol.* (2018) 15:382–96. doi: 10.1038/s41571-018-0006-2
259. Viaud S, Saccheri F, Mignot G, Yamazaki T, Daillere R, Hannani D, et al. The intestinal microbiota modulates the anticancer immune effects of cyclophosphamide. *Science.* (2013) 342:971–6. doi: 10.1126/science.1240537
260. Daillere R, Vetizou M, Waldschmitt N, Yamazaki T, Isnard C, Poirier-Colame V, et al. Enterococcus hirae and barnesiella intestinihominis facilitate cyclophosphamide-induced therapeutic immunomodulatory effects. *Immunity.* (2016) 45:931–43. doi: 10.1016/j.immuni.2016.09.009
261. Iida N, Dzutsev A, Stewart CA, Smith L, Bouladoux N, Weingarten RA, et al. Commensal bacteria control cancer response to therapy by modulating the tumor microenvironment. *Science.* (2013) 342:967–70. doi: 10.1126/science.1240527
262. Bullman S, Pedamallu CS, Sicinska E, Clancy TE, Zhang X, Cai D, et al. Analysis of Fusobacterium persistence and antibiotic response in colorectal cancer. *Science.* (2017) 358:1443–8. doi: 10.1126/science.aal5240
263. Coutinho AE, Chapman KE. The anti-inflammatory and immunosuppressive effects of glucocorticoids, recent developments and mechanistic insights. *Mol Cell Endocrinol.* (2011) 335:2–13. doi: 10.1016/j.mce.2010.04.005
264. Schadendorf D, Wolchok JD, Hodi FS, Chiarion-Sileni V, Gonzalez R, Rutkowski P, et al. Efficacy and safety outcomes in patients with advanced melanoma who discontinued treatment with nivolumab and ipilimumab

because of adverse events: a pooled analysis of randomized phase II and III trials. *J Clin Oncol.* (2017) 35:3807–14. doi: 10.1200/JCO.2017.73.2289

265. Horvat TZ, Adel NG, Dang TO, Momtaz P, Postow MA, Callahan MK, et al. Immune-related adverse events, need for systemic immunosuppression, and effects on survival and time to treatment failure in patients with melanoma treated with ipilimumab at memorial sloan kettering cancer center. *J Clin Oncol.* (2015) 33:3193–8. doi: 10.1200/JCO.2015.60.8448
266. Mahata B, Zhang X, Kolodziejczyk AA, Proserpio V, Haim-Vilmovsky L, Taylor AE, et al. Single-cell RNA sequencing reveals T helper cells synthesizing steroids de novo to contribute to immune homeostasis. *Cell Rep.* (2014) 7:1130–42. doi: 10.1016/j.celrep.2014.04.011
267. Planchard D, Popat S, Kerr K, Novello S, Smit EF, Faivre-Finn C, et al. Metastatic non-small cell lung cancer: ESMO clinical practice guidelines for diagnosis, treatment and follow-up. *Ann Oncol.* (2018) 29(Suppl. 4):iv192–237. doi: 10.1093/annonc/mdy275
268. Fuca G, Galli G, Poggi M, Lo Russo G, Proto C, Imbimbo M, et al. Modulation of peripheral blood immune cells by early use of steroids and its association with clinical outcomes in patients with metastatic non-small cell lung cancer treated with immune checkpoint inhibitors. *ESMO Open.* (2019) 4:e000457. doi: 10.1136/esmoopen-2018-000457
269. Della Corte CM, Morgillo F. Early use of steroids affects immune cells and impairs immunotherapy efficacy. *ESMO Open.* (2019) 4:e000477. doi: 10.1136/esmoopen-2018-000477
270. Vijayan D, Young A, Teng MWL, Smyth MJ. Targeting immunosuppressive adenosine in cancer. *Nat Rev Cancer.* (2017) 17:709–24. doi: 10.1038/nrc.2017.86
271. Renner K, Singer K, Koehl GE, Geissler EK, Peter K, Siska PJ, et al. Metabolic hallmarks of tumor and immune cells in the tumor microenvironment. *Front Immunol.* (2017) 8:248. doi: 10.3389/fimmu.2017.00248
272. De Rosa V, Di Rella F, Di Giacomo A, Matarese G. Regulatory T cells as suppressors of anti-tumor immunity: role of metabolism. *Cytokine Growth Factor Rev.* (2017) 35:15–25. doi: 10.1016/j.cytogfr.2017.04.001
273. Soldati L, Di Renzo L, Jirillo E, Ascierto PA, Marincola FM, De Lorenzo A. The influence of diet on anti-cancer immune responsiveness. *J Transl Med.* (2018) 16:75. doi: 10.1186/s12967-018-1448-0
274. Qu X, Tang Y, Hua S. Immunological approaches towards cancer and inflammation: a cross talk. *Front Immunol.* (2018) 9:563. doi: 10.3389/fimmu.2018.00563
275. Maccio A, Madeddu C. Blocking inflammation to improve immunotherapy of advanced cancer. *Immunology.* (2020) 159:357–64. doi: 10.1111/imm.13164
276. June CH, Warshauer JT, Bluestone JA. Is autoimmunity the Achilles' heel of cancer immunotherapy? *Nat Med.* (2017) 23:540–7. doi: 10.1038/nm.4321
277. Caspi RR. Immunotherapy of autoimmunity and cancer: the penalty for success. *Nat Rev Immunol.* (2008) 8:970–6. doi: 10.1038/nri2438
278. Mo J, Hu X, Gu L, Chen B, Khadaroo PA, Shen Z, et al. Smokers or non-smokers: who benefits more from immune checkpoint inhibitors in treatment of malignancies? An up-to-date meta-analysis. *World J Surg Oncol.* (2020) 18:15. doi: 10.1186/s12957-020-1792-4
279. Li B, Huang X, Fu L. Impact of smoking on efficacy of PD-1/PD-L1 inhibitors in non-small cell lung cancer patients: a meta-analysis. *Onco Targets Ther.* (2018) 11:3691–6. doi: 10.2147/OTT.S156421
280. Lee CK, Man J, Lord S, Cooper W, Links M, Gebski V, et al. Clinical and molecular characteristics associated with survival among patients treated with checkpoint inhibitors for advanced non-small cell lung carcinoma: a systematic review and meta-analysis. *JAMA Oncol.* (2018) 4:210–6. doi: 10.1001/jamaoncol.2017.4427
281. Abdel-Rahman O. Smoking and EGFR status may predict outcomes of advanced NSCLC treated with PD-(L)1 inhibitors beyond first line: a meta-analysis. *Clin Respir J.* (2018) 12:1809–19. doi: 10.1111/crj.12742
282. Ng TL, Liu Y, Dimou A, Patil T, Aisner DL, Dong Z, et al. Predictive value of oncogenic driver subtype, programmed death-1 ligand (PD-L1) score, and smoking status on the efficacy of PD-1/PD-L1 inhibitors in patients with oncogene-driven non-small cell lung cancer. *Cancer.* (2019) 125:1038–49. doi: 10.1002/cncr.31871
283. Kerdidani D, Magkouta S, Chouvardas P, Karavana V, Glynos K, Roumelioti F, et al. Cigarette smoke-induced emphysema exhausts early Cytotoxic CD8(+) T cell responses against nascent lung cancer cells. *J Immunol.* (2018) 201:1558–69. doi: 10.4049/jimmunol.1700700
284. Wang GZ, Zhang L, Zhao XC, Gao SH, Qu LW, Yu H, et al. The Aryl hydrocarbon receptor mediates tobacco-induced PD-L1 expression and is associated with response to immunotherapy. *Nat Commun.* (2019) 10:1125. doi: 10.1038/s41467-019-08887-7
285. Gettinger SN, Choi J, Mani N, Sanmamed MF, Datar I, Sowell R, et al. A dormant TIL phenotype defines non-small cell lung carcinomas sensitive to immune checkpoint blockers. *Nat Commun.* (2018) 9:3196. doi: 10.1038/s41467-018-05032-8
286. Inamura K, Yokouchi Y, Kobayashi M, Sakakibara R, Ninomiya H, Subat S, et al. Tumor B7-H3 (CD276) expression and smoking history in relation to lung adenocarcinoma prognosis. *Lung Cancer.* (2017) 103:44–51. doi: 10.1016/j.lungcan.2016.11.013
287. Hato SV, Khong A, de Vries IJ, Lesterhuis WJ. Molecular pathways: the immunogenic effects of platinum-based chemotherapeutics. *Clin Cancer Res.* (2014) 20:2831–7. doi: 10.1158/1078-0432.CCR-13-3141
288. Zitvogel L, Kepp O, Kroemer G. Immune parameters affecting the efficacy of chemotherapeutic regimens. *Nat Rev Clin Oncol.* (2011) 8:151–60. doi: 10.1038/nrclinonc.2010.223
289. van der Most RG, Currie AJ, Mahendran S, Prosser A, Darabi A, Robinson BW, et al. Tumor eradication after cyclophosphamide depends on concurrent depletion of regulatory T cells: a role for cycling TNFR2-expressing effector-suppressor T cells in limiting effective chemotherapy. *Cancer Immunol Immunother.* (2009) 58:1219–28. doi: 10.1007/s00262-008-0628-9
290. Kepp O, Galluzzi L, Martins I, Schlemmer F, Adjemian S, Michaud M, et al. Molecular determinants of immunogenic cell death elicited by anticancer chemotherapy. *Cancer Metastasis Rev.* (2011) 30:61–9. doi: 10.1007/s10555-011-9273-4
291. Emens LA, Middleton G. The interplay of immunotherapy and chemotherapy: harnessing potential synergies. *Cancer Immunol Res.* (2015) 3:436–43. doi: 10.1158/2326-6066.CIR-15-0064
292. Chen G, Emens LA. Chemoimmunotherapy: reengineering tumor immunity. *Cancer Immunol Immunother.* (2013) 62:203–16. doi: 10.1007/s00262-012-1388-0
293. Horn L, Mansfield AS, Szczesna A, Havel L, Krzakowski M, Hochmair MJ, et al. First-line atezolizumab plus chemotherapy in extensive-stage small-cell lung cancer. *N Engl J Med.* (2018) 379:2220–9. doi: 10.1056/NEJMoa1809064
294. Wang Y, Deng W, Li N, Neri S, Sharma A, Jiang W, et al. Combining immunotherapy and radiotherapy for cancer treatment: current challenges and future directions. *Front Pharmacol.* (2018) 9:185. doi: 10.3389/fphar.2018.00185
295. Demaria S, Golden EB, Formenti SC. Role of local radiation therapy in cancer immunotherapy. *JAMA Oncol.* (2015) 1:1325–32. doi: 10.1001/jamaoncol.2015.2756
296. Deng L, Liang H, Burnette B, Beckett M, Darga T, Weichselbaum RR, et al. Irradiation and anti-PD-L1 treatment synergistically promote antitumor immunity in mice. *J Clin Invest.* (2014) 124:687–95. doi: 10.1172/JCI67313
297. Twyman-Saint Victor C, Rech AJ, Maity A, Rengan R, Pauken KE, Stelekati E, et al. Radiation and dual checkpoint blockade activate non-redundant immune mechanisms in cancer. *Nature.* (2015) 520:373–7. doi: 10.1038/nature14292
298. Antonia SJ, Villegas A, Daniel D, Vicente D, Murakami S, Hui R, et al. Overall survival with durvalumab after chemoradiotherapy in stage III NSCLC. *N Engl J Med.* (2018) 379:2342–50. doi: 10.1056/NEJMoa1809697
299. Saha A, Chatterjee SK. Combination of CTL-associated antigen-4 blockade and depletion of CD25 regulatory T cells enhance tumour immunity of dendritic cell-based vaccine in a mouse model of colon cancer. *Scand J Immunol.* (2010) 71:70–82. doi: 10.1111/j.1365-3083.2009.02355.x
300. Gibney GT, Kudchadkar RR, DeConti RC, Thebeau MS, Czupryn MP, Tetteh L, et al. Safety, correlative markers, and clinical results of adjuvant nivolumab in combination with vaccine in resected high-risk metastatic melanoma. *Clin Cancer Res.* (2015) 21:712–20. doi: 10.1158/1078-0432.CCR-14-2468
301. Guo ZS, Liu Z, Bartlett DL. Oncolytic immunotherapy: dying the right way is a key to eliciting potent antitumor immunity. *Front Oncol.* (2014) 4:74. doi: 10.3389/fonc.2014.00074
302. Puzanov I, Milhem MM, Minor D, Hamid O, Li A, Chen L, et al. Talimogene laherparepvec in combination with ipilimumab in previously untreated,

unresectable stage IIIB-IV melanoma. *J Clin Oncol.* (2016) 34:2619–26. doi: 10.1200/JCO.2016.67.1529

303. O'Donnell JS, Massi D, Teng MWL, Mandala M. PI3K-AKT-mTOR inhibition in cancer immunotherapy, redux. *Semin Cancer Biol.* (2018) 48:91–103. doi: 10.1016/j.semcancer.2017.04.015
304. Ebert PJR, Cheung J, Yang Y, McNamara E, Hong R, Moskalenko M, et al. MAP kinase inhibition promotes T cell and anti-tumor activity in combination with PD-L1 checkpoint blockade. *Immunity.* (2016) 44:609–21. doi: 10.1016/j.immuni.2016.01.024
305. Ribas A, Lawrence D, Atkinson V, Agarwal S, Miller WH Jr., Carlino MS, et al. Combined BRAF and MEK inhibition with PD-1 blockade immunotherapy in BRAF-mutant melanoma. *Nat Med.* (2019) 25:936–40. doi: 10.1038/s41591-019-0476-5
306. Cho BC, Bahary N, Bendell J, Felip E, Johnson M, Kang Y-K, et al. Abstract CT201: phase Ib/II open-label, randomized evaluation of atezolizumab + cobimetinib vs control in MORPHEUS-NSCLC (non-small cell lung cancer), MORPHEUS-PDAC (pancreatic ductal adenocarcinoma) and MORPHEUS-GC (gastric cancer). *American Association for Cancer Research (AACR) Virtual Annual Meeting 2020.* (2020). doi: 10.1158/1538-7445.AM2020-CT201
307. Vikas P, Borcherding N, Chennamadhavuni A, Garje R. Therapeutic potential of combining PARP inhibitor and immunotherapy in solid tumors. *Front Oncol.* (2020) 10:570. doi: 10.3389/fonc.2020.00570
308. Vagia E, Viveiros P, Kang C-Y, Nelson V, Kalyan A, Kircher S, et al. Abstract CT157: phase I/Ib study of nivolumab and veliparib in patients with advanced solid tumors and lymphoma harboring mutations in selected DNA repair genes. *American Association for Cancer Research (AACR) Virtual Annual Meeting 2020.* (2020). doi: 10.1158/1538-7445.AM2020-CT157
309. Yap TA, Dhawan M, Hendifar AE, Miao M, Owonikoko TK, Quintela-Fandino M, et al. Abstract CT269: a phase 2 study of olaparib in combination with pembrolizumab in patients with previously treated advanced solid tumors with homologous recombination repair mutation (HRRm) and/or Homologous recombination repair deficiency (HDR): KEYLYNK-007. *American Association for Cancer Research (AACR) Virtual Annual Meeting 2020.* (2020). doi: 10.1158/1538-7445.AM2020-CT269
310. Wolchok JD, Saenger Y. The mechanism of anti-CTLA-4 activity and the negative regulation of T-cell activation. *Oncologist.* (2008) 13(Suppl. 4):2–9. doi: 10.1634/theoncologist.13-S4-2
311. Blake SJ, Ching AL, Kenna TJ, Galea R, Large J, Yagita H, et al. Blockade of PD-1/PD-L1 promotes adoptive T-cell immunotherapy in a tolerogenic environment. *PLoS One.* (2015) 10:e0119483. doi: 10.1371/journal.pone.0119483
312. Houot R, Schultz LM, Marabelle A, Kohrt H. T-cell-based Immunotherapy: adoptive cell transfer and checkpoint inhibition. *Cancer Immunol Res.* (2015) 3:1115–22. doi: 10.1158/2326-6066.CIR-15-0190
313. Dahlen E, Veitonmaki N, Norlen P. Bispecific antibodies in cancer immunotherapy. *Ther Adv Vaccines Immunother.* (2018) 6:3–17. doi: 10.1177/2515135518763280
314. Chen Y, Ramjiawan RR, Reiberger T, Ng MR, Hato T, Huang Y, et al. CXCR4 inhibition in tumor microenvironment facilitates anti-programmed death receptor-1 immunotherapy in sorafenib-treated hepatocellular carcinoma in mice. *Hepatology.* (2015) 61:1591–602. doi: 10.1002/hep.27665
315. Reck M, Mok TSK, Nishio M, Jotte RM, Cappuzzo F, Orlandi F, et al. Atezolizumab plus bevacizumab and chemotherapy in non-small-cell lung cancer (IMpower150): key subgroup analyses of patients with EGFR mutations or baseline liver metastases in a randomised, open-label phase 3 trial. *Lancet Respir Med.* (2019) 7:387–401. doi: 10.1016/S2213-2600(19)30084-0
316. Johnson BE, Kim TM, Hiltermann TJN, Barlesi F, Grohe C, Goto Y, et al. Abstract CT214: CANOPY-1: safety run-in results from phase (ph) 3 study of canakinumab (CAN) or placebo (PBO) in combination (comb) with pembrolizumab (PEM) plus platinum-based doublet chemotherapy (Ctx) as 1st line therapy in patients (pts) with advanced or metastatic NSCLC. *American Association for Cancer Research (AACR) Virtual Annual Meeting 2020.* (2020). doi: 10.1158/1538-7445.AM2020-CT214
317. Lee JM, Garrido P, Kim ES, Arslan C, Pujol J-L, Song Y, et al. Abstract CT192: randomized phase II study of canakinumab (CAN) or pembrolizumab (PEM) alone or in combination as neoadjuvant therapy in patients (Pts) with surgically resected (Stage IB-IIIA) non-small cell lung cancer (NSCLC): CANOPY-N. *American Association for Cancer Research (AACR) Virtual Annual Meeting 2020.* (2020). doi: 10.1158/1538-7445.AM2020-CT192
318. Mahoney KM, Rennert PD, Freeman GJ. Combination cancer immunotherapy and new immunomodulatory targets. *Nat Rev Drug Discov.* (2015) 14:561–84. doi: 10.1038/nrd4591
319. Hu-Lieskovan S, Ribas A. New combination strategies using programmed cell death 1/programmed cell death ligand 1 checkpoint inhibitors as a backbone. *Cancer J.* (2017) 23:10–22. doi: 10.1097/PPO.0000000000000246
320. Kwiatkowska D, Kluska P, Reich A. Beyond PD-1 immunotherapy in malignant melanoma. *Dermatol Ther (Heidelb).* (2019) 9:243–57. doi: 10.1007/s13555-019-0292-3
321. Forster M, Felip E, Doger B, Majem M, Carcereny E, Peguero J, et al. Abstract CT202: initial results from a phase II study (TACTI-002) in metastatic non-small cell lung or head and neck carcinoma patients receiving eftilagimod alpha (soluble lag-3 protein) and pembrolizumab. *American Association for Cancer Research (AACR) Virtual Annual Meeting 2020.* (2020). doi: 10.1158/1538-7445.AM2020-CT202
322. FIERCE Biotech *SITC18: Merck Highlights New LAG-3 and TIGIT Data. [Press Release].* (2019). Available online at: https://www.fiercebiotech.com/biotech/sitc-merck-highlights-new-lag-3-and-tigit-data (accessed September 21, 2019).
323. Bendell JC, Bedard P, Bang Y-J, LoRusso P, Hodi S, Gordon M, et al. Abstract CT302: phase Ia/Ib dose-escalation study of the anti-TIGIT antibody tiragolumab as a single agent and in combination with atezolizumab in patients with advanced solid tumors. *American Association for Cancer Research (AACR) Virtual Annual Meeting 2020.* (2020). doi: 10.1158/1538-7445.AM2020-CT302
324. Rodriguez-Abreu D, Johnson ML, Hussein MA, Cobo M, Patel AJ, Secen NM, et al. Abstract 9503: primary analysis of a randomized, double-blind, phase II study of the anti-TIGIT antibody tiragolumab (tira) plus atezolizumab (atezo) versus placebo plus atezo as first-line (1L) treatment in patients with PD-L1-selected NSCLC (CITYSCAPE). *American Society of Clinical Oncology (ASCO) Virtual Annual Meeting 2020: Journal of Clincal Oncology.* (2020). doi: 10.1200/JCO.2020.38.15_suppl.9503
325. Chen X, Song X, Li K, Zhang T. FcgammaR-binding is an important functional attribute for immune checkpoint antibodies in cancer immunotherapy. *Front Immunol.* (2019) 10:292. doi: 10.3389/fimmu.2019.00292
326. Yachnin J, Ullenhag GJ, Carneiro A, Nielsen DL, Rohrberg KS, Kvarnhammar AM, et al. Abstract CT145: a first-in-human phase 1 study in patients with advanced and/or refractory solid malignancies to evaluate the safety of ATOR-1015, a CTLA-4 x OX40 bispecific antibody. *American Association for Cancer Research (AACR) Virtual Annual Meeting 2020.* (2020). doi: 10.1158/1538-7445.AM2020-CT145
327. Postel-Vinay S, Lam VK, Ros W, Bauer TM, Hansen AR, Cho DC, et al. Abstract CT150: a first-in-human phase I study of the OX40 agonist GSK3174998 (GSK998) +/- pembrolizumab in patients (Pts) with selected advanced solid tumors (ENGAGE-1). *American Association for Cancer Research (AACR) Virtual Annual Meeting 2020.* (2020). doi: 10.1158/1538-7445.AM2020-CT150
328. Jimeno A, Gupta S, Sullivan R, Do KT, Akerley WL, Wang D, et al. Abstract CT032: a phase 1/2, open-label, multicenter, dose escalation and efficacy study of mRNA-2416, a lipid nanoparticle encapsulated mRNA encoding human OX40L, for intratumoral injection alone or in combination with durvalumab for patients with advanced malignancies. *American Association for Cancer Research (AACR) Virtual Annual Meeting 2020.* (2020). doi: 10.1158/1538-7445.AM2020-CT032

22

Use of Pralsetinib as Neoadjuvant Therapy for Non-Small Cell Lung Cancer Patient with RET Rearrangement

Ning Zhou[1,2†], Tong Li[1,2†], Maoli Liang[3†], Fan Ren[1,2], Hong Ni[1,2], Wei Liu[4], Tao Shi[5], Dongbo Xu[6], Qiusong Chen[7], Haonan Yu[7], Zuoqing Song[1,2], Lingling Zu[1,2], Shuo Li[3] and Song Xu[1,2*]*

[1] Department of Lung Cancer Surgery, Tianjin Medical University General Hospital, Tianjin, China, [2] Tianjin Key Laboratory of Lung Cancer Metastasis and Tumor Microenvironment, Lung Cancer Institute, Tianjin Medical University General Hospital, Tianjin, China, [3] Department of Respiratory and Critical Care, Tianjin Medical University General Hospital, Tianjin, China, [4] Department of Respiratory Medicine, Second Affiliated Hospital of Tianjin University of Traditional Chinese Medicine, Tianjin, China, [5] Precision Medicine Center, Tianjin Medical University General Hospital, Tianjin, China, [6] Department of Pathology, Tianjin Medical University General Hospital, Tianjin, China, [7] Department of PET/CT Diagnostic, Tianjin Medical University General Hospital, Tianjin, China

***Correspondence:**
Song Xu
xusong198@hotmail.com
Shuo Li
leasure1979@163.com

†These authors have contributed equally to this work

RET rearrangements are rare, and occur in 1%-2% of all non-small cell lung cancer (NSCLC) patients. Pralsetinib has a significant anti-tumor effect in patients with advanced NSCLC and a RET rearrangement. Previous studies have confirmed the efficiency of neoadjuvant target thorapy for NSCLC. Herein we present a case involving a female patient who was diagnosed with stage IIIA lung adenocarcinoma and harbored a KIF5B-RET rearrangement based on next-generation sequencing. Radiologic downstaging was indicated after pralsetinib treatment. Therefore, a right lower lobectomy and systemic lymphadenectomy were successfully performed. The postoperative pathologic results revealed a response rate of 74% for primary tumor and no residual viable tumor cells were observed in lymph nodes. The tumor, nodes, and metastases (TNM) stage was ypT1cN1M0. The tumor micro-environment (TME) of the primary tumor was also assessed.

Keywords: RET, pralsetinib, locally advanced (stage III) non-small cell lung cancer, neoadjuvant, targeted therapy

INTRODUCTION

The RET gene was identified as a proto-oncogene in 1985 (1). The RET gene is associated with normal embryonic development (2). RET fusions are rare, occurring in 1%-2% of all patients with non-small cell lung cancer (NSCLC) (3). Patients with RET fusions are prone to brain metastases (4). Because RET fusions occur in lung cancer, RET-targeted therapy has been attempted by clinicians. Unfortunately, the efficacy of some multi-targeted tyrosine kinase inhibitors (TKIs) was not satisfactory, including vandetanib, cabozantinib, and lenvatinib (5). Pralsetinib had a significant effect in patients with advanced NSCLC; specifically, the response rate was 61% (6). Pralsetinib was approved by the Food and Drug Administration (FDA) for treating RET fusion-positive NSCLC in

2020. Several studies have verified the availability of neoadjuvant-targeted therapy for NSCLC patients with ROS1, ALK, and epidermal growth factor receptor (EGFR) alterations (7–9); however, there are no reports regarding pralsetinib as neoadjuvant treatment for NSCLC patients with a RET rearrangement.

CASE REPORT

A 54-year-old female never-smoker was admitted to the hospital for evaluation of a non-productive cough with bloody phlegm for 1 year and persistent chest and back pain for 1 month. Enhanced computed tomography (CT) revealed a mass with a diameter of 42 mm located in the right lower lung with enlarged mediastinal and hilar lymph nodes (stations 2, 4, 7, and 10). The CT findings were confirmed by 18F-fluorodeoxyglucose (FDG) positron emission tomography (PET) as cT2bN2M0, IIIA (AJCC, 8th edition; **Figure 1**). A bronchoscopic biopsy was performed and the pathologic examination revealed that the right lung lesion was a lung adenocarcinoma. We further performed next-generation sequencing (NGS) with a 520-gene panel; a KIF5B-RET fusion was detected. Plasma ctDNA for the RET mutation was also positive with a frequency of 0.15%. After a multiple disciplinary team (MDT) discussion, the patient was diagnosed with a resectable stage IIIA lung adenocarcinoma. Based on the NGS results, we recommended neoadjuvant treatment followed by surgical resection. After obtaining informed consent from the patient, we prescribed pralsetinib at a dosage of 400 mg per day. After 1 month of treatment, a chest CT scan revealed significant shrinkage of the lung tumor (**Figure 1**). A PET-CT scan exhibited significantly decreased F18-FDG uptake in the tumor and no uptake in the hilar and mediastinal lymph nodes (**Figure 1**). In addition, the plasma ctDNA level was also tested, and we showed that the plasma ctDNA was cleared after neoadjuvant treatment (**Figure 2**). During the treatment of pralsetinib, some treatment-related adverse effects were observed, including mild edema and fatigue and moderately increased blood pressure.

Considering that radiologic downstaging was indicated, a right lower lobectomy and systemic lymphadenectomy were successfully performed 1 week after the last dose of pralsetinib (**Figure 1**). Severe adhesions were noted intraoperatively. The postoperative pathologic results showed that although the Ki67 index was significantly decreased, 26% of the tumor cells were still alive in the primary tumor bed however no residual viable tumor cells were observed in lymph nodes. Microscopically, a large number of lymphocytes were infiltrated together with some plasma cells and neutrophils. The lymphatic follicles were formed. Foam cell reactions and cholesterol crystals were observed as well as necrosis and fibrosis. To investigate the change in tumor microenvironment (TME), especially inflammatory and immune cells before and after pralsetinib neoadjuvant treatment, multiple immunohistochemistry (mIHC) staining (Genecast Biotechnology, Wuxi, Jiangsu, China) on the biopsy tissue and surgical sample was performed. The CD68+

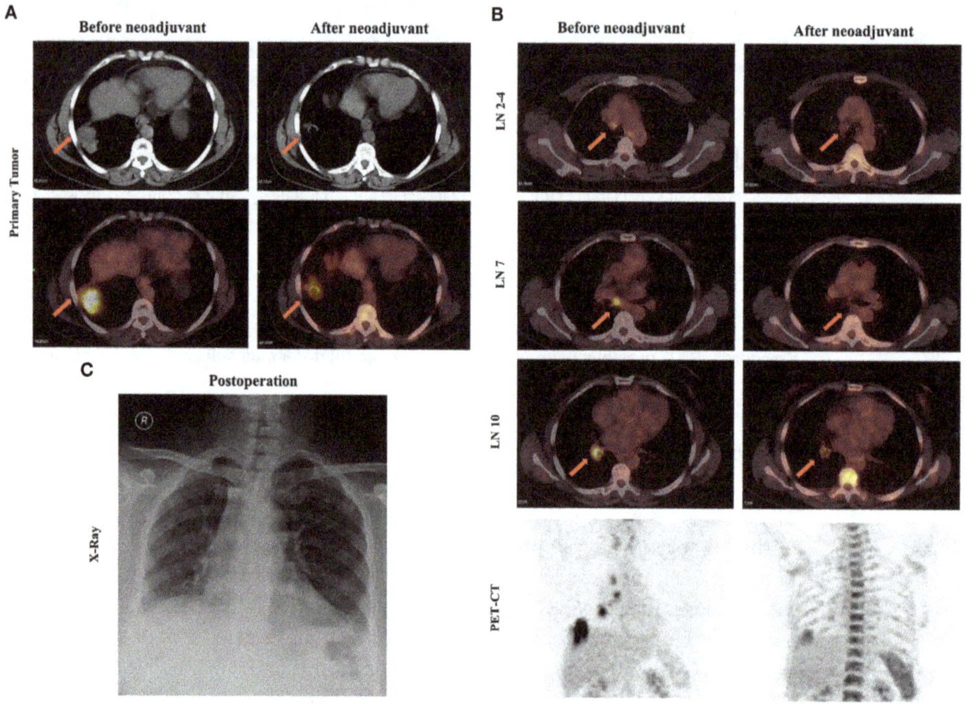

FIGURE 1 | Images before and after neoadjuvant pralsetinib treatment. **(A)** Enhanced CT and PET-CT of the primary tumor. **(B)** PET-CT of the mediastinal lymph nodes and the chest. **(C)** X-ray after surgery.

CD163+ cell population was significantly increased, whereas the proportion of CD8+ T lymphocytes was decreased (**Figure 2**). PD-L1 expression were also decreased after neoadjuvant treatment (**Figure 2**). The patient received four cycles of pemetrexed (500mg/m^2, d1) and cisplatin (75mg/m^2, d1) every 21 days in the adjuvant settings due to the unaffordable economic burden of pralsetinib.

DISCUSSION

In recent years the benefit of neoadjuvant-targeted therapies for EGFR- and ALK-driven NSCLC patients has been identified (10). To our knowledge, this is the first case of neoadjuvant pralsetinib for NSCLC patients with a RET fusion. In our case pralsetinib exhibited a significant response in a patient with NSCLC and an RET fusion and transformed the unresectable tumor into a resectable tumor; however, 26% of the tumor cells were still alive after pralsetinib neoadjuvant treatment, indicating the necessity of complete resection.

In the current study, we also performed mIHC to determine the changes in TME before and after pralsetinib neoadjuvant treatment. The staining data demonstrated that the proportion of M1 macrophages was upregulated, while the number of CD8+ tumor infiltrating lymphocytes (TILs) and the level of PD-L1 expression were decreased significantly after neoadjuvant treatment. Significant changes in other immune cells, such as natural killer (NK) cells, were not detected. The alteration of these factors indicates that the TME is less inflammatory after pralsetinib neoadjuvant treatment. A previous study suggested that high PD-L1 expression and an increased number of CD8+ TILs are related to clinical benefit in immunotherapy (11). In addition, M1 macrophages are thought to have a direct or indirect anti-tumor role (12). However, in our case, the increased proportion of M1 macrophages and decreased number of CD8+ TILs and PD-L1 expression obscured the role of immunotherapy in subsequent treatment. Further therapeutic strategies after resistance of pralsetinib treatment should be seriously considered.

In conclusion, our case, for the first time suggested that pralsetinib neoadjuvant treatment is feasible for locally advanced NSCLC patients with a RET rearrangement. This patient had an apparent radiologic downstaging after neoadjuvant treatment, which was an indication for complete resection. This case report, however, included one patient only. The role for pralsetinib in neoadjuvant treatment for locally advanced NSCLC and postoperative adjuvant-targeted therapy have not been established for early-stage NSCLC. For NSCLC patients with a RET rearrangement, additional clinical trials are

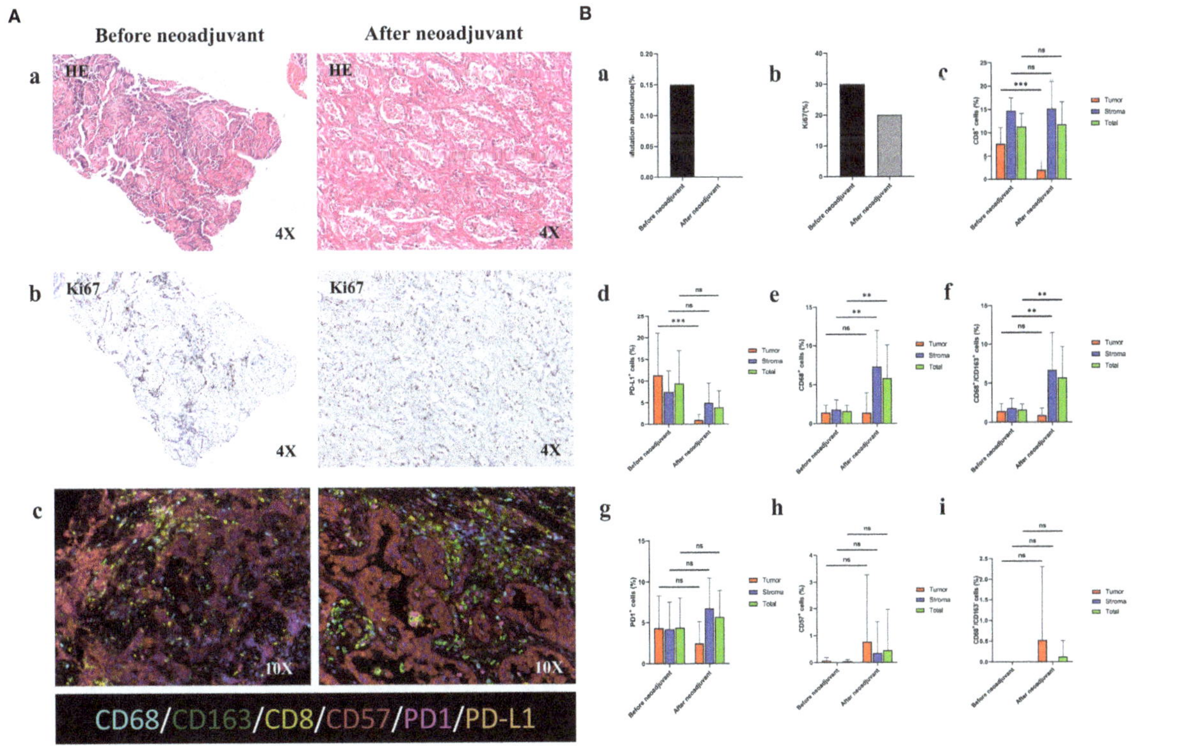

FIGURE 2 | Comprehensive pathological evaluation before and after neoadjuvant pralsetinib treatment. **(A)**. Histochemistry staining before and after neoadjuvant pralsetinib treatment. (a) Hematoxylin and eosin (HE) staining. (b) Ki67 staining. (c) Multiple immunohistochemistry staining on CD68, CD163, CD8, CD57, PD1 and PDL1. **(B)**. Quantitative analysis for plasma ctDNA and staining data. Quantitative analysis for plasma ctDNA (a), Ki67 staining (b), CD8+ (c), PD-L1+ (d), CD68+ (e), CD68+CD163+ (f), PD1+(g), CD57+ (h) and CD68+CD163 (i) cell population. **$p < 0.01$; ***$p < 0.001$; ns, not significant.

warranted to evaluate the effect of pralsetinib in locally advanced and early-stage NSCLC.

AUTHOR CONTRIBUTIONS

NZ: Data curation, Formal analysis, Writing- Original draft preparation. TL: Formal analysis, Writing- Original draft preparation. ML: Data curation, Writing- Original draft preparation. FR: Formal analysis. HN: Visualization. WL: Resources. TS: Resources. DX: Resources. QC: Resources. HY: Resources. ZS: Investigation. LZ: Investigation. SL: Conceptualization, Validation, Visualization. SX: Conceptualization, Methodology, Supervision, Writing- Reviewing and Editing. All authors contributed to the article and approved the submitted version.

REFERENCES

1. Gautschi O, Milia J, Filleron T, Wolf J, Carbone DP, Owen D, et al. Targeting RET in Patients With RET-Rearranged Lung Cancers: Results From the Global, Multicenter RET Registry. *J Clin Oncol* (2017) 35(13):1403–10. doi: 10.1200/JCO.2016.70.9352
2. Mulligan LM. RET Revisited: Expanding the Oncogenic Portfolio. *Nat Rev Cancer* (2014) 14(3):173–86. doi: 10.1038/nrc3680
3. Drilon A, Oxnard GR, Tan DSW, Loong HHF, Johnson M, Gainor J, et al. Efficacy of Selpercatinib in RET Fusion-Positive Non-Small-Cell Lung Cancer. *N Engl J Med* (2020) 383(9):813–24. doi: 10.1056/NEJMoa2005653
4. Drilon A, Lin JJ, Filleron T, Ni A, Milia J, Bergagnini I, et al. Frequency of Brain Metastases and Multikinase Inhibitor Outcomes in Patients With RET-Rearranged Lung Cancers. *J Thorac Oncol* (2018) 13:1595–601. doi: 10.1016/j.jtho.2018.07.004
5. Subbiah V, Shen T, Terzyan SS, Liu X, Hu X, Patel KP, et al. Structural Basis of Acquired Resistance to Selpercatinib and Pralsetinib Mediated by Non-Gatekeeper RET Mutations. *Ann Oncol* (2021) 32(2):261–8. doi: 10.1016/j.annonc.2020.10.599
6. Gainor JF, Curigliano G, Kim DW, Lee DH, Besse B, Baik CS, et al. Pralsetinib for RET Fusion-Positive Non-Small-Cell Lung Cancer (ARROW): A Multi-Cohort, Open-Label, Phase 1/2 Study. *Lancet Oncol* (2021) 22(7):959–69. doi: 10.1016/S1470-2045(21)00247-3
7. Zhao S, Zhu S, Lei X, Xu D, Shi T, Chen Q, et al. Use of Crizotinib as Neoadjuvant Therapy for Non-Small Cell Lung Cancers Patient With ROS1 Rearrangement: A Case Report. *Thorac Cancer* (2021) 12(20):2815–8. doi: 10.1111/1759-7714.14112
8. Zhong WZ, Chen KN, Chen C, Gu CD, Wang J, Yang XN, et al. Erlotinib Versus Gemcitabine Plus Cisplatin as Neoadjuvant Treatment of Stage IIIA-N2 EGFR-Mutant Non-Small-Cell Lung Cancer (EMERGING-CTONG 1103): A Randomized Phase II Study. *J Clin Oncol* (2019) 37(25):2235–45. doi: 10.1200/JCO.19.00075
9. Zhang C, Yan LX, Jiang BY, Wu YL, Zhong WZ. Feasibility and Safety of Neoadjuvant Alectinib in a Patient With ALK-Positive Locally Advanced NSCLC. *J Thorac Oncol* (2020) 15(6):e95–9. doi: 10.1016/j.jtho.2019.12.133
10. Blumenthal GM, Bunn PA Jr, Chaft JE, McCoach CE, Perez EA, Scagliotti GV, et al. Current Status and Future Perspectives on Neoadjuvant Therapy in Lung Cancer. *J Thorac Oncol* (2018) 13(12):1818–31. doi: 10.1016/j.jtho.2018.09.017
11. Yi M, Jiao D, Xu H, Liu Q, Zhao W, Han X, et al. Biomarkers for Predicting Efficacy of PD-1/PD-L1 Inhibitors. *Mol Cancer* (2018) 17(1):129. doi: 10.1186/s12943-018-0864-3
12. Pan Y, Yu Y, Wang X, Zhang T. Tumor-Associated Macrophages in Tumor Immunity. *Front Immunol* (2020) 11:583084. doi: 10.3389/fimmu.2020.583084

Permissions

All chapters in this book were first published by Frontiers; hereby published with permission under the Creative Commons Attribution License or equivalent. Every chapter published in this book has been scrutinized by our experts. Their significance has been extensively debated. The topics covered herein carry significant findings which will fuel the growth of the discipline. They may even be implemented as practical applications or may be referred to as a beginning point for another development.

The contributors of this book come from diverse backgrounds, making this book a truly international effort. This book will bring forth new frontiers with its revolutionizing research information and detailed analysis of the nascent developments around the world.

We would like to thank all the contributing authors for lending their expertise to make the book truly unique. They have played a crucial role in the development of this book. Without their invaluable contributions this book wouldn't have been possible. They have made vital efforts to compile up to date information on the varied aspects of this subject to make this book a valuable addition to the collection of many professionals and students.

This book was conceptualized with the vision of imparting up-to-date information and advanced data in this field. To ensure the same, a matchless editorial board was set up. Every individual on the board went through rigorous rounds of assessment to prove their worth. After which they invested a large part of their time researching and compiling the most relevant data for our readers.

The editorial board has been involved in producing this book since its inception. They have spent rigorous hours researching and exploring the diverse topics which have resulted in the successful publishing of this book. They have passed on their knowledge of decades through this book. To expedite this challenging task, the publisher supported the team at every step. A small team of assistant editors was also appointed to further simplify the editing procedure and attain best results for the readers.

Apart from the editorial board, the designing team has also invested a significant amount of their time in understanding the subject and creating the most relevant covers. They scrutinized every image to scout for the most suitable representation of the subject and create an appropriate cover for the book.

The publishing team has been an ardent support to the editorial, designing and production team. Their endless efforts to recruit the best for this project, has resulted in the accomplishment of this book. They are a veteran in the field of academics and their pool of knowledge is as vast as their experience in printing. Their expertise and guidance has proved useful at every step. Their uncompromising quality standards have made this book an exceptional effort. Their encouragement from time to time has been an inspiration for everyone.

The publisher and the editorial board hope that this book will prove to be a valuable piece of knowledge for researchers, students, practitioners and scholars across the globe.

List of Contributors

Xiaoguang Qi, Boyu Qin, Xindan Kang and Yi Hu
Department of Oncology, Chinese PLA General Hospital, Beijing, China

Chunyan Qi
Department of Health Management, Chinese PLA General Hospital, Beijing, China

Weidong Han
Department of Bio-therapeutic, Chinese PLA General Hospital, Beijing, China

Chengdi Wang, Jun Shao and Weimin Li
Department of Respiratory and Critical Care Medicine, Med-X Center for Manufacturing, National Clinical Research Center for Geriatrics, Frontiers Science Center for Disease-related Molecular Network, West China Hospital, West China School of Medicine, Sichuan University, Chengdu, China

Jiechao Ma, Shu Zhang and Zhongnan Liu
AI Lab, Deepwise Healthcare, Beijing, China

Yizhou Yu
AI Lab, Deepwise Healthcare, Beijing, China
Faculty of Engineering, The University of Hong Kong, Hong Kong, Hong Kong SAR, China

Evgeny N. Imyanitov and Alexandr O. Ivantsov
Department of Tumor Growth Biology, N.N. Petrov Institute of Oncology, St. Petersburg, Russia
Department of Clinical Genetics, St.-Petersburg Pediatric Medical University, Saint Petersburg, Russia

Ilya V. Tsimafeyeu
Institute of Oncology, Hadassah Moscow, Moscow, Russia

Zhimin Zhang and Bicheng Zhang
Cancer Center, Renmin Hospital of Wuhan University, Wuhan, China

Yanyan Gu
Department of Nutrition, Changzheng Hospital, Second Military Medical University, Shanghai, China

Xiaona Su, Wei Guan, Jungang Ma, Jia Luo, Juan He, Mingying Geng and Chuan Chen
Cancer Center, Daping Hospital, Army Medical University (Third Military Medical University), Chongqing, China

Jing Bai, Xuefeng Xia and Yanfang Guan
Geneplus-Beijing Institute, Beijing, China

Cheng Shen
Department of Thoracic Surgery, Daping Hospital, Army Medical University (Third Military Medical University), Chongqing, China

Karam Khaddour
Department of Medicine, Rosalind Franklin University of Medicine and Science, McHenry, IL, United States
Department of Medicine, Division of Hematology and Oncology, University of Illinois at Chicago, Chicago, IL, United States

Sandra L. Gomez-Perez
Department of Clinical Nutrition, Rush University Medical Center, Chicago, IL, United States

Nikita Jain
Department of Medicine, Rosalind Franklin University of Medicine and Science, McHenry, IL, United States

Jyoti D. Patel
Division of Hematology/Oncology, Feinberg School of Medicine, Northwestern University, Robert H. Lurie Comprehensive Cancer Center, Chicago, IL, United States

Yanis Boumber
Division of Hematology/Oncology, Feinberg School of Medicine, Northwestern University, Robert H. Lurie Comprehensive Cancer Center, Chicago, IL, United States
Institute of Fundamental Medicine and Biology, Kazan Federal University, Kazan, Russia

Yinqi Zhang
Zhongshan School of Medicine, Sun Yat-Sen University, Guangzhou, ChinaWW
Department of Minimally Invasive Interventional Therapy, Sun Yat-Sen University Cancer Center, Guangzhou, China

Chengqi Gao and Penghui Zhou
State Key Laboratory of Oncology in South China, Collaborative Innovation Center of Cancer Medicine, Sun Yat-Sen University, Guangzhou, China

Fei Cao, Ying Wu, Xue Han, Zhiyu Qiu, Weijun Fan and Lujun Shen
Department of Minimally Invasive Interventional Therapy, Sun Yat-Sen University Cancer Center, Guangzhou, China
State Key Laboratory of Oncology in South China, Collaborative Innovation Center of Cancer Medicine, Sun Yat-Sen University, Guangzhou, China

Shuanggang Chen
Department of Oncology, Yuebei People's Hospital, Shantou University Medical College, Shaoguan, China

Jingqin Mo
Zhongshan School of Medicine, Sun Yat-Sen University, Guangzhou, China

Kamila Wojas-Krawczyk
Department of Pneumonology, Oncology and Allergology, Medical University of Lublin, Lublin, Poland

Tomasz Kubiatowski
Department of Clinical Oncology, Saint John of Dukla Oncology Centre of the Lublin Region, Lublin, Poland

Jianfeng Peng
Department of Radiation Oncology, Shandong Cancer Hospital Affiliated to Shandong First Medical University, Jinan, China

Xianguang Zhao and Xiangjiao Meng
Department of Radiation Oncology, Shandong Cancer Hospital, Jinan, China

Kaikai Zhao
Department of Radiation Oncology, The First Affiliated Hospital of China Medical University, Shenyang, China
Department of Radiation Oncology, Yantai Affiliated Hospital of Binzhou Medical University, Yantai, China

Zhenlin Yang, He Tian, Zheng Zhou, Fenglong Bie, Renda Li, Yue Peng, Guangyu Bai, Lei Liu, Tao Fan, Chu Xiao, Yujia Zheng, Chunxiang Li, Shugeng Gao and Jie He
Department of Thoracic Surgery, National Cancer Center/National Clinical Research Center for Cancer/Cancer Hospital, Chinese Academy of Medical Sciences, Peking Union Medical College, Beijing, China

Jiachen Xu and Jie Wang
Department of Medical Oncology, National Cancer Center/National Clinical Research Center for Cancer/Cancer Hospital, Chinese Academy of Medical Sciences, Peking Union Medical College, Beijing, China

Junhui Yang
Genetron Health (Beijing) Co. Ltd., Beijing, China

Yanhua Tian
Department of Thoracic Surgery/Head & Neck Medical Oncology, The University of Texas (UT) MD Anderson Cancer Center, Houston, TX, United States

Ying Chen
Department of Thoracic Surgery I, The Third Affiliated Hospital of Kunming Medical University (Yunnan Cancer Hospital, Yunnan Cancer Center), Kunming, China

Bo Zheng
Department of Pathology, National Cancer Center/National Clinical Research Center for Cancer/Cancer Hospital, Chinese Academy of Medical Sciences, Peking Union Medical College, Beijing, China

Liang Zhao, Kaili Fu, Jinluan Li, Yaqing Dai and Qin Lin
Department of Radiation Oncology, The First Affiliated Hospital of Xiamen University, Teaching Hospital of Fujian Medical University, Xiamen, China

Peiqiong Chen, Yuhuan Wang and Yanzhen Zhuang
Department of Pathology, The First Affiliated Hospital of Xiamen University, Teaching Hospital of Fujian Medical University, Xiamen, China

Long Sun and Haojun Chen
Department of Nuclear Medicine & Minnan PET Center, The First Affiliated Hospital of Xiamen University, Teaching Hospital of Fujian Medical University, Xiamen, China

Bin Liu, Ziyu Wang, Meng Gu, Cong Zhao and Teng Ma
Department of Cellular and Molecular Biology, Beijing Chest Hospital, Capital Medical University, Beijing Tuberculosis and Thoracic Tumor Research Institute, Beijing, China

Jinghui Wang
Department of Medical Oncology, Beijing Chest Hospital, Capital Medical University, Beijing Tuberculosis and Thoracic Tumor Research Institute, Beijing, China

Teng Li, Shouzheng Wang, Yiying Guo, Puyuan Xing and Junling Li
Department of Medical Oncology, National Cancer Center/National Clinical Research Center for Cancer/Cancer Hospital, Chinese Academy of Medical Sciences and Peking Union Medical College, Beijing, China

Xiaocong Pang
Department of Pharmacy, Peking University First Hospital, Beijing, China

Junyun Wang
CAS Key Laboratory of Genome Sciences and Information, Beijing Institute of Genomics, Chinese Academy of Sciences/China National Center for Bioinformation, Beijing, China
Research Institute, GloriousMed Clinical Laboratory (Shanghai) Co., Ltd., Shanghai, China

Ning He
Research Institute, GloriousMed Clinical Laboratory (Shanghai) Co., Ltd., Shanghai, China

Sameh Daher, Yaacov R. Lawrence, Damien Urban, Rossie Navon, Raya Leibowitz, Teodor Gottfried, Amir Onn and Jair Bar
Thoracic Cancer Unit, Institute of Oncology, Sheba Medical Center, Tel HaShomer, Israel

Elizabeth Dudnik and Nir Peled
Thoracic Cancer Unit, Davidoff Cancer Center, Rabin Medical Center, Petah Tikva, Israel

Ekaterina Hanovich
Institute of Oncology, Shamir Medical Center, Zerifin, Israel

Ariel Hammerman and Erez Battat
Department of Pharmaceutical Technology Assessment, Clalit Health Services Headquarters, Tel Aviv, Israel

Haiyi Deng, Xinqing Lin, Xiaohong Xie, Yilin Yang, Liqiang Wang, Jianhui Wu, Ming Liu, Zhanhong Xie, Yinyin Qin and Chengzhi Zhou
State Key Laboratory of Respiratory Disease, National Clinical Research Centre for Respiratory Disease, Guangzhou Institute of Respiratory Health, First Affiliated Hospital, Guangzhou Medical University, Guangzhou, China

Yi Zheng, Cheng Xiang, Yaguang Han, Qiang Zhen, Yiyi Zhao, Miao Zhang and Yan Zhang
Department of Oncology, Shijiazhuang People's Hospital, Shijiazhuang, China

Shiying Hao
Department of Cardiothoracic Surgery, Standford University, Stanford, CA, United States

Yanhong Shang
Department of Oncology, Affiliated Hospital of Hebei University, Baoding, China

Mohammed Safi, Abdullah Al-Danakh, Feng Ping, Xiu Shan and Jiwei Liu
Department of Oncology, First Affiliated Hospital of Dalian Medical University, Dalian, China

Ravindran Kanesvaran
National Cancer Center Singapore, Singapore General Hospital, Singapore, Singapore

Mohammed Alradhi
Department of Urology, Second Affiliated Hospital of Dalian Medical University, Dalian, China

Najeeb Al-Sabai
Dalian Medical University, Medical School, Dalian, China

Shao Feng and Zhang Qiang
Department of Thoracic Surgery, Nanjing Chest Hospital, The Affiliated Brain Hospital of Nanjing Medical University, Nanjing, China

Cheng Wanwan and Fang Shencun
Department of Respiratory Medicine, Nanjing Chest Hospital, The Affiliated Brain Hospital of Nanjing Medical University, Nanjing, China

Zeng Zhaozhun and Xie Yuewu
Medical Oncology Scientific Group of the Central Medical Department, Jiangsu Hansoh Pharmaceutical Group Co., Ltd., Shanghai, China

Jiamao Lin and Haiyong Wang
Department of Internal Medicine Oncology, Shandong Cancer Hospital and Institute, Shandong First Medical University and Shandong Academy of Medical Sciences, Jinan, China

Xiaohui Wang
Research Service Office, Shandong Liaocheng People's Hospital, Liaocheng, China

Chenyue Zhang
Department of Integrated Oncology, Fudan University Shanghai Cancer Center, Shanghai, China

Shuai Bu
Research Department, The Second Affiliated Hospital of Shandong University of Traditional Chinese Medicine, Jinan, China

Chenglong Zhao
Department of Pathology, Shandong Cancer Hospital and Institute, Shandong First Medical University and Shandong Academy of Medical Sciences, Jinan, China

Xiang Li, Shi Yan, Yaqi Wang, Chao Lv, Shaolei Li, Yue Yang and Nan Wu
Key Laboratory of Carcinogenesis and Translational Research (Ministry of Education), Department of Thoracic Surgery II, Peking University Cancer Hospital & Institute, Beijing, China

Jichun Yang
Central Laboratory, The Second Affiliated Hospital of Kunming Medical University, Kunming, China

Jun Zhao and Minglei Zhuo
Key Laboratory of Carcinogenesis and Translational Research (Ministry of Education), Department I of Thoracic Oncology, Peking University Cancer Hospital & Institute, Beijing, China

Longyao Zhang, Linpeng Zheng and Jianguo Sun
Cancer Institute, Xinqiao Hospital, Army Medical University, Chongqing, China

Qiao Yang
Department of Ultrasound, The 941Hospital of the Chinese People's Liberation Army (PLA) Joint Logistic Support Force, Xining, China

Fen Wang
Guangdong Provincial Key Laboratory of Translational Medicine in Lung Cancer, Guangdong Provincial People's Hospital, Guangdong Academy of Medical Sciences, School of Medicine, Guangdong Lung Cancer Institute, South China University of Technology, Guangzhou, China
Shenzhen Key Laboratory of Gastrointestinal Cancer Translational Research, Department of Oncology, Cancer Institute of Shenzhen-PKU-HKUST Medical Center, Peking University Shenzhen Hospital, Shenzhen, China

Shubin Wang
Shenzhen Key Laboratory of Gastrointestinal Cancer Translational Research, Department of Oncology, Cancer Institute of Shenzhen-PKU-HKUST Medical Center, Peking University Shenzhen Hospital, Shenzhen, China

Qing Zhou
Guangdong Provincial Key Laboratory of Translational Medicine in Lung Cancer, Guangdong Provincial People's Hospital, Guangdong Academy of Medical Sciences, School of Medicine, Guangdong Lung Cancer Institute, South China University of Technology, Guangzhou, China

Ning Zhou, Tong Li, Fan Ren, Hong Ni, Zuoqing Song, Lingling Zu and Song Xu
Department of Lung Cancer Surgery, Tianjin Medical University General Hospital, Tianjin, China
Tianjin Key Laboratory of Lung Cancer Metastasis and Tumor Microenvironment, Lung Cancer Institute, Tianjin Medical University General Hospital, Tianjin, China

Maoli Liang and Shuo Li
Department of Respiratory and Critical Care, Tianjin Medical University General Hospital, Tianjin, China

Wei Liu
Department of Respiratory Medicine, Second Affiliated Hospital of Tianjin University of Traditional Chinese Medicine, Tianjin, China

Tao Shi
Precision Medicine Center, Tianjin Medical University General Hospital, Tianjin, China

Dongbo Xu
Department of Pathology, Tianjin Medical University General Hospital, Tianjin, China

Qiusong Chen and Haonan Yu
Department of PET/CT Diagnostic, Tianjin Medical University General Hospital, Tianjin, China

Index

www.ingramcontent.com/pod-product-compliance
Lightning Source LLC
LaVergne TN
LVHW082146200926
848484LV00008B/2111
* 9 7 9 8 8 8 7 4 0 5 7 0 4 *